DUKE'S
ANESTHESIA

SECRETS

DUKE'S
ANESTHESIA
SECRETS

Dedicated to Renee, My Wonderful Wife and Companion, to Dr. Philip Mehler,
and to the Many Contributors to Anesthesia Secrets.

James C. Duke

To my wife Molly, thank you for all your love and support, and to my Mom, Dad and brother
for always being there for me.

Brian M. Keech

DEDICATION TO DR. DUKE, MD, MBA

This dedication is for Dr. James Duke, co-editor of this fifth edition of *Anesthesia Secrets* and also editor of the previous four editions of this text. Sadly, Dr. Duke recently passed after a two-year struggle with a brain tumor.

Dr. Duke, or Jim as he was known at Denver Health, was a superbly talented anesthesiologist both for complicated elective cases as well as for those critically injured trauma patients seen at Denver Health, where Dr. Duke worked the last 20 years of his almost three-decade career. In addition, while at Denver Health, he quickly distinguished himself as someone who was passionate about quality of care, process improvement and patient safety. Soon after joining Denver Health, he was appointed Associate Director of the Anesthesia Department, a position he admirably held until his medical retirement in 2013.

Moreover, his leadership skills earned him an appointment to the Denver Health Medical Executive Committee, for which he held the role of Secretary of the Medical Staff, and ultimately was appointed President of the Medical Staff, which he held until his retirement.

Dr. Duke was a superb educator, beloved and respected by the hundreds of students and residents with whom he interacted during his career. His assiduous dedication to the *Anesthesia Secrets* text is a testament to his commitment to medical education.

Dr. Duke was a true "renaissance" man. He was an affable person, with impeccable tastes in clothing, food, motorcycles, and gardening. His subtle southern drawl was a perfect complement to his overall persona.

Jim will be sorely missed. His contribution to Denver Health and its anesthesia department, to the next generation of medical professionals, and to humanity are unassailable and indeed most impressive. The legacy he has formally established with the *Anesthesia Secrets* text will continue to be impactful for many generations to come and will keep him in our collective memories for many years forthwith.

Philip S. Mehler, MD, FACP, FAED
Glassman Professor of Medicine
University of Colorado
Denver Health Medical Center and
The University of Colorado
Denver, CO

CONTENTS

SECTION 7   SPECIAL ANESTHETIC CONSIDERATIONS

CONTRIBUTORS

Rita Agarwal, MD
Professor of Anesthesiology, Director of
Pediatric Education, Department of
Anesthesiology, University of Colorado,
Aurora, CO
Pediatric Anesthesiology Program Director,
Anesthesiology, Children's Hospital
Colorado, Aurora, CO

Benjamin Atwood, MD
Anesthesia Resident, Department of
Anesthesia, Critical Care and Pain
Medicine, Massachusetts General Hospital,
Boston, MA
Clinical Fellow in Anesthesia, Harvard
Medical School, Boston, MA

Daniel R. Beck, MD, MS
Assistant Professor, Cardiothoracic
Anesthesiologist, Department of
Anesthesiology, University of Colorado,
Veterans Affairs Medical Center,
Denver, CO

Bethany Benish, MD
Assistant Professor of Anesthesiology,
Department of Anesthesiology, University
of Colorado, Aurora, CO
Attending Anesthesiologist, Department of
Anesthesiology, Denver Health Medical
Center, Denver, CO

Mark Chandler, MD
Assistant Professor, University of
Colorado Health Sciences Center,
Aurora, CO
Anesthesiologist, Department of
Anesthesiology, Denver Health Medical
Center, Denver, CO

Christopher Ciarallo, MD, FAAP
Assistant Professor, Department of
Anesthesiology, University of Colorado
School of Medicine, Aurora, CO
Director of Pediatric Anesthesiology,
Department of Anesthesiology, Denver
Health Medical Center, Denver, CO
Pediatric Anesthesiologist, Anesthesiology,
Children's Hospital Colorado, Aurora, CO

Rachel D. Clopton, MD
Fellowship, Pediatric Anesthesia, Children's
Hospital Colorado, University of Colorado
Hospital, Aurora, CO

Mary DiMiceli, MD
OB Anesthesiology Fellow, Obstetric
Anesthesia, Vanderbilt University Hospital,
Nashville, TN

James C. Duke, MD, MBA (Deceased)
Associate Director, Retired, Anesthesiology,
Denver Health Medical Center,
Denver, CO

Matthew J. Fiegel, BA, MD
Associate Professor, Anesthesiology,
University of Colorado Hospital,
Aurora, CO

Jacob Friedman, MD
Assistant Professor, Department of
Anesthesiology, University of Colorado
Health Sciences Center, Aurora, CO
Staff Anesthesiologist, Department of
Anesthesiology, Denver Veteran's Affairs
Hospital, Denver, CO

Robert Friesen, MD
Professor, Anesthesiology, Children's Hospital
Colorado, Aurora, CO
Professor, Department of Anesthesiology,
University of Colorado School of Medicine,
Denver, CO

Andrea J. Fuller, MD
Assistant Professor of Anesthesiology,
University of Colorado Health Sciences
Center, Aurora, CO

James B. Haenel, RRT
Surgical Critical Care Specialist, Surgery,
Denver Health Medical Center, Denver, CO

Michelle Dianne Herren, MD
Pediatric Anesthesiologist, Department of
Anesthesiology, University of Colorado
Hospital, Aurora, CO
Pediatric Anesthesiologist, Denver Health
Medical Center, Denver, CO
Pediatric Anesthesiologist, Children's Hospital
Colorado, Aurora, CO

Daniel J. Janik, MD
Associate Professor, Department of
  Anesthesiology, University of Colorado
  School of Medicine, Aurora, CO
Co-director Intraoperative Neuromonitoring,
  Anesthesiology, University of Colorado
  Hospital, Aurora, CO

Gillian E. Johnson, MD
Anesthesiologist, Pikes Peak Anesthesia,
  Colorado Springs, CO

Jeffrey L. Johnson, MD
Assistant Professor of Surgery, University
  of Colorado Health Sciences Center,
  Aurora, CO
Director, Surgical Intensive Care, Denver
  Health Medical Center, Denver, CO

Alma N. Juels, MD
Assistant Professor, Department of
  Anesthesiology, University of Colorado,
  Aurora, CO
Attending Physician, Department of
  Anesthesiology, Denver Health Medical
  Center, Denver, CO

Rachel M. Kacmar, MD
Assistant Professor, Department of
  Anesthesiology, University of Colorado,
  Aurora, CO

Brian M. Keech, MD, FAAP
Staff Anesthesiologist, Denver Health
  Medical Center, Denver, CO
Assistant Professor of Anesthesiology,
  University of Colorado School of Medicine,
  Denver, CO

Michael Kim, BA, DO
Anesthesia Resident, Anesthesiology,
  University of Colorado Health Sciences
  Center, Aurora, CO

Renee Kolte-Edwards, MD
Anesthesiologist, Anesthesiology, Altru
  Health System, Grand Forks, ND

Jason P. Krutsch, MD
Associate Professor, Pain Medicine Fellowship
  Site Director, Department of
  Anesthesiology, University of Colorado,
  Denver, CO

Sunil Kumar, MD, FFARCS
Assistant Professor, Department of
  Anesthesiology, University of Colorado
  Health Sciences Center, Aurora, CO
Anesthesiologist, Department of
  Anesthesiology, Denver Health Medical
  Center, Denver, CO

Philip R. Levin, MD
Clinical Professor, Department of
  Anesthesiology, David Geffen School of
  Medicine at UCLA, Los Angeles, CA

Ana M. Lobo, MD, MPH
Assistant Professor of Anesthesiology,
  Department of Anesthesiology, Yale New
  Haven Hospital, New Haven, CT

Christopher M. Lowry, MD
Assistant Professor of Medicine, Department
  of Cardiology, University of Colorado,
  Aurora, CO
Director of Cardiac Electrophysiology,
  Department of Cardiology, Denver Health
  Medical Center, Denver, CO
Staff Electrophysiologist, Department of
  Cardiology, University of Colorado
  Hospital, Aurora, CO

Howard Miller, MD
Associate Director, Anesthesiology, Denver
  Health Medical Center, Denver, CO
Associate Professor, Department of
  Anesthesiology, University of Colorado
  School of Medicine, Aurora, CO

Aaron Murray, MD
Assistant Professor, Department of
  Anesthesiology, University of Colorado
  Health Sciences Center, Aurora, CO
Anesthesiologist, Department of
  Anesthesiology, Denver Health Medical
  Center, Denver, CO

Malcolm Packer, MD
Associate Professor of Anesthesiology,
  Department of Anesthesiology, University
  of Colorado Denver, CO
Attending Anesthesiologist, Department of
  Anesthesiology, Denver Health and
  Hospitals Authority; Children's Hospital
  Colorado, Aurora, CO

Gurdev S. Rai, MD
Chief, Anesthesia, Eastern Colorado Health
  Care System/Denver Veterans Affairs
  Medical Center, Denver, CO
Assistant Professor, Department of Anesthesia,
  University of Colorado, Aurora, CO

Prairie N. Robinson, MD
Anesthesiology Resident, University of
  Colorado Health Sciences Center,
  Aurora, CO

Olivia Romano, MD
Assistant Professor, Department of
  Anesthesiology, University of Colorado
  Anschutz Medical Campus, Aurora, CO

Michael M. Sawyer, MD
Assistant Professor of Anesthesiology,
 Department of Anesthesiology, University
 of Colorado Health Hospital Association,
 Denver, CO

Lawrence I. Schwartz, MD
Associate Professor, Department of
 Anesthesiology, Children's Hospital
 Colorado, University of Colorado,
 Aurora, CO

Tamas Seres, MD
Associate Professor, Department of
 Anesthesiology, University of Colorado,
 Aurora, CO

Robert Slover, MD
Director of Pediatrics, The Barbara Davis
 Center for Diabetes, University of
 Colorado, Aurora, CO

Robin Slover, MD
Associate Professor, Department of
 Anesthesiology, University of Colorado,
 Aurora, CO
Medical Director, Pain Consultation Services,
 Anesthesiology, Children's Hospital
 Colorado, Aurora, CO

Laurie M. Steward, MD
Pediatric Anesthesiologist and Senior
 Instructor, Department of Anesthesiology,
 Children's Hospital Colorado, Aurora, CO

Mark Twite, MA, MB, BChir, FRCP
Director of Pediatric Cardiac Anesthesia,
 Department of Anesthesiology, Children's
 Hospital and University of Colorado,
 Aurora, CO

Ronald Valdivieso, MD
Associate Professor, Department of
 Anesthesiology, University of Colorado,
 Aurora, CO

Nathaen Weitzel, MD
Associate Professor, Department of
 Anesthesiology, University of Colorado,
 Aurora, CO

Barbara Wilkey, MD
Assistant Professor, Department of
 Anesthesiology, University of Colorado,
 Aurora, CO

Jennifer Zieg, MD
Senior Instructor, Anesthesiology, Children's
 Hospital Colorado, University of Colorado
 Hospital, Aurora, CO

PREFACE

In this fifth edition of *Anesthesia Secrets*, the goal continues to be concise presentation of a wide range of topics important to anyone interested in anesthesiology. My goal has always been not to merely offer a few words suitable for the sake of familiarity, but to provide appropriate depth to allow readers to integrate the concerns of this field into their wider knowledge of medicine in general. It is my hope for medical students that both rotating through the anesthesia clinical services elective and reviewing Anesthesia Secrets contributes to their decision to enter this esteemed profession.

I am humbled by the reception *Anesthesia Secrets* has received since the first edition was published in 1996. I take it as an affirmation that my contributors and I have a good idea of the important concepts in the field, as much as they can be described in a text of this size. I thank my contributors for this edition and all previous editions. Over the years my contributors have gone on to successful careers across the country, yet their imprint remains throughout. Although they may no longer be listed as authors, they nonetheless have my thanks.

And to you, the reader, thank you for making *Anesthesia Secrets* a part of your educational program.

James C. Duke, MD, MBA

It has been an honor for me to work with Dr. Jim Duke and the contributors of the now rightly named, *Duke's Anesthesia Secrets*, FIFTH EDITION. From using this series as a medical student, resident, fellow and now attending anesthesiologist, I can attest to its excellence. Whether used as a quick reference for the most salient topics in anesthesiology, or as a starting point for more in-depth study, its quality is unmatched.

Thank you for choosing *Duke's Anesthesia Secrets*, FIFTH EDITION as your study aid. I hope you enjoy using it as much as we have enjoyed preparing it for you.

Brian M. Keech, MD, FAAP

TOP 100 SECRETS

These secrets are 100 of the top board alerts. They summarize the concepts, principles, and most salient details of anesthesiology.

1. A preoperative visit by an informative and reassuring anesthesiologist provides useful psychological preparation and calms the patient's fears and anxiety before anesthesia. The choice of premedication depends on the physical and mental status of the patient, whether the patient is an inpatient or outpatient, whether the surgery is elective or emergent, and whether the patient has a history of postoperative nausea and vomiting.

2. "All that wheezes is not asthma." Also consider mechanical airway obstruction, congestive heart failure, allergic reaction, pulmonary embolus, pneumothorax, aspiration, and endobronchial intubation.

3. Under most circumstances, peri-induction hypotension responds best to intravenous fluid. Estimating volume status requires gathering as much clinical information as possible because any single variable may be misleading. Always look for supporting information. Replace intraoperative fluid losses with isotonic fluids.

4. Thorough airway examination and identification of the patient with a potentially difficult airway are of paramount importance. The "difficult-to-ventilate, difficult-to-intubate" scenario must be avoided if possible.

5. For the elective case, fasting guidelines include:

Clear liquids (water, clear juices)	2 hours
Nonclear liquids (Jello, breast milk)	4 hours
Light meal or snack (crackers, toast, liquid)	6 hours
Full meal (fat containing, meat)	8 hours

6. Increasing the delivered concentration of anesthetic, increasing the fresh gas flow, increasing alveolar ventilation, and using nonlipid-soluble anesthetics increase speed of onset of volatile anesthetics.

7. Obese patients may be difficult to ventilate and difficult to intubate. Backup strategies should always be considered and readily available before airway management begins.

8. Infants may be difficult to intubate because they have a more anterior larynx, relatively large tongues, and a floppy epiglottis. The narrowest part of the larynx is below the vocal cords at the cricoid cartilage.

9. The semiclosed circuit using a circle system is the most commonly used anesthesia circuit. Components include an inspiratory limb, expiratory limb, unidirectional valves, a CO_2 absorber, a gas reservoir bag, and a pop-off valve on the expiratory limb.

10. Advantages of a circle system include conservation of heat and moisture, the ability to use low flows of fresh gas, and the ability to scavenge waste gases. Disadvantages include multiple sites for disconnection and high compliance.

11. Local anesthetic agents are either aminoesters or aminoamides. The two classes of agents differ in their allergic potential and method of biotransformation.

12. Termination of effect of intravenous anesthetics is through redistribution, not biotransformation and breakdown. Benzodiazepines and opioids have synergistic effects with intravenous induction agents, requiring adjustment in dosing.

13. Chronic pain is best treated by using multiple therapeutic modalities, including physical therapy, psychological support, pharmacologic management, and rational use of more invasive procedures such as nerve blocks and implantable technologies. Neuropathic pain is usually less responsive to opioids than pain originating from nociceptors.

14. The most common complications from epidural analgesia are hypotension, inadequate analgesia requiring replacement or manipulation, pruritus, nausea/vomiting, and shivering, with less common but potentially detrimental complications being post–dural puncture headache (PDPH), high/total spinal, intrathecal (IT) or intravenous (IV) catheter placement, systemic toxicity and nerve injury.

15. Definitive treatment of preeclampsia is immediate delivery, but mainstay of management is blood pressure control and seizure prophylaxis with β blocker or vasodilators and magnesium sulfate, respectively.

16. Anesthesiologists should be aware of patients at high risk for postpartum hemorrhage or uterine atony and prepare accordingly—type and cross and have blood to transfuse readily available.

17. Most elective thoracic surgical procedures in adults using one-lung ventilation (OLV) can be achieved using a left double-lumen endotracheal tube (DLT). Right DLTs and bronchial blockers are more difficult to place and more likely to move during surgery, requiring repositioning with a fiber-optic bronchoscope (FOB). The initiation of OLV stops all ventilation to one lung, which would create a 50% right-to-left shunt and relative hypoxemia if perfusion were unchanged. Methods to improve oxygenation during OLV include increasing fractionalized inspired oxygen concentration (FiO_2), adding positive end-expiratory pressure (PEEP) to the dependent lung, adding continuous positive airway pressure to the nondependent lung, adjusting tidal volumes, and clamping the blood supply to the nonventilated lung.

18. When somatosensory-evoked potentials (SSEPs) are monitored during spine surgery, avoid exceeding 1 minimal alveolar concentration (MAC) of volatile anesthetic to maximize the effectiveness of signal acquisition.

19. During prolonged spine surgery in the prone position, use a combination of colloid and crystalloid for fluid replacement to help avoid ischemic optic neuropathy.

20. Patients on β blockers should take them on the day of surgery and continue them perioperatively. Because the receptors are upregulated, withdrawal may precipitate hypertension, tachycardia, and myocardial ischemia. Rarely are β blockers initiated the day of surgery. Clonidine should be continued.

21. Even mild hypothermia has a negative influence on patient outcome, increasing rates of wound infection, delaying healing, increasing blood loss, and increasing cardiac morbidity threefold.

22. O-negative blood is the *universal donor* for packed red blood cells; for plasma it is AB positive.

23. Not all elderly patients need an extensive preoperative workup; tailor it to their underlying illnesses and invasiveness of the surgery. Patients with Alzheimer disease may become more confused and disoriented with preoperative sedation.

24. Basal function of most organ systems is relatively unchanged by the aging process per se, but the functional reserve and ability to compensate for physiologic stress are reduced. In general, anesthetic requirements are decreased in geriatric patients. There is an increased potential for a wide variety of postoperative complications in the elderly, and postoperative cognitive dysfunction is arguably the most common.

25. Pregnant patients can pose airway management problems because of airway edema, large breasts that make laryngoscopy difficult, full stomachs rendering them prone to

aspiration, and rapid oxygen desaturation caused by decreased functional residual capacity.

26. Normal saline, when administered in large quantities, produces a hyperchloremic metabolic acidosis; the associated base deficit may lead the provider to conclude incorrectly that the patient continues to be hypovolemic.

27. There is no set hemoglobin/hematocrit level at which transfusion is required. The decision should be individualized to the clinical situation, taking into consideration the patient's health status. If blood is needed in an emergency, type O–packed cells (best is O-negative) and/or type-specific blood may be used.

28. The most common intraoperative bleeding diathesis is dilutional thrombocytopenia. In general, this is not seen until significant blood loss has occurred and has been replaced with IV crystalloid and blood products that do not contain platelets.

29. Thromboelastography (TEG) is a dynamic point of care test of clotting that can help distinguish between surgical and non-surgical bleeding. It can identify specific deficiencies of coagulation factors, fibrinogen and platelets, and can detect plasmin dysregulation and abnormal clot breakdown.

30. The primary treatment for disseminated intravascular coagulation (DIC) is to treat the underlying medical condition.

31. Forced vital capacity (FVC), forced expiratory volume in 1 second (FEV_1), the FEV_1/FVC ratio, and the flow between 25% and 75% of the FVC (mean maximal flow [MMF_{25-75}]) are the most clinically helpful indices obtained from spirometry. No single pulmonary function test result absolutely contraindicates surgery.

32. Common opioid side effects include nausea, pruritus, bradycardia, urinary retention, and respiratory depression.

33. Appropriate dosing of intravenous anesthetics requires considering intravascular volume status, comorbidities, age, and chronic medications.

34. Ketamine is the best induction agent for patients with hypovolemic trauma as long as there is no risk for increased intracranial pressure (ICP). It is also a good agent for patients with active bronchospastic disease.

35. Propofol is the least likely of all induction agents to result in nausea and vomiting. Termination of the effects of intravenous anesthetics is by redistribution, not biotransformation and breakdown.

36. Metabolism of relaxants is more important than pharmacologic reversal for termination of relaxant effect. Train-of-four assessment is highly subjective and has been demonstrated repeatedly to underestimate residual neuromuscular blockade. It may be a best practice to administer reversal agents to all patients receiving nondepolarizing relaxants. Leave clinically weak patients intubated and support respirations until the patient can demonstrate return of strength.

37. Lipid solubility, pK_a, and protein binding of the local anesthetics determine their potency, onset, and duration of action, respectively.

38. Vasopressin has a role in blood pressure maintenance in septic shock, cardiogenic shock, and other shock states.

39. Low-dose dopamine is ineffective for prevention and treatment of acute renal failure and for protection of the gut. Dopamine is not an effective treatment for septic shock. The best way to maintain renal function during surgery is to ensure an adequate intravascular volume, maintain cardiac output, and avoid drugs known to decrease renal perfusion.

40. The risk of clinically significant aspiration pneumonitis in healthy patients having elective surgery is very low. Many patients require little or no premedication. Routine use of pharmacologic agents to alter the volume or pH of gastric contents is unnecessary.

41. American College of Cardiology/American Heart Association guidelines for cardiac testing are the current gold standard for preoperative cardiac assessment. However, the most important component of the preanesthetic evaluation is a thorough, accurate and focused history and physical examination.

42. The four active cardiac conditions that will likely result in surgical cancellation to assess cardiac evaluation and treatment are unstable coronary syndrome, decompensated heart failure, significant cardiac arrhythmias, and severe valvular disease.

43. Postoperative blindness is increasing in frequency, but it is unclear exactly which patients are at risk. Although not a guarantee to prevent this complication, during lengthy spine procedures in the prone position, intravascular volume, hematocrit, and perfusion pressure should be maintained.

44. The most common postoperative nerve injury is ulnar neuropathy. It is most commonly found in men older than 50 years, is delayed in presentation, is not invariably prevented by padding, and is multifactorial in origin.

45. Oxygenation and ventilation are separate processes, and pulse oximetry does not assess adequacy of ventilation. Treat the patient, not the symptom!

46. Trends in central venous pressures (CVPs) are more valuable than isolated values and should always be evaluated in the context of the patient's scenario.

47. The systolic blood pressure in the radial artery may be as much as 20 to 50 mm Hg higher than the pressure in the central aorta.

48. Awareness is most likely in cases where minimal anesthetic is administered, such as in cardiopulmonary bypass, hemodynamic instability, trauma, and fetal delivery.

49. Symptoms of awareness can be nonspecific, and the use of neuromuscular blockade increases the risk of unrecognized awareness.

50. Even mild hypothermia has a negative influence on patient outcome, increasing wound infection rates, increasing nitrogen loss, delaying healing, increasing blood loss, and increasing hospitalization as well as cardiac morbidity. Hypothermia is dissatisfying in postoperative patients. The best method to treat hypothermia is use of forced-air warming blankets. Warm all fluids and blood products. Cover all body surfaces possible, including the head, to further reduce heat loss.

51. Patients with suspected sleep apnea should be managed in the same way patients with diagnosed sleep apnea are managed. Supplemental oxygen, regular checks, and oxygen saturations are the best standards for treatment.

52. Patients with excellent exercise capacity, even in the presence of ischemic heart disease, will be able to tolerate the stresses of noncardiac surgery. The ability to climb two or three flights of stairs without significant symptoms (angina, dyspnea) is usually an indication of adequate cardiac reserve.

53. β-Blocker therapy significantly decreases the postoperative mortality rate of patients with high cardiac risk after noncardiac surgery so it should be established whenever it is indicated, as well as before surgery.

54. Diastolic dysfunction can cause primarily heart failure in the presence of normal ejection fraction (EF) or it can be secondary in systolic heart failure with low EF with increased left atrial (LA) pressure. Different types of diastolic dysfunction need different types of fluid and hemodynamic management.

55. The most common cause of perioperative mortality is cardiac disease. Postoperative renal failure also has an important impact on outcome.

56. In the normal brain, cerebral blood flow varies directly with the cerebral metabolic rate. Inhalational agents are said to *uncouple* this relationship in that they decrease

the cerebral metabolic rate while concurrently dilating cerebral blood vessels and increasing cerebral blood flow.

57. The key to subarachnoid hemorrhage (SAH) management is early diagnosis and surgical treatment within 72 hours. Vasospasm should be treated with hypertensive, hypervolemic, hemodilution (HHH) therapy. None of the methods of monitoring cerebral blood flow during carotid endarterectomy (CEA) has been demonstrated to improve outcome, and none has gained widespread acceptance as the monitor of choice.

58. Patients for planned pulmonary resections absolutely require pulmonary function tests to ensure that more lung is not resected than is compatible with life. Injudicious resections may create a ventilator-dependent patient.

59. Mechanical ventilation settings for patients with acute respiratory disease syndrome (ARDS) or acute lung injury (ALI) include tidal volume at 6 to 8 ml/kg of ideal body weight and limiting plateau pressures to <30 cm H_2O. PEEP should be adjusted to prevent end-expiratory collapse.

60. Hypoxia, hypercarbia, and acidosis worsen pulmonary artery pressure (PAP). Vasopressin increases systemic vascular resistance (SVR) without increasing PAP. Norepinephrine increases SVR to a greater extent than it increases pulmonary vascular resistance (PVR), so it is also useful in pulmonary artery hypertension (PAH).

61. Patients with liver disease commonly have an increased volume of distribution, necessitating an increase in initial dose requirements.

62. Although the portal vein supplies up to 75% of total hepatic blood flow, only 45% to 55% of the oxygen requirements are provided by this part of the circulation. Because of the large hepatic reserve, significant impairment of physiologic function must occur before clinical signs and symptoms of hepatic failure become evident.

63. Patients undergoing cardiac or aortic surgery are particularly at risk for developing postoperative renal insufficiency.

64. Preoperative renal risk factors (increased creatinine and a history of renal dysfunction), left ventricular dysfunction, advanced age, jaundice, and diabetes mellitus are predictive of postoperative renal dysfunction.

65. The majority of renal function tests are neither sensitive nor specific in predicting perioperative renal dysfunction and are affected by many variables common to the perioperative environment. The best way to maintain renal function during surgery is to ensure an adequate intravascular volume, maintain cardiac output, and avoid drugs known to decrease renal perfusion.

66. Malignant hyperthermia (MH) is a hypermetabolic disorder that presents in the perioperative period after exposure to inhalational agents or succinylcholine. The sine qua non of MH is an unexplained rise in end-tidal carbon dioxide in a patient with unexplained tachycardia. A temperature rise is a late feature. Patients with a history of, or susceptibility to, MH must receive anesthesia with a nontriggering agent. The anesthesiologist must have a heightened awareness of MH, have prepared the anesthetic machine, and have the MH cart in the room.

67. Chronic alcoholics may have cardiomyopathy and dysrhythmias, may be predisposed to aspiration, and may have diminished pulmonary function. They may have impaired synthetic liver function (important screening tests are albumin and prothrombin time). Alcohol withdrawal may cause seizures.

68. Cocaine sensitizes the cardiovascular system to the effects of endogenous catecholamines. Ketamine and pancuronium potentiate the cardiovascular toxicity of cocaine and should be avoided.

69. Patients with diabetes have a high incidence of coronary artery disease with an atypical or silent presentation. Maintaining perfusion pressure, controlling heart rate, conducting continuous ECG observation, and maintaining a high index of suspicion

during periods of refractory hypotension are key considerations. The goal for insulin management during surgery is to maintain glucose between 120 and 200 mg/dl.

70. Perioperatively mild to moderate hypothyroidism is of little concern even for elective surgery. Patients with severe, symptomatic hypothyroidism should be treated before surgery. MAC of volatile anesthetics is unchanged in both hypothyroid and hyperthyroid states. Thyroid storm may mimic malignant hyperthermia.

71. Chronic exogenous glucocorticoid therapy should not be discontinued abruptly. Doing so may precipitate acute adrenocortical insufficiency.

72. Morbidly obese patients have numerous systemic disorders and physiologic challenges, including restrictive lung disease, obstructive sleep apnea, coronary artery disease, diabetes, hypertension, cardiomegaly, pulmonary hypertension, and delayed gastric emptying. Safe anesthetic practice requires preparation for diagnosis, monitoring, and emergent treatment of any of these conditions.

73. Obese patients often have obstructive sleep apnea (OSA), requiring appropriate diagnosis and care, especially in the postoperative period.

74. The major causes of anaphylactic reactions in the operating room are muscle relaxants and latex allergy. Concerning latex allergy, proper preparation of the operating room environment is critical. Schedule at-risk patients as the first surgical cases of the day. Latex- and nonlatex-containing supplies should be clearly identified and the former avoided. Powdered gloves should be avoided. Health care workers are at increased risk for latex hypersensitivity. Avoid the use of powdered gloves whenever possible and be alert for the development of symptoms that might signify latex allergy.

75. The initial management of a trauma patient requires attention to the ABCs: airway, breathing, and circulation. Ensuring numerous large-gauge intravenous sites for resuscitation is a priority.

76. Precipitous cardiovascular collapse may be caused by unrecognized sources of bleeding, cardiac tamponade, tension pneumothorax, or air embolism. Unstable, hemorrhaging patients should receive O-negative, type-specific, or crossmatched blood if still unstable after resuscitation with 2 liters of balanced crystalloid solution.

77. Massive transfusion protocols now mandate aggressive administration of plasma and platelets as well as red blood cells, usual in a 1:1:1 ratio. The triad of hypothermia, acidosis, and coagulopathy is highly lethal; in this scenario, damage-control surgical principles should be considered and long operative periods avoided.

78. The initial goal of resuscitation in burn patients is to correct hypovolemia. Burns cause a generalized increase in capillary permeability with loss of significant fluid and protein into interstitial tissue. There should be a low threshold for elective intubation in burn patients suspected of having inhalation injury.

79. Infants may be difficult to intubate because they have a more anterior larynx, relatively large tongues, and a floppy epiglottis. The narrowest part of the larynx has been found to be below the vocal cords at the cricoid cartilage. Children desaturate more rapidly than do adults because of increased metabolic rate, increased dead space, inefficient chest wall mechanics, and, in neonates, immature alveoli.

80. Physiologic alterations in patients during pregnancy include increases in cardiac output, heart rate, plasma volume, minute ventilation, and oxygen consumption; decreases in SVR; dilutional anemia; loss of functional residual capacity (FRC); and a hypercoagulable state.

81. Uterine atony is the most common cause of postpartum hemorrhage and often results in substantial blood loss.

82. Obesity and diabetes mellitus increase the parturients' risk for development of preeclampsia, preterm labor and delivery, painful labor, fetal macrosomia, and operative delivery, for which a well-functioning, early placed epidural will increase success for safe delivery and avoid risks for potential general anesthesia.

83. Basal function of most organ systems is relatively unchanged by the aging process, but the functional reserve and ability to compensate for physiologic stress are reduced.

84. There is increased potential for a wide variety of postoperative complications in the elderly; postoperative cognitive dysfunction (POCD) is arguably the most common.

85. Administering anesthesia to a patient undergoing magnetic resonance imaging (MRI) poses unique challenges. Any ferromagnetic object can become a projectile and all equipment, including gas cylinders, must be nonferrous.

86. In the pacemaker coding system, the first letter refers to the chamber paced, the second letter to the chamber in which sensing occurs, the third letter to the responses to sensing in chambers, and the fourth letter to rate responsiveness.

87. Loss of afferent sensory and motor stimulation renders a patient sensitive to sedative medications secondary to deafferentation. For the same reason neuraxial anesthesia decreases the MAC of volatile anesthetics.

88. The correct use of peripheral nerve block (PNB) can decrease the incidence of perioperative complications such as pain, nausea, vomiting, and other opioid side effects caused by the decreased use of such drugs.

89. OLV can be achieved with DLTs, bronchial blockers, and standard single-lumen endotracheal tubes. A malpositioned tube or bronchial blocker is suggested by an acute increase in ventilator pressures and hypoxemia. During OLV, protective ventilation strategies include low-tidal volume ventilation (6 ml/kg), PEEP 5 cm H_2O, limited peak airway pressures, and permissive hypercapnia. Methods to improve oxygenation during OLV include increasing FiO_2, checking DLT and bronchial blocker placement, applying PEEP to the ventilated lung and continuous positive airway pressure (CPAP) to the nonventilated lung, asking the surgeon to restrict pulmonary blood flow to the nonventilated lung, and returning to two-lung ventilation.

90. If ICP is high, as evidenced by profound changes in mental status or radiologic evidence of cerebral swelling, avoid volatile anesthetics and opt instead for a total intravenous anesthetic technique.

91. If ICP is high, as evidenced by profound changes in mental status or radiologic evidence of cerebral swelling, avoid volatile anesthetics and opt instead for a total intravenous anesthetic technique. Measures to acutely decrease ICP include elevation of the head of the bed; hyperventilation ($PaCO_2$ 25 to 30 mm Hg); diuresis (mannitol and/or furosemide); and minimized intravenous fluid. In the setting of elevated ICP, avoid ketamine and nitrous oxide. Preexisting cerebral vasospasm may be worsened by systemic hypotension during surgery.

92. Chronic pain is best treated using multiple therapeutic modalities. These include physical therapy, psychological support, pharmacologic management, and the rational use of more invasive procedures such as nerve blocks and implantable technologies.

93. Measures to acutely decrease ICP include elevation of the head of the bed; hyperventilation ($PaCO_2$ 25 to 30 mm Hg); diuresis (mannitol and/or furosemide); and minimized intravenous fluid. In the setting of elevated ICP, avoid ketamine and nitrous oxide.

94. Pulmonary catheterization has not been shown to improve outcome in all patient subsets.

95. Malignant hyperthermia is an inherited disorder that presents in the perioperative period after exposure to inhalational agents and/or succinylcholine. Dantrolene is a mainstay of therapy. Discontinue volatile anesthetic and ask for HELP!

96. Perioperative glucocorticoid supplementation should be considered for patients receiving exogenous steroids.

97. Pulmonary catheterization has not been shown to improve outcome in all patient subsets.

98. Patients with diabetes have a high incidence of coronary artery disease with an atypical or silent presentation.

99. From about 24 hours after injury until the burn has healed, succinylcholine may cause hyperkalemia because of proliferation of extrajunctional neuromuscular receptors. Hyperkalemia is a contraindication.

100. Patients with liver disease commonly have an increased volume of distribution, necessitating an increase in initial dose requirements. However, because the drug metabolism may be reduced, smaller doses are subsequently administered at longer intervals.

1 BASICS OF PATIENT MANAGEMENT

AUTONOMIC NERVOUS SYSTEM

James C. Duke, MD, MBA

1. **Describe the autonomic nervous system.**
   The autonomic nervous system (ANS) is a network of nerves and ganglia that controls involuntary physiologic actions and maintains internal homeostasis and stress responses. The ANS innervates structures within the cardiovascular, pulmonary, endocrine, exocrine, gastrointestinal, genitourinary, and central nervous systems (CNS) and influences metabolism and thermal regulation. The ANS is divided into two parts: the sympathetic (SNS) and parasympathetic (PNS) nervous systems. The effects of SNS stimulation are widespread across the body. In contrast, PNS stimulation tends to produce localized, discrete effects. The SNS and PNS generally have opposing effects on end-organs, with either the SNS or the PNS exhibiting a dominant tone at rest and without exogenous stimulating events (Table 1-1). In general, the function of the PNS is homeostatic, whereas stimulation of the SNS prepares the organism for some stressful event (this is often called the fight-or-flight response).

> ## KEY POINTS: AUTONOMIC NERVOUS SYSTEM
>
> 1. Patients on β-blockers should take them on the day of surgery and continue them perioperatively. Because the receptors are upregulated, withdrawal may precipitate hypertension, tachycardia, and myocardial ischemia. Rarely are β-blockers initiated the day of surgery.
> 2. Clonidine should also be continued perioperatively because of concerns for rebound hypertension.
> 3. Indirect-acting sympathomimetics (e.g., ephedrine) depend on norepinephrine release to be effective. Norepinephrine-depleted states will not respond to ephedrine administration.
> 4. Under most circumstances, peri-induction hypotension responds best to intravenous fluid administration and the use of direct-acting sympathomimetics such as phenylephrine.
> 5. Orthostatic hypotension is common after surgery and may be caused by the use of any or all anesthetic agents and lying supine for extended periods. It is necessary to be cognizant of this potential problem when elevating a patient's head after surgery or even when moving the patient from the operating room table to a chair (e.g., procedures requiring only sedation and monitoring).

2. **Review the anatomy of the SNS.**
   Preganglionic sympathetic neurons originate from the intermediolateral columns of the thoracolumbar spinal cord. These myelinated fibers exit via the ventral root of the spinal nerve and synapse with postganglionic fibers in paravertebral sympathetic ganglia, unpaired prevertebral ganglia, or a terminal ganglion. Preganglionic neurons may ascend or descend the sympathetic chain before synapsing. Preganglionic neurons stimulate nicotinic cholinergic postganglionic neurons by releasing acetylcholine. Postganglionic adrenergic neurons synapse at targeted end-organs and release norepinephrine (Figure 1-1).

3. **Elaborate on the location and names of the sympathetic ganglia. Practically speaking, what is the importance of knowing the name and location of these ganglia?**
   Easily identifiable paravertebral ganglia are found in the cervical region (including the stellate ganglion) and along thoracic, lumbar, and pelvic sympathetic trunks. Prevertebral ganglia are named in relation to major branches of the aorta and include the celiac, superior and inferior mesenteric, and renal ganglia. Terminal ganglia are located close to the organs that they serve. The practical significance of knowing the location of some of these ganglia is that local anesthetics can be injected in the region of these structures to ameliorate sympathetically mediated pain.

Table 1-1. Autonomic Dominance Patterns at Effector Sites

SYMPATHETIC NERVOUS SYSTEM	PARASYMPATHETIC NERVOUS SYSTEM
Arterioles	Sinoatrial node
Veins	Gastrointestinal tract
Sweat glands	Uterus
Urinary bladder	
Salivary glands	
Iris	
Ciliary muscle	

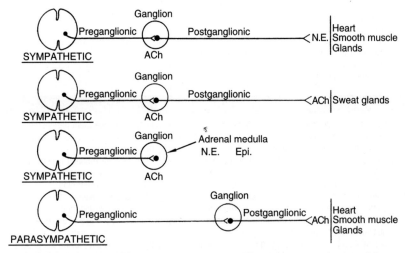

Figure 1-1. Neuronal anatomy of the autonomic nervous system with respective neurotransmitters. *Ach,* Acetylcholine; *Epi.,* epinephrine; *NE,* norepinephrine. *(Moss J, Glick D: The autonomic nervous system. In Miller RD, editor: Miller's anesthesia, ed 7, Philadelphia, 2010, Churchill-Livingstone, p. 347.)*

4. **Describe the postganglionic adrenergic receptors of the SNS and the effects of stimulating these receptors.**
   There are alpha-1 (α_1), alpha-2 (α_2), beta-1 (β_1), and beta-2 (β_2) adrenergic receptors. The α_1, α_2, and β_2 receptors are postsynaptic and are stimulated by the neurotransmitter norepinephrine. The α_2 receptors are presynaptic, and stimulation inhibits release of norepinephrine, reducing overall the autonomic response. Molecular pharmacologists have further subdivided these receptors, but this is beyond the scope of this discussion. Dopamine stimulates postganglionic dopaminergic receptors, classified as D1 and D2. The response to receptor activation in different sites is described in Table 1-2.

5. **Review the anatomy and function of the PNS.**
   Preganglionic parasympathetic neurons originate from cranial nerves III, VII, IX, and X and sacral segments 2-4. Preganglionic parasympathetic neurons synapse with postganglionic neurons close to the targeted end-organ, creating a more discrete physiologic effect. Both preganglionic and postganglionic parasympathetic neurons release acetylcholine; these cholinergic receptors are subclassified as either nicotinic or muscarinic. The response to cholinergic stimulation is summarized in Table 1-3.

Table 1-2. End-Organ Effects of Adrenergic Receptor Stimulation

RECEPTOR	ORGAN	RESPONSE
β_1	Heart	Increases heart rate, contractility, and conduction velocity
Fat cells	Lipolysis	
β_2	Blood vessels	Dilation
Bronchioles	Dilation	
Uterus	Relaxation	
Kidneys	Renin secretion	
Liver	Gluconeogenesis, glycogenolysis	
Pancreas	Insulin secretion	
α_1	Blood vessels	Constriction
Pancreas	Inhibits insulin release	
Intestine, bladder	Relaxation but constriction of sphincters	
α_2	Presynaptic nerve endings	Inhibits norepinephrine release
Dopamine-1	Blood vessels	Dilates renal, coronary, and splanchnic vessels
Dopamine-2	Presynaptic endings	Inhibits norepinephrine release
Central nervous system	Psychic disturbances	

Table 1-3. End-Organ Effects of Cholinergic Receptor Stimulation

RECEPTOR	ORGAN	RESPONSE
Muscarinic	Heart	Decreased heart rate, contractility, conduction velocity
Bronchioles	Constriction	
Salivary glands	Stimulates secretion	
Intestine	Contraction and relaxation of sphincters, stimulates secretions	
Bladder	Contraction and relaxation of sphincters	
Nicotinic	Neuromuscular junction	Skeletal muscle contraction
Autonomic ganglia	SNS stimulation	

SNS, Sympathetic nervous system.

6. **What are catecholamines? Which catecholamines occur naturally? Which are synthetic?**
   Catecholamines are hydroxy-substituted phenylethylamines and stimulate adrenergic nerve endings. Norepinephrine, epinephrine, and dopamine are naturally occurring catecholamines, whereas dobutamine and isoproterenol are synthetic catecholamines.

7. **Review the synthesis of dopamine, norepinephrine, and epinephrine.**
   The amino acid tyrosine is actively transported into the adrenergic presynaptic nerve terminal cytoplasm, where it is converted to dopamine by two enzymatic reactions: hydroxylation of tyrosine by tyrosine hydroxylase to dopamine and decarboxylation of dopamine by aromatic L-amino acid decarboxylase. Dopamine is transported into storage vesicles, where it is hydroxylated by dopamine β-hydroxylase to norepinephrine. Epinephrine is synthesized in the adrenal medulla from norepinephrine through methylation by phenylethanolamine N-methyltransferase (Figure 1-2).

8. **How is norepinephrine metabolized?**
   Norepinephrine is removed from the synaptic junction by reuptake into the presynaptic nerve terminal and metabolic breakdown. Reuptake is the most important mechanism and allows reuse of the neurotransmitter. The enzyme monoamine oxidase (MAO) metabolizes norepinephrine within the neuronal cytoplasm; both MAO and catecholamine O–methyltransferase (COMT) metabolize the neurotransmitter at extraneuronal sites. The important metabolites are 3-methoxy-4-hydroxymandelic acid, metanephrine, and normetanephrine.

9. **Describe the synthesis and degradation of acetylcholine.**
   The cholinergic neurotransmitter acetylcholine (ACh) is synthesized within presynaptic neuronal mitochondria by esterification of acetyl coenzyme A and choline by the enzyme choline acetyltransferase; it is stored in synaptic vesicles until release. After release, ACh is principally metabolized by acetylcholinesterase, a membrane-bound enzyme located in the synaptic junction. Acetylcholinesterase is also located in other nonneuronal tissues such as erythrocytes.

10. **What are sympathomimetics?**
    Sympathomimetics are synthetic drugs with vasopressor and chronotropic effects similar to those of catecholamines. They are commonly used in the operating room to reverse the circulatory depressant effects of anesthetic agents by increasing blood pressure and heart rate; they also temporize the effects of hypovolemia while fluids are administered. They are effective during both general and regional anesthesia.

11. **Review the sympathomimetics commonly used in the perioperative environment.**
    Direct-acting sympathomimetics are agonists at the targeted receptor, whereas indirect-acting sympathomimetics stimulate release of norepinephrine. Sympathomimetics may be mixed in their actions, having both direct and indirect effects. Practically speaking, phenylephrine (direct acting) and ephedrine (mostly indirect acting) are the sympathomimetics commonly used perioperatively. Also, epinephrine, dopamine, and norepinephrine may be used perioperatively and most often by infusion since their effects on blood pressure, heart rate, and myocardial oxygen consumption can be profound.

12. **Discuss the effects of phenylephrine and review common doses of this medication.**
    Phenylephrine stimulates primarily α_1 receptors, resulting in increased systemic vascular resistance and blood pressure. Larger doses stimulate α_2 receptors. Reflex bradycardia may be a response to increasing systemic vascular resistance. Usual intravenous doses of phenylephrine range between 50 and 200 mcg. Phenylephrine may also be administered by infusion at 10 to 20 mcg/min.

13. **Discuss the effects of ephedrine and review common doses of this medication. Give some examples of medications that contraindicate the use of ephedrine and why.**
    Ephedrine produces norepinephrine release, stimulating mostly α_1 and β_1 receptors; the effects resemble those of epinephrine although they are less intense. Increases in systolic blood pressure, diastolic blood pressure, heart rate, and cardiac output are noted. Usual intravenous doses of ephedrine are between 5 and 25 mg. Repeated doses demonstrate diminishing response known as *tachyphylaxis*, possibly because of exhaustion of norepinephrine supplies or receptor blockade. Similarly, an inadequate response to ephedrine may be the result of already depleted norepinephrine stores. Ephedrine should not be used when the patient is taking drugs that prevent reuptake of norepinephrine

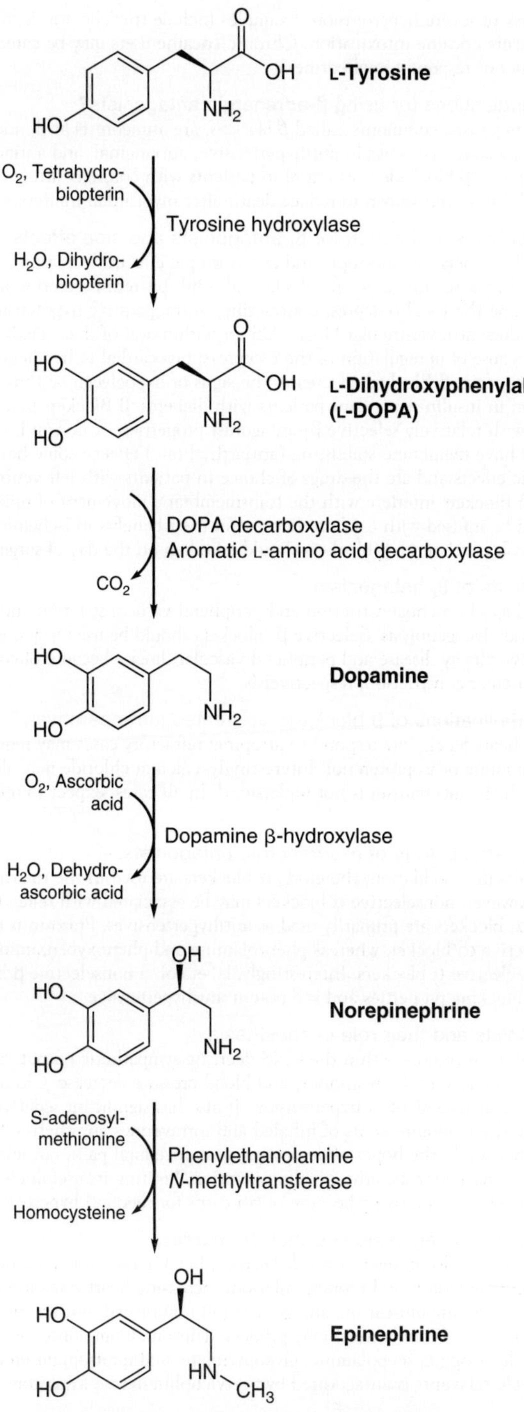

Figure 1-2. The catecholamine synthetic pathway. (*From* http://www.answers.com/topic/epinephrine.)

because of the risk of severe hypertension. Examples include tricyclic antidepressants, MAO inhibitors, and acute cocaine intoxication. Chronic cocaine users may be catecholamine depleted and may not respond to ephedrine.

14. **What are the indications for using β-adrenergic antagonists?**
β-Adrenergic antagonists, commonly called *β blockers*, are antagonists at β_1 and β_2 receptors. β Blockers are mainstays in antihypertensive, antianginal, and antiarrhythmic therapy. Perioperative β blockade is essential in patients with coronary artery disease, and the use of atenolol has been shown to reduce death after myocardial infarction.

15. **Review the mechanism of action for β_1 antagonists and side effects.**
β_1 Blockade produces negative inotropic and chronotropic effects, decreasing cardiac output and myocardial oxygen requirements. β_1 Blockers also inhibit renin secretion and lipolysis. Because volatile anesthetics also depress contractility, intraoperative hypotension is a risk. β Blockers can produce atrioventricular block. Abrupt withdrawal of these medications is not recommended because of upregulation of the receptors; myocardial ischemia and hypertension may occur. β Blockade decreases the signs of hypoglycemia; thus, it must be used with caution in insulin-dependent patients with diabetes. β Blockers may be cardioselective, with relatively selective β_1-antagonist properties, or noncardioselective. Some β blockers have membrane-stabilizing (antiarrhythmic) effects; some have sympathomimetic effects and are the drugs of choice in patients with left ventricular failure or bradycardia. β Blockers interfere with the transmembrane movement of potassium; thus, potassium should be infused with caution. Because of their benefits in ischemic heart disease and the risk of rebound, β blockers should be taken on the day of surgery.

16. **Review the effects of β_2 antagonism.**
β_2 Blockade produces bronchoconstriction and peripheral vasoconstriction and inhibits insulin release and glycogenolysis. Selective β_1 blockers should be used in patients with chronic or reactive airway disease and peripheral vascular disease because of concerns for bronchial and vascular constriction, respectively.

17. **How might complications of β blockade be treated intraoperatively?**
Bradycardia and heart block may respond to atropine; refractory cases may require the β_2 agonism of dobutamine or isoproterenol. Interestingly, calcium chloride may also be effective, although the mechanism is not understood. In all cases, expect to use larger than normal doses.

18. **Describe the pharmacology of α-adrenergic antagonists.**
α_1 Blockade results in vasodilation; therefore, α blockers are used in the treatment of hypertension. However, nonselective α blockers may be associated with reflex tachycardia. Thus, selective α_1 blockers are primarily used as antihypertensives. Prazosin is the prototypical selective α_1 blocker, whereas phentolamine and phenoxybenzamine are examples of nonselective α blockers. Interestingly, labetalol, a nonselective β blocker, also has selective α_1-blocking properties and is a potent antihypertensive.

19. **Review α_2 agonists and their role in anesthesia.**
When stimulated, α_2 receptors within the CNS decrease sympathetic output. Subsequently, cardiac output, systemic vascular resistance, and blood pressure decrease. Clonidine is an α_2 agonist used in the management of hypertension. It also has significant sedative qualities. It decreases the anesthetic requirements of inhaled and intravenous anesthetics. It has also been used intrathecally in the hopes of decreasing postprocedural pain, but unacceptable hypotension is common after intrathecal administration, limiting its usefulness. Clonidine should be continued perioperatively because of concerns for rebound hypertension.

20. **Discuss muscarinic antagonists and their properties.**
Muscarinic antagonists, also known as *anticholinergics*, block muscarinic cholinergic receptors, producing mydriasis and bronchodilation, increasing heart rate, and inhibiting secretions. Centrally acting muscarinic antagonists (all nonionized, tertiary amines with the ability to cross the blood-brain barrier) may produce delirium. Commonly used muscarinic antagonists include atropine, scopolamine, glycopyrrolate, and ipratropium bromide. When the effect of muscle relaxants is antagonized by acetylcholinesterase inhibitors, muscarinic

antagonists must be administered to avoid the risk of profound bradycardia, heart block, and asystole. Glycopyrrolate is a quaternary ammonium compound, cannot cross the blood-brain barrier, and therefore lacks CNS activity. When inhaled, ipratropium bromide produces bronchodilation.

21. **What is the significance of autonomic dysfunction? How might you tell if a patient has autonomic dysfunction?**

    The term that is used currently is *dysautonomia*. Patients with autonomic dysfunction, also called autonomic failure, tend to have severe hypotension pre- and intraoperatively. Evaluation of changes in orthostatic blood pressure and heart rate is a quick and effective way of assessing autonomic dysfunction. If the ANS is intact, an increase in heart rate of 15 beats/min and a decrease of 10 to 20 mm Hg in diastolic blood pressure are expected when changing position from supine to sitting. Autonomic dysfunction is suggested whenever there is a loss of heart rate variability, whatever the circumstances. Autonomic dysfunction includes vasomotor, bladder, bowel, and sexual dysfunction. Response to medications may also be manifestations of autonomia. Additional signs include blurred vision, reduced or excessive sweating, dry or excessively moist eyes and mouth, cold or discolored extremities, incontinence or incomplete voiding, diarrhea or constipation, and impotence. Diabetics and chronic alcoholics are also patient groups well known to demonstrate autonomic dysfunction.

22. **What is a pheochromocytoma, and what are its associated symptoms? How is pheochromocytoma diagnosed?**

    A pheochromocytoma is a catecholamine-secreting tumor composed of chromaffin tissue, producing either norepinephrine or epinephrine. Most are intraadrenal, but some are extraadrenal (within the bladder wall is common), and about 10% are malignant. Signs and symptoms include paroxysms of hypertension, syncope, headache, palpitations, flushing, and sweating. Pheochromocytoma is confirmed by detecting elevated levels of plasma and urinary catecholamines and their metabolites, including vanillylmandelic acid, normetanephrine, and metanephrine.

23. **Review the preanesthetic and intraoperative management of pheochromocytoma patients.**

    These patients are markedly volume depleted and at risk for severe hypertensive crises. It is essential that before surgery, α blockade and rehydration should first be instituted. The α_1 antagonist phenoxybenzamine is commonly administered orally. β Blockers are often administered once α blockade is achieved and should never be given first because unopposed α_1 vasoconstriction results in severe, refractory hypertension. Labetalol may be the β blocker of choice since it also has α-blocking properties.

    Intraoperatively intraarterial monitoring is required since fluctuations in blood pressure may be extreme. Manipulation of the tumor may result in hypertension. Intraoperative hypertension is managed by infusing the α blocker phentolamine or vasodilator nitroprusside. Once the tumor has been removed, hypotension is a risk, and fluid administration and administration of the α agonist phenylephrine may be necessary. Central venous pressure monitoring will assist with volume management.

SUGGESTED READINGS

Mustafa HI, Fessel JP, Barwise J, et al: Dysautonomia. Perioperative implications, Anesthesiology 116:205–215, 2012.

Neukirchen M, Kienbaum P: Sympathetic nervous system. Evaluation and importance for clinical general anesthesia, Anesthesiology 109:1113–1131, 2008.

CHAPTER 2

RESPIRATORY AND PULMONARY PHYSIOLOGY

Barbara Wilkey, MD

1. **Describe the lung volumes and capacities.**
   - Tidal volume (V_T) = volume of gas inspired and passively expired during normal breathing
   - Residual volume (RV) = volume of gas remaining in the lung after maximal exhalation
   - Expiratory reserve volume (ERV) = volume of gas that can be maximally exhaled with the lungs and chest at rest
   - Inspiratory reserve volume (IRV) = volume of gas that can be maximally inhaled at the inspiratory peak of the tidal volume
   - Total lung capacity (TLC) = IRV + V_T + ERV + RV
   - Vital capacity (VC) = IRV + V_T + ERV
   - Inspiratory capacity (IC) = IRV + V_T
   - Functional residual capacity (FRC) = ERV + RV

2. **What is the FRC? What factors affect FRC?**
   The FRC is the volume in the lungs at the end of passive expiration. The FRC is determined by opposing forces of the expanding chest wall and the elastic recoil of the lung. A normal FRC = 1.7–3.5 L.
   FRC is increased by:
   - Body size (FRC increases with height)
   - Age (FRC increases slightly with age)
   - Certain lung diseases, including asthma and chronic obstructive pulmonary disease (COPD).
   FRC is decreased by:
   - Sex (women have a 10% decrease in FRC when compared with men)
   - Diaphragmatic muscle tone (individuals with paralyzed diaphragms have less FRC when compared with normal individuals)
   - Posture (FRC greatest standing > sitting > prone > lateral > supine)
   - Certain lung disease where elastic recoil is diminished (e.g., interstitial lung disease, thoracic burns, and kyphoscoliosis).
   - Increased abdominal pressure (e.g., obesity, ascites)

3. **What is closing capacity? What factors affect the closing capacity? What is the relationship between closing capacity and FRC?**
   Closing capacity is the point during expiration when small airways begin to close. In young individuals, with average body mass index, closing capacity is approximately half the FRC when upright and approximately two thirds of the FRC when supine.
   Closing capacity increases with age and is equal to FRC in the supine individual at approximately 44 years and in the upright individual at approximately 66 years. Whereas the FRC is dependent on position, the closing capacity is independent of position. Closing capacity increases with increasing intraabdominal pressure, age, decreased pulmonary blood flow, and pulmonary parenchymal disease that decreases compliance.

4. **What is the clinical consequence of a decreased FRC and an increased closing capacity?**
   Patients with a decreased functional residual capacity and/or increased closing capacity will become hypoxic faster after induction of apnea than those with normal volumes.

5. **Discuss the factors that affect the resistance to gas flow. What is laminar and turbulent gas flow?**

   The resistance to flow can be separated into the properties of the tube and the properties of the gas. At low flow, or laminar flow (nonobstructed breathing), the viscosity is the major property of the gas that affects flow. Clearly, the major determining factor in resistance is the radius of the tube. This can be shown by the Hagen-Poiseuille relationship: $R = (8 \times L \times \mu) / (\pi \times r^4)$, where R is resistance, L is the length of the tube, μ is the viscosity, and r is the radius of the tube. At higher flow rate (in obstructed airways and in heavy breathing), the flow is turbulent. At these flows, the major determinants of resistance to flow are the density of the gas, ρ and the radius of the tube, r: $R \propto \rho/r^5$.

   In a ventilated patient, normal resistance is 1 to 8 cm H_2O/L per second.

6. **Discuss the impact and determinants of flow qualities.**

   Laminar flow is the most efficient flow type for oxygen delivery. With turbulent flow, a greater change in pressure must be achieved to obtain the same flow. The Reynolds number (Re) is a dimensionless number associated with delineation of turbulent versus laminar flow. A lower Re is associated with laminar flow, and a higher Re is associated with turbulent flow. $Re = 2rv\rho/\eta$, where r is radius of the tube, v is velocity, ρ is gas density, and η is viscosity.

7. **How does gas flow resistance apply to clinical practice?**

   Patients who are intubated must move air through a smaller radius than their normal airway, as the endotracheal tube has a smaller diameter than the airway in which it is placed. Because of this higher airway resistance, spontaneous respiration in an intubated patient requires greater work of breathing. This work of breathing can be overcome with pressure support through a ventilator. Pressure support allows the patient to trigger spontaneous ventilation; however, the ventilator provides enough positive pressure to overcome the resistance of the endotracheal tube.

8. **Discuss clinical interventions that may mitigate turbulent flow.**

   As noted earlier, with airway obstruction there can be transition from laminar flow to turbulent flow. If this obstruction is due to airway edema, racemic epinephrine delivered via inhalation may shrink the mucosal tissue thereby increasing the airway radius and decreasing the Reynolds number.

   Another option to overcome increased airway resistance in turbulent flow situations due to airway obstruction is changing gas density. Helium is a noncombustible gas; it is insoluble in human tissue and has a very low density. When helium and oxygen are combined, the result is a gas with a similar viscosity to air, but a much lower density. This reduces the Reynolds number and sways the equation toward laminar flow. Traditionally, this mixture has been 70% helium and 30% oxygen.

9. **Discuss dynamic and static compliance.**

   Compliance describes the elastic properties of the lung. It is a measure of the change in volume of the lung when pressure is applied. The lung is an elastic body that exhibits elastic hysteresis. When lung is rapidly inflated and held at a given volume, the pressure peaks and then exponentially falls to a plateau pressure. The volume change of the lung per the initial peak pressure change is the dynamic compliance. The volume change per the plateau pressure represents the static compliance of the lung. Dynamic compliance includes the resistive forces in the lungs.

   In a ventilated individual, normal compliance is 57 to 85 ml/cm H_2O per second.

10. **What are some commonly seen clinical conditions that can change compliance and resistance?**

    Acute respiratory disease syndrome (ARDS) and cardiogenic pulmonary edema tend to result in elevated resistance and decreased compliance. COPD tends to cause an elevated compliance and resistance.

11. **How does surface tension affect the forces in the small airways and alveoli?**

    Laplace's law describes the relationship between pressure (P), tension (T), and the radius (R) of a bubble and can be applied to the alveoli: $P = 2 T / R$.

As the radius decreases, the pressure increases. In a lung without surfactant present, as the alveoli decrease in size, the pressure is higher in small alveoli, causing gas to move from the small to larger airways, collapsing in the process. Surfactant, a phospholipid substance produced in the lung by type II alveolar epithelium, reduces the surface tension of the small airways, thus decreasing the pressure as the airways decrease in size. This important substance helps keep the small airways open during expiration.

12. **What clinical scenarios might result in an absolute or relative surfactant deficiency?**
The classic example of absolute surfactant deficiency is that of the premature newborn, leading to respiratory distress syndrome. One can also acquire a relative surfactant deficiency. This may be seen in conditions such as ARDS, many forms of obstructive lung disease, respiratory infection, idiopathic pulmonary fibrosis, and lung transplantation.

13. **Review the different zones of West in the lung with regard to perfusion and ventilation.**
West described three areas of perfusion in an upright lung and a fourth area was later added. Beginning at the apices, they are
- Zone 1: Alveolar pressure (P_{Alv}) exceeds pulmonary artery pressure (P_{pa}) and pulmonary venous pressure (P_{pv}), leading to ventilation without perfusion (alveolar dead space) ($P_{Alv} > P_{pa} > P_{pv}$).
- Zone 2: Pulmonary arterial pressure exceeds alveolar pressure, but alveolar pressure still exceeds venous pressure ($P_{pa} > P_{Alv} > P_{pv}$). Blood flow in zone 2 is determined by arterial-alveolar pressure difference.
- Zone 3: Pulmonary venous pressure exceeds alveolar pressure, and flow is determined by the arterial-venous pressure difference ($P_{pa} > P_{pv} > P_{Alv}$).
- Zone 4: Interstitial pressure ($P_{interstitium}$) is greater than venous and alveolar pressures; thus, flow is determined by the arterial-interstitial pressure difference ($P_{pa} > P_{interstitium} > P_{pv} > P_{Alv}$). Zone 4 should be minimal in a healthy patient.

A change from upright to supine position increases pulmonary blood volume by 25% to 30%, thus increasing the size of larger numbered West zones.

14. **What is the alveolar gas equation and what is the normal alveolar pressure at sea level on room air?**
The alveolar gas equation is used to calculate the alveolar oxygen partial pressure.

$$P_AO_2 = F_iO_2(P_b - P_{H2O}) - P_aCO_2/Q$$

where P_AO_2 is the alveolar oxygen partial pressure, F_iO_2 is the fraction of inspired oxygen, P_b is the barometric pressure, P_{H2O} is the partial pressure of water, P_aCO_2 is the partial pressure of carbon dioxide, and Q is the respiratory quotient, dependent on metabolic activity and diet and is considered to be about 0.825. At sea level, the alveolar partial pressure (P_AO_2) is

$$P_AO_2 = 0.21(760 - 47) - 40/0.8 = 99.7.$$

15. **Using the above equation, would room air P_AO_2 be lower or higher in Denver, CO (elevation 5280 ft), compared with Gainesville, FL (elevation near sea level)?**
Room air is equivalent in Gainesville and Denver, but the partial pressure of Gainesville, compared with Denver, increases the oxygen partial pressure.

16. **What are the causes of hypoxemia?**
- Low inspired oxygen concentration (FiO_2): To prevent delivery of hypoxic gas mixtures during an anesthetic, oxygen concentration alarms are present on the anesthesia machine and will render the anesthetist alert to make the proper intervention and increase the amount of oxygen to the patient.
- Hypoventilation: Patients under general anesthesia may be incapable of maintaining an adequate minute ventilation, due to muscle relaxants or the ventilatory depressant effects of anesthetic agents. Hypoventilation is a common problem postoperatively, but an adequate oxygenation saturation may be confirmed by pulse oximetry. Worsening hypercarbia from hypoventilation can be masked by increasing the inspired oxygen

concentration. Always deliver the least amount of oxygen necessary and evaluate the patient if oxygen saturation is inadequate.

- Shunt: Sepsis, liver failure, arteriovenous malformations, pulmonary emboli, and right-to-left cardiac shunts may create sufficient shunting to result in hypoxemia. As shunted blood is not exposed to alveoli, hypoxemia caused by a shunt cannot be overcome by increasing FiO_2.
- Ventilation-perfusion (V/Q) mismatch: Ventilation and perfusion of the alveoli in the lung ideally have close to a 1-to-1 relationship, promoting efficient oxygen exchange between alveoli and blood. When alveolar ventilation and perfusion to the lungs are unequal (V/Q mismatching), hypoxemia results. Causes of V/Q mismatching include atelectasis, lateral decubitus positioning, bronchial intubation, bronchospasm, pneumonia, mucus plugging, pulmonary contusion, and adult respiratory distress syndrome. Hypoxemia due to V/Q mismatching can usually be overcome by increasing FiO_2.
- Diffusion defects: Efficient O_2 exchange depends on a healthy interface between the alveoli and the bloodstream. Advanced pulmonary disease and pulmonary edema may have associated diffusion impairment.

KEY POINTS: CAUSES OF HYPOXEMIA

1. Low inspired oxygen tension
2. Alveolar hypoventilation
3. Right-left shunting
4. V/Q mismatch
5. Diffusion abnormality

17. **Discuss V/Q mismatch.**
In the normal individual, alveolar ventilation (V) and perfusion (Q) vary throughout the lung anatomy. In the ideal situation, V and Q are equal, and V/Q = 1. In shunted lung, the perfusion is greater than the ventilation, creating areas of lung where blood flow is high, but little gas exchange occurs. In dead space lung, ventilation is far greater than perfusion, creating areas of lung where gas is delivered, but little blood flow and gas exchange occurs. Both situations can cause hypoxemia. In the case of dead space, increasing the FiO_2 will potentially increase the hemoglobin oxygen saturation, whereas in cases of shunt, it will not. In many pathologic situations, both extremes coexist within the lung.

18. **How can general anesthesia worsen V/Q mismatch?**
Under general anesthesia, FRC is reduced by approximately 400 ml in an adult. The supine position decreases FRC another 800 ml. A large enough decrease in FRC may bring end-expiratory volumes or even the entire tidal volume to levels below the closing volume (the volume at which small airways close). When small airways begin to close, atelectasis and low V/Q areas develop.

19. **Define anatomic, alveolar, and physiologic dead space.**
Physiologic dead space (V_D) is the sum of anatomic and alveolar dead space. Anatomic dead space is the volume of lung that does not exchange gas. This includes the nose, pharynx, trachea, and bronchi. This is about 2 ml/kg in the spontaneously breathing individual and is the majority of physiologic dead space. Endotracheal intubation will decrease the total anatomic dead space. Alveolar dead space is the volume of gas that reaches the alveoli but does not take part in gas exchange because the alveoli are not perfused. In healthy patients, alveolar dead space is negligible.

20. **How is V_D/V_T calculated?**
V_D/V_T is the ratio of the physiologic dead space to the tidal volume, is usually about 33%, and is determined by the following formula:

$$V_d/V_t = [(\text{alveolar } PCO_2 - \text{expired } PCO_2)] / \text{alveolar } PCO_2$$

Alveolar PCO_2 is calculated using the alveolar gas equation, and expired PCO_2 is the average PCO_2 in an expired gas sample.

21. **Describe the pulmonary circulation.**
The pulmonary circulation is a low-resistance, high-flow system, and accounts for approximately 450 ml of blood. Blood is supplied to the lungs through the pulmonary and bronchial arteries. Blood in the pulmonary arteries, partially deoxygenated, flows through the hilum of the lungs with a mean arterial pressure of 15 mm Hg, then onto the bronchial divisions to the more peripheral oxygen exchange units of the lung. Here the vessels rapidly decrease in size and increase in cross-sectional area, as capillaries, where they surround the alveoli and participate in gas exchange. From there, they coalesce into veins, traversing through the interlobular septae back to the hilum, and drain into the pulmonary veins and left atria of the heart, where the mean pressure is 5 mm Hg. The bronchial arteries supply 1% to 2% of the lungs with oxygen and arise from the thoracic aorta. They supply blood to the supportive tissue and bronchi, eventually emptying into the pulmonary veins, thus accounting for a 1% to 2% physiologic shunt.

22. **Define absolute shunt. How is the shunt fraction calculated?**
Absolute shunt is defined as blood that reaches the arterial system without passing through ventilated regions of the lung. The fraction of cardiac output that passes through a shunt is determined by the following equation:

$$Qs/Qt = (CiO_2 - CaO_2) / (CiO_2 - CvO_2),$$

where Qs is the physiologic shunt blood flow per minute, Qt is the cardiac output per minute, CiO_2 is the ideal arterial oxygen concentration when $V/Q = 1$, CaO_2 is arterial oxygen content, and CvO_2 is mixed venous oxygen content. It is estimated that 2% to 5% of cardiac output is normally shunted through post-pulmonary shunts, thus accounting for the normal alveolar-arterial oxygen gradient (A-a gradient). Post-pulmonary shunts include thebesian, bronchial, mediastinal, and pleural veins.

23. **What is hypoxic pulmonary vasoconstriction?**
Hypoxic pulmonary vasoconstriction (HPV) is a local response of pulmonary arterial smooth muscle that decreases blood flow in the presence of low alveolar oxygen pressure, helping to maintain normal V/Q relationships by diverting blood from underventilated areas. HPV is inhibited by volatile anesthetics and vasodilators but is not affected by intravenous anesthesia.

24. **Calculate arterial and venous oxygen content (CaO_2 and CvO_2).**
CaO_2 (ml O_2/dl) is calculated by summing the oxygen bound to hemoglobin (Hgb) and the dissolved oxygen of blood:

$$\text{Oxygen content} = 1.34 \times [Hgb] \times SaO2 + (PaO_2 \times 0.003),$$

where 1.34 is the O_2 content per gram hemoglobin, SaO_2 is the hemoglobin saturation, [Hgb] is the hemoglobin concentration, and PaO_2 is the arterial oxygen concentration.
If [Hgb] = 15 gm/dl, arterial saturation = 96%, and PaO_2 = 90 mm Hg, mixed venous saturation = 75%, and PvO_2 = 40 mm Hg, then

$$CaO_2 = (1.34 \text{ ml } O_2/\text{gm Hgb} \times 15 \text{ gm Hgb/dl} \times 0.96) + (90 \times 0.003) = 19.6 \text{ ml } O_2/\text{dl}$$

and

$$CvO_2 = (1.34 \text{ ml } O_2/\text{gm Hgb} \times 15 \text{ gm Hgb/dl} \times 0.75) + (40 \times 0.003) = 15.2 \text{ ml } O_2/\text{dl}.$$

25. **What factors alter oxygen consumption?**
Factors increasing oxygen consumption include hyperthermia (including malignant hyperthermia), hypothermia with shivering, hyperthyroidism, pregnancy, sepsis, burns, pain, and pheochromocytoma. Factors decreasing oxygen consumption include hypothermia without shivering, hypothyroidism, neuromuscular blockade, and general anesthesia.

26. Discuss a clinical scenario in which an anesthesiologist might have to consider shunting, oxygen delivery, oxygen consumption, and hypoxic pulmonary vasoconstriction.

    One lung ventilation is a classic example. How much hypoxemia an individual can experience is directly related to oxygen delivery and consumption.

27. How is CO_2 transported in the blood?

    CO_2 exists in three forms in blood: dissolved CO_2 (7%), bicarbonate ions (HCO_3^-) (70%), and combined with hemoglobin (23%).

28. How is PCO_2 related to alveolar ventilation?

    The partial pressure of CO_2 (PCO_2) is inversely related to the alveolar ventilation and is described by the equation $PCO_2 = (VCO_2/V_{alveolar})$, where VCO_2 is total CO_2 production and $V_{alveolar}$ is the alveolar ventilation (minute ventilation less the dead space ventilation). In general, minute ventilation and PCO_2 are inversely related.

KEY POINTS: USEFUL PULMONARY EQUATIONS

1. Alveolar gas partial pressure: $P_AO_2 = F_iO_2 (P_b - P_{H_2O}) - P_aCO_2/Q$
2. Oxygen content of blood: $C_aO_2 = 1.34 \times [Hgb] \times SaO_2 + (PaO_2 \times 0.003)$
3. Resistance of laminar flow through a tube: $R = (8 \times L \times \mu)/(\pi \times r^4)$
4. Resistance of turbulent flow through a tube: $R \propto \rho/r^5$
5. Calculation of shunt fraction: $Qs/Qt = (CiO_2 - CaO_2) / (CiO_2 - CvO_2)$

29. What effects do inhalational anesthetics have on ventilation?

    Volatile anesthetics greatly attenuate the ventilatory response to hypercarbia and hypoxemia.

30. Where is the respiration center located?

    The respiratory center is located bilaterally in the medulla and pons. Three major centers contribute to respiratory regulation. The dorsal respiratory center is mainly responsible for inspiration, the ventral respiratory center for both expiration and inspiration, and the pneumotaxic center helps control the breathing rate and pattern. A chemosensitive area also exists in the brainstem just beneath the ventral respiratory center. This area responds to changes in cerebrospinal fluid (CSF) pH, sending corresponding signals to the respiratory centers. Anesthetics cause repression of the respiratory centers of the brainstem.

31. How do carbon dioxide and oxygen act to stimulate and repress breathing?

    Carbon dioxide (indirectly) or hydrogen ions (directly) work on the chemosensitive area in the brainstem. Oxygen interacts with the peripheral chemoreceptors located in the carotid and aortic bodies. During hypercapnic and hypoxic states, the brainstem is stimulated to increase minute ventilation, while the opposite is true for hypocapnia and normoxia. Carbon dioxide is, by far, more influential in regulating respiration than is oxygen.

SUGGESTED READINGS

Barash PG, Cullen BF, Stoelting RK, editors: Clinical anesthesia, ed 5, Philadelphia, 2006, Lippincott Williams & Wilkins, pp 790–812.

Gentile MA, Davies JD: Bedside monitoring of pulmonary function. In Vincent J, Abraham E, Moore FA, et al, editors: Textbook of critical care, ed 6, Philadelphia, 2011, Saunders, pp 279–287.

Hite RD: Surfactant deficiency in adults, Clin Pulm Med 9:39–45, 2002.

Reuben AD, Harris AR: Heliox for asthma in the emergency department: a review of the literature, Emerg Med J 21:131–135, 2004.

Wilson WC, Benumof JL: Respiratory physiology and respiratory function during anesthesia. In Miller RD, editor: Miller's anesthesia, ed 6, Philadelphia, 2005, Churchill Livingstone, pp 679–722.

CHAPTER 3

BLOOD GAS AND ACID-BASE ANALYSIS

James C. Duke, MD, MBA

1. **What are the normal arterial blood gas (ABG) values in a healthy patient breathing room air at sea level?**
   See Table 3-1.

2. **What information does ABG provide?**
   ABG provides an assessment of the following:
   - **Oxygenation** (PaO_2). The PaO_2 is the amount of oxygen dissolved in the blood and therefore provides initial information on the efficiency of oxygenation.
   - **Ventilation** ($PaCO_2$). The adequacy of ventilation is inversely proportional to the $PaCO_2$ so that, when ventilation increases, $PaCO_2$ decreases, and when ventilation decreases, $PaCO_2$ increases.
   - **Acid-base status** (pH, HCO_3^-, and base deficit). A plasma pH >7.4 indicates alkalemia, and a pH <7.35 indicates acidemia. Despite a normal pH, an underlying acidosis or alkalosis may still be present.

3. **How is the regulation of acid-base balance traditionally described?**
   Acid-base balance is traditionally explained using the Henderson-Hasselbalch equation, which states that changes in HCO_3^- and $PaCO_2$ determine pH as follows:

   $$pH = pK + \log[HCO_3 / 0.03 \times PaCO_2]$$

   To prevent a change in pH, any increase or decrease in the $PaCO_2$ should be accompanied by a compensatory increase or decrease in the HCO_3^-. The importance of other physiologic nonbicarbonate buffers was later recognized and partly integrated into the base deficit and the corrected anion gap, both of which aid in interpreting complex acid-base disorders.

KEY POINTS: MAJOR CAUSES OF AN ANION GAP METABOLIC ACIDOSIS

Elevated anion gap metabolic acidosis is caused by accumulation of unmeasured anions:
- Lactic acid
- Ketones
- Toxins (ethanol, methanol, iron, salicylates, ethylene glycol, propylene glycol)
- Uremia

4. **What are the common acid-base disorders and their compensation?**
   See Table 3-2.

5. **How do you calculate the degree of compensation?**
   See Table 3-3.

6. **What are the common causes of respiratory acid-base disorders?**
   - **Respiratory alkalosis:** Sepsis, hypoxemia, anxiety, pain, and central nervous system lesions
   - **Respiratory acidosis:** Drugs (residual anesthetics, residual neuromuscular blockade, benzodiazepines, opioids), asthma, emphysema, obesity-hypoventilation syndromes, central nervous system lesions (infection, stroke), and neuromuscular disorders

Table 3-1. Arterial Blood Gas Values at Sea Level

pH	7.36–7.44
$PaCO_2$	33–44 mm Hg
PaO_2	75–105 mm Hg
HCO_3	20–26 mmol/L
BD (base deficit)	+3 to −3 mmol/L
SaO_2	95%–97%

Table 3-2. Major Acid-Base Disorders and Compensatory Mechanisms*

PRIMARY DISORDER	PRIMARY DISTURBANCE	PRIMARY COMPENSATION
Respiratory acidosis	↑ $PaCO_2$	↑ HCO_3
Respiratory alkalosis	↓ $PaCO_2$	↓ HCO_3
Metabolic acidosis	↓ HCO_3	↓ $PaCO_2$
Metabolic alkalosis	↑ HCO_3	↑ $PaCO_2$

*Primary compensation for metabolic disorders is achieved rapidly through respiratory control of CO_2, whereas primary compensation for respiratory disorders is achieved more slowly as the kidneys excrete or absorb acid and bicarbonate. Mixed acid-base disorders are common.

Table 3-3. Calculating the Degree of Compensation*

PRIMARY DISORDER	RULE
Respiratory acidosis (acute)	HCO_3^- increases $0.1 \times (PaCO_2 - 40)$ pH decreases $0.008 \times (PaCO_2 - 40)$
Respiratory acidosis (chronic)	HCO_3^- increases $0.4 \times (PaCO_2 - 40)$
Respiratory alkalosis (acute)	HCO_3^- decreases $0.2 \times (40 - PaCO_2)$ pH increases $0.008 \times (40 - PaCO_2)$
Respiratory alkalosis (chronic)	HCO_3^- decreases $0.4 \times (40 - PaCO_2)$
Metabolic acidosis	$PaCO_2$ decreases 1 to $1.5 \times (24 - HCO_3^-)$
Metabolic alkalosis	$PaCO_2$ increases 0.25 to $1 \times (HCO_3^- - 24)$

*Compensatory mechanisms never overcorrect for an acid-base disturbance; when ABG analysis reveals apparent overcorrection, the presence of a mixed disorder should be suspected.
Data from Schrier RW: Renal and electrolyte disorders, ed 3, Boston, 1986, Little, Brown.

7. What are the major buffering systems of the body?
   Bicarbonate, albumin, intracellular proteins, and phosphate are the major buffering systems. The extracellular bicarbonate system is the fastest to respond to pH change but has less total capacity than the intracellular systems, which account for 60% to 70% of the chemical buffering of the body. Hydrogen ions are in dynamic equilibrium with all buffering systems of the body. CO_2 molecules also readily cross cell membranes and keep both intracellular and extracellular buffering systems in dynamic equilibrium. In addition, CO_2 has the advantage of excretion through ventilation.

8. What organs play a major role in acid-base balance?
   • The lungs are the primary organ involved in rapid acid-base regulation. Carbon dioxide produced in the periphery is transported to the lung, where the low carbon dioxide

tension promotes conversion of bicarbonate to carbon dioxide, which is then eliminated. The respiratory regulatory system can increase and decrease minute ventilation to compensate for metabolic acid-base disturbances.

- The kidneys control acid-base balance by eliminating fixed acids; kidneys also control the elimination of electrolytes, bicarbonate, ammonia, and water.
- The liver is involved in multiple reactions that result in the production or metabolism of acids.
- The gastrointestinal tract secretes acidic solutions in the stomach and absorbs water and other electrolytes in the small and large intestines. This can have a profound effect on acid-base balance.

9. **What is meant by pH?**
pH is the negative logarithm of the hydrogen ion concentration ($[H^+]$). pH is a convenient descriptor for *power of hydrogen*. Normally the $[H^+]$ in extracellular fluid is 40 nmol/L, a very small number. By taking the negative log of this value, we obtain a pH of 7.4, a much simpler way to describe $[H^+]$. The pH of a solution is determined by a pH electrode that measures the $[H^+]$.

10. **Why is pH important?**
pH is important because hydrogen ions react highly with cellular proteins, altering their function. Avoiding acidemia and alkalemia by tightly regulating hydrogen ions is essential for normal cellular function. Deviations from normal pH suggest that normal physiologic processes are in disorder and the causes should be determined and treated.

11. **List the major consequences of acidemia.**
Severe acidemia is defined as blood pH <7.20 and is associated with the following major effects:
- Impairment of cardiac contractility, cardiac output, and the response to catecholamines
- Susceptibility to recurrent arrhythmias and lowering of the threshold for ventricular fibrillation
- Arteriolar vasodilation resulting in hypotension
- Vasoconstriction of the pulmonary vasculature, leading to increased pulmonary vascular resistance
- Hyperventilation (a compensatory response)
- Confusion, obtundation, and coma
- Insulin resistance
- Inhibition of glycolysis and adenosine triphosphate synthesis
- Hyperkalemia as potassium ions are shifted extracellularly

12. **List the major consequences of alkalemia.**
Severe alkalemia is defined as blood pH >7.60 and is associated with the following major effects:
- Increased cardiac contractility until pH >7.7, when a decrease is seen
- Refractory ventricular arrhythmias
- Coronary artery spasm/vasoconstriction
- Vasodilation of the pulmonary vasculature, leading to decreased pulmonary vascular resistance
- Hypoventilation (which can frustrate efforts to wean patients from mechanical ventilation)
- Cerebral vasoconstriction
- Neurologic manifestations such as headache, lethargy, delirium, stupor, tetany, and seizures
- Hypokalemia, hypocalcemia, hypomagnesemia, and hypophosphatemia
- Stimulation of anaerobic glycolysis and lactate production

13. **Is the HCO_3 value on the ABG the same as the CO_2 value on the chemistry panel?**
No. The HCO_3^- is a calculated value, whereas the CO_2 is a measured value. Because the CO_2 is measured, it is thought to be a more accurate determination of HCO_3^-. The ABG HCO_3^- is calculated using the Henderson-Hasselbalch equation and the measured values of

pH and $PaCO_2^-$. In contrast, a chemistry panel reports a measured serum carbon dioxide content (CO_2), which is the sum of the measured bicarbonate (HCO_3^-) and carbonic acid (H_2CO_3). The CO_2 is viewed as an accurate determination of HCO_3^- because HCO_3^- concentration in blood is about 20 times greater than the H_2CO_3 concentration; thus, H_2CO_3 is only a minor contributor to the total measured CO_2.

14. **What is the base deficit (BD)? How is it determined?**
The BD (or base excess) is the amount of base (or acid) needed to titrate a serum pH back to normal at 37°C while the $PaCO_2$ is held constant at 40 mm Hg. The BD represents only the metabolic component of an acid-base disorder. The ABG analyzer derives the BD from a nomogram based on the measurements of pH, HCO_3^-, and the nonbicarbonate buffer hemoglobin. Although the BD is determined in part by the nonbicarbonate buffer hemoglobin, it is criticized because it is derived from a nomogram and assumes normal values for other important nonbicarbonate buffers such as albumin. Thus, in a hypoalbuminemic patient, the BD should be used with caution since it may conceal an underlying metabolic acidosis.

15. **What is the anion gap?**
The anion gap (AG) estimates the presence of unmeasured anions. Excess inorganic and organic anions that are not readily measured by standard assays are termed *unmeasured anions*. The AG is a tool used to further classify a metabolic acidosis as an AG metabolic acidosis (elevated AG) or a non-AG metabolic acidosis (normal AG). This distinction narrows the differential diagnosis. The AG is the difference between the major serum cations and anions that are routinely measured:

$$AG = Na^+ - (HCO_3^- + Cl^-)$$

A normal value is 12 mEq/L ± 4 mEq/L. When unmeasured acid anions are present, they are buffered by HCO_3^-, thereby decreasing the HCO_3^- concentration. According to the previous equation, this decrease in HCO_3^- will increase the AG. Keep in mind that hypoalbuminemia has an alkalinizing effect that lowers the AG, which may mask an underlying metabolic acidosis caused by unmeasured anions. This pitfall can be avoided by correcting the AG when evaluating a metabolic acidosis in a hypoalbuminemic patient:

$$Corrected\ AG = observed\ AG + 2.5 \times (normal\ albumin - observed\ albumin)$$

KEY POINTS: MAJOR CAUSES OF A NON–ANION GAP METABOLIC ACIDOSIS

Non–anion gap metabolic acidosis results from loss of Na^+ and K^+ or accumulation of Cl^-. The result of these processes is a decrease in HCO_3^-.
- Iatrogenic administration of hyperchloremic solutions (hyperchloremic metabolic acidosis)
- Alkaline gastrointestinal losses
- Renal tubular acidosis
- Ureteric diversion through ileal conduit
- Endocrine abnormalities

16. **List the common causes of a metabolic alkalosis.**
Metabolic alkalosis is commonly caused by vomiting, volume contraction (diuretics, dehydration), alkali administration, and endocrine disorders.

17. **List the common causes of elevated and nonelevated AG metabolic acidosis.**
- Nonelevated AG metabolic acidosis is caused by iatrogenic administration of hyperchloremic solutions (hyperchloremic metabolic acidosis), alkaline gastrointestinal losses, renal tubular acidosis, or ureteric diversion through ileal conduit. Excess administration of normal saline is a cause of hyperchloremic metabolic acidosis.
- Elevated AG metabolic acidosis is caused by accumulation of lactic acid or ketones, poisoning from toxins (e.g., ethanol, methanol, salicylates, ethylene glycol, propylene glycol), or uremia.

18. Describe a stepwise approach to acid-base interpretation.
    - Check the pH to determine acidemia or alkalemia.
    - If the patient is breathing spontaneously, use the following rules:
      - If the PCO_2 is increased and the pH is <7.35, the primary disorder is most likely a respiratory acidosis.
      - If the PCO_2 is decreased and the pH >7.40, the primary disorder is most likely a respiratory alkalosis.
      - If the primary disorder is respiratory, determine if it is acute or chronic.
      - If the PCO_2 is increased and the pH is >7.40, the primary disorder is most likely a metabolic alkalosis with respiratory compensation.
      - If the PCO_2 is decreased and the pH <7.35, the primary disorder is most likely a metabolic acidosis with respiratory compensation.
    - Metabolic disorders can also be observed by analyzing the base excess or BD. If there is a metabolic acidosis, calculate the AG and determine if the acidosis is a non-AG or AG acidosis, remembering to correct for hypoalbuminemia.
      - If the patient is mechanically ventilated or if the acid-base disorder doesn't seem to make sense, check electrolytes and albumin, and consider calculating the strong ion difference (SID). Also consider the clinical context of the acid-base disorder (e.g., iatrogenic fluid administration, massive blood resuscitation, renal failure, liver failure, diarrhea, vomiting, gastric suctioning, toxin ingestion). This may require further testing, including measuring urine electrolytes, serum, and urine osmolality, and identifying ingested toxins.

SUGGESTED READINGS

Casaletto JJ: Differential diagnosis of metabolic acidosis, Emerg Med Clin North Am 23:771–787, 2005.

Corey HE: Stewart and beyond: new models of acid-base balance, Kidney Int 64:777–787, 2003.

Kraut JA, Madias NE: Serum anion gap: its uses and limitations in clinical medicine, Clin J Am Soc Nephrol 2:162–174, 2007.

Morris CG, Low J: Metabolic acidosis in the critically ill. Part 1. Classification and pathophysiology, Anaesthesia 63:294–301, 2008.

Morris CG, Low J: Metabolic acidosis in the critically ill. Part 2. Cause and treatment, Anaesthesia 63:396–411, 2008.

Rastegar A: Use of the $\Delta AG/\Delta HCO_3^-$ ratio in the diagnosis of mixed acid-base disorders, J Am Soc Nephrol 18:2429–2431, 2007.

VOLUME REGULATION, VOLUME DISTURBANCES, AND FLUID REPLACEMENT

James C. Duke, MD, MBA

1. **Describe the functionally distinct compartments of body water, using a 70-kg patient for illustration.**

   Accurate estimations are difficult because ordinarily ideal body weight (IBW) is used as a basis for calculation. Obesity is rampant in U.S. society, making accurate estimations difficult. Figure 4-1 estimates body water compartments in a patient with an IBW of 70 kg.

2. **Describe the dynamics of fluid distribution between the intravascular and interstitial compartments.**

   The intravascular and interstitial fluid spaces compose the extracellular fluid and are in dynamic equilibrium, governed by hydrostatic and oncotic forces. Under normal circumstances, the capillary hydrostatic pressure produces an outward movement of fluid, whereas the capillary oncotic pressure results in resorption. The sum of the forces leads to an egress of fluids from arterioles; about 90% of the fluid returns into the venules. The remainder of the fluid is subsequently returned to the circulation via the lymphatic system.

3. **How are body water and tonicity regulated?**

   Antidiuretic hormone (ADH) is a primary mechanism; it circulates unbound in plasma, has a half-life of roughly 20 minutes, and increases production of cyclic adenosine monophosphate in the distal collecting tubules of the kidney. Tubular permeability to water increases, resulting in conservation of water and sodium and production of concentrated urine. Stimuli for the release of ADH include the following:

   - Hypothalamic osmoreceptors have an osmotic threshold of about 289 mOsm/kg. Above this level, ADH release is stimulated.
   - Hypothalamic thirst center neurons regulate conscious desire for water and are activated by an increase in plasma sodium of 2 mEq/L, an increase in plasma osmolality of 4 mOsm/L, and loss of potassium from thirst center neurons and angiotensin II.
   - Aortic baroreceptors and left atrial stretch receptors respond to volume depletion and stimulate hypothalamic neurons.

4. **Discuss the synthesis of ADH.**

   ADH, or vasopressin, is synthesized in the supraoptic and paraventricular nuclei of the hypothalamus. It is transported attached to carrier proteins down the pituitary stalk in secretory granules into the posterior pituitary gland (neurohypophysis). There it is stored and released into the capillaries of the neurohypophysis in response to stimuli from the hypothalamus. ADH-producing neurons receive efferent innervation from osmoreceptors and baroreceptors.

5. **List conditions that stimulate and inhibit release of ADH.**

   See Table 4-1.

6. **What is diabetes insipidus (DI)?**

   DI is caused by a deficiency of ADH synthesis, impaired release of ADH from the neurohypophysis (neurogenic DI), or renal resistance to ADH (nephrogenic DI). The result is excretion of large volumes of dilute urine, which, if untreated, leads to dehydration, hypernatremia, and serum hyperosmolality. The usual test for DI is cautious fluid restriction. The inability to decrease and concentrate urine suggests the diagnosis, which may be

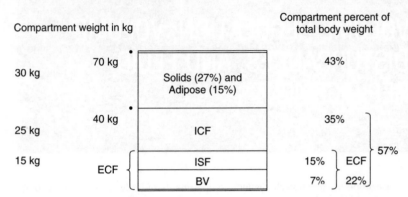

Figure 4-1. Body water compartments in a patient with an ideal body weight of 70 kg. *BV*, Blood volume; *ECF*, extracellular fluid; *ICF*, intracellular fluid; *ISF*, interstitial fluid.

Table 4-1. Conditions that Stimulate and Inhibit Release of Anti-Diuretic Hormone (ADH)

	STIMULATES ANTI-DIURETIC HORMONE RELEASE	INHIBITS ANTI-DIURETIC HORMONE RELEASE
Normal physiologic states	Hyperosmolality Hypovolemia Upright position β-Adrenergic stimulation Pain and emotional stress Cholinergic stimulation	Hypo-osmolality Hypervolemia Supine position α-Adrenergic stimulation
Abnormal physiologic states	Hemorrhagic shock Hyperthermia Increased intracranial pressure Positive airway pressure	Excess water intake Hypothermia
Medications	Morphine Nicotine Barbiturates Tricyclic antidepressants Chlorpropamide	Ethanol Atropine Phenytoin Glucocorticoids Chlorpromazine
Results	Oliguria, concentrated urine	Polyuria, dilute urine

confirmed by plasma ADH measurements. Administration of aqueous vasopressin tests the response of the renal tubule. If the osmolality of plasma exceeds that of urine after mild fluid restriction, the diagnosis of DI is suggested.

7. List causes of DI.
   See Table 4-2.

8. Discuss alternative treatments for DI.
   Available preparations of ADH include pitressin tannate in oil, administered every 24 to 48 hours; aqueous pitressin, 5 to 10 units intravenously or intramuscularly every 4 to 6 hours; desmopressin (DDAVP), 10 to 20 units intranasally every 12 to 24 hours; or aqueous vasopressin, 100 to 200 mU/hr. Incomplete DI may respond to thiazide diuretics or chlorpropamide (which potentiates endogenous ADH).

Table 4-2. Causes of Diabetes Insipidus

VASOPRESSIN DEFICIENCY (NEUROGENIC DIABETES INSIPIDUS)	VASOPRESSIN INSENSITIVITY (NEPHROGENIC DIABETES INSIPIDUS)
Familial (autosomal-dominant)	Familial (X-linked recessive)
Acquired	Acquired
Idiopathic	Pyelonephritis
Craniofacial, basilar skull fractures	Post renal obstruction
Craniopharyngioma, lymphoma, metastasis	Sickle cell disease and trait
Granuloma (sarcoidosis, histiocytosis)	Amyloidosis
Central nervous system infections	Hypokalemia, hypercalcemia
Sheehan syndrome, cerebral aneurysm, cardiopulmonary bypass	Sarcoidosis
Hypoxic brain injury, brain death	Lithium

Because the patient is losing water, administration of isotonic solutions may cause hypernatremia; in addition, excessive vasopressin causes water intoxication. Measurement of plasma osmolality, urine output, and osmolality is indicated when vasopressin is infused.

KEY POINTS: FLUIDS AND VOLUME REGULATION

1. Estimating volume status requires gathering as much clinical information as possible because any single variable may be misleading. Always look for supporting information.
2. Replace intraoperative fluid losses with isotonic fluids.
3. Normal saline, when administered in large quantities, produces a hyperchloremic metabolic acidosis; the associated base deficit may lead the provider to conclude incorrectly that the patient continues to be hypovolemic.
4. Hypotension is a late finding in acute hypovolemia because sympathetic tone will increase vascular tone to maintain cardiac output.

9. **Define the syndrome of inappropriate ADH release. What is the primary therapy?**
   Hypotonicity caused by the nonosmotic release of ADH, which inhibits renal excretion of water, typifies the syndrome of inappropriate antidiuretic hormone (SIADH) release. Three criteria must be met to establish the diagnosis of SIADH:
   1. The patient must be euvolemic or hypervolemic.
   2. The urine must be inappropriately concentrated (plasma osmolality <280 mOsm/kg, urine osmolality >100 mOsm/kg).
   3. Renal, cardiac, hepatic, adrenal, and thyroid function must be normal.
   The primary therapy for SIADH is water restriction. Postoperative SIADH is usually a temporary phenomenon and resolves spontaneously. Chronic SIADH may require the addition of demeclocycline, which blocks the ADH-mediated water resorption in the collecting ducts of the kidney.

10. **What disorders are associated with SIADH?**
    Central nervous system events are frequent causes, including acute intracranial hypertension, trauma, tumors, meningitis, and subarachnoid hemorrhage. Pulmonary causes are also common, including tuberculosis, pneumonia, asthma, bronchiectasis, hypoxemia, hypercarbia, and positive-pressure ventilation. Malignancies may produce ADH-like compounds. Adrenal insufficiency and hypothyroidism also have been associated with SIADH.

11. **What is aldosterone? What stimulates its release? What are its actions?**
Aldosterone, a mineralocorticoid, is responsible for the precise control of sodium excretion. A decrease in systemic or renal arterial blood pressure, hypovolemia, or hyponatremia leads to release of renin from the juxtaglomerular cells of the kidney. Angiotensinogen, produced in the liver, is converted by renin to angiotensin I. In the bloodstream, angiotensin I is converted to angiotensin II, and the zona glomerulosa of the adrenal cortex is then stimulated to release aldosterone. An additional effect of angiotensin II is vasoconstriction. Aldosterone acts on the distal renal tubules and cortical collecting ducts, promoting sodium retention. In addition to hyponatremia and hypovolemia, stimuli for aldosterone release include hyperkalemia, increased levels of adrenocorticotropic hormone, and surgical stimulation.

12. **How much fluid is appropriate to administer during a surgical procedure?**
Use of such poorly quantifiable features such as insensible fluid loss and third-space fluid migration has led to over-resuscitation and fluid balances in excess of what is necessary. In fact, arbitrary fluid administration may lead to complications, delay recovery, and prolong hospitalization.
Concerning outcomes of fluid resuscitation in intraabdominal surgery, it has been observed that patients with restrictive fluid maintenance (4 ml/kg/hr) had better outcomes when compared to patients receiving liberal fluid resuscitation (12 ml/kg/hr). Outcomes were improved overall when fluid administration was restrictive; these improved outcomes included more rapid return of bowel function, increased hematocrit and serum albumin, and earlier discharge from hospitalization. Similarly, there is also good evidence that fluid restriction is limited in patients having thoracotomy and lung resections because of concern for postoperative pulmonary edema. Elective neurosurgical procedures and hepatic resections also require judicious fluid administration. The viability of myocutaneous flaps and bowel reanastomosis is impaired in the setting of excess edema.
Recently, measurements of cardiac volumes (not pressures) or aortic flow through Doppler visualization are becoming increasingly measured, and increased use is expected as the technology expands. The goal is optimizing, not maximizing, intravascular volumes.

13. **Review the composition of crystalloid solutions.**
Fluid resuscitation in the operating room is accomplished with isotonic fluids since intraoperative losses include both salts and water. Thus, only relatively isotonic fluids are listed. Patients requiring replacement of maintenance fluids are usually treated with hypotonic fluids because their losses are predominantly free water, but this is uncommon intraoperatively. Although normal saline is the preferred crystalloid to dilute packed red blood cells, administering large quantities results in hyperchloremic metabolic acidosis caused by dilution of bicarbonate (Table 4-3).

14. **Are there distinct advantages to using colloids to resuscitate a patient?**
There is ongoing debate over the use of colloids versus crystalloids. Colloid advocates claim that, because these solutions have an intravascular space half-life of 3 to 6 hours (much greater than crystalloids), they are superior resuscitation fluids. When compared with crystalloids in a controlled fashion, colloids have not been shown to improve outcomes. Further, in cases in which capillary permeability increases (e.g., burns, sepsis, trauma), colloids accumulate extracellularly, pulling other fluids along because of the osmotic gradient, resulting in extracellular edema. Finally, colloid solutions may lead to allergic reactions.

Table 4-3. Most Common Intraoperative Balanced Crystalloid Solutions

OSMOLALITY*	Na	Cl⁻	K	Ca²	Mg²	LACTATE	ACETATE	GLUCONATE
NS	308	154	154					
LR	273	120	109	4	3	28		
Plasma-Lyte	294	140	98	5	3	27	23	

*Osmolality is measured in mOsm/L; other substances are measured in mEq/L.
LR, Lactated Ringer solution; NS, normal saline.

Although only a third to a fourth of a liter of crystalloid remains in the intravascular space, if given in sufficient quantities (replacing losses in a ratio of 3–4 to 1), crystalloids are excellent resuscitation fluids. It should be noted that dehydrated patients suffer from fluid losses in both intracellular and extracellular compartments, and crystalloids will replete both compartments.

15. Review the colloidal solutions that are available.

There are two albumin preparations, 5% and 25%. Preparation methods eliminate the possibility of infection. The 5% solution has a colloid osmotic pressure of about 20 mm Hg, which is the approximate colloid osmotic pressure under normal circumstances. The 25% solution (also called *salt-poor* albumin) obviously has a colloid osmotic pressure of about five times the normal situation. If intravascular volume is depleted but extracellular volume is greatly expanded, this excess colloid osmotic pressure will draw fluid from the interstitium into the vascular space.

Hydroxyethyl starch in a 6% solution (dissolved in either normal saline or lactated Ringer solution) is another colloid preparation. The heterogeneous preparation contains polymerized molecules with molecular weights of between 20,000 and 100,000 daltons. Metabolized by amylase, it accumulates in the reticuloendothelial system and is renally excreted. Partial thromboplastin time is increased. It has dilutional effects on clotting factors, and the hetastarch molecules can move into organizing fibrin clot. Thus, coagulation can be impaired. It is recommended that not more than 20 ml/kg be administered. The preparation dissolved in lactated Ringer solution is thought to have lesser effects on coagulation, perhaps because it is less heterogeneous in molecular weight dispersion. There are no effects on crossmatching of blood.

Dextrans are water-soluble, polymerized glucose molecules. Two preparations are available (dextran 40 and 70), and the molecular weights of the respective solutions are 40 and 70 kilodaltons. Anaphylactic and anaphylactoid reactions and inhibition of platelet adhesiveness have been noted. Crossmatching of blood may be difficult (Table 4-4).

16. Is albumin suitable for volume replacement?

In the perioperative environment, there are few indications for use of albumin for volume replacement or normalization of serum albumin, not to mention its use is expensive. In fact, some studies have demonstrated adverse outcomes with its use, including patients with traumatic brain injury or in patients with multi-organ failure due to critical illness. Nonetheless, inappropriate use has been determined to be greater than 50% in both adult and pediatric patients.

17. What is the normal range for serum osmolality?

Different sources quote different ranges, but in general, normal serum osmolality ranges between 285 and 305 mOsm/L. A quick rough estimate is to double the sodium concentration. A more accurate estimate of osmolality can be obtained using the following equation:

$$2 \times [Na] + Glucose/18 + BUN/2.8,$$

where the values in the brackets are the concentrations of the substances (sodium in mEq/L, glucose and BUN in g/L).

Table 4-4. Commonly Administered Colloids	
COLLOID	**BENEFITS AND RISKS**
Albumin (5% or 25%)	Expensive; allergic reactions; question its use where there is a loss of capillary integrity
Hetastarch	Currently constituted in either NS or LR; administer less than 20 ml/kg to avoid antiplatelet effects; renally excreted; increases serum amylase
Dextran (40 or 70)	Anaphylactic reactions; interferes with platelet function and crossmatching; increases hepatic transaminases

LR, Lactated Ringer solution; *NS*, normal saline.

18. **What situations might be appropriate for the use of hypertonic saline?**
    Hypertonic saline (usually 3%) has been used successfully during aortic reconstructions and extensive cancer resections; for hypovolemic shock, slow correction of symptomatic chronic hyponatremia, increased intracranial pressure; and to reduce peripheral edema after major fluid resuscitations. Its success in resuscitation remains under investigation.

19. **What is meant by third-space losses? What are the effects of such losses?**
    In certain clinical conditions such as major intraabdominal operations, hemorrhagic shock, burns, and sepsis, patients develop fluid requirements that are not explained by externally measurable losses. Losses are internal, a temporary sequestration of intravascular fluid into a functionless *third space*, which may not readily participate in the dynamic fluid exchanges at the microcirculatory level. The volume of this internal loss is proportional to the degree of injury, and its composition is similar to plasma or interstitial fluid. The creation of the third space necessitates further fluid infusions to maintain intravascular volume, adequate cardiac output, and perfusion, and third-space fluids will persist until the patient's primary problem has resolved.

20. **Is blood pressure a good sign of hypovolemia?**
    Blood pressure is not significantly affected until approximately 30% of blood volume is lost. Early compensatory mechanisms, including peripheral vasoconstriction and tachycardia, may mask significant volume loss.

21. **What clinical findings support a diagnosis of hypervolemia?**
    The patient may have rales on lung auscultation, frothy secretions in the endotracheal tube, edematous mucous membranes, polyuria, and peripheral edema. Like hypovolemia, hypervolemia is best diagnosed when a constellation of findings, and not just a single finding, is present.

SUGGESTED READINGS

Boldt J: Use of albumin: an update, Br J Anaesth 104:276–284, 2010.

Chappel D, Jacob M, Hofmann-Kiefer K, et al: A rational approach to perioperative fluid management, Anesthesiology 109:723–740, 2008.

Ellison DH, Berl T: The syndrome of inappropriate antidiuresis, N Engl J Med 356:2064–2072, 2007.

Grocott MPW, Mythen MG, Gan TJ: Perioperative fluid management and clinical outcomes in adults, Anesth Analg 100:1093–1106, 2005.

Nisanevich V, Felsenstein I, Almogy G, et al: Effect of intraoperative fluid management on outcome after intraabdominal surgery, Anesthesiology 103:25–32, 2005.

ELECTROLYTES

James C. Duke, MD, MBA

1. **What is a normal sodium concentration? What degree of hyponatremia is acceptable to continue with a planned elective procedure?**
   A normal sodium level is between 135 and 145 mEq/L. Generally a sodium level of 130 mEq/L will not result in cancellation of a planned procedure as long as the patient is not symptomatic and hyponatremia is not an expected result of the procedure. Recognizing hyponatremia should prompt an investigation of the cause. Whether the investigation should take priority over the surgery depends on the urgency of the procedure and an overall assessment of the patient's condition.

2. **How is hyponatremia classified?**
   Hyponatremia may occur in the presence of hypotonicity, normal tonicity, or hypertonicity; thus it is important to measure serum osmolality to determine the cause of hyponatremia. Assessment of volume status is also important in determining the cause. An excess of total body water is more common than a loss of sodium in excess of water. Table 5-1 summarizes causes and treatment of hyponatremia.

3. **How should acute hyponatremia be treated?**
   The rate at which hyponatremia develops and the presence of symptoms determine the aggressiveness of treatment. If hyponatremia has developed quickly, the patient may develop nausea, vomiting, visual disturbances, muscle cramps, weakness, hypertension, bradycardia, confusion, apprehension, agitation, obtundation, or seizures; usually the sodium content is found to be less than 125 mEq/L. The aggressiveness of treatment depends on the extent of symptoms.
   In the simplest cases, fluid restriction may be sufficient. Administration of loop diuretics may also be indicated. Severe neurologic symptoms require careful administration of hypertonic (3%) saline. The dose of 3% saline (513 mEq Na/L) is determined as follows:

   $$\text{Dose (mEq)} = (\text{Weight in kg}) \times (140 - \text{measured sodium concentration in mEq/L}) \times 0.6$$

   Correction should occur slowly, with serial sodium concentrations measured. For serum sodium concentrations below, correct at a rate of about 1 mEq/L/hr. Once a concentration of 125 mEq/L has been achieved, the likelihood of continued severe neurologic symptoms will diminish. It should be noted that aggressive correction may result in central pontine myelinolysis.
   Seizures require securing a protected airway, oxygenation, ventilation, and perhaps administration of anticonvulsants, although seizures are usually self-limited.

4. **Is there a subset of patients who may tend to have residual neurologic sequelae from a hyponatremic episode?**
   Females of reproductive age, and especially during menstruation, have been noted to be at greatest risk for residual sequelae. There may be an estrogen-related impairment of the adaptive ability of the brain in the setting of hyponatremia.

5. **What may cause acute hyponatremia in the operating room?**
   Administration of hypotonic fluids or absorption of sodium-poor irrigants may result in hyponatremia. Such irrigants are used to facilitate transurethral resection of the prostate or distend the uterus during hysteroscopies. However, isotonic fluids are used increasingly in these settings when bipolar electrical cautery is used for the surgical procedure. Thus hyponatremia as a consequence of these procedures has been observed with decreasing frequency. Some surgeons may still prefer monopolar cautery because the resection is more rapid. In this instance a hypotonic irrigation fluid is used to prevent dispersal of the electrical current; in such a scenario, hyponatremia is a risk. The most common cause of

Table 5-1. Causes of Hyponatremia

TOTAL SODIUM CONTENT	CAUSES	TREATMENT (ALWAYS TREAT UNDERLYING DISORDER)
Decreased	Diuretics (including osmotic diuretics); renal tubular acidosis; hypoaldosteronism; salt-wasting nephropathies; vomiting; diarrhea	Restore fluid and sodium deficits with isotonic saline
Normal	SIADH; hypothyroidism; cortisol deficiency	Water restriction
Increased	Congestive heart failure; cirrhosis; nephrotic syndrome	Water restriction, loop diuretics

SIADH, Syndrome of inappropriate antidiuretic hormone.

Table 5-2. Causes of Hypernatremia

TOTAL SODIUM CONTENT	CAUSES	TREATMENT (ALWAYS TREAT UNDERLYING DISORDER)
Decreased	Osmotic diuresis; increased insensible losses	First restore intravascular volume with isotonic fluids; then correct Na with hypotonic fluids
Normal	Diabetes insipidus (neurogenic nephrogenic); diuretics; renal failure	Correct water loss with hypotonic fluids
Increased	Excessive Na administration (NaHCO$_3$; 3% NaCl); hyperaldosteronism	Slowly correct fluid deficits with D$_5$W, loop diuretics

postoperative hyponatremia is syndrome of inappropriate antidiuretic hormone secretion and subsequent water retention.

6. **Discuss hypernatremia and its causes.**
Hypernatremia is less common than hyponatremia and is always associated with hypertonicity. Hypernatremia can be associated with either low, normal, or high total body sodium content. Frequently hypernatremia is the result of decreased access to free water, as in elderly or debilitated patients with impaired thirst and decreased oral intake. Other causes include a lack of antidiuretic hormone (diabetes insipidus) and an excess sodium intake (either parenterally or intravenously such as with administration of sodium bicarbonate or 3% sodium chloride). Table 5-2 lists causes and treatment for each category.

7. **What problems does hypernatremia pose for the anesthesiologist?**
Most often hypernatremia is associated with fluid deficits, and the hypovolemia poses the greater challenge to the anesthesiologist. Complicating this, fluid deficits must be corrected slowly so that cellular edema does not develop. Generally elective surgery should be delayed if serum sodium levels exceed 150 mEq/L. Hypernatremia increases minimal alveolar concentration.

8. **Review hypokalemia and its causes.**
A serum level of less than 3.5 mEq/L defines hypokalemia. Hypokalemia may be the result of total body loss of potassium (gastrointestinal and renal), transcellular shifts in potassium, or inadequate intake. Diuretics frequently cause hypokalemia, as do gastrointestinal losses and renal tubular acidosis. β-Adrenergic agonists, insulin, and alkalosis (respiratory and metabolic) shift potassium to the intracellular space. Hypokalemia is not uncommon in

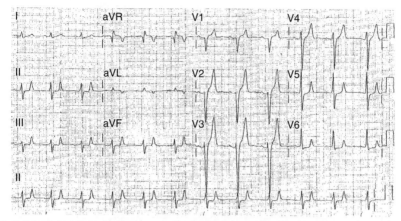

Figure 5-1. This ECG was obtained from a patient with hypokalemia (3.2 mmol/L). Note the prominent U wave after the T wave in the precordial leads V2-6. There is often TU fusion with hypokalemia, creating a broad T wave and an increase in the measured QT interval. Polymorphic ventricular tachycardia may result from hypokalemia.

pregnant women receiving tocolytic therapy or in patients requiring inotropic support because β-agonists are used in both instances.

9. **What are the risks of hypokalemia?**

   Hypokalemia produces electrocardiogram abnormalities (ST-segment and T-wave depression and onset of U waves) and cardiac arrhythmias (often premature ventricular contractions and atrial fibrillation) (Figure 5-1). It also impairs cardiac contractility. These cardiac abnormalities are usually not seen until serum K decreases to 3 mEq/L. Hypokalemia is especially worrisome in patients taking digitalis or with ischemic heart disease or preexisting arrhythmias. Hypokalemia renders muscles weak and sensitive to muscle relaxants. However, there are no definitive data that suggest that patients having surgery with potassium levels as low as 2.6 mEq/L have adverse outcomes.

10. **A patient takes diuretics and is found to have a potassium level of 3 mEq/L. Why not give the patient enough potassium to restore the serum level to normal?**

    The total body deficit of potassium, primarily an intracellular cation, is not reflected by serum concentrations. A patient with a serum potassium of 3 mEq/L may have a total body potassium deficit of 100 to 200 mEq. Rapid attempts to correct hypokalemia poorly address the problem and have resulted in cardiac arrest. Hypokalemic patients without the risk factors previously discussed who are not undergoing major thoracic, vascular, or cardiac procedures can tolerate modest hypokalemia (certainly 3 mEq/L and possibly as low as 2.8 mEq/L).

11. **If potassium is administered, how much should be administered and how fast should it be administered?**

    Potassium should be administered at a rate no greater than 0.5 to 1 mEq/L. As a safety measure, no more than 20 mEq of potassium, diluted in a carrier and run through a controlled infusion pump, should be connected into a patient's intravenous lines at any one time.

12. **Define hyperkalemia and review its symptoms.**

    Hyperkalemia is defined as serum concentration greater than 5.5 mEq/L. Hyperkalemia may produce profound weakness. Cardiac conduction manifestations include enhanced automaticity and repolarization. T waves become peaked, and there is PR interval and QRS prolongation and an increased risk for severe ventricular arrhythmias (Figure 5-2).

13. **What are some causes of hyperkalemia?**

    Hyperkalemia may be either acute or chronic in etiology and secondary to increased intake, decreased excretion, or intracellular shifts related to acid-base status. Hyperkalemia

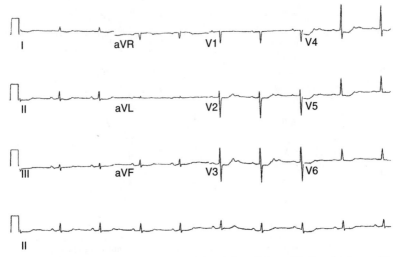

Figure 5-2. This ECG was obtained from a patient with hyperkalemia (9.2 mmol/L). Note the sharp peaking of T waves, broadening of the QRS complex, and diminished P-wave amplitude.

may be iatrogenic (e.g., potassium supplementation, potassium-containing medications) and associated with massive transfusion, metabolic acidosis, and renal failure (acute and chronic); it may also occur after massive tissue trauma or rhabdomyolysis. Medications that may cause hyperkalemia include angiotensin antagonists and receptor blockers, potassium-sparing diuretics (spironolactone and triamterene), and succinylcholine.

14. **Describe the patterns of hyperkalemia observed after the administration of succinylcholine.**
    Mild hyperkalemia (an increase of approximately 0.5 mEq/L) occurs after routine administration of succinylcholine, but susceptible patients may experience life-threatening hyperkalemia. Examples of such patients include those with chronic spinal cord or denervation injuries, head injuries, and unhealed significant burns, and patients who have been immobile (e.g., patients in intensive care). I am aware of an otherwise healthy patient who experienced hyperkalemic cardiac arrest after administration of succinylcholine. His only risk factor was that he was a hospitalized prisoner chained to the bed day after day.

15. **A patient with chronic renal failure requires an arteriovenous fistula for hemodialysis. Potassium is measured as 7 mEq/L. What are the risks of general anesthesia?**
    Hyperkalemia greater than 6 mEq/L should be corrected before elective procedures. Usually dialysis is the treatment. Always consider hyperkalemia when a patient with renal failure suffers cardiac arrest.

16. **How is hyperkalemia treated?**
    Emergent treatment of hyperkalemia is threefold. Treat cardiotoxicity with intravenous calcium chloride. Potassium can be quickly shifted intracellularly by hyperventilation, β-adrenergic stimulation (e.g., β-agonist nebulizer), sodium bicarbonate, and insulin (if insulin is given, one should consider glucose supplementation). Bodily excretion of potassium is more time-consuming but is accomplished using diuretics, Kayexalate, and dialysis.

17. **What are the major causes and manifestations of hypocalcemia?**
    The major causes of hypocalcemia are hypoparathyroidism, hyperphosphatemia, vitamin D deficiency, malabsorption, rapid blood transfusion (chelated by citrate), pancreatitis, rhabdomyolysis, and fat embolism. Hypocalcemia is a concern after thyroidectomy if no

parathyroid tissue is left, and the patient may develop laryngeal spasms and stridor. This must be differentiated from other causes of postoperative stridor, including wound hematoma and injury to the recurrent laryngeal nerves. Hypocalcemia also impairs cardiac contractility, resulting in hypotension, a not uncommon event during massive transfusion. Patients may also be confused.

KEY POINTS: ELECTROLYTES

1. Rapid correction of electrolyte disturbances may be as dangerous as the underlying electrolyte disturbance.
2. Electrolyte disturbances cannot be corrected without treating the underlying cause.
3. Acute hyperkalemia is life threatening and is associated with ventricular tachycardia and fibrillation. It should always be suspected when cardiac collapse follows succinylcholine administration or in any patient with chronic renal disease.
4. When other causes have been ruled out, persistent and refractory hypotension in trauma or other critically ill patients may be caused by hypocalcemia or hypomagnesemia.

18. How is hypocalcemia treated?

Treatment of acute hypocalcemia is straightforward: administer calcium chloride. Volume to volume, this provides more calcium than the gluconate preparation. Always remember to address the primary disturbance.

19. Review normal levels of serum magnesium (Mg) and abnormal magnesium levels and the roles of magnesium.

Magnesium is the fourth most common essential ion with many fundamental cellular roles. A typical serum magnesium level is 1.3–2.2 mEq/L.

20. Does hypomagnesemia pose a problem for the anesthesiologist?

Hypomagnesemia is effective in the management of preeclampsia and torsades de pointes and is increasingly recognized in patients with gastrointestinal losses and critically ill patients, often in association with hypokalemia and hypophosphatemia. It is common in alcoholic patients. Hypokalemia cannot be corrected unless hypomagnesemia is also treated. Patients with hypomagnesemia have increased susceptibility to muscle relaxants and may be weak after surgery, including having respiratory insufficiency. They may have impaired cardiac contractility and dysrhythmias. Trauma patients having massive blood resuscitations may also become hypomagnesemic, and such patients should be administered magnesium chloride, 1 to 2 g, if dysrhythmias develop or refractory hypotension ensues. Ninety-five percent of magnesium is renally resorbed.

21. Hyperchloremia has been increasingly recognized after administration of what *standard* resuscitation fluid?

Hyperchloremia is associated with massive resuscitation with normal saline and with metabolic acidosis caused by dilution of sodium bicarbonate, and it should be part of the differential diagnosis of metabolic acidosis in this setting. Besides after trauma, it has been noted during aortic, gynecologic, and cardiopulmonary bypass surgeries and during the management of sepsis.

Suggested Readings

Bagshaw SM, Townsend DR, McDermid RC: Disorders of sodium and water balance in hospitalized patients, Can J Anesth 56:151–167, 2009.

Elliott MJ, Ronksley PE, Clase CM, et al: Management of patients with acute hyperkalemia, CMAJ 182:1631–1635, 2010.

Handy JM, Soni N: Physiological effects of hyperchloraemia and acidosis, Br J Anaesth 101:141–150, 2008.

Herroeder S, Schönherr ME, De Hert SG, et al: Magnesium—essentials for anesthesiologists, Anesthesiology 114:971–993, 2011.

Palmer BF: Approach to fluid and electrolyte disorders and acid-base problems, Prim Care Clin Pract 35:195–213, 2008.

CHAPTER 6

TRANSFUSION THERAPY

James C. Duke, MD, MBA

1. **How would knowledge of oxygen delivery impact the decision to transfuse?**
   A transfusion would be indicated when oxygen delivery falls to a critical level (DO_{2crit}) and oxygen consumption (VO_2) needs are not met. Recall that DO_2 is a function of cardiac output (CO) and the arterial oxygen content (CaO_2). Arterial oxygen content is a function of arterial oxygen saturation, the oxygen-carrying capacity of hemoglobin, and the hemoglobin concentration. Oxygen dissolved in blood provides a minimal oxygen contribution to that bound to hemoglobin.

   Ordinarily DO_2 exceeds VO_2 by a factor of four (800 to 1200 ml/min vs. 200 to 300 ml/min). Thus the extraction ratio ($O_2ER = VO_2/DO_2$) is 20% to 30%. As long as DO_2 exceeds VO_2, VO_2 is "supply independent." However, below DO_{2crit}, VO_2 becomes "supply dependent," creating a situation in which end-organs are at risk for ischemia. It is at this point that a transfusion is clearly indicated.

2. **At what point is DO_{2crit} reached? What are our surrogate measures for DO_{2crit}?**
   As long as the patient is euvolemic, DO_{2crit} is not reached until hemoglobin decreases to about 3.5 g/dl. Also important is pulmonary function suitable to deliver oxygen to the circulation. It should be mentioned that the DO_{2crit} is modified by the patient's oxygen requirements above baseline (e.g., catabolic states such as sepsis, burns, trauma, etc.) and the presence of end-organ disease such as coronary artery disease.

   Given that in the course of normal operating room conditions, technology for measuring DO_{2crit} is generally unavailable, other variables are used to determine whether the patient is transfused. These include hypotension, tachycardia, urine output, the presence of lactic acidosis, signs of myocardial ischemia (new ST-segment depression >0.1 mV, new ST-segment elevation >0.2 mV, regional wall motion abnormalities by echocardiography), and low mixed venous oxygen saturation (<50% and requires pulmonary artery catheterization and newer developing technology to determine).

3. **What are the physiologic adaptations to acute normovolemic anemia?**
   During surgery, acute blood loss is usually replaced with crystalloid solutions and, if in sufficient volume, results in acute normovolemic hemodilution. Compensatory changes include sympathetic stimulation, resulting in tachycardia and increased cardiac output. Decreased viscosity reduces afterload, increases preload, and improves flow at the capillary level. Since capillary flow is not maximal under resting conditions, capillary recruitment is an adaptive mechanism as well. In addition, there is redistribution of blood to the tissues that are oxygen supply dependent (e.g., heart and brain) and oxygen extraction is increased.

   It is important to note that myocardial oxygen extraction is high under normal circumstances; thus the reserve is less. The heart is dependent on increasing blood flow to increase oxygen delivery, and the significance of this becomes clear in coronary artery disease. A failure for acute normovolemic anemia to deliver oxygen in excess of consumption is another argument in favor of blood transfusion.

4. **Historically, a hemoglobin level of 10 g/dl (hematocrit of 30) was used as a transfusion trigger. Why is this no longer an accepted practice?**
   In patients with coronary artery disease having signs of myocardial ischemia, this level of hemoglobin might be appropriate. Otherwise, it has come to be viewed as a liberal transfusion trigger. Recall that in an otherwise normal situation, DO_{2crit} has not been reached until hemoglobin decreases to 3.5 g/dl.

5. **What are the risks of transfusion?**
   The risks include contracting an infectious disease through transfusion, transfusion reactions, and the immunomodulatory effects of transfusion.

6. **What infectious diseases can be contracted from a transfusion and how significant is that risk?**

At this point in time, the blood supply is as safe as it has ever been, with risks of contracting hepatitis or human immunodeficiency virus (HIV) in a developed nation estimated at 1 in 2.4 million units transfused. Donated blood is tested for hepatitis B (hepatitis B core antigen), hepatitis C (hepatitis C antibody), syphilis, HIV, human T-cell lymphotropic virus, West Nile virus, and cytomegalovirus. Because of improvements in testing, the window between donation and seroconversion is becoming increasingly narrow.

However, there are new infectious risks, including contracting prion-mediated diseases (variant Creutzfeldt-Jakob disease [vCJD]), parasitic diseases (Chagas disease, malaria), and avian flu. There are concerns that severe acute respiratory syndrome will eventually be spread through the blood supply. The risks of these diseases vary with the geographic locality. For instance, malaria is a greater risk in undeveloped countries (as is HIV); the only known cases of contraction of vCJD through transfusion are in the United Kingdom.

Because platelets are stored at a higher temperature (20°C to 22°C) than red blood cells (4°C) or other blood products, platelets are the blood component at greatest risk for bacterial infection. However, testing for sepsis in platelet units is improving, and the risk will likely decrease over time.

7. **Review the major transfusion-related reactions.**
   - **Hemolytic transfusion reactions** caused by ABO incompatibility are most commonly caused by clerical errors and transfusion of the wrong unit. Mistransfusion is thought to occur with a frequency between 1:14,000 and 1:18,000. Most reactions occur during or shortly after a transfusion. Clinical manifestations include fever; chills; chest, flank, and back pain; hypotension; nausea; flushing; diffuse bleeding; oliguria or anuria; and hemoglobinuria. General anesthesia may mask some of the clinical manifestations, and hypotension, hemoglobinuria, and diffuse bleeding may be the only signs. Signs of a severe hemolytic reaction might be missed while the patient is under general anesthesia or attributed to another cause.
   - **Anaphylactic reactions** are caused by binding of IgE; present with bronchospasm, edema, redness, and hypotension; and require urgent treatment with epinephrine, fluid infusions, corticosteroids and antihistamines, and other therapies as indicated by severity and progression of symptoms.
   - **Febrile reactions** may be an early sign of hemolytic transfusion reaction (but other symptoms should be present) or bacterial contamination of the blood product. Febrile nonhemolytic transfusion reactions usually occur in patients who have had prior transfusions; headache, nausea, and malaise are associated symptoms. The reaction is caused by leukocyte antibodies, and leukocyte-depleted red blood cells may be indicated for these patients. Antipyretics may decrease the symptoms if given before the transfusion; meperidine may decrease the severity of chills.
   - **Transfusion-related acute lung injury (TRALI)** is in the top three of the most commonly occurring transfusion-related deaths, having a mortality of 50%. A form of noncardiogenic pulmonary edema, TRALI is also immune related and is usually noted within 6 to 12 hours after transfusion. Symptoms include hypoxia, dyspnea, fever, and pulmonary edema; treatment is supportive.
   - **Urticarial reactions** secondary to mast cell degranulation do not require that the transfusion be stopped; antihistamines may be given.
   - These transfusion reactions are compared in Table 6-1.

8. **What are the current standards for the length of storage of blood? What is a blood storage lesion?**

Federal regulation requires that at least 70% of transfused red blood cells survive 24 hours after CPDA-1 (citrate phosphate dextrose adenosine) and for 42 days when AS-1 (Adsol) or AS-3 (Nutrice) is added.

As stored blood ages, *storage lesions* develop. They include reduction in red cell deformability; free circulating lipids; altered red cell adhesiveness; depletion of adenosine triphosphate stores; and reduction in 2,3-diphosphoglycerate (2,3-DPG), which decreases the ability of the hemoglobin dissociation curve to shift to the right, which enhances

Table 6-1. Differential Diagnosis of Transfusion-Related Acute Lung Injury*

DIAGNOSTIC ENTITY	ONSET	MAJOR SIGNS AND SYMPTOMS	DIFFERENTIATING FEATURES
Transfusion-related acute lung injury (TRALI)	Minutes to hours	Dyspnea, respiratory distress, hypoxemia, cyanosis, pulmonary edema, fever, tachycardia	Noncardiogenic pulmonary edema, frequent fever
Anaphylactic or anaphylactoid reaction	Minutes to hours	Bronchospasm, respiratory distress, hypotension, cyanosis, generalized erythema and urticaria, mucous membrane edema	Rash, urticaria, and edema present; hypotension and bronchospasm prominent
Bacterial contamination of blood products	Minutes	Fever, rigors, hypotension, and vascular collapse	Fever, rigors, and vascular collapse predominant; most common with platelets
Hemolytic transfusion reaction	Minutes	Fever, rigors, hypotension, hemoglobinuria, disseminated intravascular coagulation	Usually with red blood cell transfusion, hemolysis

*Symptoms may be missed while under general anesthesia, and differential diagnosis should be expanded to include common intraoperative problems.
Reprinted with permission from Boshkov LK: Transfusion-related acute lung injury and the ICU. Crit Care Clin 21:479–495, 2005.

peripheral oxygen release. Proinflammatory cytokines accumulate and, even after 2 weeks, are capable of significantly priming neutrophils for an exacerbated inflammatory response.

9. **Is there convincing evidence that the effect of a transfusion on immune function is harmful?**
Much of the evidence for immune modulation and infection related to transfusion is retrospective in nature and, as such, suffers from a failure to control for confounding variables. There are insufficient numbers of randomized, controlled studies of sufficient power, and the studies that do exist have been conducted on critically ill patients, not in the perioperative setting (perhaps with the exception of patients having coronary bypass). As such, there are no definitive recommendations at this time. However, a few points are worthy of discussion.
The Transfusion Requirements in Critical Care trial was sufficiently powered to evaluate the impact of transfusion on outcome. The groups under study were divided into a restrictive transfusion (hemoglobin trigger of 7 g/dl, targeting a hemoglobin level between 7 and 9 g/dl) and a liberal transfusion group (hemoglobin transfusion trigger of 10 g/dl, targeting a hemoglobin level of 10 to 12 g/dl). Thirty-day mortality was lower in the restrictive transfusion group, although a statistical significance was not found. However, if the patients were subdivided by acuity of illness, results would show that fewer acutely ill patients in the restrictive transfusion group had lower 30-day mortality.
Other prospective studies are less convincing in their findings, but there are overlapping transfusion triggers, and the patient populations differ. Some observational studies have found that the number of transfused units is an independent risk factor for mortality and increased length of stay. In sum, the final word on the impact of transfusion on mortality has yet to be written. Many countries now routinely perform leukoreduction on donated blood out of concern for the impact of transfusion on the recipient's immune function.

10. **Review the features of TRALI.**

Recently TRALI has been identified as the leading cause of transfusion-related deaths in the United States. It is estimated that 1 in 5000 transfusions will result in TRALI. All blood components have resulted in TRALI, including packed erythrocytes, random donor platelets, single donor (apheresis) platelets, fresh frozen plasma, and cryoprecipitate. However, the cellular components have a greater association with TRALI. Even autologous blood has resulted in TRALI, suggesting that there may be some storage lesion contributing to its etiology.

Although donor antibodies have been shown to be present in many TRALI series, their presence is neither necessary nor sufficient to result in TRALI. It is now believed that TRALI is multifactorial and a two-event subtype of acute lung injury. Because of some associated conditions, the recipient has a high level of inflammatory mediators (e.g., cytokines), primed white blood cells, and pulmonary endothelium. The administered blood product provides the second event, through classic antibody-antigen coupling of the lipid products or other cytokines generated during storage of the blood products. The primed white blood cells are activated to release substances such as superoxides that damage the pulmonary endothelium.

11. **What conditions may predispose a patient to TRALI?**

Some conditions that have been associated with TRALI include sepsis, organ ischemia, massive transfusion, extracorporeal circulation, malignancies, recent surgical procedures, aspiration of gastric contents, near-drowning, pneumonia, long-bone fractures, burns, pulmonary contusion, and disseminated intravascular coagulation. However, the patient must be ill enough to require a transfusion. Close monitoring and judicious transfusion are indicated.

12. **Discuss the criteria for diagnosis of TRALI.**

- Acute onset: often occurring in less than 2 hours after a transfusion and usually less than 6 hours
- Pulmonary arterial occlusion pressure ≤18 mm Hg or lack of clinical evidence of left atrial overload (i.e., the problem is noncardiogenic pulmonary edema)
- Bilateral infiltrates observed on chest radiograph
- Hypoxemia with a ratio of PaO_2/FiO_2 ≤300 mm Hg regardless of the level of positive end-expiratory pressure, or oxygen saturation ≤90% on room air
- No acute lung injury prior to transfusion

13. **What treatments are available for TRALI?**

If the patient experiences deterioration in oxygenation during transfusion, the transfusion should be discontinued and the remainder of the transfused blood returned to the laboratory for analysis. Of course, some other form of transfusion injury besides TRALI may be taking place.

Therapy is supportive, continuing to treat the patient's other medical problems (which may have been the priming event for TRALI). Diuresis and steroid administration are contraindicated, but aggressive pulmonary support is necessary. If further transfusions are needed, it is wise to use blood products that have a reduced likelihood of having inflammatory mediators, including leukoreduced packed erythrocytes, packed units less than 14 days old, washed erythrocytes, or, in the case of platelets, apheresis units less than 3 days old.

14. **Review the ABO and Rh blood genotypes and the associated antibody patterns.**

Blood type is determined by two alleles of three types: O, A, and B. A and B refer to antigens on the red blood cell surface. An individual can have either A or B, both A and B, or neither (blood type O). If an individual does not have the type A antigen, over time anti-A antibodies (also known as *agglutinins*) form. A patient with type AB blood has both antigens and will form no agglutinins. Individuals with type O blood have no antigen and develop both A and B antibodies (Table 6-2). The antibodies are primarily immunoglobulin (Ig)M or IgG. Acute hemolytic reactions are caused by complement activation and release of proteolytic enzymes that digest the red cell membrane.

People with type O blood have neither A nor B antigens (agglutinogens) on their cell surface. These cells cannot be agglutinated by antibodies (agglutinins) that may be present in a transfusion recipient's blood. Thus type O blood is known as the *universal donor* for red

Table 6-2. Blood Types and Their Constituent Antigens and Antibodies

BLOOD GENOTYPES	BLOOD TYPE	ANTIGENS (AGGLUTINOGENS)	ANTIBODIES (AGGLUTININS)
OO	O	None*	Anti-A and anti-B
OA or AA	A	A	Anti-B
OB or BB	B	B	Anti-A
AB	AB	A and B	None†

*The absence of agglutinogens makes the O-packed cells the universal packed cell donor.
†The absence of agglutinins makes AB plasma the universal plasma donor.

Table 6-3. Crossmatch and Compatibility

DEGREE OF CROSSMATCH	CHANCE OF COMPATIBLE TRANSFUSION
ABO-Rh type only	99.8%
ABO-Rh type + antibody screen	99.94%
ABO-Rh type + antibody screen crossmatch	99.95%

blood cells. Patients with type AB blood have both classes of antigens (agglutinogens) and therefore do not form A or B antibodies (agglutinins). Because there are no antibodies in the plasma, type AB patients are universal donors for plasma.

There are six common antigens in the Rh system; the presence of the *D* antigen is what is most commonly referred to as *Rh positive*. The Rh blood type system is slightly different because Rh agglutinins rarely form spontaneously. Usually massive exposure, as from a prior transfusion, is necessary to stimulate their formation. An Rh-negative patient can receive Rh-positive blood in an emergency situation, although antibodies will form in some patients, and there may be a delayed, usually mild, hemolytic transfusion reaction. However, after receiving Rh-positive blood, the Rh-negative patient will be Rh sensitized and can have a more significant transfusion reaction if exposed to Rh-positive blood at a later date.

15. **What is the difference between a type and screen and a crossmatch?**
The patient's blood is typed for ABO and Rh group by placing his or her red cells with commercially available anti-A and anti-B reagents and reverse typing the patient's serum against A and B reagent cells. A screen for antibodies involves placing the patient's serum with specially selected red cells containing all relevant blood group antigens. In a crossmatch the patient's serum is also incubated with a small quantity of red cells from the proposed donor unit to verify in vitro compatibility. A crossmatch also detects more unique antibodies (Table 6-3).

16. **What type of blood should be used in an emergency situation?**
Transfusions in emergency situations do not allow time for a complete crossmatch. Under these circumstances the fastest choice is to use type O, Rh-negative uncrossmatched blood. If more than two units of type O blood are given to patients who are type A or B, type O blood should continue to be administered until testing of the patient's blood has been ensured. Type-specific, uncrossmatched blood would be the next choice, followed by type-specific, partially crossmatched blood, and finally, fully crossmatched blood.

17. **What are some of the complications of massive blood transfusion?**
Massive transfusion is defined as the administration of more than one blood volume within several hours. Complications include:
• Coagulopathy secondary to dilutional thrombocytopenia, lack of labile coagulation factors V and VIII, and disseminated intravascular coagulation

- Metabolic disturbances associated with banked blood, including hyperkalemia, hypocalcemia (citrate toxicity), acidosis, and impaired oxygen delivery caused by reduced 2,3-DPG
- Hypothermia. It has been found that mild hypothermia (34°C to 36°C) increases blood loss by 16% and increases the relative risk for transfusion by 22%. Hypothermia impairs platelet function and proteins of the coagulation cascade.

18. **If a major transfusion reaction is suspected, how should it be managed?**
    - Stop the transfusion immediately and remove the blood tubing.
    - Alert the blood bank and send a recipient and donor blood specimen for compatibility testing.
    - Treat hypotension aggressively with intravenous fluids and pressor agents.
    - Maintain urine output with intravenous hydration. Mannitol and loop diuretics are used on occasion, but caution must be used to avoid creating hypovolemia with diuresis.
    - Massive hemolysis can result in hyperkalemia. Follow serum potassium levels and continuously monitor the electrocardiogram for electrocardiographic signs of hyperkalemia.
    - Disseminated intravascular coagulation may occur. The best treatment is identifying and treating the underlying cause. Follow prothrombin, partial thromboplastin, fibrinogen, and D-dimer levels.
    - Check urine and plasma hemoglobin levels and verify hemolysis with direct antiglobulin (Coombs) test, bilirubin, and plasma haptoglobin levels.
    - The availability of thromboelastography is increasing and is very useful for assessing coagulation disturbances.

19. **What alternatives are there to transfusion of donor blood?**
    - Autologous transfusion (the collection and reinfusion of the patient's own blood). It should be noted that only about 55% of pre-donated units are returned to the patient. The patient scheduled for autologous transfusion still runs the risk of clerical errors and bacterial infection. There is also a report of a patient who received an autologous transfusion developing TRALI.
    - Preoperative use of erythropoietin to stimulate erythrocyte production. Erythropoietin stimulates erythrocyte production in 5 to 7 days and has been shown to reduce use of allogeneic blood in patients with renal insufficiency and anemia of chronic disease and when transfusion is refused.
    - Intraoperative collection and reinfusion of blood lost during surgery
    - Intraoperative isovolemic hemodilution (the reduction of hematocrit or hemoglobin by withdrawal of blood and simultaneous intravascular replacement with crystalloids)
    - Use of hemoglobin solutions

20. **What are the limitations, advantages, and disadvantages of alternative hemoglobin solutions?**
    The benefits of alternatives to erythrocyte transfusion include a lack of antigenicity, possible unlimited availability, no disease transmission risk, long storage life, and better rheologic properties. Two types of oxygen-carrying solutions have been developed:
    - Perfluorocarbon emulsions that have a high gas-dissolving capacity for oxygen
    - Hemoglobin-based oxygen carriers
        This discussion focuses on the latter. Such compounds are manufactured from human recombinant hemoglobin, outdated human blood, or bovine blood. The stromal components of erythrocytes are removed, and the hemoglobin molecule polymerized or liposome encapsulated to prevent rapid renal excretion and nephrotoxicity. Cell-free hemoglobin solutions have two major problems. First, they have low concentrations of 2,3-DPG. The lack of 2,3-DPG shifts the oxyhemoglobin dissociation curve to the left, the affinity of hemoglobin for oxygen increases, and oxygen cannot be off-loaded at the tissue level. Second, they are nitric oxide scavengers and produce excessive vasoconstriction. Pulmonary hypertension and myocardial ischemia are risks; in fact, reports of death from myocardial infarction have delayed release of these solutions for general use. These solutions also result in platelet activation; release of proinflammatory mediators; methemoglobinemia; and, because of their color, interference with laboratory tests.

KEY POINTS: TRANSFUSION THERAPY

1. There is no set hemoglobin/hematocrit level at which transfusion is required. The decision should be individualized to the clinical situation, taking into consideration the patient's health status.
2. If blood is needed in an emergency, type O–packed cells (O-negative is best) and/or type-specific blood may be used.
3. Numerous transfusion-related reactions are possible, and vigilance while administering under anesthesia is essential because many of the classic signs and symptoms might be missed in a draped patient under general anesthesia.

WEBSITE

American Society of Anesthesiologists: http://www.asahq.org

SUGGESTED READINGS

American Society of Anesthesiologists Task Force on Perioperative Blood Transfusions: Practice guidelines for perioperative blood transfusion and adjuvant therapies, Anesthesiology 105:198–208, 2006.

Hebert PC, Tinmouth A, Corwin H: Anemia and red cell transfusion in critically ill patients, Crit Care Med 31(Suppl):S672–S677, 2003.

Madjdpour C, Spahn DR: Allogeneic red blood cell transfusions: efficiency, risks, alternatives and indications, Br J Anaesth 98:33–42, 2005.

Rajagopalan S, Mascha E, Na J, et al: The effects of mild perioperative hypothermia on blood loss and transfusion requirement, Anesthesiology 108:71–77, 2008.

Spahn DR, Kocian R: Artificial O_2 carriers: status in 2005, Curr Pharm Des 11:4099–4114, 2005.

Triulzi DJ: Transfusion-related acute lung injury. Current concepts for the clinician, Anesth Analg 108:770–776, 2009.

COAGULATION

Jason P. Krutsch, MD

CHAPTER 7

1. How can you identify a patient at risk for bleeding?

Preoperative evaluation includes history, physical examination, and appropriate lab testing. Questions about bleeding disorders (e.g., tendency to form large hematomas after minor trauma, severe bleeding while brushing teeth) and bleeding after previous surgical procedures (e.g., dental extractions, tonsillectomy) are important. Prior surgery without transfusion suggests the absence of an inherited coagulation disorder. Review of medications is necessary to identify medications with anticoagulant potential (e.g., nonsteroidal antiinflammatory drugs [NSAIDs], antiplatelet drugs, and anticoagulants). Coagulation studies may confirm a clinical suspicion that the patient has a bleeding disorder. No evidence supports the value of preoperative coagulation studies in asymptomatic patients.

2. What processes form the normal hemostatic mechanism?

Three intertwined processes ensure that blood remains in a liquid state until vascular injury occurs: primary hemostasis, secondary hemostasis, and fibrinolysis.

3. Describe primary hemostasis.

Within seconds of vascular injury, platelets become activated and adhere to the subendothelial collagen layer of the denuded vessel via glycoprotein receptors; this interaction is stabilized by von Willebrand factor (vWF). Collagen and epinephrine activate phospholipases A and C in the platelet plasma membrane, resulting in formation of thromboxane A2 (TXA2) and degranulation, respectively. TXA2 is a potent vasoconstrictor that promotes platelet aggregation. Platelet granules contain adenosine diphosphate (ADP), TXA2, vWF, factor V, fibrinogen, and fibronectin. ADP alters the membrane glycoprotein IIb/IIIa, facilitating the binding of fibrinogen to activated platelets. Thus a platelet plug is constructed and reinforced.

4. Review secondary hemostasis.

Secondary hemostasis involves the formation of a fibrin clot. The fibrin network binds and strengthens the platelet plug. Fibrin can be formed via two pathways (intrinsic and extrinsic) and involves activation of circulating coagulation precursors. Regardless of which pathway is triggered, the coagulation cascade results in the conversion of fibrinogen to fibrin.

5. What are the intrinsic and extrinsic coagulation pathways?

Traditionally these two pathways have been viewed as separate mechanisms that merge after the formation of activated factor X (Figure 7-1). This rigid division has lost absolute validity because of the crossover of many factors. For instance, factor VIIa can activate factor IX, but factors IXa, Xa, thrombin, and XIIa can activate factor VII. However, the classic two-pathway model is still useful for the interpretation of in vitro coagulation studies.

The intrinsic pathway occurs within the blood vessel and is triggered by the interaction between subendothelial collagen with circulating factor XII, high-molecular-weight kininogen, and prekallikrein. Platelet phospholipid (platelet factor 3 [PF3]) serves as a catalyst to this pathway. The extrinsic pathway begins with the release of tissue thromboplastin (factor III) from the membranes of injured cells.

6. Explain fibrinolysis.

The fibrinolytic system is activated simultaneously with the coagulation cascade and functions to maintain the fluidity of blood during coagulation. It also serves in clot lysis once tissue repair begins. When a clot is formed, plasminogen is incorporated and then converted to plasmin by tissue plasminogen activator (tPA) and fragments of factor XII.

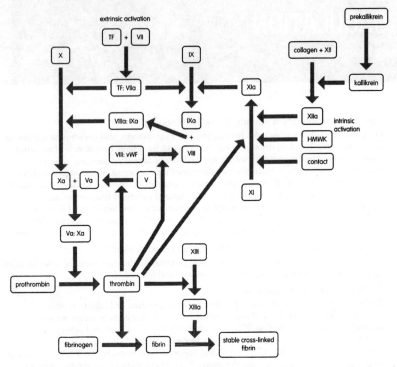

Figure 7-1. The clotting cascade, including intrinsic and extrinsic pathways. The roman numerals indicate the different clotting factors. The letter "a" indicates the activated form. *HMWK*, High-molecular-weight heparin; *TF*, tissue factor; *vWF*, von Willebrand factor. (*From Griffin J, Arif S, Mufti A: Crash course: immunology and hematology, ed 2, St. Louis, 2004, Mosby.*)

Endothelial cells release tPA in response to thrombin. Plasmin degrades fibrin and fibrinogen into small fragments. These fibrin degradation products possess anticoagulant properties because they compete with fibrinogen for thrombin; they are normally cleared by the monocyte-macrophage system.

7. **Why doesn't blood coagulate in normal tissues?**
   Coagulation is limited to injured tissue by localization of platelets to the site of injury and maintenance of normal blood flow in noninjured areas. The monocyte-macrophage system scavenges activated coagulation factors in regions of normal blood flow. Normal vascular endothelium produces prostacyclin (prostaglandin I_2); it is a potent vasodilator that inhibits platelet activation and helps confine primary hemostasis to the injured area. In addition, antithrombin III, proteins C and S, and tissue factor pathway inhibitor are coagulation inhibitors that are normally present in plasma. Antithrombin III complexes with and deactivates circulating coagulation factors (except factor VIIa). Protein C inactivates factors Va and VIIIa; protein S augments the activity of protein C. Finally, tissue factor pathway inhibitor antagonizes factor VIIa.

8. **What is an acceptable preoperative platelet count?**
   A normal platelet count is 150,000 to 440,000/mm^3. Thrombocytopenia is defined as a count of <150,000/mm^3. Intraoperative bleeding can be severe with counts of 40,000 to 70,000/mm^3, and spontaneous bleeding usually occurs at counts <20,000/mm^3. The minimal recommended platelet count before surgery is 75,000/mm^3. However, qualitative differences in platelet function make it unwise to rely solely on platelet count. Thrombocytopenic

patients with accelerated destruction but active production of platelets have relatively less bleeding than patients with hypoplastic disorders at a given platelet count.

Assessment of preoperative platelet function is further complicated by lack of correlation between bleeding time or any other test of platelet function and a tendency for increased intraoperative bleeding. However, normal bleeding times range from 4 to 9 minutes, and a bleeding time >1.5 times normal (>15 minutes) is considered significantly abnormal.

9. **List the causes of platelet abnormalities.**

Thrombocytopenia
- Dilution after massive blood transfusion
- Decreased platelet production caused by malignant infiltration (e.g., aplastic anemia, multiple myeloma), drugs (e.g., chemotherapy, cytotoxic drugs, ethanol, hydrochlorothiazide), radiation exposure, or bone-marrow depression after viral infection
- Increased peripheral destruction caused by hypersplenism, disseminated intravascular coagulation (DIC), extensive tissue and vascular damage after extensive burns, or immune mechanisms (e.g., idiopathic thrombocytopenic purpura, drugs such as heparin, autoimmune diseases)

Qualitative platelet disorders
- Inherited (e.g., von Willebrand disease)
- Acquired (uremia, cirrhosis, medications [e.g., aspirin, NSAIDs])

10. **How does aspirin act as an anticoagulant?**

Primary hemostasis is controlled by the balance between the opposing actions of two prostaglandins: TXA2 and prostacyclin. Depending on the dose, salicylates produce a differential effect on prostaglandin synthesis in platelets and vascular endothelial cells. Lower doses preferentially inhibit platelet cyclooxygenase, impeding production of TXA2 and inhibiting platelet aggregation. The effect begins within 2 hours of ingestion. Because platelets lack a cell nucleus and cannot produce protein, the effect lasts for the entire life of the platelet (7 to 10 days). NSAIDs have a similar but more transient effect than aspirin, lasting for only 1 to 3 days after cessation of use.

11. **Review the properties of factor VIII.**

Factor VIII is a large protein complex of two noncovalently bound factors: vWF (factor VIII:vWF) and factor VIII antigen. Factor VIII:vWF is necessary for both platelet adhesion and formation of the hemostatic plug through regulation and release of factor VIII antigen. In von Willebrand disease, there is a decrease of both factor VIII antigen and factor VIII:vWF.

KEY POINTS: COAGULATION

1. An outpatient with a bleeding diathesis usually can be identified through history (including medications) and physical examination. Preoperative coagulation studies in asymptomatic patients are of little value.
2. In vivo, coagulation is initiated primarily by contact of factor VII with extravascular tissue.
3. The most common intraoperative bleeding diathesis is dilutional thrombocytopenia.
4. The primary treatment for DIC is to treat the underlying medical condition.
5. Thromboelastography is a dynamic test of clotting and can be as useful as all other clotting tests combined.

12. **How does vitamin K deficiency affect coagulation?**

Four clotting factors (II, VII, IX, and X) are synthesized by the liver. Each factor undergoes vitamin K–dependent carboxylation to bind to the phospholipid surface. Without vitamin K, the factors are produced but are not functional. The extrinsic pathway is affected first by vitamin K deficiency because the factor with the shortest half-life is factor VII, found only in the extrinsic pathway. With further deficiency, both extrinsic and intrinsic pathways are affected.

The warfarin-like drugs compete with vitamin K for binding sites on the hepatocyte. Administration of subcutaneous vitamin K reverses the functional deficiency in 6 to 24 hours. With active bleeding or in emergency surgery, fresh frozen plasma (FFP) can be administered for immediate hemostasis.

13. **How does heparin act as an anticoagulant?**
Heparin is a polyanionic mucopolysaccharide that accelerates the interaction between antithrombin III and the activated forms of factors II, X, XI, XII, and XIII, effectively neutralizing each. The half-life of heparin's anticoagulant effect is about 90 minutes in a normothermic patient. Patients with reduced levels of antithrombin III are resistant to the effect of heparin. Heparin may also affect platelet function and number through an immunologically mediated mechanism.

14. **Give a general description of the different coagulation tests.**
The basic difference between the intrinsic and extrinsic pathways is the phospholipid surface on which the clotting factors interact before merging at the common pathway. Either platelet phospholipid (intrinsic pathway) or tissue thromboplastin (extrinsic pathway) can be added to the patient's plasma, and the time taken for clot formation is measured. Less than 30% of normal factor activity is required for the tests to be affected. The tests are also prolonged in the setting of decreased fibrinogen concentration (<100 mg/dl) and dysfibrinogenemias. The partial thromboplastin time (PTT), activated partial thromboplastin time (aPTT), and activated clotting time (ACT) measure intrinsic and common pathways.

15. **What does PTT measure?**
PTT measures the clotting ability of all factors in the intrinsic and common pathways except factor XIII. Partial thromboplastin is substituted for platelet phospholipid and eliminates platelet variability. Normal PTT is about 40 to 100 seconds; >120 seconds is abnormal.

16. **Describe aPTT.**
Maximal activation of the contact factors (XII and XI) eliminates the lengthy natural contact activation phase and results in more consistent and reproducible results. An activator is added to the test tube before addition of partial thromboplastin. Normal aPTT is 25 to 35 seconds.

17. **How is ACT measured?**
Fresh whole blood (providing platelet phospholipid) is added to a test tube already containing an activator. The automated ACT is widely used to monitor heparin therapy in the operating room. The normal range is 90 to 120 seconds.

18. **What is the prothrombin time?**
Prothrombin time (PT) measures the extrinsic and common pathways. Tissue thromboplastin is added to the patient's plasma. The test varies in sensitivity and response to oral anticoagulant therapy whether measured as PT in seconds or simple PT ratio ($PT_{patient}/PT_{normal}$), where "normal" is the mean normal PT value of the laboratory test system. Normal PT is 10 to 12 seconds.

19. **Explain the international normalized ratio.**
The international normalized ratio (INR) was introduced to improve the consistency of oral anticoagulant therapy. INR is calculated as ($PT_{patient}/PT_{normal-ISI}$), where ISI is the international sensitivity index assigned to the test system. The recommended therapeutic ranges for standard oral anticoagulant therapy and high-dose therapy, respectively, are INR values of 2 to 3 and 2.5 to 3.5.

20. **What are the indications for administering FFP?**
When microvascular bleeding is noted and PT or PTT exceeds 1.5 the control value, FFP should be considered. The usual dose is 10 to 15 ml/kg. FFP will also reverse the anticoagulant effects of warfarin (5 to 8 ml/kg). (Administration of vitamin K will have the same result but will take 6 to 12 hours to become effective.) Volume expansion is not an indication for FFP.

21. **What is cryoprecipitate? When should it be administered?**

Cryoprecipitate is the cold-insoluble white precipitate formed when FFP is thawed. It is removed by centrifugation, refrozen, and thawed immediately before use. Cryoprecipitate contains factor VIII, vWF, fibrinogen, and factor XIII. It is used to replace fibrinogen, factor VIII deficiencies, and factor XIII deficiencies. It has been used to treat von Willebrand disease (unresponsive to desmopressin) and hemophilia. There is now a purified factor VIII concentrate more appropriate for use in these selected problems. One unit of cryoprecipitate per 10 kg of body weight will increase fibrinogen levels by 50 mg/dl. Because cryoprecipitate lacks factor V, for the treatment of DIC, FFP is also necessary.

22. **What is DIC?**

DIC is usually seen in clinical situations in which clotting pathways are activated by circulating phospholipid, leading to thrombin generation, but the usual mechanisms preventing unbalanced thrombus formation are impaired. The fibrinolytic system is activated, and plasmin begins to cleave fibrinogen and fibrin into fibrin degradation products (FDPs). DIC is not a disease entity but rather a clinical complication of other problems:

- Obstetric conditions (e.g., amniotic fluid embolism, placental abruption, retained fetus syndrome, eclampsia, saline-induced abortion)
- Septicemia and viremia (e.g., bacterial infections, cytomegalovirus, hepatitis, varicella, human immunodeficiency virus)
- Disseminated malignancy and leukemia
- Transfusion reactions, crush injury, tissue necrosis, and burns
- Liver disease (e.g., obstructive jaundice, acute hepatic failure)

23. **What tests are used for the diagnosis of DIC?**

There is no one diagnostic test. More often than not, both PT and PTT are elevated, and platelet count is reduced. Hypofibrinogenemia is common. In 85% to 100% of patients, FDPs are elevated. One measured form of FDP is the D-dimer. D-dimer is a neoantigen formed by the action of thrombin in converting fibrinogen to cross-linked fibrin. It is specific for FDPs formed from the digestion of cross-linked fibrin by plasmin.

24. **Describe the treatment of DIC.**

The most important measure is to treat the underlying disease process. Often specific blood components are depleted and require repletion based on tests of coagulation. Occasionally, if bleeding persists despite conventional treatment, antifibrinolytic therapy with ε-aminocaproic acid should be considered, but only if the intravascular coagulation process is under control and residual fibrinolysis continues.

25. **What is recombinant factor VIIa (NovoSeven)?**

Factor VIIa complexes with tissue factor to activate factors IX and X. Factor Xa subsequently aids in the conversion of prothrombin to thrombin, which leads to the activation of fibrinogen to fibrin. The beneficial effects of recombinant factor VIIa have been demonstrated in the settings of hemophilia, liver transplantation, major trauma, intracerebral hemorrhage, gastrointestinal bleeding, cardiac surgery, and warfarin-induced bleeding when traditional approaches to the bleeding patient have proved to be marginally effective or noneffective.

26. **Discuss the basic principles of thromboelastography.**

The thromboelastography (TEG) measures the viscoelastic properties of blood as it is induced to clot in a low shear environment resembling venous flow, providing some measure of clot strength and stability, including the time to initial clot formation, the acceleration phase, strengthening, retraction, and clot lysis. A sample of celite-activated whole blood is placed into a prewarmed cuvette. A suspended piston is then lowered into the cuvette that rotates back and forth. The forming clot transmits its movement on to the suspended piston. A weak clot stretches and delays the arc movement of the piston and is graphically expressed as a narrow TEG. Conversely, a strong clot will move the piston simultaneously in proportion to the movements of the cuvette, creating a thick TEG.

Characteristic Thromboelastograph Tracings

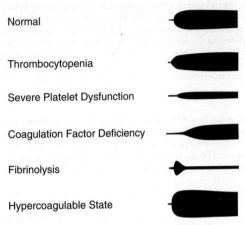

Normal

Thrombocytopenia

Severe Platelet Dysfunction

Coagulation Factor Deficiency

Fibrinolysis

Hypercoagulable State

Figure 7-2. Typical thromboelastography pattern and variables measured as normal values and examples of some abnormal tracings. (*From DeCastro M: Evaluation of the coagulation system. In Faust RJ, editor: Anesthesiology reviews, ed 3, New York, 2002, Churchill Livingstone, p 352.*)

27. **Discuss the parameters measured by thromboelastography.**
    There are five parameters of the TEG tracing: R, k, alpha angle, MA, and MA60 (Figure 7-2).
    - R: Period of time from the initiation of the test to initial fibrin formation
    - k: Time from the beginning of clot formation until the amplitude of TEG reaches 20 mm, representing the dynamics of clot formation
    - Alpha angle: Angle between the line in the middle of the TEG tracing and the line tangential to the developing body of the tracing, representing the kinetics of fibrin cross-linking
    - MA (maximum amplitude): Reflects the strength of the clot, which depends on the number and function of platelets and their interaction with fibrin
    - MA60: Measures the rate of amplitude reduction 60 minutes after MA, representing the stability of the clot (Figure 7-2)

WEBSITE
International Scientific Publications: http://www.ispub.com

SUGGESTED READINGS
Drummond JC, Petrovitch CT: Hemostasis and hemotherapy. In Barash PG, Cullen BF, Stoelting RK, editors: Clinical anesthesia, ed 5, Philadelphia, 2006, Lippincott, Williams & Wilkins, pp 221–240.
Wenker O, Wojciechowski Z, Sheinbaum R, et al: Thromboelastography, Internet J Anesthesiol 1(3): 1997.

AIRWAY MANAGEMENT

James C. Duke, MD, MBA

CHAPTER 8

1. **List several indications for endotracheal intubation.**
   - General anesthesia, but there are alternatives to endotracheal intubation
   - Positive-pressure ventilation
   - Protecting the respiratory tract from aspiration of gastric contents
   - Surgical procedures in which the anesthesiologist cannot easily control the airway (e.g., prone, sitting, or lateral decubitus procedures)
   - Situations in which neuromuscular paralysis has been instituted
   - Surgical procedures within the chest, abdomen, or cranium
   - When intracranial hypertension must be treated
   - Protecting a healthy lung from a diseased lung to ensure its continued performance (e.g., hemoptysis, empyema, pulmonary abscess)
   - Severe pulmonary and multisystem injury associated with respiratory failure (e.g., severe sepsis, airway obstruction, hypoxemia, and hypercarbia of various etiologies)

2. **Review objective measures suggesting the need to perform endotracheal intubation.**
   These objective measures are often used for patients in critical care settings, not necessarily perioperatively. But they also are useful in determining which patients should not be extubated after surgery.
   - Respiratory rate >35 breaths/min
   - Vital capacity <5 ml/kg in adults and 10 ml/kg in children
   - Inability to generate a negative inspiratory force of 20 mm Hg
   - Arterial partial pressure of oxygen (PaO_2) <70 mm Hg on 40% oxygen
   - Alveolar-arterial (A-a) gradient >350 mm Hg on 100% O_2
   - Arterial partial pressure of carbon dioxide ($PaCO_2$) >55 mm Hg (except in chronic retainers)
   - Dead space (V_D/V_T) >0.6

3. **What historical information might be useful in assessing a patient's airway?**
   Patients should be questioned about adverse events related to previous airway management episodes. For instance, have they ever been informed by an anesthesiologist that they had an airway management problem (e.g., "difficult to ventilate, difficult to intubate")? Have they had a tracheostomy or other surgery or radiation about the face and neck? Have they sustained significant burns to these areas? Do they have obstructive sleep apnea, snoring, or temporomandibular joint (TMJ) dysfunction? Acromegalic patients are difficult intubations. Review of prior anesthetic records is always helpful. Children with Down syndrome may have atlantoaxial instability and have risks associated endotracheal intubation. Flexion-extension radiographs are recommended prior to planned intubation.

4. **Describe the physical examination of the oral cavity.**
   Examine the mouth and oral cavity, noting the extent and symmetry of opening (three fingerbreadths is optimal), the health of the teeth (loose, missing, or cracked teeth should be documented), and the presence of dental appliances. Prominent buck teeth may interfere with the use of a laryngoscope. The size of the tongue should be noted (large tongues rarely make airway management impossible, only more difficult), as should the arch of the palate (high-arched palates have been associated with difficulty in visualizing the larynx).

5. **Review the Mallampati classification.**
   The appearance of the posterior pharynx may predict difficulty in laryngoscopy and visualization of the larynx. Meta-analysis of pertinent studies has revealed that, when used alone, the Mallampati test has limited accuracy for predicting the difficult airway. Thus it is clear that a comprehensive airway examination, not just a Mallampati classification, is

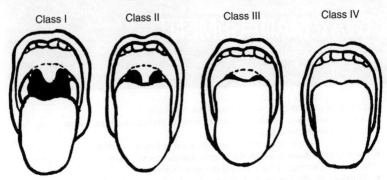

Figure 8-1. Mallampati classification of the oropharynx.

necessary to identify patients who may be difficult to intubate. This classification also does not address the issue of ease of mask ventilation, but patients with Mallampati class III or IV airways are subject to increased airway trauma during airway management.

Mallampati has organized patients into classes I to IV based on the visualized structures (Figure 8-1). Visualization of fewer anatomic structures (particularly classes III and IV) is associated with difficult laryngeal exposure. With the patient *sitting upright*, mouth fully open, and tongue protruding, classification is based on visualization of the following structures:

- Class I: Pharyngeal pillars, entire palate, and uvula are visible.
- Class II: Pharyngeal pillars and soft palate are visible, with visualization of the uvula obstructed by the tongue.
- Class III: Soft palate is visible, but pharyngeal pillars and uvula are not visualized.
- Class IV: Only the hard palate is visible; the soft palate, pillars, and uvula are not visualized.

Compared to laboring women, post-labor women have a deterioration in Mallampati classification. This could be of importance if the women's childbirth changed from active labor to general surgery for cesarean delivery.

6. **What is the next step after examination of the oral cavity?**
   After examination of the oral cavity is completed, attention is directed at the size of the mandible and quality of TMJ function. A short mandible (shorter than three fingerbreadths) as measured from the mental process to the prominence of the thyroid cartilage (thyromental distance) suggests difficulty in visualizing the larynx. Patients with TMJ dysfunction may have asymmetry or limitations in opening the mouth and popping or clicking. Manipulation of the jaw in preparation for laryngoscopy may worsen symptoms after surgery. It is curious that some patients with TMJ dysfunction have greater difficulty opening the mouth after anesthetic induction and neuromuscular paralysis than when they are awake and cooperative.

7. **Describe the examination of the neck.**
   Evidence of prior surgeries (especially tracheostomy) or significant burns is noted. Does the patient have abnormal masses (e.g., hematoma, abscess, cellulitis or edema, lymphadenopathy, goiter, tumor, soft-tissue swelling) or tracheal deviation? A short or thick neck may prove problematic. A neck circumference of greater than 18 inches has been reported to be associated with a difficult airway. Large breasts (e.g., a parturient) may make using the laryngoscope itself difficult, and short-handled laryngoscope handles have been developed with this in mind.

   It is also important to have the patient demonstrate the range of motion of the head and neck. Preparation for laryngoscopy requires extension of the neck to facilitate visualization. Elderly patients and patients with cervical fusions may have limited motion. Furthermore, patients with cervical spine disease (disk disease or cervical instability, as in rheumatoid arthritis) may develop neurologic symptoms with motion of the neck. Radiologic views of the neck in flexion and extension may reveal cervical instability in such patients.

It is my experience that the preoperative assessment of range of motion in patients with prior cervical spine surgery does not equate well with their mobility after they have been anesthetized and paralyzed, suggesting that in this patient group wariness is the best policy, and advanced airway techniques, as will be described, should be considered.

Particularly in patients with pathology of the head and neck, such as laryngeal cancer, it is valuable to know the results of nasolaryngoscopy performed by otolaryngologists. (This is always the case in ear, nose, and throat surgery—never assume anything. Always work closely and preemptively with the surgeon to determine how the airway should be managed.) Finally, if history suggests dynamic airway obstruction (as in intrathoracic or extrathoracic masses), pulmonary function tests, including flow-volume loops, may alert the clinician to the potential for loss of airway once paralytic agents are administered.

8. **Discuss the anatomy of the larynx.**
The larynx, located in adults at cervical levels 4 to 6, protects the entrance of the respiratory tract and allows phonation. It is composed of three unpaired cartilages (thyroid, cricoid, and epiglottis) and three paired cartilages (arytenoid, corniculate, and cuneiform). The thyroid cartilage is the largest and most prominent, forming the anterior and lateral walls. The cricoid cartilage is shaped like a signet ring, faces posteriorly, and is the only complete cartilaginous ring of the laryngotracheal tree. The cricothyroid membrane connects these structures anteriorly. The epiglottis extends superiorly into the hypopharynx and covers the entrance of the larynx during swallowing. The corniculate and cuneiform pairs of cartilages are relatively small and do not figure prominently in the laryngoscopic appearance of the larynx or in its function. The arytenoid cartilages articulate on the posterior aspect of the larynx and are the posterior attachments of the vocal ligaments (or vocal cords). Identification of the arytenoid cartilages may be important during laryngoscopy. In a patient with an *anterior* airway, the arytenoids may be the only visible structures. Finally, the vocal cords attach anteriorly to the thyroid cartilage.

9. **Describe the innervation and blood supply to the larynx.**
The superior and recurrent laryngeal nerves, both branches of the vagus nerve, innervate the larynx. The superior laryngeal nerves decussate into internal and external branches. The internal branches provide sensory innervation of the larynx above the vocal cords, whereas the external branches provide motor innervation to the cricothyroid muscle, a tensor of the vocal cords. The recurrent laryngeal nerves provide sensory innervation below the level of the cords and motor innervation of the posterior cricoarytenoid muscles, the only abductors of the vocal cords. The glossopharyngeal or ninth cranial nerve provides sensory innervation to the vallecula (the space anterior to the epiglottis) and the base of the tongue.

Arteries that supply the larynx include the superior laryngeal (a branch of the superior thyroid artery) and inferior laryngeal (a branch of the inferior thyroid artery). Venous drainage follows the same pattern as the arteries; there is also ample lymphatic drainage.

10. **Summarize the various instruments available to facilitate oxygenation.**
Oxygen supplementation is always a priority when patients are sedated or anesthetized. Devices range from nasal cannulas, face tents, and simple masks to masks with reservoirs and masks that can be used to deliver positive-pressure ventilation. Their limitation is the oxygen concentration that can be delivered effectively.

11. **What are the benefits of oral and nasal airways?**
Oral airways are usually constructed of hard plastic; they are available in numerous sizes and shaped to curve behind the tongue, lifting it off the posterior pharynx. The importance of these simple devices cannot be overstated because the tongue is the most frequent cause of airway obstruction, particularly in obtunded patients. Nasal airways (*trumpets*) can be gently inserted down the nasal passages into the nasopharynx and are better tolerated than oral airways in awake or lightly anesthetized patients. However, epistaxis is a risk.

12. **How are laryngoscopes used?**
Laryngoscopes are usually left-handed tools designed to facilitate visualization of the larynx. Short handles work best for obese patients or those with thick chests or large breasts. Laryngoscope blades come in various styles and sizes. The most commonly used blades include the curved Macintosh and the straight Miller blades. The curved blades are inserted

into the vallecula, immediately anterior to the epiglottis, which is literally flipped out of the visual axis to expose the laryngeal opening. The Miller blade is inserted past the epiglottis, which is simply lifted out of the way of laryngeal viewing.

13. **What structures must be aligned to accomplish visualization of the larynx?**
   To directly visualize the larynx, it is necessary to align the oral, pharyngeal, and laryngeal axes. To facilitate this process, elevating the head on a small pillow and extending the head at the atlanto-occipital axes are necessary (Figure 8-2).

14. **What is a GlideScope?**
   Different laryngoscope blades have been discussed, and it should be no surprise that various arrangements of laryngoscope handles and blades have been developed. The GlideScope video laryngoscope (Verathon, Inc., Bothell, WA) has a one-piece rigid plastic handle and curved blade; at the tip of the blade is not only the light but a camera eye. The image is transmitted to a screen at bedside. By using the GlideScope, it has not been necessary to align the three axes as discussed in the prior question. Thus the patient might easily be intubated with the neck in a neutral position. In addition, in patients in whom, on conventional laryngoscopy, the laryngeal aperture is anterior to the visual axis, the GlideScope facilitates visualization of the larynx and endotracheal intubation. The GlideScope has proven to be an outstanding addition to the airway management armamentarium.

KEY POINTS: AIRWAY MANAGEMENT

1. A thorough airway examination and identification of the patient with a potentially difficult airway are of paramount importance.
2. The *difficult-to-ventilate, difficult-to-intubate* scenario must be avoided if possible.
3. An organized approach, as reflected in the American Society of Anesthesiologists' (ASAs') difficult airway algorithm, is necessary and facilitates high-quality care for patients with airway management difficulties.

---

15. **What endotracheal tubes are available?**
   Endotracheal tubes come in a multitude of sizes and shapes. They are commonly manufactured from polyvinyl chloride, with a radiopaque line from top to bottom; standard-size connectors for anesthesia circuits or resuscitation bags; a high-volume, low-pressure cuff and pilot balloon; and a hole in the beveled, distal end (the Murphy eye). Internal diameter ranges from 2 to 10 mm in half-millimeter increments. Endotracheal tubes may be reinforced with wire, designed with laser applications in mind, or unusually shaped so they are directed away from the surgical site (oral or nasal RAE tubes). Endotracheal tubes can produce tracheal trauma, including cough, sore throat, hoarseness, and blood-streaked expectorant. Laryngeal edema, laryngeal ulceration, and subglottic stenosis have also been reported.

16. **What are laryngeal mask airways?**
   Laryngeal mask airways (LMAs) maintain a patent airway during anesthesia when endotracheal intubation is neither required nor desired (e.g., asthmatic patients, professional singers in the local opera company). Increasingly LMAs are being substituted for endotracheal tubes. They are an important part of the management of difficult airways and patients can be intubated through a well-placed LMA.

17. **What other airway management devices are available?**
   Light wands may be useful for blind intubation of the trachea. The technique is termed *blind* because the laryngeal opening is not seen directly. When light is well transilluminated through the neck (the jack-o'-lantern effect), the end of the endotracheal tube is at the entrance of the larynx, and the tube can be threaded off the wand and into the trachea in a blind fashion. Gum elastic bougies are flexible, somewhat malleable stylets with an anteriorly directed, bent tip that may be useful for intubating a tracheal opening anterior to

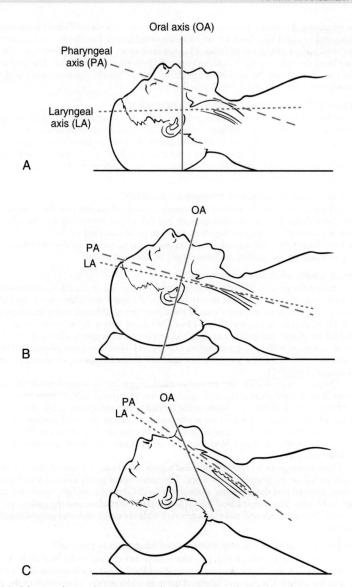

Figure 8-2. Schematic diagram demonstrating the head position for endotracheal intubation. **A,** Successful direct laryngoscopy for exposure of the glottic opening requires alignment of the oral, pharyngeal, and laryngeal axes. **B,** Elevation of the head about 10 cm with pads below the occiput and with the shoulders remaining on the table aligns the laryngeal and pharyngeal axes. **C,** Subsequent head extension at the atlanto-occipital joint creates the shortest distance and most nearly straight line from the incisor teeth to glottic opening. *(From Gal TJ: Airway management. In Miller RD, editor: Miller's anesthesia, ed 6, Philadelphia, 2005, Churchill Livingstone, p 1622.)*

the visual axis. Fiberoptic endoscopy is commonly used to facilitate difficult intubations and allows endotracheal tube insertion under direct visualization. Finally, the trachea may be intubated using a retrograde technique. In simplistic terms, a long Seldinger-type wire is introduced through a catheter that punctures the cricothyroid membrane. The wire is directed superiorly and brought out through the nose or mouth, and an endotracheal tube is threaded over the wire and lowered into the trachea.

18. **Describe the indications for an awake intubation.**
If the physical examination leaves in question the ability to ventilate and intubate once the patient is anesthetized and paralyzed, consideration should be given to awake intubation. Patients with a previous history of difficult intubation, acute processes that compromise the airway (e.g., soft-tissue infections of the head and neck, hematomas, mandibular fractures, or other significant facial deformities), morbid obesity, or cancer involving the larynx are reasonable candidates for awake intubation.

19. **How is the patient prepared for awake intubation?**
A frank discussion with the patient is necessary because patient safety is the priority. The anticipated difficulty of airway management and the risks of proceeding with anesthesia without previously securing a competent airway must be conveyed in clear terms. Despite our best efforts to provide topical anesthesia and sedation, sometimes the procedure is uncomfortable for the patient, and this should be discussed as well.

20. **How is awake intubation performed?**
In preparing the patient, administration of glycopyrrolate, 0.2 to 0.4 mg 30 minutes before the procedure, is useful to reduce secretions. Many clinicians also administer nebulized lidocaine to provide topical anesthesia of the entire airway, although many techniques are available to provide airway anesthesia. Once the patient arrives in the operating suite, standard anesthetic monitors are applied and supplemental oxygen is administered. The patient is sedated with appropriate agents (e.g., opioid, benzodiazepine, propofol). The level of sedation is titrated so the patient is not rendered obtunded, apneic, or unable to protect the airway (Table 8-1).

The route of intubation may be oral or nasal, depending on surgical needs and patient factors. If nasal intubation is planned, nasal and nasopharyngeal mucosa must be anesthetized; vasoconstrictor substances are applied to prevent epistaxis. Often nasal trumpets with lidocaine ointment are gently inserted to dilate the nasal passages. A transtracheal injection of lidocaine is often performed via needle puncture of the cricothyroid membrane. Nerve blocks are also useful to provide topical anesthesia (see the following question).

Once an adequate level of sedation and topical anesthesia is achieved, the endotracheal tube is loaded on the fiberoptic endoscope. The endoscope is gently inserted into the chosen passage, directed past the epiglottis, through the larynx, into the trachea, visualizing tracheal rings and carina. The endotracheal tube is passed into the trachea, and the endoscope is removed. Breath sounds and end-tidal carbon dioxide are confirmed, and general anesthesia is begun.

21. **What nerve blocks are useful when awake intubation is planned?**
The glossopharyngeal nerve, which provides sensory innervation to the base of the tongue and the vallecula, may be blocked by transmucosal local anesthetic injection at the base of the tonsillar pillars. The superior laryngeal nerve provides sensory innervation of the larynx above the vocal cords and may be blocked by injection just below the greater cornu of the hyoid. Care must be taken to aspirate before injection because this is carotid artery territory. Many clinicians are reluctant to block the superior laryngeal nerves and perform a transtracheal block in patients with a full stomach because all protective airway reflexes are lost. Such patients are unable to protect themselves from aspiration if gastric contents are regurgitated.

22. **What is a difficult mask ventilation?**
Difficult mask ventilation (DMV) was described by the ASA (2003) as "a situation that develops when it is not possible for the unassisted anesthesiologist to maintain the oxygen saturation of >90% using 100% oxygen and positive pressure ventilation, or to prevent

Table 8-1. Useful Medications for Awake Intubations

MEDICATION	PURPOSE	DOSE	ROUTE
Glycopyrrolate	Antisialagogue	0.2–0.4 mg	IV or IM
Midazolam	Sedation/amnesia	1–4 mg	IV
Fentanyl	Analgesic	50–250 mcg	IV
Cocaine	Topical anesthesia and vasoconstriction	40–160 mg	Intranasal
1% Phenylephrine	Vasoconstriction	Spray	Intranasal
2% Viscous lidocaine	Topical anesthesia	5–20 ml	Orally
Cetacaine spray	Topical anesthesia	2–4 sprays	Orally
Lidocaine 1%–4%	Airway anesthesia	2–3 ml	Transtracheal or nerve block
Dexmedetomidine	Sedation		0.5–1.0 micrograms/kg IV

IM, Intramuscular; IV, intravenous.

saturation <90% using 100% oxygen and positive pressure ventilation, or to prevent or reverse signs of inadequate ventilation." (p. 1272)

23. **What are predictors of difficult mask ventilation? Why is this important?**
There is much focus on intubation and predictors of difficult intubation. It should be recognized that the ability to mask-ventilate a patient is equally and perhaps more important than the ability to intubate. For instance, if it is determined at the time of intubation that perhaps a patient is impossible to intubate by conventional laryngoscopy, if the patient's oxygen saturations can be maintained through mask ventilation, the situation remains under a degree of control while help and additional airway management tools are summoned. However, if you have a patient who is difficult to intubate and ventilate, the situation is not under control, and the patient is at risk for hypoxic injury.
    Between 1% and 2% of patients will be difficult to ventilate. Predictors of difficult mask ventilation include limitations in mandibular protrusion; a thyromental distance less than 6 cm; advanced age (older than 57 years in one study); abnormal neck anatomy; sleep apnea, snoring; body mass index of 30 kg/m² or greater; and the presence of a beard. A beard may make mask ventilation difficult, but it may also hide a small thyromental distance. Some men may choose to wear a beard because they don't care for their weak chin facies, which is another way of saying that they have a small thyromental distance.

24. **The patient has been anesthetized and paralyzed, but the airway is difficult to intubate. Is there an organized approach to handling this problem?**
The patient who is difficult to ventilate and intubate is quite possibly the most serious problem faced by anesthesiologists because hypoxic brain injuries and cardiac arrest are real possibilities in this scenario. It has been established that persistent failed intubation attempts are associated with death. Although a thorough history and physical examination are likely to identify the majority of patients with difficult airways, unanticipated problems occasionally occur. Only through preplanning and practiced algorithms are such situations managed optimally. The ASA has prepared a difficult airway algorithm (Figure 8-3) to assist the clinician. The relative merits of different management options (surgical vs. nonsurgical airway, awake vs. postinduction intubation, spontaneous vs. assisted ventilation) are weighed. Once these decisions have been made, primary and alternative strategies are laid out to assist in stepwise management. This algorithm deserves close and repeated inspection before the anesthesiologist attempts to manage such problems. This is no time for heroism; if intubation or ventilation is difficult, call for help.
    It is always wise to consider the merits of regional anesthesia to avoid a known or suspected difficult airway. However, in patients with a difficult airway, the use of regional anesthesia does not relieve the anesthesiologist of some planning for airway difficulties.

1. Assess the likelihood and clinical impact of basic management problems:
   A. Difficult Ventilation
   B. Difficult Intubation
   C. Difficulty with Patient Cooperation or Consent
   D. Difficult Tracheostomy

2. Actively pursue opportunities to deliver supplemental oxygen throughout the process of difficult airway management

3. Consider the relative merits and feasibility of basic management choices:

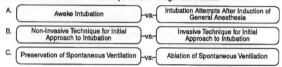

   A. Awake Intubation —vs.— Intubation Attempts After Induction of General Anesthesia
   B. Non-Invasive Technique for Initial Approach to Intubation —vs.— Invasive Technique for Initial Approach to Intubation
   C. Preservation of Spontaneous Ventilation —vs.— Ablation of Spontaneous Ventilation

4. Develop primary and alternative strategies:

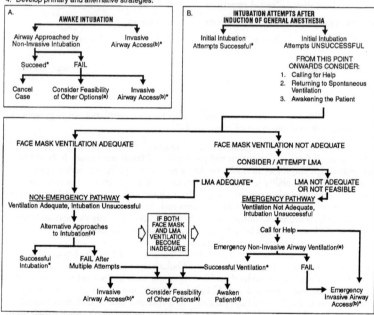

* Confirm ventilation, tracheal intubation, or LMA placement with exhaled CO$_2$

a. Other options include (but are not limited to): surgery utilizing face mask or LMA anesthesia, local anesthesia infiltration or regional nerve blockade. Pursuit of these options usually implies that mask ventilation will not be problematic. Therefore, these options may be of limited value if this step in the algorithm has been reached via the Emergency Pathway.

b. Invasive airway access includes surgical or percutaneous tracheostomy or cricothyrotomy.

c. Alternative non-invasive approaches to difficult intubation include (but are not limited to): use of different laryngoscope blades, LMA as an intubation conduit (with or without fiberoptic guidance), fiberoptic intubation, intubating stylet or tube changer, light wand, retrograde intubation, and blind oral or nasal intubation.

d. Consider re-preparation of the patient for awake intubation or canceling surgery.

e. Options for emergency non-invasive airway ventilation include (but are not limited to): rigid bronchoscope, esophageal-tracheal combitube ventilation, or transtracheal jet ventilation.

Figure 8-3. Management of the difficult airway. LMA, Laryngeal mask airway. (*From the American Society of Anesthesiologists.*)

Death and central nervous system injuries remain the leading cause of adverse outcomes in the perioperative setting. However, it has been noted through analysis of closed medicolegal claims that the incidence of these injuries has decreased since these algorithms and advanced airway techniques were introduced.

25. **Describe the technique of transtracheal ventilation and its limitations.**
Transtracheal ventilation is a temporizing measure if mask ventilation becomes inadequate. A catheter (12- or 14-G) is inserted through the cricothyroid membrane and then connected to a jet-type (Sanders) ventilator capable of delivering oxygen under pressure.

The gas is delivered intermittently by a handheld actuator. The duration of ventilation is best assessed by watching the rise and fall of the chest; an inspiratory to expiratory ratio of 1:4 seconds is recommended. Usually oxygenation improves rapidly; however, patients frequently cannot expire fully, perhaps because of airway obstruction, and can develop increased intrathoracic pressures, putting them at risk for barotrauma or decreased cardiac output. Carbon dioxide retention limits the duration of the usefulness of the technique.

26. **What are criteria for extubation?**
The patient should be awake and responsive with stable vital signs. Adequate reversal of neuromuscular blockade must be established as demonstrated by sustained head lift. In equivocal situations, negative inspiratory force should exceed 20 mm Hg (see Question 2).

27. **What is rapid-sequence induction? Which patients are best managed in this fashion?**
It is easiest to appreciate the distinctions of rapid-sequence induction (RSI) if an induction under non–rapid-sequence conditions is understood. Ordinarily the patient has fasted for at least 6 to 8 hours and is not at risk for pulmonary aspiration of gastric contents. The patient is preoxygenated, and an anesthetic induction agent is administered. Once it is established that the patient can be mask-ventilated satisfactorily, a muscle relaxant is given. The patient is then mask-ventilated until complete paralysis is ensured by nerve stimulation. Laryngoscopy and endotracheal intubation are undertaken, and the case proceeds.

In contrast, RSI is undertaken in patients who are thought to be at risk for pulmonary aspiration of gastric contents. Patients with full stomachs are at risk; other risk factors include pregnancy, diabetes, pain, opioid analgesics, recent traumatic injury, intoxication, and pathologic involvement of the gastrointestinal tract such as small bowel obstruction. Patients with full stomachs should be premedicated with agents that reduce the acidity and volume of gastric contents, such as histamine-2 receptor blockers (ranitidine, cimetidine), nonparticulate antacids (Bicitra or Alka-Seltzer), or gastrokinetics (metoclopramide).

28. **How is RSI performed?**
The goal of RSI is to secure and control the airway rapidly. The patient is preoxygenated. An induction agent is administered, followed quickly by a rapid-acting relaxant, either succinylcholine or larger doses of rocuronium. Simultaneously an assistant applies pressure to the cricoid cartilage (the only complete cartilaginous ring of the respiratory tract), which closes off the esophagus and prevents entry of regurgitated gastric contents into the trachea and lungs. Known as the Sellick maneuver, such pressure is maintained until the airway is protected by tracheal intubation.

29. **What is the purpose of preoxygenation before the induction of anesthesia?**
Preoxygenation is an important part of any general anesthetic. Inspired room air contains approximately 21% O_2, with the remainder being mostly nitrogen (N_2). Not many people can go more than a few minutes without ventilation before desaturation occurs. If patients breathe 100% oxygen for several minutes, they may not desaturate for up to 3 to 5 minutes because the functional residual capacity (FRC) of the lung has been completely washed of N_2 and filled with O_2.

30. **Anesthesiologists routinely deliver 100% oxygen for a few minutes before extubation. What is the logic behind this action, and why might an FiO_2 of 80% be better?**
Patients emerging from general anesthesia may develop airway obstruction or disorganized breathing patterns. A 5-minute period of inspiring 100% oxygenation is sufficient to fill the patient's FRC with 100% oxygen, establishing a depot of oxygen in case airway obstruction or other respiratory difficulties accompany extubation. Unfortunately, 100% oxygen promotes atelectasis, reducing the surface area available for gas exchange and causing intrapulmonary shunting. Although an FiO_2 of 0.8 appears to prevent atelectasis, it is not clear whether the small increase in atelectasis associated with breathing 100% oxygen is of clinical importance. Until this is demonstrated, the best practice is to administer 100% oxygen before extubation.

WEBSITE

American Society of Anesthesiologists: http://www.asahq.org

SUGGESTED READINGS

American Society of Anesthesiologists: Practice guidelines for management of the difficult airway: an updated report by the ASA Task Force on Management of the Difficult Airway, Anesthesiology 98:1269–1277, 2003.

Benjamin B, Holinger LD: Laryngeal complications of endotracheal intubation, Ann Otol Rhinol Laryngol 117:1–20, 2008.

Hodali BS, Chandrasekhar S, Bulich LN: Airway changes during labor and delivery, Anesthesiology 108:357–362, 2008.

Kheterpal S, Han R, Tremper K, et al: Incidence and predictors of difficult and impossible mask ventilation, Anesthesiology 105:885–891, 2006.

Kheterpal S, Martin L, Shanks AM, et al: Prediction and outcomes of impossible mask ventilation, Anesthesiology 110:891–897, 2009.

Liu J, Zhang X, Gong W, et al: Correlations between controlled endotracheal tube cuff pressure and postprocedural complications: a multicenter study, Anesth Analg 111:1133–1137, 2010.

Peterson GM, Domino KB, Caplan RA, et al: Management of the difficult airway: a closed claims analysis, Anesthesiology 103:33–39, 2005.

PULMONARY FUNCTION TESTING

James C. Duke, MD, MBA

CHAPTER 9

1. **What are pulmonary function tests, and how are they used?**

   The term *pulmonary function test (PFT)* refers to a standardized measurement of a patient's airflow, lung volumes, and diffusing capacity for inspired carbon monoxide (DLCO). These values are always reported as a percentage of a predicted normal value, which is calculated based on the age and height of the patient. Used in combination with the history, physical examination, blood gas analysis, and chest radiograph, PFTs facilitate the classification of respiratory disease into obstructive, restrictive, or mixed disorder.

2. **What is the benefit of obtaining PFTs?**

   The primary goal of preoperative pulmonary function testing, also called *spirometry*, is to recognize patients at high or prohibitive risk for postoperative pulmonary complications. Abnormal PFTs identify patients who will benefit from aggressive perioperative pulmonary therapy and those in whom surgery should be avoided entirely. However, no single test or combination of tests will definitively predict which patients will develop postoperative pulmonary complications.

3. **What are recognized risk factors for postoperative pulmonary complications?**

   - Age >70 years
   - Obesity
   - Upper abdominal or thoracic surgery
   - History of lung disease
   - Greater than 20-pack/year history of smoking
   - Resection of an anterior mediastinal mass

4. **Describe standard lung volumes.**

   The tidal volume (TV) is the volume of air inhaled and exhaled with each normal breath. Inspiratory reserve volume (IRV) is the volume of air that can be maximally inhaled beyond a normal TV. Expiratory reserve volume (ERV) is the maximal volume of air that can be exhaled beyond a normal TV. Residual volume (RV) is the volume of air that remains in the lung after maximal expiration (Figure 9-1).

5. **What are the lung capacities?**

   Lung capacities are composed of two or more lung volumes:
   - Total lung capacity (TLC) is the sum of IRV, tidal volume (TV), ERV, and RV.
   - Vital capacity (VC) is the sum of IRV, TV, and ERV.
   - Inspiratory capacity (IC) is the sum of IRV and TV.
   - Functional residual capacity (FRC) is the volume of air in the lung at the end of a normal expiration and is the sum of RV and ERV (see Figure 9-1).

6. **What are the measures of pulmonary function and their significance?**

   These are effort dependent and require a motivated patient (see Figure 9-2).
   - Forced expiratory volume in 1 second (FEV_1)
   - Forced vital capacity (FVC)
   - The ratio of FEV_1 and FVC, or FEV_1/FVC ratio. The FVC may be normal or decreased as a result of respiratory muscle weakness or dynamic airway obstruction.
   - Forced expiratory flow at 25% to 75% of FVC (FEF_{25-75}). A decreased FEF_{25-75} reflects collapse of the small airways and is a sensitive indicator of early airway obstruction.

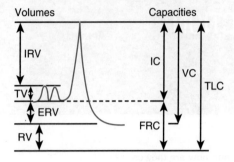

Figure 9-1. Subdivisions of lung volumes and capacities. *ERV*, Expiratory reserve volume; *FRC*, functional residual capacity; *IC*, inspiratory capacity; *IRV*, inspiratory reserve volume; *RV*, residual volume; *TLC*, total lung capacity; *TV*, tidal volume; *VC*, vital capacity.

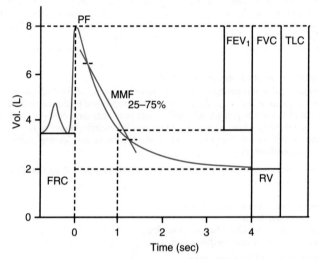

Figure 9-2. Spirogram. *FEV$_1$*, Forced expiratory volume in 1 second; *FRC*, functional residual capacity; *FVC*, forced vital capacity; *MMF*, mean maximal flow; *RV*, residual volume; *TLC*, total lung capacity.

7. **Review obstructive airway disease and the associated PFT abnormalities.**
   Obstructive airway diseases include asthma, chronic bronchitis, emphysema, cystic fibrosis, and bronchiolitis. These diseases involve airways distal to the carina and exhibit diminished expiratory airflow:
   - FEV$_1$, FEV$_1$/FVC ratio, and FEF$_{25-75}$ are the most significant clinically observed spirometry results and are below predicted values.
   - FVC may be normal or decreased as a result of respiratory muscle weakness or dynamic airway collapse with subsequent air trapping. See Table 9-1 and Table 9-2.

8. **What is the diffusing capacity for the single-breath diffusion capacity (DLCO), and what causes abnormal DLCO?**
   DLCO is dependent on membrane diffusion capacity and the underlying pulmonary vasculature. Therefore, it is a measure of functioning alveolar capillary units. Patients with obstructive, interstitial, or pulmonary vascular disease may have decreased DLCO.

9. **Describe age-related changes with pulmonary function.**
   There is loss of static recoil, chest wall stiffening, and a diminished total alveolar surface area. Work of breathing increases and overall, pulmonary reserve is lessened.

Table 9-1. Alterations in Measures of Lung Function in Obstructive Lung Disease

MEASURE	ASTHMA	BRONCHITIS	EMPHYSEMA
TLC	Increased	Normal or increased	Increased
VC	Normal or decreased	Normal or decreased	Normal or decreased
RV	Increased	Increased	Increased
FRC	Increased	Increased	Increased
DLCO	No change or increased	No change or decreased	Decreased
FEV_1	Decreased	Decreased	Decreased

DLCO, Diffusing capacity for inspired carbon monoxide; FEV_1, forced expiratory volume in 1 second; FRC, functional residual capacity; RV, residual volume; TLC, total lung capacity; VC, vital capacity. *Adapted from Taylor AE et al: Clinical respiratory physiology, Philadelphia, 1989, Saunders.*

Table 9-2. Severity of Obstructive and Restrictive Airway Diseases as Measured by FEV_1/FVC and TLC*

MEASURE OF PULMONARY FUNCTION	NORMAL	MILD	MODERATE	SEVERE
FEV_1/FVC	>73%	61%–73%	51%–60%	<50%
TLC	>81%	66%–80%	51%–65%	<50%

*Percentages are of predicted values.
FEV_1, Forced expiratory volume in 1 second; FVC, forced vital capacity; TLC, total lung capacity.

10. **What is the impact of age-related changes on anesthesia and surgery?**
    Fluid resuscitation, especially when in excess of needs, may result in pulmonary failure. Other contributors to failure include excessive opioids and residual neuromuscular blockade. Regional anesthetic techniques may benefit a patient with diminished pulmonary reserve.

11. **Review restrictive lung disorders and their associated PFT abnormalities.**
    Disorders that result in decreased lung volumes include abnormal chest cage configuration, respiratory muscle weakness, loss of alveolar air space (e.g., pulmonary fibrosis, pneumonia), and encroachment of the lung space by disorders of the pleural cavity (e.g., effusion, tumor). The characteristic restrictive pattern is a reduction in lung volumes, particularly TLC and VC. Airflow rates can be normal or increased.

12. **What is a flow-volume loop, and what information does it provide?**
    Using routine spirometric values, flow-volume loops assist in identifying the anatomic location of airway obstruction. Forced expiratory and inspiratory flow at 50% of FVC (FEF_{50} and FIF_{50}) are shown in Figure 9-3. Note that expiratory flow is represented above the x-axis, whereas inspiratory flow is represented below the axis. In a normal flow-volume loop, the FEF_{50}/FIF_{50} ratio is 1.

13. **What are the characteristic patterns of the flow-volume loop in a fixed airway obstruction, variable extrathoracic obstruction, and intrathoracic obstruction?**
    Upper airway lesions (e.g., tracheal stenosis) are fixed when there is a plateau during both inspiration and expiration. The FEF_{50}/FIF_{50} ratio remains unchanged. An extrathoracic obstruction occurs when the lesion (e.g., tumor) is located above the sternal notch and is characterized by a flattening of the flow-volume loop during inspiration. The flattening of the loop represents no further increase in airflow because the mass causes airway collapse. The FEF_{50}/FIF_{50} ratio is >1. An intrathoracic obstruction is characterized by a flattening of the expiratory loop of a flow-volume loop, and the FEF_{50}/FIF_{50} ratio is <1. The lesion causes airway collapse during expiration (Figure 9-4).

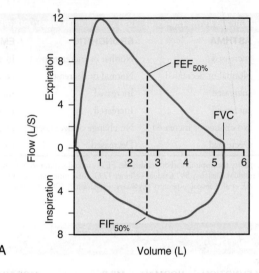

A

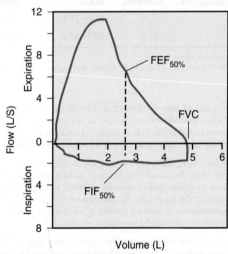

B

Figure 9-3. Idealized flow-volume loop. *EXP*, Expiratory; *FEF50*, expiratory flow at 50% of forced vital capacity; *FIF50*, inspiratory flow at 50% of forced vital capacity; *FVC*, forced vital capacity; *RV*, residual volume; *TLC*, total lung capacity. (Flow in L/sec is abbreviated V.) *(From Harrison RA: Respiratory function and anesthesia. In Barash PG, Cullen BF, Stoelting RK, editors: Clinical anesthesia, Philadelphia, 1989, Lippincott, pp 877–994, with permission.)*

14. **What is the value of measuring flow-volume loops in a patient with an anterior mediastinal mass?**

Injudicious anesthetic induction and paralysis in patients with an anterior mediastinal mass (e.g., lymphoma, thymoma, thyroid mass) may result in an inability to ventilate the patient and cardiovascular collapse caused by compression of the tracheobronchial tree, vena cava, pulmonary vessels, or heart. The change from spontaneous negative-pressure respirations to assisted positive-pressure ventilation is a significant factor in this collapse. The preoperative evaluation of flow-volume loops in sitting and supine positions helps to assess potentially

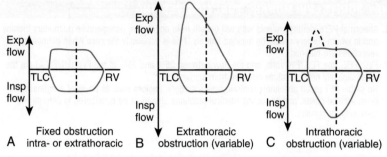

Figure 9-4. Flow-volume loops in a fixed, extrathoracic, and intrathoracic airway obstruction. The hashmarks represent flow at 50% of vital capacity. *Exp,* Expiratory; *Insp,* inspiratory; *RV,* residual volume; *TLC,* total lung capacity. (*From Kryger M, Bode F, Antic R, et al: Diagnosis of obstruction of the upper and central airways. Am J Med 61:85–93, 1976.*)

Table 9-3. Pulmonary Function Criteria Suggesting Increased Risk for Abdominal and Thoracic Surgery

MEASURE OF PULMONARY FUNCTION	ABDOMINAL	THORACIC
FVC	<70% predicted	<70% predicted or <1.7 L
FEV_1	<70% predicted	<2 L,* <1 L,† <0.6 L‡
FEV_1/FVC	<65%	<35%
MVV	<50% predicted	<50% predicted or <28 L/min
RV	<47% predicted	
DLCO	<50%	
VO_2	<15 ml/kg/min	

*Pneumonectomy.
†Lobectomy.
‡Segmentectomy.
DLCO, Diffusing capacity for inspired carbon monoxide; FEV_1, forced expiratory volume in 1 second; FVC, forced vital capacity; MVV, maximal voluntary ventilation; RV, residual volume; VO_2, oxygen consumption.
Data from Gass GD, Olsen GN: Preoperative pulmonary function testing to predict postoperative morbidity and mortality. Chest 89:127–135, 1986.

obstructive lesions of the airway and identify patients in whom alternative management may be indicated.

15. **What are the effects of surgery and anesthesia on pulmonary function?**
    All patients undergoing general anesthesia and surgical procedures (particularly in the thorax and upper abdomen) exhibit changes in pulmonary function that promote postoperative pulmonary complications. For instance, VC is reduced to approximately 40% of preoperative values and remains depressed for at least 10 to 14 days after open cholecystectomy. Upper abdominal procedures result in a decrease in FRC within 10 to 16 hours; FRC gradually returns to normal by 7 to 10 days. The normal pattern of ventilation is also altered, with decreased sigh breaths and decreased clearance of secretions.

16. **What PFT values predict increased perioperative pulmonary complications after abdominal or thoracic surgery?**
    See Table 9-3.

KEY POINTS: PULMONARY FUNCTION TESTING

1. Abnormal PFTs identify patients who will benefit from aggressive perioperative pulmonary therapy and in whom surgery should be avoided entirely. This is especially the case when pulmonary resections are planned.
2. FVC, FEV_1, the FEV_1/FVC ratio, and the flow between 25% and 75% of the FVC (MMF_{25-75}) are the most clinically helpful indices obtained from spirometry.
3. No single PFT result absolutely contraindicates surgery. Factors such as physical examination, arterial blood gases, and coexisting medical problems also must be considered in determining suitability for surgery.

SUGGESTED READINGS

Gal TJ: Pulmonary function testing. In Miller RD, editor: Miller's anesthesia, ed 6, Philadelphia, 2005, Churchill Livingstone, pp 999–1016.

Sprung J, Gajic O, Warner DO: Review article: age related alterations in respiratory function—anesthetic considerations, Can J Anaesth 53:1244–1257, 2006.

Wanger J, Clausen JL, Coates A, et al: Standardization of the measurement of lung volumes, Eur Respir J 26:511–522, 2005.

VOLATILE ANESTHETICS

Michelle D. Herren, MD

CHAPTER 10

1. **What are the properties of an ideal anesthetic gas?**

   An ideal anesthetic gas would be predictable in onset and emergence; provide muscle relaxation, cardiostability, and bronchodilation; not trigger malignant hyperthermia or other significant side effects (such as nausea and vomiting); be inflammable; undergo no transformation within the body; and allow easy estimation of concentration at the site of action.

2. **What are the chemical structures of the more common anesthetic gases? Why do we no longer use the older ones?**

   Isoflurane, desflurane, and sevoflurane are the most commonly used volatile anesthetics. As the accompanying molecular structures demonstrate, they are substituted halogenated *ethers*, except halothane, a substituted halogenated *alkane*. Many older anesthetic agents had unfortunate properties and side effects such as flammability (cyclopropane and fluroxene), slow induction (methoxyflurane), hepatotoxicity (chloroform and fluroxene), nephrotoxicity (methoxyflurane), and the theoretic risk of seizures (enflurane) (Figure 10-1).

3. **How are the potencies of anesthetic gases compared?**

   The potency of anesthetic gases is compared using minimal alveolar concentration (MAC), which is the concentration at 1 atmosphere that abolishes motor response to a painful stimulus (i.e., surgical incision) in 50% of patients. Of note, 1.3 MAC is required to abolish this response in 99% of patients. Other definitions of MAC include the MAC-BAR, which is the concentration required to block autonomic reflexes to nociceptive stimuli (1.7 to 2 MAC), and the MAC-awake, the concentration required to block appropriate voluntary reflexes and measure perceptive awareness (0.3 to 0.5 MAC). MAC appears to be consistent across species lines. The measurement of MAC assumes that alveolar concentration directly reflects the partial pressure of the anesthetic at its site of action and equilibration between the sites.

4. **What factors may influence MAC?**

   The highest MACs are found in infants at 6 to 12 months of age; MACs decrease with both increasing age and prematurity. For every Celsius degree drop in body temperature, MAC decreases approximately 2% to 5%. Hyponatremia, opioids, barbiturates, α_2 blockers, calcium channel blockers, acute alcohol intoxication, and pregnancy decrease MAC. Hyperthermia, chronic alcoholism, and central nervous system (CNS) stimulants (cocaine) increase MAC. Factors that do not affect MAC include hypocarbia, hypercarbia, gender, thyroid function, and hyperkalemia. MAC is additive. For example, nitrous oxide potentiates the effects of volatile anesthetics.

5. **Define *partition coefficient*. Which partition coefficients are important?**

   A partition coefficient describes the distribution of a given agent at equilibrium between two substances at the same temperature, pressure, and volume. Thus the blood-to-gas coefficient describes the distribution of anesthetic between blood and gas at the same partial pressure. A higher blood-to-gas coefficient correlates with a greater concentration of anesthetic in blood (i.e., a higher solubility). Therefore a greater amount of anesthetic is taken into the blood, which acts as a reservoir for the agent, reducing the alveolar concentration and thus slowing the rate of induction. Equilibration is relatively quick between alveolar and brain anesthetic partial pressure in insoluble volatile anesthetics. The alveolar concentration ultimately is the principal factor in determining onset of action.

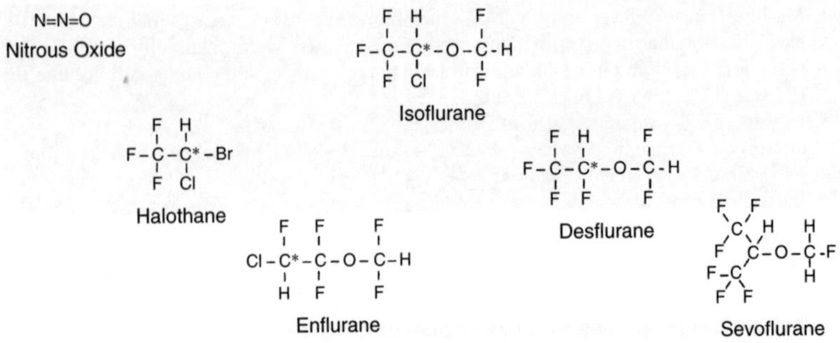

N=N=O
Nitrous Oxide

Isoflurane

Halothane

Enflurane

Desflurane

Sevoflurane

Figure 10-1. Molecular structures of contemporary gaseous anesthetics.

Table 10-1. Physical Properties of Contemporary Anesthetic Gases

	ISOFLURANE	DESFLURANE	HALOTHANE	NITROUS OXIDE	SEVOFLURANE
Molecular weight	184.5	168	197.5	44	200
Boiling point (°C)	48.5	23.5	50.2	−88	58.5
Vapor pressure (mm Hg)	238	664	241	39,000	160
Partition Coefficients at 37°C					
Blood to gas	1.4	0.42	2.3	0.47	0.69
Brain to blood	2.6	1.2	2.9	1.7	1.7
Fat to blood	45	27	60	2.3	48
Oil to gas	90.8	18.7	224	1.4	47.2
MAC (% of 1 atm)	1.15	6	0.77	104	1.7

atm, Atmosphere; *MAC*, minimum alveolar concentration.

Other important partition coefficients include brain to blood, fat to blood, liver to blood, and muscle to blood. Except for fat to blood, these coefficients are close to 1 (equally distributed). Fat has partition coefficients for different volatile agents of 30 to 60 (i.e., anesthetics continue to be taken into fat for quite some time after equilibration with other tissues) (Table 10-1).

6. Review the evolution in hypothesis as to how volatile anesthetics work.
   • At the turn of the century Meyer and Overton independently observed that an increasing oil-to-gas partition coefficient correlated with anesthetic potency. The Meyer-Overton lipid solubility theory dominated for nearly half a century before it was modified.
   • Franks and Lieb found that an amphophilic solvent (octanol) correlated better with potency than lipophilicity and concluded that the anesthetic site must contain both polar and nonpolar sites.

- Modifications of Meyer and Overton's membrane expansion theories include the excessive volume theory, in which anesthesia is created when polar cell membrane components and amphophilic anesthetics synergistically create a larger cell volume than the sum of the two volumes together.
- In the critical volume hypothesis, anesthesia results when the cell volume at the anesthetic site reaches a critical size. These theories rely on the effects of membrane expansion on and at ion channels.
- Early 19th-century theories oversimplify the mechanism of anesthetic action and have been abandoned for the following reasons: volatile anesthetics lead to only mild perturbations in lipids, and the same changes can be reproduced by changes in temperature without leading to behavioral changes; also, variations in size, rigidity, and location of the anesthetic in the lipid bilayer are similar to those in compounds that do not have anesthetic activity, which implies that specific receptors are involved.
- Newer accepted theories propose distinct molecular targets and anatomic sites of action rather than nonspecific actions on cell volume or wall. Volatile anesthetics are thought to enhance inhibitory receptors on ion channels, including γ-aminobutyric acid (GABA) type A and glycine receptors. Blockade of excitatory ion channels are also a feature and mediated through excitation of NMDA (N-methyl-D-aspartate) receptors.
- There is also evidence supporting an inhibitory effect on excitatory channels such as neuronal nicotinic and glutamate receptors.
- Most likely the actions of immobilization and amnesia are caused by separate mechanisms at different anatomic sites. At the spinal cord level, anesthetics lead to suppression of nociceptive motor responses and are responsible for immobilization of skeletal muscle. Supraspinal effects on the brain are responsible for amnesia and hypnosis. The thalamus and midbrain reticular formation are more depressed than other regions of the brain. Amnesia, awareness, and immobility are not guaranteed in all cases, especially when the patient has received muscle relaxants.

7. **What factors influence speed of induction?**

Factors that increase alveolar anesthetic concentration speed onset of volatile induction:
- Increasing the delivered concentrations of anesthetic
- High flow within the breathing circuit
- Increasing minute ventilation
- Factors that decrease alveolar concentration slow onset of volatile induction:
- Increase in cardiac output
- Decreased minute ventilation
- High anesthetic lipid solubility
- Low flow within the breathing circuit

8. **What is the second gas effect? Explain diffusion hypoxia.**

In theory this phenomenon should speed the onset of anesthetic induction. Because nitrous oxide is insoluble in blood, its rapid absorption from alveoli results in an abrupt rise in the alveolar concentration of the accompanying volatile anesthetic. However, even at high concentrations (70%) of nitrous oxide, this effect accounts for only a small increase in concentration of volatile anesthetic. Recent studies have yielded conflicting results as to whether this phenomenon is valid. When nitrous oxide is discontinued abruptly, its rapid diffusion from the blood to the alveolus decreases the oxygen tension in the lung, leading to a brief period of decreased oxygen concentration known as *diffusion hypoxia*. Administering 100% oxygen at the end of a case can mitigate this.

9. **Should nitrous oxide be administered to patients with pneumothorax? Are there other conditions in which nitrous oxide should be avoided?**

Although nitrous oxide has a low blood-to-gas partition coefficient, it is 20 times more soluble than nitrogen (which comprises 79% of atmospheric gases). Thus nitrous oxide can diffuse 20 times faster into closed spaces than it can be removed, resulting in expansion of pneumothorax, bowel gas, or air embolism or in an increase in pressure within noncompliant cavities such as the cranium or middle ear (Figure 10-2).

KEY POINTS: VOLATILE ANESTHETICS

1. Speed of onset of volatile anesthetics is increased by increasing the delivered concentration of anesthetic, increasing the fresh gas flow, increasing alveolar ventilation, and using nonlipid-soluble anesthetics.
2. Volatile anesthetics lead to a decrease in tidal volume and an increase in respiratory rate, resulting in a rapid, shallow breathing pattern.
3. MAC is decreased by old age or prematurity, hyponatremia, hypothermia, opioids, barbiturates, α_2 blockers, calcium channel blockers, acute alcohol intoxication, and pregnancy.
4. MAC is increased by hyperthermia, chronic alcoholism, and CNS stimulants (e.g., cocaine).
5. The physiologic response to hypoxia and hypercarbia is blunted by volatile anesthetics in a dose-dependent fashion.
6. Because of its insolubility in blood and rapid egress into air-filled spaces, nitrous oxide should not be used in the setting of pneumothorax, bowel obstruction, or pneumocephalus or during middle ear surgery.
7. Degradation of desflurane and sevoflurane by desiccated absorbents may lead to CO production and poisoning.
8. Nitrous oxide toxicity is a rare but real threat in substance abusers, patients with vitamin B_{12} deficiencies, and possibly unborn fetuses because of impaired methionine synthesis and results in neurologic sequelae.

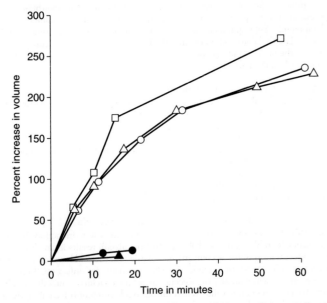

Figure 10-2. Increase in intrapleural gas volume on administration of nitrous oxide (*open squares, circles, and triangles*) as opposed to change in volume on administration of oxygen, plus halothane (*filled triangles and filled circles*). (Redrawn from Eger EI II, Saidman LJ: Hazards of nitrous oxide anesthesia in bowel obstruction and pneumothorax, Anesthesiology 26:61–68, 1965.)

10. **Describe the ventilatory effects of the volatile anesthetics.**
    Delivery of anesthetic gases results in dose-dependent depression of ventilation mediated directly through medullary centers and indirectly through effects on intercostal muscle function. Minute volume decreases secondary to reductions in tidal volume, although rate appears generally to increase in a dose-dependent fashion. Ventilatory drive in response to

hypoxia can be easily abolished at 1 MAC and attenuated at lower concentrations. Increasing the delivered anesthetic concentration also attenuates the ventilatory response to hypercarbia.

11. **What effects do volatile anesthetics have on hypoxic pulmonary vasoconstriction, airway caliber, mucociliary function, and intracranial pressure?**
    Hypoxic pulmonary vasoconstriction (HPV) is a locally mediated response of the pulmonary vasculature to decreased alveolar oxygen tension and serves to match ventilation to perfusion. Inhalational agents decrease this response.

    All volatile anesthetics appear to decrease airway resistance by a direct relaxing effect on bronchial smooth muscle and by decreasing the bronchoconstricting effect of hypocapnia. The bronchoconstricting effects of histamine release also appear to be decreased when an inhalational anesthetic is administered.

    Mucociliary clearance appears to be diminished by volatile anesthetics, principally through interference with ciliary beat frequency. The effects of dry inhaled gases, positive-pressure ventilation, and high inspired oxygen content also contribute to ciliary impairment.

    Malignant hyperthermia has been thought a stimulant for malignant hyperthermia.

    Volatile anesthetics increase intracranial blood flow and may increase intracranial pressure (ICP). Use of an intravenous anesthetic may be preferred to volatile anesthetics when increasing ICP may impair effective intracranial blood flow.

12. **What effects do volatile anesthetics have on circulation?**
    See Table 10-2.

13. **Which anesthetic agent is most associated with cardiac dysrhythmias?**
    Halothane has been shown to increase the sensitivity of the myocardium to epinephrine, resulting in premature ventricular contractions and tachydysrhythmias. The mechanism may be related to the prolongation of conduction through the His-Purkinje system, which facilitates the reentrant phenomenon and β_1-adrenergic receptor stimulation within the heart. Compared with adults, children undergoing halothane anesthesia appear to be relatively resistant to this sensitizing effect, although halothane has been shown to have a cholinergic, vagally induced bradycardic effect in children.

Table 10-2. Circulatory Effects of Contemporary Anesthetic Gases

	ISOFLURANE/ DESFLURANE	SEVOFLURANE	HALOTHANE	NITROUS OXIDE
Cardiac output	0	0	–*	+
Heart rate	++/0	0	0	+
Blood pressure	—*	—*	–*	0
Stroke volume	–*	–*	–*	—
Contractility	—*	—*	—*	–*
Systemic vascular resistance	—	—	0	0
Pulmonary vascular resistance	0	0	0	+
Coronary blood flow	+	+	0	0
Cerebral blood flow	+	+	++	0
Muscle blood flow	+	+	–	0
Catecholamine levels	0	0	0	0

*, Dose-dependent; +, increase; ++, large increase; 0, no change; –, decrease; —, large decrease.

14. **Discuss the biotransformation of volatile anesthetics and the toxicity of metabolic products.**

    For the most part, oxidative metabolism occurs within the liver via the cytochrome P-450 system and to a lesser extent within the kidneys, lungs, and gastrointestinal tract. Desflurane and isoflurane are metabolized less than 1%, whereas halothane is metabolized more than 20% by the liver. Under hypoxic conditions, halothane may undergo reductive metabolism, producing metabolites that may cause hepatic necrosis. Halothane hepatitis is secondary to an autoimmune hypersensitivity reaction.

    Fluoride is another potentially toxic product of anesthetic metabolism. Fluoride-associated renal dysfunction has been linked to the use of methoxyflurane and greatly contributed to the withdrawal of methoxyflurane from the market. The fluoride produced by sevoflurane has not been implicated in renal dysfunction, perhaps because sevoflurane is not as lipid soluble as methoxyflurane and the time of exposure (fluoride burden) is much less.

    Soda lime can also degrade sevoflurane. One of the metabolic by-products is a vinyl ether known as *Compound A*. Compound A has been shown to be nephrotoxic to rats, but no organ dysfunction in association with clinical use in humans has been noted. Compound A may accumulate during longer cases, low-flow anesthesia, and dry absorbent and with high sevoflurane concentrations. Anesthesia machines left on over the weekend with persistent gas flow desiccate the absorbent and make CO formation a possibility.

15. **Review the effects of CO_2 absorbents on volatile anesthetic by-products.**

    Desflurane, much more than any other volatile anesthetic, has been associated with the production of carbon monoxide (CO). There are a number of key conditions. The volatile compound must contain a difluoromethoxy group (desflurane, enflurane, and isoflurane). This group interacts with the strongly alkaline and desiccated CO_2 absorbent. A base-catalyzed proton abstraction forms a carbanion that can either be reprotonated by water to regenerate the original anesthetic or form CO when the absorbent is dry. Because of the greater opportunity to dry the absorbent out, the incidence of CO exposure is highest in the first case of the day, when machines have not been used for some time, or when fresh gas flow has been left on for a protracted period of time. The prior conditions are often found to be most significant on the first day of the week (e.g., mostly Mondays) if the machine has not been used during the weekend. Absorbents should be changed routinely despite lack of apparent color change, and moisture levels should be monitored.

    Potassium hydroxide (KOH)–containing absorbents are the stronger alkalis and result in greater CO production. From greatest to least, KOH-containing absorbents are Baralyme (4.6%) > classic soda lime (2.6%) > new soda lime (0%) > calcium hydroxide lime (Amsorb) (0%). Choice of volatile anesthetic also determines the amount of CO produced, and at equiMAC concentrations desflurane > enflurane > isoflurane. Sevoflurane, once thought to be innocent, has recently been implicated as well when exposed to dry absorbent (especially KOH-containing). This leads to CO production and a rapid increase in absorbent temperature, generation of formic acid leading to severe airway irritation, and a lower effective circuit concentration of delivered sevoflurane compared with that of vaporizer dial concentration.

16. **Which anesthetic agent has been shown to be teratogenic in animals? Is nitrous oxide toxic to humans?**

    Nitrous oxide administered to pregnant rats in concentrations greater than 50% for over 24 hours has been shown to increase skeletal abnormalities. The mechanism is probably related to the inhibition of methionine synthetase; the mechanism may also be secondary to the physiologic effects of impaired uterine blood flow by nitrous oxide. Although, due to ethical reasons, this is not possible to study in humans, it may be prudent to limit the use of nitrous oxide in pregnant women.

    Several surveys have attempted to quantify the relative risk of operating room personal exposure to nonscavenged anesthetic gases. Pregnant women were reported to have a 30% increased risk of spontaneous abortion and a 20% increased risk for congenital abnormalities. However, responder bias and failure to control for other exposure hazards may account for some of these findings.

    Nitrous oxide can be toxic to humans because of its ability to prevent cobalamin (vitamin B_{12}) to act as a coenzyme for methionine synthase. Toxic effects (e.g., myelinopathies, spinal cord degeneration, altered mental status, paresthesias, ataxia, weakness, spasticity) generally are seen in persons abusing nitrous oxide for long periods of time. Other patients may be disposed to toxicity during routine nitrous-based anesthetics, including pernicious anemia and vitamin B_{12} deficiency. Patients having surgery where 70% nitrous oxide was used for over 2 hours have been shown to have more postoperative complications, including atelectasis, fever, pneumonia, and wound infections. It seems prudent then to limit the use of nitrous oxide in longer procedures.

SUGGESTED READINGS

Campagna JA, Miller KE, Forman SA: Mechanisms of actions of inhaled anesthetics, N Engl J Med 348:2110–2124, 2003.

Coppens MJ, Versichelen LFM, Rolly G, et al: The mechanism of carbon monoxide production by inhalational agents, Anaesthesia 61:462–468, 2006.

Eger EI II, Saidman LJ: Hazards of nitrous oxide anesthesia in bowel obstruction and pneumothorax, Anesthesiology 26:61–68, 1965.

McKay RE: Inhaled anesthetics. In Miller RD, Pardo MC, editors: Basics of anesthesia, ed 6, Philadelphia, 2011, Elsevier Saunders, pp 78–98.

Myles PS, Leslie K, Chan MTV, et al: Avoidance of nitrous oxide for patients undergoing major surgery, Anesthesiology 107:221–231, 2007.

Sanders RD, Weimann J, Maze M: Biologic effects of nitrous oxide, Anesthesiology 109:707–722, 2008.

CHAPTER 11

OPIOIDS

Christopher L. Ciarallo, MD

1. **What is an opiate? An opioid? A narcotic?**

   Opiates are analgesic and sedative drugs that contain opium or an opium derivative from the poppy plant (*Papaver somniferum*). Opiates include opium, morphine, and codeine. An opioid is any substance with morphine-like activity that acts as an agonist or antagonist at an opioid receptor. Opioids may be exogenous or endogenous (such as the endorphins) and may be natural, derived, or completely synthetic. The term *narcotic* is not specific for opioids and refers to any substance with addictive potential that induces analgesia and sedation.

2. **What are endogenous opioids?**

   The endorphins, enkephalins, and dynorphins are the three classes of endogenous peptides that are derived from prohormones and are functionally active at opioid receptors. Although their physiologic roles are not completely understood, they appear to modulate nociception. Endorphins are not limited to the central nervous system (CNS) and may even be expressed by activated leukocytes. A fourth class, the nociceptins, is currently being investigated.

3. **Differentiate opioid tolerance, dependence, and abuse.**

   Tolerance is a diminution in the physiologic effects of a substance resulting from repeated administration. *Dependence* may be physical or psychological and refers to the repeated use of a substance to avoid withdrawal symptoms. Tolerance may be necessary to establish the diagnosis of dependence. *Abuse* refers to the habitual use of a substance despite adverse consequences, including social and interpersonal problems.

4. **Name the opioids commonly used in the perioperative setting, their trade names, equivalent morphine doses, half-lives, and chemical classes.**

   See Table 11-1.

5. **Describe the various opioid receptors and their effects.**

   See Table 11-2.

6. **What is an opioid agonist-antagonist?**

   Drugs such as pentazocine, butorphanol, buprenorphine, and nalbuphine were initially thought to be μ-receptor antagonists and κ-receptor agonists. However, they are now classified as μ- and κ-receptor partial agonists. These drugs provide analgesia, but with less euphoria and risk of dependence as compared with pure agonists. Agonist-antagonists, in general, cause less respiratory depression than do agonists and may reverse the respiratory depression and pruritus caused by pure agonists.

7. **Explain the mechanism of action, duration, and side effects of the opioid antagonist naloxone.**

   Naloxone is a μ-, κ-, and δ-receptor antagonist that will reverse the effects of agonist drugs. The peak effect occurs within 1 to 2 minutes of intravenous administration. The duration of action is between 30 and 60 minutes and may be shorter than the duration of the offending opioid agonist. Incremental doses of 0.5–1 mcg/kg should initially be used to reverse respiratory depression in order to minimize side effects, such as acute opioid withdrawal, severe hypertension, ventricular dysrhythmias, or pulmonary edema.

8. **Describe the various routes of administration of opioids.**

   Typical routes of administration include oral, intravenous, intramuscular, epidural, subarachnoid, and rectal. Intranasal, nebulized, and subcutaneous may also be utilized. Lipophilic opioids (such as fentanyl) are also available in transdermal, transmucosal, and sublingual formulations.

Table 11-1. Comparison of Commonly Used Opioids

GENERIC NAME	TRADE NAME	EQUIPOTENT IV/IM (MG)	EQUIPOTENT PO (MG)	PLASMA HALF-LIFE (HR)	CHEMICAL CLASS
Morphine	Roxanol	10	30	2	Phenanthrene
Morphine CR	MS-Contin	—	30	15	Phenanthrene
Diacetylmorphine	Heroin	5	45–60	0.5	Phenanthrene
Alfentanil	Alfenta	1	—	1.5	Phenylpiperidine
Fentanyl	Sublimaze	0.1	—	3–4	Phenylpiperidine
Sufentanil	Sufenta	0.01–0.02	—	2.5–4	Phenylpiperidine
Remifentanil	Ultiva	0.04	—	9 min	Phenylpiperidine
Hydromorphone	Dilaudid	1.3–2	7.5	2–3	Phenanthrene
Oxymorphone	Opana	1	10	7–9	Phenanthrene
Meperidine	Demerol	75	300	3–4	Phenylpiperidine
Methadone (Acute) (Chronic)	Dolophine	10 2–4	20 2–4	15–40	Diphenylheptane
Codeine	Tylenol #3*	130 IM	200	2–4	Phenanthrene
Hydrocodone	Vicodin, Lortab*	—	30	4	Phenanthrene
Oxycodone	Percocet*	—	20	4–5	Phenanthrene
Oxycodone Sr	OxyContin	—	20	5–6.5	Phenanthrene
Tramadol	Ultram	100	120–150	5–7	Cyclohexanol

*Opioid compounded with acetaminophen.
CR, Controlled release; SR, sustained release.

Table 11-2. Opioid Receptor Subtypes

OPIOID RECEPTOR SUBTYPE	AGONISTS	AGONIST RESPONSE
Mu-1 (μ-1)	Enkephalin Beta-endorphin Phenanthrenes Phenylpiperidines Methadone	Supraspinal analgesia Euphoria Miosis Urinary retention
Mu-2 (μ-2)	Enkephalin Beta-endorphin Phenanthrenes Phenylpiperidines Methadone	Spinal analgesia Respiratory depression Bradycardia Constipation Dependence
Kappa (κ)	Dynorphin Butorphanol Levorphanol Nalbuphine Oxycodone	Spinal analgesia (Kappa-1) Supraspinal analgesia (Kappa-2) Dysphoria Sedation
Delta (δ)	Enkephalin Deltorphin Sufentanil	Spinal analgesia (Delta-1) Supraspinal analgesia (Delta-2) Respiratory depression Urinary retention Dependence
Nociceptin/orphanin FQ (N/OFQ)	Nociceptin/OFQ	Spinal analgesia Supraspinal hyperalgesia

Modified from Stoelting RK, Miller RD: Basics of anesthesia, ed 4, New York, 2000, Churchill Livingstone, p 71; Al-Hashimi M, Scott WM, Thompson JP, et al: Opioids and immune modulation: more questions than answers. Br J Anaesth 111:80–88, 2013.

9. **What are the typical side effects of opioids?**
   Opioid side effects include respiratory depression, nausea and vomiting, pruritus, cough suppression, urinary retention, and biliary tract spasm. Some opioids may induce histamine release and cause hives, bronchospasm, and hypotension. Intravenous opioids may cause abdominal and chest wall rigidity. Most opioids, with the notable exception of meperidine, produce a dose-dependent bradycardia.

10. **Which opioids are associated with histamine release?**
    Parenteral doses of meperidine, morphine, and codeine have been associated with histamine release and resultant cutaneous reactions and hypotension. The incidence and severity, at least with morphine, appear to be dose dependent.

11. **Describe the mechanism of opioid-induced nausea.**
    Opioids bind directly to opioid receptors in the chemotactic trigger zone (CTZ) in the area postrema of the medulla and stimulate the vomiting center. They exert a secondary effect by sensitizing the vestibular system. The incidence of nausea and vomiting is similar for all opioids and appears irrespective of the route of administration.

12. **List the non-opioid receptors that contribute to opioid-induced nausea and vomiting.**
    Pharmacologic agents such as glucocorticoids, benzodiazepines, and propofol are also antiemetic, but their mechanisms of action and functional receptors have not been identified (see Table 11-3).

Table 11-3. Antiemetic Drugs and Their Chemical Receptors

CHEMICAL RECEPTOR	ABBREVIATION	PHARMACOLOGIC ANTAGONIST
Dopamine	D_2	Haloperidol Droperidol Prochlorperazine Olanzapine Metoclopramide*
Histamine	H_1	Promethazine Diphenhydramine
Serotonin	$5\text{-}HT_3$	Ondansetron Dolasetron Palonosetron Granisetron
Acetylcholine	ACh	Scopolamine
Tachykinin	NK-1	Aprepitant
Cannabinoid	CB_1	Dronabinol

*Ineffective for prevention of postoperative nausea and vomiting at 10-mg dose.

13. **What are the considerations when administering systemic opioids to a breastfeeding mother?**
    All opioids are transferred to various degrees into human breast milk. Surprisingly, very few reports of opioid-induced toxicity in breastfeeding infants exist. Clinical toxicology recommendations include the following:
    - Avoid opioids or doses that induce maternal sedation, as maternal CNS depression has a high correlation with infant CNS depression.
    - Infants less than 2 months old represent the majority of case reports, and newborns in the first few weeks of life appear to be at highest risk for opioid-induced toxicity.
    - Codeine appears to have an increased rate of complications and should be avoided for long-term therapy.
    - Oxycodone is highly transferred and is associated with a 20% incidence of infant CNS depression.
    - Methadone is poorly transferred and appears safe to use in breastfeeding mothers.
    - Breast milk should be discarded (i.e., "pump and dump") in circumstances involving maternal CNS depression or vulnerable infants (e.g., preterm or afflicted by an underlying medical condition).

14. **What is methylnaltrexone, and what potential role does it have in opioid therapy?**
    Methylnaltrexone is a peripheral opioid receptor antagonist derived from naltrexone. It is a charged, polar molecule that is unable to cross the blood-brain barrier. Methylnaltrexone is approved in the United States for palliative care use in the treatment of opioid-induced constipation. A related drug, alvimopan, has been approved in an oral form for the treatment of postoperative ileus after bowel resection.

15. **Describe the cardiovascular effects of opioids.**
    As a group, opioids have minimal effects on the cardiovascular system. With the exception of meperidine, they cause a dose-dependent bradycardia through vagal nucleus stimulation. Other than the myocardial depressant activity of meperidine, opioids have minimal inotropic effect on the myocardium. Some opioids may induce histamine release and significantly reduce systemic vascular resistance (SVR), but most effect only a moderate reduction of SVR, even at anesthetic doses.

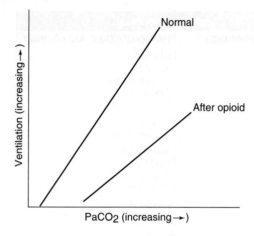

Figure 11-1. Ventilatory response to $PaCO_2$ in the presence of opioids.

Table 11-4. Commonly Used Intravenous Opioids

OPIOID	ONSET (MIN)	PEAK EFFECT (MIN)	DURATION (HR)
Fentanyl	1–3	3–5	0.5–1
Morphine	5–15	20–30	2–4
Hydromorphone	5–10	15–30	1–3

16. Describe the typical respiratory pattern and ventilatory response to carbon dioxide in the presence of opioids.
   Opioids reduce alveolar ventilation in a dose-dependent manner. They slow the respiratory rate and may cause periodic breathing or apnea. Graphically, opioids shift the alveolar ventilatory response to carbon dioxide curve down and to the right. Accordingly, for a given arterial carbon dioxide level, the alveolar ventilation will be reduced in the presence of opioids. Furthermore, an increase in arterial carbon dioxide will not stimulate an appropriate increase in ventilation. Opioids also impair the hypoxic ventilatory drive (Figure 11-1).

17. Describe the analgesic onset, peak effect, and duration of intravenous fentanyl, morphine, and hydromorphone.
   See Table 11-4.

18. Explain how fentanyl can have a shorter duration of action but a longer elimination half-life than morphine.
   Elimination half-lives correspond with duration of action in a single-compartment pharmacokinetic model. Lipophilic opioids, such as fentanyl, are better represented by a multi-compartment model, as redistribution plays a much larger role than elimination in determining their duration of action.

19. Explain the concept of context-sensitive half-time and its relevance to opioids.
   Context-sensitive half-time is the time required for a 50% reduction in the plasma concentration of a drug after termination of a constant infusion. This time is determined by both elimination and redistribution, and it varies considerably as a function of infusion duration for commonly used opioids (Figure 11-2).

20. Explain why morphine may cause prolonged ventilatory depression in patients with renal failure.
   Five to ten percent of a morphine dose will be excreted unchanged in the urine. The remainder is primarily conjugated in the liver as morphine-3-glucuronide (50%–75%) and

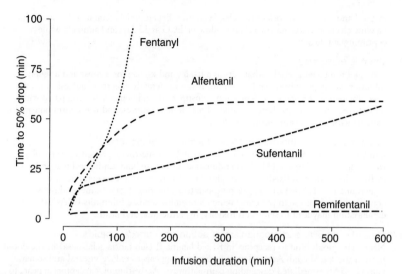

Figure 11-2. Context-sensitive half-times of commonly used opioids as a function of infusion duration. (*Adapted from Egan TD, Lemmens HJM, Fiset P, et al: The pharmacokinetics of the new short-acting opioid remifentanil (GI87084B) in healthy adult male volunteers.* Anesthesiology 79:881, 1993.)

morphine-6-glucuronide (10%), of which 90% is renally excreted. Morphine-3-glucuronide is inactive, but morphine-6-glucuronide is approximately 100 times more potent than morphine as a μ-receptor agonist.

21. **Which opioids may be associated with seizure activity in patients with renal failure?**
Hydromorphone and meperidine. Rarely, the metabolites hydromorphone-3-glucuronide and normeperidine can accumulate in renal failure and promote myoclonus and seizures.

22. **What is remifentanil and how does it differ from other opioids?**
Remifentanil is an ultra-short-acting opioid with duration of 5 to 10 minutes and a context-sensitive half-time of 3 minutes. It contains an ester moiety and is metabolized by nonspecific plasma esterases. Although remifentanil is most commonly administered as a continuous infusion, it has been used as an intravenous bolus to facilitate intubation, but it may induce bradycardia, chest-wall rigidity, and involuntary glottic closure. Remifentanil has been shown to induce hyperalgesia and acute opioid tolerance, and its use should be questioned in patients with chronic pain syndromes.

23. **Describe the metabolism of codeine.**
Codeine is metabolized by cytochrome P-450 2D6 (CYP2D6) and undergoes demethylation to morphine. Genetic polymorphisms in the CYP2D6 gene lead to patient stratification into poor metabolizers, extensive metabolizers, and ultra-fast metabolizers. Poor metabolizers may obtain marginal analgesia from codeine, whereas ultra-fast metabolizers may have up to 50% higher plasma concentrations of morphine and morphine-6-glucuronide than the extensive metabolizers. Ultra-fast metabolizers may be at significant risk of opioid intoxication and apnea with typical perioperative doses of codeine.

24. **What are some particular concerns with methadone dosing?**
As methadone has a particularly long and variable half-life, repeated dosing may lead to excessive plasma levels, particularly on days 2 through 4 after initiating therapy. Methadone acts both as an agonist at μ-opioid receptors and as an antagonist at the N-methyl-D-aspartate (NMDA) receptor. NMDA-receptor antagonism may potentiate the μ-receptor effects and prevent opioid tolerance. Finally, methadone may prolong the electrocardiographic QT

interval and increase the risk of torsades de pointes. Expert panel recommendations include a baseline electrocardiogram (ECG) and follow-up ECG at 30 days and annually while continuing methadone.

25. **What is tramadol?**
    Tramadol is a codeine analog that acts as a μ-, δ-, and κ-receptor agonist and a reuptake inhibitor of norepinephrine and serotonin. It is a moderately effective analgesic with a lower incidence of respiratory depression, constipation, and dependence compared with other μ-receptor agonists. Rarely, tramadol may induce seizures, and it is contraindicated in patients with a preexisting seizure disorder.

26. **What are some of the unique characteristics of meperidine?**
    Unlike other opioids, meperidine has some weak local anesthetic properties, particularly when administered neuraxially. Meperidine does not cause bradycardia and may induce tachycardia, perhaps related to its atropine-like structure. As a κ-receptor agonist, meperidine may be used to suppress postoperative shivering. Notably, meperidine is contraindicated for use in patients taking monoamine oxidase inhibitors (MAOIs), as the combination may lead to serotonin toxicity, hyperthermia, and death.

27. **Describe the site and mechanism of action of neuraxial opioids.**
    Neuraxial opioids bind to receptors in Rexed lamina II (substantia gelatinosa) in the dorsal horn of the spinal cord. Activation of μ-receptors appears to reduce visceral and somatic pain via GABA-mediated descending pain pathways. Activation of κ receptors appears to reduce visceral pain via inhibition of substance P. The effect of δ receptors is not entirely elucidated but appears minimal in some animal models.

28. **Are opioid receptors exclusively in the CNS?**
    No. Peripheral opioid receptors exist on primary afferent neurons, but they are functionally inactive under normal conditions. Tissue inflammation may induce opioid receptor upregulation and signaling efficiency.

29. **Discuss the effect of lipid solubility on neuraxial opioid action.**
    Lipophilic opioids (such as fentanyl) diffuse across spinal membranes more rapidly than do hydrophilic opioids. As a result, lipophilic opioids have a more rapid onset of analgesia. However, they also diffuse across vascular membranes more readily, typically resulting in increased serum concentrations and a shorter duration of action. Hydrophilic opioids (such as morphine and hydromorphone) achieve greater cephalocaudal spread when administered into the epidural or subarachnoid space. They attain broader analgesic coverage than do lipophilic opioids but may result in delayed respiratory depression following cephalad spread to the brainstem.

30. **Discuss the incidence and evolution of respiratory depression following neuraxial morphine administration.**
    The incidence of respiratory depression ranges from 0.01% to 7% following intrathecal morphine and from 0.08% to 3% following epidural morphine. The respiratory depression may be biphasic with an early presentation at 30 to 90 minutes and a delayed presentation between 6 and 18 hours after neuraxial administration. The delayed respiratory depression is likely due to cephalad spread within the CSF and direct brainstem penetration (specifically, inhibition of the neurokinin-1 receptors in the medullary pre-Bötzinger complex). As a result, the American Society of Anesthesiologists recommends monitoring respiratory rate, depth of respiration, oxygenation, and level of consciousness every hour for 12 hours and then every 2 hours for the subsequent 12 hours following a single injection of neuraxial morphine.

31. **Describe the advantages of combining local anesthetics and opioids in neuraxial analgesia.**
    Despite their analgesic benefits, epidural local anesthetics have troublesome side effects, such as motor blockade and systemic hypotension. Epidural opioids are burdened with causing pruritus and nausea. Combined, opioids and local anesthetics function in a synergistic manner to provide analgesia with attenuated side effects.

32. **What is DepoDur® and how is it different from other neuraxial opioids?**
DepoDur® is an opioid agonist that consists of lipid-based particles with internal morphine vesicles (Depofoam®). It is approved only for single-dose epidural use and may provide up to 48 hours of analgesia. Except for the epidural test dose, DepoDur® may not be coadministered with local anesthetics because of the risk of accelerated morphine release. No other medication may be dosed within the epidural space for 48 hours after DepoDur® administration.

33. **Describe the controversial influence of opioids in cancer recurrence or metastasis.**
Opioids inhibit cell-mediated and humoral immunity, and the effects are agent specific. For example, morphine inhibits the toll-like receptor (TLR) on macrophages, while fentanyl depresses natural killer (NK) cell activity. Codeine, methadone, morphine, remifentanil, and fentanyl are stronger modulators than hydromorphone, oxycodone, hydrocodone, buprenorphine, or tramadol. In cell lines and animal models, this immunomodulation results in increased tumor growth or metastasis and appears to be μ-opioid receptor mediated. Opioids also induce angiogenesis and stimulate vascular endothelial growth factor (VEGF) receptors. However, the in vitro results remain controversial. Ongoing, prospective outcome studies in humans are comparing opioid to regional analgesia in the surgical management of breast, prostate, lung, and colorectal tumors.

KEY POINTS: OPIOIDS

1. Common opioid side effects include nausea, pruritus, bradycardia, urinary retention, and respiratory depression.
2. Morphine and meperidine should be used with caution in patients with renal failure because of the risk of prolonged ventilatory depression and seizures, respectively.
3. Neuraxial opioids and local anesthetics act synergistically to provide analgesia with reduced side effects.
4. Naloxone should be titrated in incremental doses for opioid-induced respiratory depression and may require repeated dosing for reversal of long-acting opioid agonists.
5. Opioids may be used with caution in breastfeeding mothers if maternal sedation is minimized and the exposure to infants less than 2 months old is limited.
6. Opioid equianalgesic conversions are approximations, and they do not account for incomplete opioid cross-tolerance.
7. Opioids inhibit cell-mediated and humoral immunity and may be implicated in cancer recurrence or metastasis.

SUGGESTED READINGS

American Society of Anesthesiologists Task Force on Neuraxial Opioids: Practice guidelines for the prevention, detection and management of respiratory depression associated with neuraxial opioid administration, Anesthesiology 110:218–230, 2009.
Coda BA: Opioids. In Barash PG, Cullen BF, Stoelting RK, editors: Clinical anesthesia, ed 5, Philadelphia, 2006, Lippincott Williams & Wilkins.
Crawford MW, Hickey C, Zaarour C, et al: Development of acute opioid tolerance during infusion of remifentanil for pediatric scoliosis surgery, Anesth Analg 102:1662–1667, 2006.
Fukuda K: Intravenous opioid anesthetics. In Miller RD, editor: Anesthesia, ed 6, Philadelphia, 2005, Elsevier.
Gillman PK: Monoamine oxidase inhibitors, opioid analgesics and serotonin toxicity, Br J Anaesth 95:434–441, 2005.
Heaney A, Buggy DJ: Can anaesthetic and analgesic techniques affect cancer recurrence or metastasis? Br J Anaesth 109:i17–i28, 2012.
Hendrickson RG, McKeown NJ: Is maternal opioid use hazardous to breast-fed infants? Clin Toxicol 50:1–14, 2012.
Kirchheiner J, Schmidt H, Tzvetkov M, et al: Pharmacokinetics of codeine and its metabolite morphine in ultra-rapid metabolizers due to CYP2D6 duplication, Pharmacogenomics J 7:257–265, 2007.
Krantz MJ, Martin J, Stimmel B, et al: QTc interval screening in methadone treatment: the CSAT consensus guideline, Ann Intern Med 2008. [Epub ahead of print].

Moss J, Rosow CE: Development of peripheral opioid antagonists: new insights into opioid effects, Mayo Clin Proc 83:1116–1130, 2008.

Reisine T, Pasternak G: Opioid analgesics and antagonists. In Hardman JG, Limbird LE, editors: Goodman and Gilman's The pharmacological basis of therapeutics, ed 9, New York, 1996, McGraw-Hill.

Sachs HC, Committee on Drugs: The transfer of drugs and therapeutics into human breast milk: an update on selected topics, Pediatrics 132:e796–e809, 2013.

Smith HS: Peripherally-acting opioids, Pain Physician 11:S121–S132, 2008.

Viscusi ER, Martin G, Hartrick CT, et al: Forty-eight hours of postoperative pain relief after total hip arthroplasty with a novel, extended-release epidural morphine formulation, Anesthesiology 103:1014–1022, 2005.

INTRAVENOUS ANESTHETICS AND BENZODIAZEPINES

Olivia B. Romano, MD

CHAPTER 12

1. **What qualities would the ideal intravenous induction agent possess?**

   The ideal agent would be lipophilic, have a rapid and smooth onset and recovery, producing amnesia, analgesia, and hypnosis with minimal hemodynamic or respiratory effects. It would be water soluble, nonpainful, and nontoxic to veins and tissues with few enduring side effects, few interactions with other medications, and rarely occurring hypersensitivity reactions.

2. **List the commonly used induction agents and their properties. Compare their cardiovascular effects.**

   - Etomidate is an imidazole derivative with selective γ-aminobutyric acid (GABA)$_A$ receptor modulation noted for its hemodynamic stability. Cardiac output (CO) and contractility are preserved with only a mild decrease in mean arterial pressure (MAP). Side effects include pain on injection, nausea and vomiting, myoclonus, seizures, and adrenal suppression.

   - Propofol is a GABA$_A$ receptor agonist that results in a more profound decrease in MAP compared with thiopental. This is due to a combination of arterial and venous vasodilation, baroreceptor inhibition (no reflex tachycardia), and a mild decrease in myocardial contractility. It is administered by bolus dosing or infusion.

   - Ketamine inhibits N-methyl-D-aspartate (NMDA) receptors, causing dissociative anesthesia with profound analgesia. It is purported to be a direct myocardial depressant, but its sympathomimetic effects usually result in an overall increased CO, MAP, and heart rate (HR).

   - Midazolam is the principal benzodiazepine used perioperatively. Benzodiazepines provide anxiolysis, sedation, amnesia, and in high doses unconsciousness through GABA$_A$ receptor activation and potentiation. Midazolam has minimal myocardial depression. There is no effect on MAP or CO; HR may increase slightly.

   - Opioids are morphine-like drugs used for analgesia and adjunctively in induction. High doses of most opioids have a vagolytic effect, producing bradycardia. The exception is meperidine, which has sympathomimetic effects that produce tachycardia. A decreased MAP may be noted secondary to bradycardia, vasodilation, blockade of sympathetic response, and histamine release (especially evident with morphine and meperidine). In general, meperidine has fallen into disfavor in the anesthesia environment. An exception, meperidine 25 mg, is used regularly to treat postoperative shivering not caused by hypothermia.

     Larger doses of multiple classes of induction agents and sedation medications may result in undesirable hemodynamic effects. Hence, a preferred technique requires multiple medications used in smaller doses. This is termed *balanced anesthesia* and takes advantage of the synergism of these agents while minimizing the potential adverse effects of each. Muscle relaxants ordinarily are also portions of balanced anesthesia. The effects of intravenous anesthetics terminate through redistribution as opposed to metabolism (Table 12-1 and Table 12-2).

3. **Describe the properties of propofol.**

   Diisopropylphenol, or propofol, has become a highly preferred intravenous anesthetic. It may be administered by bolus or intravenous dosing. Hemodynamic effects have been described. Lipid soluble agents such as soybean oil, lecithin, and glycerol are used in

Table 12-1. Dosing Guidelines for Anesthetic Induction and Sedation*

AGENT	CLASS	DOSE FOR ANESTHETIC INDUCTION	DOSE FOR SEDATION
Sodium thiopental	Barbiturate	3–6 mg/kg IV	0.5–1.5 mg/kg IV
Ketamine	Phencyclidine derivative	1–2 mg/kg IV 2–4 mg/kg IM	0.2–0.5 mg/kg IV
Etomidate	Imidazole derivative	0.2–0.5 mg/kg IV	Inappropriate use
Propofol	Substituted phenol	1–2.5 mg/kg IV bolus 50–200 mcg/kg/min infusion	25–100 mcg/kg/min IV
Midazolam	Benzodiazepine	0.1–0.4 mg/kg IV	0.01–0.1 mg/kg IV

*Doses of medications should be adjusted for intravascular volume status, comorbidities, and other medications. IM, Intramuscular; IV, intravenous.

Table 12-2. Cardiovascular Effects of Induction Agents

AGENT	MAP	HR	SVR	CO	CONTRACTILITY	VENODILATION
Ketamine	++	++	+	+	+ or −*	0
Midazolam	0 to −	0 to +	0 to −	0 to −	0 to −	+
Propofol	−	+	−	0	−	+
Etomidate	0	0	0	0	0	0

*The effect of ketamine depends on patient's catecholamine levels.
CO, Cardiac output; HR, heart rate; MAP, mean arterial pressure; SVR, systemic vascular resistance; ++, increases significantly; +, increases; 0, no effect; −, decreases.

propofol emulsions. These agents are prone to bacterial infection and require sterile management and administration within a few hours to avoid such infection to the patient.

4. **How do induction agents affect respiratory drive?**
   All intravenous induction agents, with the exception of ketamine, produce dose-dependent respiratory depression manifested by decreased tidal volume, decreased minute ventilation, decreased response to hypoxia, and a rightward shift in the carbon dioxide response curve, culminating in hypoventilation or apnea.

5. **Describe the properties of ketamine.**
   Ketamine is an NMDA receptor antagonist that is chemically related to phencyclidine and causes a dose-dependent dissociative state and unconsciousness. It is a potent analgesic but its amnestic ability is weak. Concurrent administration of a benzodiazepine may decrease the incidence of adverse sensory effects.
      Ketamine causes a centrally mediated increase in sympathetic outflow, resulting in tachycardia, increased CO, and increased MAP. However, ketamine has direct myocardial depressant effects that tend not to be manifest because of overriding sympathetic stimulation. Therefore, in catecholamine-depleted states, the myocardial depressant effects may be unmasked. Ketamine is considered an ideal induction agent in patients with conditions such as shock, significant hypovolemia, and cardiac tamponade.
      Other desirable side effects include bronchodilation and preserved respiratory drive. Undesirable side effects include increased cerebral blood flow and cerebral metabolic rate, increased oral secretions, and potentially unpleasant psychotomimetic reactions.

6. **Discuss concerns over the use of etomidate in the critically ill patient.**
   Etomidate causes adrenal suppression by a dose-dependent inhibition of the enzyme 11-β-hydroxylase in the cortisol synthesis pathway. Clinically significant adrenal suppression

and increased morbidity and mortality have been documented in critically ill patients and those with septic shock after receiving even a single dose of etomidate. However, the stable hemodynamic properties of etomidate make it a desirable induction agent for patients with shock. Hydrocortisone supplementation may mitigate the adrenosuppressive effects of etomidate in these patients, but study results are contradictory.

KEY POINTS: INTRAVENOUS ANESTHETICS AND BENZODIAZEPINES

1. Appropriate dosing of intravenous anesthetics requires consideration of intravascular volume status, comorbidities, age, and chronic medications.
2. Benzodiazepines and opioids have synergistic effects with intravenous induction agents, requiring adjustment in dosing.
3. Ketamine is the best induction agent for hypovolemic trauma patients as long as there is no risk for increased intracranial pressure. It is also a good agent for patients with active bronchospastic disease.
4. Propofol is the least likely of all induction agents to result in nausea and vomiting.
5. Termination of the effects of intravenous anesthetics is by redistribution, not biotransformation and breakdown.

---

7. **Describe propofol infusion syndrome (PRIS).**
First described in 1990, PRIS occurs in critically ill patients receiving high-dose propofol infusions over long periods of time (higher than 4 mg/kg/hr for longer than 48 hours). Incidence is 1.1% in the adult intensive care and occurs at a median of 3 days. Risk factors include severe head injuries, sepsis, high exogenous or endogenous catecholamine and glucocorticoid levels, low carbohydrate to high lipid intake, and inborn errors of fatty acid oxidation. Critically ill children are at the highest risk. Common presenting features include new-onset metabolic acidosis and cardiac dysfunction. Other manifestations include rhabdomyolysis, renal failure, hypertriglyceridemia, and possible death. PRIS is thought to be secondary to impairment of mitochondrial oxidative phosphorylation and free fatty acid utilization, leading to lactic acidosis and myocyte necrosis. Currently propofol is not approved for use in the pediatric intensive care unit for sedation and should not be used in adults without regular creatine kinase, lactate, and triglyceride monitoring.

8. **What are some contraindications to the use of propofol?**
Because it is water insoluble, propofol is constituted with soy oil and egg lecithin; thus patients with allergies to eggs and soy products should not receive this medication. Propofol crosses the placenta and may be associated with neonatal depression. It has cardiodepressant effects; thus patients with cardiomyopathies and hypovolemia may not be ideal candidates. Finally consider the advisability of its use in patients with disorders of lipid metabolism such as primary hyperlipoproteinemia, diabetic hyperlipidemia, and pancreatitis.

9. **What would be an appropriate induction agent for a 47-year-old healthy male with a parietal lobe tumor scheduled for craniotomy and tumor excision?**
Propofol is an agent that preserves cerebral perfusion pressure without increasing cerebral blood flow. Ketamine should be avoided because it increases cerebral blood flow, cerebral metabolic rate ($CRMO_2$), and intracranial pressure.

10. **Describe the mechanism of action of benzodiazepines.**
GABA is the primary inhibitory neurotransmitter of the central nervous system, and its receptor is found in postsynaptic nerve endings. The GABA receptor is composed of two α subunits and two β subunits. The α subunits are the binding sites for benzodiazepines, the β subunits are the binding sites for GABA, and a chloride ion channel is located in the center.
    Benzodiazepines produce their effects by enhancing the binding of GABA to its receptor. GABA activates the chloride ion channel, which hyperpolarizes the neuron and thereby inhibits it.
    Benzodiazepines are metabolized in the liver by microsomal oxidation and glucuronidation and should be used with caution in the elderly. The potency, onset, and

duration of action of benzodiazepines depend on their lipid solubility. Onset of action is achieved by rapid distribution to the vessel-rich brain. Termination of effect occurs as the drug is redistributed to other parts of the body.

11. **What benzodiazepines are commonly administered intravenously?**
    - **Midazolam** is lipid soluble and therefore has the most rapid onset and shortest duration of action. Unlike other benzodiazepines, midazolam is both lipid soluble and water soluble and therefore can be manufactured without the pain-inducing solvent propylene glycol. It has a single metabolite with minimal activity. It is by far the most common benzodiazepine used perioperatively.
    - **Diazepam** is slightly slower in onset. It has a long elimination half-life and two active metabolites that may prolong sedation.
    - **Lorazepam** is the least lipid soluble and therefore is the slowest in onset and longest in duration of action. It also has a long elimination half-life.

12. **How should oversedation induced by benzodiazepines be managed?**
    As a first principle, always provide supportive care. Open the airway and mask-ventilate if needed. Assess the adequacy of the circulation. Second, administer the benzodiazepine antagonist flumazenil. Flumazenil works by competitive inhibition, reversing sedation and respiratory depression in a dose-dependent fashion. Onset is rapid and peaks within 1 to 3 minutes. It should be titrated to effect by administering doses of 0.2 mg intravenously for a maximum dose of 3 mg. It should be used with caution, if at all, in patients with a history of seizure disorder or a history of benzodiazepine use.

13. **What do you tell the nurses who will monitor this patient about possible side effects of flumazenil?**
    The elimination half-life of midazolam is 2 to 3 hours, whereas the elimination half-life of flumazenil is 1 hour, so resedation is a risk. Flumazenil may be repeated or administered as an infusion at 0.5–1 mg/hr.

SUGGESTED READINGS

Annane D: ICU physicians should abandon the use of etomidate! Intensive Care Med 31:325–326, 2005.
Bloomfield R, Noble DW: Etomidate and fatal outcome—even a single bolus dose may be detrimental for some patients, Br J Anaesth 97:116–117, 2006.
Wong JM: Propofol infusion syndrome, Am J Ther 17:487–491, 2010.

MUSCLE RELAXANTS AND MONITORING OF RELAXANT ACTIVITY

CHAPTER 13

James C. Duke, MD, MBA

1. **Describe the anatomy of the neuromuscular junction.**
   A motor nerve branches near its terminus, losing myelin to branch farther and come into closer contact with the junctional area of the muscle surface. Within the most distal aspect of the motor neuron, vesicles containing the neurotransmitter acetylcholine (ACh) can be found. The terminal neuron and muscle surface are loosely approximated with protein filaments, and this intervening space is known as the junctional cleft. Also contained within the cleft is extracellular fluid and acetylcholinesterase, the enzyme responsible for metabolizing ACh. The postjunctional motor membrane is highly specialized and invaginated, and the shoulders of these folds are rich in ACh receptors (Figure 13-1).

2. **What is the structure of the ACh receptor?**
   The ACh receptor is contained within the motor cell membrane and consists of five glycoprotein subunits: two α and one each of β, δ, and ϵ. These are arranged in a cylindric fashion; the center of the cylinder is an ion channel. ACh binds to the α subunits.

3. **With regard to neuromuscular transmission, list all locations for ACh receptors.**
   ACh receptors are found in several areas:
   - About 5 million ACh receptors per neuromuscular junction (NMJ) are located on the postjunctional motor membrane.
   - Prejunctional receptors are present and influence the release of ACh. The prejunctional and postjunctional receptors have different affinities for ACh.
   - Extrajunctional receptors are located throughout the skeletal muscle in relatively low numbers owing to suppression of their synthesis by normal neural activity. In cases of traumatized skeletal muscle or denervation injuries, these receptors proliferate.

4. **When and where are there unsafe succinylcholine (SCH) receptors? What is the effect of SCH on extrajunctional receptors?**
   Denvervation states upregulate NMJs. Pathologic states where denervation has been noted include upper and lower motor neuron disease, strokes, prolonged use of muscle relaxants or immobilization, burns, and severe infections. Any of these extrajunctional receptors are susceptible to SCH and can produce uncontrolled and severe hyperkalemia, enough to create serious dysrhythmias, enough to begin resuscitation.

5. **Review the steps involved in normal neuromuscular transmission.**
   A nerve action potential is transmitted, and the nerve terminal is depolarized.
   ACh is released from storage vesicles at the nerve terminal. Enough ACh is released to bind 500,000 receptors.
   ACh molecules bind to the α subunits of the ACh receptor on the postjunctional membrane, generating a conformational change and opening receptor channels. Receptors do not open unless both α receptors are occupied by ACh (a basis for the competitive antagonism of nondepolarizing relaxants).
   Sodium and calcium flow through the open receptor channel generating an end-plate potential.
   When between 5% and 20% of the receptor channels are open and a threshold potential is reached, a muscle action potential (MAP) is generated.

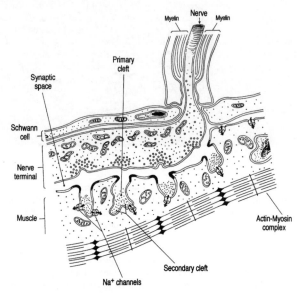

Figure 13-1. The neuromuscular junction. *(From Kandel ER, Schwartz JH, Jessel TM, editors:* Principles of neural science, *ed 3, New York, 1991, Elsevier, p 136.)*

Propagation of the MAP along the muscle membrane leads to muscle contraction. The rapid hydrolysis of ACh by acetylcholinesterase (true cholinesterase) within the synaptic cleft return the NMJ to a nondepolarized, resting state, and the ACh receptors are closed.

6. **What are the benefits and risks of using muscle relaxants?**
By interfering with normal neuromuscular transmission, these drugs paralyze skeletal muscle and can be used to facilitate endotracheal intubation, assist with mechanical ventilation, and optimize surgical conditions. Only occasionally are they used to reduce the metabolic demands of breathing and facilitate the treatment of raised intracranial pressure (ICP). Because they paralyze all respiratory muscles, they are dangerous drugs to use in the unintubated patient unless the caregiver is trained in airway management.

7. **How are muscle relaxants classified?**
   - Depolarizing relaxants: SCH is two molecules of ACh bound together, a competitive agonist at the NMJ, and the only depolarizing relaxant available clinically. As such, SCH binds to the α subunits of the ACh receptor. After binding, SCH can open the ion channel and depolarize the end plate. Although SCH, like ACh, binds only briefly to the receptor, it is not hydrolyzed in the synaptic cleft by acetylcholinesterase. In fact, SCH molecules may unbind and rebind receptors repeatedly. SCH must diffuse away and be broken down in the plasma by enzymes called plasma- or pseudocholinesterase, and time for clearance from the body is an accurate measure of its duration of effect.
   - Nondepolarizing relaxants: These drugs are competitive antagonists to ACh at the postsynaptic membrane. They need only bind to one of the two α subunits to prevent opening of the ionic pore. There are numerous noncompetitive agonists.

8. **What are the indications for using SCH?**
SCH provides the most rapid onset and termination of effect of any neuromuscular blocker currently available. Its onset is 60 to 90 seconds, and the duration of effect is only 5 to 10 minutes. When the patient has a full stomach and is at risk for pulmonary aspiration of gastric contents, rapid paralysis and airway control are priorities, and SCH is often the drug

indicated. (Rocuronium, when given in large doses, also has an SCH-like onset of action, although a prolonged duration of effect would contraindicate its use in patients likely to be difficult to ventilate or intubate.) Patients at risk for full stomachs include those with diabetes mellitus, hiatal hernia, obesity, pregnancy, severe pain, bowel obstructions, and trauma.

9. **If SCH works so rapidly and predictably, why not use it all the time?**
   SCH has numerous side effects:
   - SCH stimulates both nicotinic and muscarinic cholinergic receptors. Stimulation of muscarinic receptors within the sinus node results in numerous bradyarrhythmias, including sinus bradycardia, junctional rhythms, ventricular escape, and asystole.
   - SCH is a trigger for malignant hyperthermia.
   - Prolonged exposure of the receptors to SCH results in persistent open receptor channel and ionic fluxes through the ion pore, known as *phase II* or *desensitization blockade.* Normal depolarization/repolarization is not possible until SCH is metabolized.
   - In patients ambulatory soon after surgery, random generalized muscle contractions (fasciculations) have been associated with painful myalgias. Whether pretreating with a subparalyzing dose of a nondepolarizing relaxant before SCH is effective in reducing myalgias continues to be a matter of debate.
   - SCH increases ICP. The etiology is not completely understood, but it is known that a subparalyzing dose of a nondepolarizing relaxant before SCH administration reduces the increase in ICP; thus perhaps fasciculations are the cause of the increase in ICP.
   - In the presence of immature extrajunctional receptors, administration of SCH may result in severe hyperkalemia and malignant ventricular arrhythmias. Extrajunctional receptors are normally suppressed by activity. Any condition that decreases motor-nerve activity results in a proliferation of these receptors. Examples include spinal cord and other denervation injuries, upper and lower motor neuron disease, closed head injuries, burns, neuromuscular diseases, and even prolonged immobility.
   - SCH increases intraocular pressure (IOP). There is a theoretic risk for the use of SCH in patients with open eye injury (i.e., extrusion of extraocular contents). However, the increases in IOP are modest, and from a clinical perspective extrusion of ocular contents has not been observed. Certainly if a nondepolarizing agent is administered instead of SCH and the patient is intubated before optimal intubating conditions, coughing on the endotracheal tube (called *bucking*) increases IOP significantly and puts the patient at risk for extruding ocular contents.

10. **Can SCH be used safely in patients in end-stage renal disease (ESRD)? Define hyperkalemia.**
    Hyperkalemia is defined as K >5.5 mEq/L) Classically, SCH administration creates an increase in serum K by 0.5 to 1.0 mEq/L. The magnitude of SCH-induced hyperkalemia is independent of ESRD. Furthermore, patients with ESRD are accustomed to fluxes in serum K, especially when they periodically receive renal dialysis. Dysrhythmias associated with acute rises in serum K in patients with ESRD are thought to be uncommon, and use of SCH in these patients is safe.

11. **How do mature and immature ACh receptors differ?**
    Mature ACh receptors are also known as *innervated* or *ε-containing* receptors (because of the ε subunit within the ACh receptor. They are tightly clustered at the NMJ and are responsible for normal neuromuscular activation. Immature receptors, also known as *fetal, extrajunctional,* or *γ receptors,* differ from the mature receptors in that they are present during fetal development and suppressed by normal activity, are dispersed across the muscular membrane rather than localized at the NMJ, and have a γ-, not an ε, subunit as part of the receptor. The half-life of mature receptors is about 2 weeks, whereas the half-life of immature receptors is less than 24 hours. The immature receptors depolarize more easily in the presence of ACh or SCH and thus are more prone to release potassium. Also, once depolarized, immature receptors tend to stay open longer. Immature receptors are upregulated in the presence of denervation injuries, burns, and the like. This also exaggerates the potential for hyperkalemia when SCH is administered.

12. **Differentiate between qualitative and quantitative deficiencies in pseudocholinesterase**
Pseudocholinesterase is produced in the liver and circulates in the plasma. Quantitative deficiencies of pseudocholinesterase are observed in liver disease, pregnancy, malignancies, malnutrition, collagen vascular disease, and hypothyroidism; they slightly prolong the duration of blockade with SCH. However, from a practical standpoint, the increase in duration of SCH is probably not clinically important.

There may also be qualitative deficiencies in pseudocholinesterase (i.e., the activity of the enzyme is impaired). These are genetic diseases and, as such, can be present in heterozygotic or homozygotic forms. The most common form is called dibucaine-resistant cholinesterase deficiency and refers to the laboratory test that characterizes it. When added to the serum under study, dibucaine inhibits normal plasma cholinesterase by 80%, whereas the atypical plasma cholinesterase is inhibited by only 20%. Therefore a patient with normal pseudocholinesterase is assigned a dibucaine number of 80. If a patient has a dibucaine number of 40 to 60, that patient is heterozygous for this atypical pseudocholinesterase and will have a moderately prolonged and usually clinically insignificant block with SCH. If a patient has a dibucaine number of 20, he or she is homozygous for atypical plasma cholinesterase and will have an extremely prolonged block with SCH.

13. **Review the properties of nondepolarizing muscle relaxants.**
Nondepolarizing relaxants are competitive antagonists at the NMJ and are classified by their duration of action (short-, intermediate-, and long-acting). The doses, onset, and duration of effect are described in Table 13-1.

14. **Review the metabolism of nondepolarizing neuromuscular blockers.**
- Aminosteroid relaxants (e.g., pancuronium, vecuronium, pipecuronium, and rocuronium) are diacetylated in the liver, and their action may be prolonged in the presence of hepatic dysfunction. Vecuronium and rocuronium also have significant biliary excretion, and their action may be prolonged with extrahepatic biliary obstruction.
- Relaxants with significant renal excretion include tubocurarine, metocurine, doxacurium, pancuronium, and pipecuronium.

Table 13-1. Properties of Nondepolarizing Muscle Relaxants

RELAXANT	ED$_{95}$* (MG/KG)	INTUBATING DOSE (MG/KG)	ONSET AFTER INTUBATING DOSE (MINUTES)	DURATION[†] (MINUTES)
Short-acting				
Mivacurium	0.08	0.2	1–1.5	15–20
Rocuronium	0.3	0.6	2–3	30
Intermediate-acting				
Rocuronium[‡]	0.3	1.2	1	60
Vecuronium	0.05	0.15–0.2	1.5	60
Atracurium	0.23	0.75	1–1.5	45–60
Cisatracurium	0.05	0.2	2	60–90
Long-acting				
Pancuronium	0.07	0.08–0.12	4–5	90
Pipecuronium	0.05	0.07–0.85	3–5	80–90
Doxacurium	0.025	0.05–0.08	3–5	90–120

*Dose expected to reduce single-twitch height by 95%.
[†]Duration measured as return of twitch to 25% of control.
[‡]Rocuronium, when administered in a dose of 1.2 mg/kg, has an onset similar to that of succinylcholine, although the duration is significantly longer.

- Atracurium is unique in that it undergoes spontaneous breakdown at physiologic temperatures and pH (Hofmann elimination) as well as ester hydrolysis, and thus it is ideal for use in patients with compromised hepatic or renal function.
- Mivacurium, like SCH, is metabolized by pseudocholinesterase.

15. Describe common side effects of nondepolarizing neuromuscular blockers
Histamine release is most significant with *d*-tubocurarine but is also noted with mivacurium, atracurium, and doxacurium. The amount of histamine released is frequently dose related. Cisatracurium does not seem to cause significant histamine release. Tachycardia is usually a side effect of pancuronium because of ganglionic stimulation and vagolysis.

16. Review medications that potentiate the actions of muscle relaxants.
- Volatile anesthetics produce central nervous system depression, increased blood flow to muscle (and the delivery of relaxant molecules), and desensitization of the postjunctional membrane.
- Local anesthetics affect the prejunctional, postjunctional, and motor membranes, depressing normal functions at all these sites.
- Calcium channel and β-adrenergic blockers impair ion transport, but the clinical significance at the NMJ is probably not important.
- Antibiotics, and most notably aminoglycosides, appear to have negative prejunctional and postjunctional effects. Penicillin and cephalosporins do not affect relaxant activity.
- Magnesium inhibits the release and the depolarizing effect of ACh and decreases muscle fiber excitability. Lithium also potentiates neuromuscular blockade.
- Long-term use of steroids results in a myopathy and also has some effect on the NMJ, particularly when muscle relaxants have been used for a prolonged period.
- Dantrolene depresses skeletal muscle directly and impairs excitation-contraction.

17. What clinical conditions potentiate the actions of neuromuscular blockers?
Respiratory acidosis, metabolic alkalosis, hypothermia, hypokalemia, hypercalcemia, and hypermagnesemia potentiate blockade. Hepatic or renal dysfunction also increases the duration of action of relaxants.

18. Discuss important characteristics of a nerve stimulator.
A nerve stimulator should be capable of delivering single-twitch stimulation at 0.1 Hz (1 stimulus every 10 seconds), train of four (TOF) at 2 Hz (2 per second), and tetanic stimulation at 50 Hz (50 per second). The black electrode of the stimulator is negatively charged, and the red electrode is positively charged. The black electrode depolarizes the membrane, and the red electrode hyperpolarizes the membrane. Although stimulation is possible wherever the electrodes are placed, maximal twitch height occurs when the negative electrode is placed in closest proximity to the nerve.

19. List the different patterns of stimulation.
- Single stimulus
- TOF stimulation
- Tetanic stimulation
- Posttetanic facilitation and posttetanic count
- Double-burst (DB) stimulation

20. Which is the simplest mode of stimulation?
Single stimulus is the simplest mode of stimulation. It consists of the delivery of single impulses separated by at least 10 seconds. It is of limited clinical use.

21. Which mode is most commonly used to assess degree of blockade? How is it done?
TOF stimulation is the most common modality used to assess degree of blockade. Four stimuli are delivered at a frequency of 2 Hz (2 per second), and the ratio of the amplitude of the fourth to the first response in a train (T4:T1) ratio estimates the degree of block. The four twitches of the TOF disappear in reverse order as the degree of blockade deepens. The fourth twitch of the TOF disappears when 75% to 80% of the receptors are occupied, the third twitch disappears at 85% occupancy, the second twitch disappears at 85% to 90% occupancy, and the first twitch disappears at 90% to 95% occupancy. However, there is

accumulating evidence that visual or tactile evaluation of the TOF response is inadequate for evaluating neuromuscular function because it has been demonstrated repeatedly that, even with experienced practitioners, subjective TOF estimations correlate poorly with true TOF fade. Recently there has been a call for more objective measures of return of motor function such as acceleromyography, strain-gauge monitoring, and electromyography.

KEY POINTS: MUSCLE RELAXANTS

1. Metabolism of relaxants is more important than pharmacologic reversal for termination of relaxant effect.
2. Train-of-four assessment is highly subjective and has been repeatedly demonstrated to underestimate residual neuromuscular blockade.
3. It may be a best practice to administer reversal agents to all patients receiving nondepolarizing relaxants.
4. Leave clinically weak patients intubated and support respirations until the patient can demonstrate return of strength.

---

22. **What is tetanic stimulation?**

Tetanic stimulation consists of repetitive, high-frequency stimulation at frequencies of 50 Hz or greater. Loss of contraction during tetanic stimulation, known as *tetanic fade*, is a sensitive indicator of residual neuromuscular blockade. Tetanus stimulates the release of ACh from the prejunctional membrane, decreasing the validity of further nerve stimulation for upward of 30 minutes, leading to overestimating the return of neuromuscular function. A tetanic stimulus is painful.

23. **Explain posttetanic facilitation and posttetanic count.**

This mode of stimulation is useful during periods of intense neuromuscular blockade (when there is no response to TOF stimulation) and extends our range of monitoring. It provides an indication as to when recovery of a single twitch is anticipated and thus when reversal of neuromuscular blockade is possible. An application of a 50-Hz stimulus for 5 seconds is followed in 3 seconds by repetitive single twitches at 1 Hz. The number of twitches observed is inversely related to the degree of blockade.

24. **What is double-burst stimulation?**

DB stimulation appears to be more sensitive than TOF stimulation for detecting small degrees of residual neuromuscular blockade. DB involves the application of an initial burst of three 0.2-ms impulses at 50 Hz followed by an identical stimulation in 750 ms. The magnitude of the responses to double burst is approximately three times greater than that of TOF stimulation, thus making it easier to assess degree of fade present.

25. **What is acceleromyography?**

There is concern that the visual and tactile qualities of conventional TOF stimulation and assessments of strength such as 5-second head lift are not sufficiently quantitative to detect all instances of residual neuromuscular blockade. The operating concept is, as force is proportional to acceleration, acceleration measured during TOF stimulation will be proportional to muscular force generated. Acceleromyography is thought to provide comparatively more quantitative information about TOF stimulation, and there is growing evidence that acceleromyography should be routinely used to reduce the risk of residual weakness and adverse postoperative events.

26. **Which nerves can be chosen for stimulation?**

Any easily accessible nerve may be used, but the most common nerve stimulated is the ulnar nerve. Contraction of the adductor pollicis muscle of the thumb is observed. The ophthalmic branch of the facial nerve may also be stimulated, monitoring the contraction of the orbicularis oculi muscle. Stimulating the peroneal nerve near the fibular head results in dorsiflexion of the ankle. Stimulating the posterior tibial nerve and ankle results in plantar flexion of the big toe.

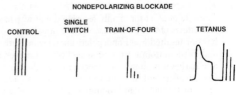

Figure 13-2. Response to nondepolarizing muscle relaxant blockade. *(From Bevan DR, Bevan JC, Donati F: Muscle relaxants in clinical anesthesia, Chicago, 1988, Year Book, pp 49–70.)*

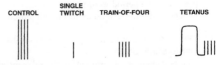

Figure 13-3. Response to depolarizing muscle relaxant blockade. *(From Bevan DR, Bevan JC, Donati F: Muscle relaxants in clinical anesthesia, Chicago, 1988, Year Book, pp 49–70.)*

27. **What are the characteristic responses to the various patterns of stimulation produced by nondepolarizing agents?**
   - Repetitive stimulation (TOF or tetanus) is associated with fade in the muscle response.
   - Following a tetanic stimulus, response to subsequent stimulations is increased (posttetanic facilitation). This may be caused by increased prejunctional ACh release or increased sensitivity at the end plate (Figure 13-2).

28. **Summarize the characteristic responses to the various patterns of stimulation produced by depolarizing relaxants (SCH).**
   The single-twitch, TOF, and tetanus amplitudes are uniformly decreased at any level of blockade. There is lack of fade in response to TOF and tetanus and lack of posttetanic facilitation. A desensitization or phase II blockade may develop with prolonged exposure to SCH. Phase II blockade has the same twitch characteristics as nondepolarizing blockade (Figure 13-3).

29. **For surgical purposes, based on nerve stimulation, what is adequate muscular relaxation?**
   Adequate relaxation is generally present when one to two twitches of the TOF response are present, correlating with 80% depression of single-twitch height. However, volatile anesthetics, other medications, and the patient's underlying health also affect strength, and under these conditions lighter levels of blockade may be satisfactory. Variation in the degree of blockade may be unappreciated by non-anesthesia providers.

30. **How might relaxant activity be terminated?**
   There may be competitive agonism at the NMJ, as when acetylcholinesterase inhibitors are administered to prevent metabolism of ACh, increasing the concentration of ACh at the NMJ. Alternatively, the relaxant might migrate away from its site of action, suggesting that there is a concentration gradient favoring this. Such a concentration gradient is commonly created through metabolism of the relaxant. However, selective binding of relaxant molecules is a pharmacologic alternative that is emerging in clinical practice. The first of this class of drugs likely to become commonly available is sugammadex.

31. **Review the properties of sugammadex.**
   Sugammadex is a modified cyclodextrin that forms extremely tight water-soluble complexes with relaxants having steroidal nuclei (rocuronium > vecuronium ≫ pancuronium). The cyclodextrin molecule is doughnut shaped; the relaxant is bound within the doughnut hole, roughly speaking; and the dissociation rate is very low. Binding of the relaxant molecule to sugammadex creates a concentration gradient away from the NMJ. Its efficacy does not depend on renal excretion of the cyclodextrin-relaxant complex. Sugammadex appears to be relatively free of side effects. Sugammadex has no effect on acetylcholinesterase or any other cholinergic receptors.

32. How might sugammadex alter anesthetic practice?

The role of SCH for rapidly securing the airway has been discussed, as have the numerous side effects of SCH. Pharmacologic innovation in development of muscle relaxants per se has not resulted in a nondepolarizing relaxant with quick-onset, short duration of action and freedom from worrisome side effects. However, sugammadex may provide a useful alternative if it allows the caregiver to administer rocuronium in rapid paralysis doses (≈1.2 mg/kg) and have an avenue for pharmacologic antagonism soon after dosing of the relaxant through tight binding of circulating relaxant molecules. In fact, the use of sugammadex after rocuronium dosing may provide faster onset-offset profile than SCH given at 1 mg/kg and eliminate the need to ever administer anticholinesterase medications. Finally, it should be mentioned that elimination of residual neuromuscular blockade in the postoperative period would be of definite clinical benefit. Sugammadex has no muscarinic effects. It is effective on aminosteroid muscle relaxants but not benzylisoquinolines.

33. Discuss the appropriate time to reverse neuromuscular blockade based on nerve stimulation.

The best method of terminating the relaxant effect is to dose sparingly and allow the relaxant to be metabolized. Recall that only one of the α subunits of the postjunctional receptor needs be occupied by a relaxant molecule to inhibit function, whereas two molecules of ACh are necessary to stimulate the receptor; thus, even though the nondepolarizing relaxants are competitive antagonists, the receptor dynamics favor the relaxants. With these caveats, neuromuscular blockade can be reversed when there is at least one twitch with TOF stimulation. However, this still reflects a very deep level of blockade, and the clinician should monitor the patient closely for clinical signs of inadequate return of strength. The greater the TOF when reversed, the better. It is also important to remember that recent tetanic stimuli will result in overestimating the TOF.

34. Review the acetylcholinesterase inhibitors commonly used to antagonize nondepolarizing blockade.

Acetylcholinesterase inhibitors prevent the breakdown of acetylcholinesterase, increasing the amount of ACh available at the NMJ. Neostigmine, 25 to 70 mcg/kg, and edrophonium, 0.5 to 1 mg/kg, are commonly used for this purpose perioperatively. Edrophonium also stimulates the prejunctional membrane, increasing release of ACh. These medications contain positively charged quaternary ammonium groups, are water soluble, and are renally excreted.

35. Review important side effects of acetylcholinesterase administration.

Increasing the available ACh at the NMJ (a nicotinic receptor) also stimulates muscarinic cholinergic receptors. Of particular concern is the effect on cardiac conduction. Unopposed muscarinic effects impair sinus-node conduction, resulting in sinus bradycardia, junctional rhythms, and, in the extreme, asystole. To prevent the muscarinic effects, anticholinergics are administered in concert with the acetylcholinesterase. Glycopyrrolate, 7 to 15 mcg/kg, is coadministered with neostigmine, and atropine, 7 to 10 mcg/kg, is coadministered with edrophonium so the onset of anticholinergic activity is appropriately timed with the onset of acetylcholinesterase inhibition.

36. Should all patients who receive nondepolarizing relaxants be reversed?

There is mounting evidence that residual neuromuscular blockade and clinical weakness occur with disturbing frequency, even when the patient has received only one dose of an intermediate-duration nondepolarizing relaxant. These residual effects have been noted even 2 hours after a single dose. Part of the problem appears to be subjective misinterpretations of full return of TOF, as discussed earlier. It appears that routine reversal of all patients might be a prudent practice. How sugammadex changes anesthetic practice remains to be determined.

37. Review the clinical signs associated with return of adequate strength.

See Table 13-2.

Table 13-2. Tests of Return of Neuromuscular Function

TEST	RESULTS	PERCENTAGE OF RECEPTORS OCCUPIED
Tidal volume	>5 ml/kg	80
Single twitch	Return to baseline	75–80
Train of four	No fade	70–75
Sustained tetanus (50 Hz, 5 seconds)	No fade	70
Vital capacity	>20 ml/kg	70
Double-burst stimulation	No fade	60–70
Sustained tetanus (100 Hz, 5 seconds)	No fade	50
Inspiratory force	>−40 cm H_2O	50
Head lift	Sustained 5 seconds	50
Hand grip	Return to baseline	50
Sustained bite	Sustained clenching of a tongue depressor	50

38. A patient appears weak after pharmacologic reversal of neuromuscular blockade. What factors should be considered?
   - Has enough time elapsed to observe peak reversal effect?
   - Was blockade so intense that reversal is not possible?
   - Is your twitch monitor functioning, and are leads well placed?
   - Are body temperature, acid-base status, and electrolyte status normal?
   - Hypothermia potentiates neuromuscular blockade, as does acidosis, hypokalemia, hypocalcemia, and hypermagnesemia. Is the patient receiving medications that potentiate neuromuscular blockade?
   - What is the patient's renal and hepatic function?
   - Importantly, if the patient is weak, do not extubate. Time usually cures all that ails.

SUGGESTED READINGS

Fagerlund MJ, Eriksson LI: Current concepts in neuromuscular transmission, Br J Anesth 103:108–114, 2009.
Hemmerling TM, Le N: Brief review: Neuromuscular monitoring: an update for clinician, Can J Anaesth 54:58–72, 2007.
Hirsch NP: Neuromuscular junction in health and disease, Br J Anaesth 99:132–138, 2007.
Martyn JAJ, Richtsfeld M: Succinylcholine-induced hyperkalemia in acquired pathologic states, Anesthesiology 104:158–169, 2006.
Murphy GS, Szokol JW, Marymont JH, et al: Intraoperative acceleromyographic monitoring reduces the risk of residual neuromuscular blockade and adverse respiratory events in the postanesthesia care unit, Anesthesiology 109:363–364, 2008.
Naguib M: Sugammadex: Another milestone in clinical neuromuscular pharmacology, Anesth Analg 104:575–581, 2007.
Schow AJ, Lubarsky DA, Olson RP, et al: Can succinylcholine be used safely in hyperkalemic states? Anesth Analg 95:119–122, 2002.

CHAPTER 14

LOCAL ANESTHETICS

Sunil Kumar, MD, and James C. Duke, MD, MBA

1. **What role do local anesthetics play in the practice of anesthesiology?**
   As local anesthetics reversibly block nerve conduction, they are used to provide regional anesthesia for surgery and postoperative analgesia for painful surgical procedures. Local anesthetics given intravenously attenuate the pressor response to tracheal intubation, decrease coughing during intubation and extubation, and are antiarrhythmic.

2. **How are local anesthetics classified?**
   - **Aminoesters:** Esters are local anesthetics, the intermediate chain of which forms an ester link between the aromatic and amine groups. Commonly used ester local anesthetics include procaine, chloroprocaine, cocaine, and tetracaine (Figure 14-1).
   - **Aminoamides:** Amides are local anesthetics with an amide link between the aromatic and amine groups. Commonly used amide anesthetics include lidocaine, prilocaine, mepivacaine, bupivacaine, levobupivacaine, ropivacaine, and etidocaine.

3. **How are local anesthetics metabolized?**
   Esters undergo hydrolysis by pseudocholinesterases found principally in plasma. Amides undergo enzymatic biotransformation primarily in the liver. The lungs may also extract lidocaine, bupivacaine, and prilocaine from circulation. Chloroprocaine is least likely to produce sustained elevation in blood levels because of very rapid hydrolysis in the blood. Risk of toxicity to esters is increased in patients with atypical pseudocholinesterase and severe liver disease and in neonates. Liver disease or decreases in liver blood flow as may occur in patients with congestive heart failure or during general anesthesia can decrease the metabolism of aminoamides.

4. **How are impulses conducted in nerve cells?**
   Transmission of impulses depends on the electrical gradient across the nerve membrane, which in turn depends on the movement of sodium (Na) and potassium (K) ions. Application of a stimulus of sufficient intensity leads to a change in membrane potential (from −90 mV to −60 mV), subsequent depolarization of the nerve, and propagation of the impulse. Depolarization is caused by inflow of Na ions from the extracellular to the intracellular space. Repolarization is caused by outflow of K ions from the intracellular to the extracellular space. The Na-K pump restores equilibrium in the nerve membrane after completion of the action potential.

5. **What is the mechanism of action of local anesthetics?**
   The cascade of events (Figure 14-2) is as follows:
   - Diffusion of the unionized (base) form across the nerve sheath and membrane
   - Reequilibration between the base and cationic forms in the axoplasm
   - Binding of the cation to a receptor site inside of the Na channel, resulting in its blockade and consequent inhibition of Na conductance

6. **Your patient states that he was told he is allergic to Novocain, which he received for a tooth extraction. Should you avoid using local anesthetics in this patient?**
   Probably not. Allergy to local anesthetics is rare despite frequent use of local anesthetics. Less than 1% of adverse reaction to local anesthetics is true allergy. Most reactions labeled as allergy are probably one of the following: vasovagal response, systemic toxicity, or systemic effects of epinephrine. True allergy would be suggested by history of rash, bronchospasm, laryngeal edema, hypotension, elevation of serum tryptase, and positive intradermal testing.

   Esters produce metabolites related to *p*-aminobenzoic acid and are more likely to produce allergic reactions than are amide local anesthetics. Allergic reactions following use

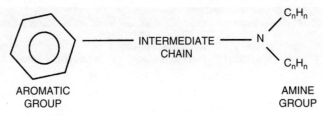

Figure 14-1. Structure of ester and amide local anesthetics.

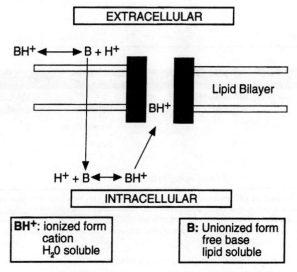

Figure 14-2. Mechanism of action of local anesthetics.

of local anesthetics may also be caused by methylparaben or other preservatives in commercial preparations of local anesthetics. There is no cross-sensitivity between classes of local anesthetics. Therefore patients known to be allergic to ester local anesthetics could receive amide local anesthetics. Caution is still warranted in case the patient is allergic to the preservative that may be common to both classes of drugs.

7. **What determines local anesthetic potency?**
   The higher the solubility, the greater the potency (Table 14-1). This relationship is more clearly seen in isolated nerve than in clinical situations when factors such as vasodilation and tissue redistribution response to various local anesthetics influence the duration of local anesthetic effect. For example, high lipid solubility of etidocaine results in profound nerve blockade in isolated nerve. Yet, in clinical epidural use, etidocaine is considerably sequestered in epidural fat, leaving a reduced amount of etidocaine available for neural blockade.

8. **What factors influence the duration of action of local anesthetics?**
   The greater the protein binding, the longer the duration of action. The duration of action is also influenced by peripheral vascular effects of the local anesthetics. For example, lidocaine, prilocaine, and mepivacaine provide anesthesia of similar duration in an isolated nerve. However, lidocaine is a more potent vasodilator, increasing absorption and

Table 14-1. Local Anesthetic Potency

AGENT	LIPID SOLUBILITY	RELATIVE POTENCY	PROTEIN BINDING (%)	DURATION	pKa	ONSET TIME
Procaine	<1	1	5	Short	8.9	Slow
2-Chloroprocaine	>1	3	—	Short	8.7	Very quick
Mepivacaine	1	1.5	75	Medium	7.7	Quick
Lidocaine	3	2	65	Medium	7.9	Quick
Bupivacaine	28	8	95	Long	8.1	Moderate
Tetracaine	80	8	85	Long	8.5	Slow
Ropivacaine	14	8	94	Long	8.1	Moderate

Table 14-2. Maximum Safe Doses of Local Anesthetics*

DRUG	MAXIMUM DOSE (mg/kg)	DRUG	MAXIMUM DOSE (mg/kg)
Procaine	7	Mepivacaine	5
Chloroprocaine	8–9	Bupivacaine	2.5
Tetracaine	1.5 (topical)		
Lidocaine	5 or 7 (with epinephrine)		

*These doses are based on subcutaneous administration and apply only to single-shot injections. Continuous infusions of local anesthetic, as might occur over several hours during labor epidural anesthesia, allow a greater total dose of anesthetic before toxic plasma levels are reached. Maximum safe dose is also influenced by vascularity of the tissue bed and whether epinephrine is added to the local anesthetic.

metabolism of the drug, thus resulting in a shorter clinical blockade than that produced by prilocaine or mepivacaine.

9. **What determines local anesthetic onset time?**
   Degree of ionization: the closer the pKa of the local anesthetic is to tissue pH, the more rapid the onset time will be. pKa is defined as the pH at which the ionized and unionized forms exist in equal concentrations. Because all local anesthetics are weak bases, those with pKa that lies near physiologic pH (7.4) will have more molecules in the unionized, lipid-soluble form. At physiologic pH, less than 50% of the drug exists in unionized form. As mentioned, the unionized form must cross the axonal membrane to initiate neural blockade. The latency of a local anesthetic can also be shortened by using a higher concentration and carbonated local anesthetic solutions to adjust the local pH.

10. **How does the onset of anesthesia proceed in a peripheral nerve block?**
    Conduction blockade proceeds from the outermost (mantle) to the innermost (core) nerve bundles. Generally speaking, mantle fibers innervate proximal structures, and core fibers innervate distal structures. This accounts for early block of more proximal areas, and muscle weakness may appear before the sensory block if motor fibers are more peripheral.

11. **What are the maximum safe doses of various local anesthetics?**
    See Table 14-2.

12. **Which regional anesthetic blocks are associated with the greatest degree of systemic vascular absorption of local anesthetic?**
    Intercostal nerve block > caudal > epidural > brachial plexus > sciatic-femoral > subcutaneous. Because the intercostal nerves are surrounded by a rich vascular supply, local

anesthetics injected into this area are more rapidly absorbed, thus increasing the likelihood of achieving toxic levels.

13. **Why are epinephrine and phenylephrine often added to local anesthetics? What cautions are advisable regarding the use of these drugs?**
These drugs cause local tissue vasoconstriction, limiting uptake of the local anesthetic into the vasculature and thus prolonging its effects and reducing its toxic potential (see Question 14). Epinephrine, usually in 1:200,000 concentration, is also a useful marker of inadvertent intravascular injection. Epinephrine is contraindicated for digital blocks or other areas with poor collateral circulation. Systemic absorption of epinephrine may also cause hypertension and cardiac dysrhythmias, and caution is advised in patients with ischemic heart disease, hypertension, preeclampsia, and other conditions in which such responses may be undesirable.

14. **How does a patient become toxic from local anesthetics? What are the clinical manifestations of local anesthetic toxicity?**
Systemic toxicity is caused by elevated plasma local anesthetic levels, most often a result of inadvertent intravascular injection and, less frequently, a result of systemic absorption of local anesthetic from the injection site. Toxicity involves the cardiovascular and central nervous systems. Because the central nervous system (CNS) is generally more sensitive to the toxic effects of local anesthetics, it is usually affected first. The manifestations are presented below in chronologic order:
- CNS toxicity: light-headedness, tinnitus, perioral numbness, confusion
- Muscle twitching, auditory and visual hallucinations
- Tonic-clonic seizure, unconsciousness, respiratory arrest
- Cardiotoxicity: less common but can be fatal
- Hypertension, tachycardia
- Decreased contractility and cardiac output, hypotension
- Sinus bradycardia, ventricular dysrhythmias, circulatory arrest

15. **Is the risk of cardiotoxicity the same with various local anesthetics?**
There have been multiple case reports of cardiac arrest and electrical standstill after bupivacaine administration, many associated with difficult resuscitation. The cardiotoxicity of more potent drugs such as bupivacaine and ropivacaine differs from that of lidocaine in the following manner:
- The ratio of the dosage required for irreversible cardiovascular collapse and the dosage that produces CNS toxicity is much lower for bupivacaine than for lidocaine.
- Pregnancy, acidosis, and hypoxia increase the risk of cardiotoxicity with bupivacaine.
- Cardiac resuscitation is more difficult following bupivacaine-induced cardiovascular collapse. It may be related to the lipid solubility of bupivacaine, which results in slow dissociation of this drug from cardiac sodium channels (fast-in, slow-out). By contrast, recovery from less lipid-soluble lidocaine is rapid (fast-in, fast-out).
   In an effort to minimize the risk of cardiac toxicity in the event of an accidental intravascular injection, the use of bupivacaine in concentrations greater than 0.5% should be avoided, especially in obstetric epidural anesthesia. For postoperative analgesia, bupivacaine concentrations of 0.25% generally provide excellent effect.

KEY POINTS: LOCAL ANESTHETICS

1. Local anesthetic agents are either aminoesters or aminoamides. The two classes of agents differ in their allergic potential and method of biotransformation.
2. Lipid solubility, pKa, and protein binding of the local anesthetics determine their potency, onset, and duration of action, respectively.
3. Local anesthetic–induced CNS toxicity manifests with excitation, followed by seizures, then loss of consciousness, whereas hypotension, conduction blockade, and cardiac arrest are signs of local anesthetic cardiovascular toxicity.
4. Bupivacaine has the highest risk of producing severe cardiac dysrhythmias and irreversible cardiovascular collapse. Use of more than 0.5% concentration should be avoided, especially in obstetric epidurals.

16. **How will you prevent and treat systemic toxicity?**
    - Most reactions can be prevented by careful selection of dose and concentration, use of test dose with epinephrine, incremental injection with frequent aspiration, monitoring patient for signs of intravascular injection, and judicious use of benzodiazepine to raise the seizure threshold.
    - Tonic-clonic seizures can quickly lead to hypoxia and acidosis, and acidosis worsens the toxic effects. A patent airway and adequate ventilation with 100% oxygen should be ensured.
    - If seizures develop, small doses of intravenous diazepam (0.1 mg/kg) or thiopental (1 to 2 mg/kg) may terminate the seizure. Short-acting muscle relaxants may be indicated for ongoing muscle activity or to facilitate intubation if necessary.
    - Cardiovascular collapse with refractory ventricular fibrillation or asystole following local anesthetics, particularly bupivacaine or ropivacaine, can be extremely difficult to resuscitate. Bradycardia may precede the arrhythmias previously described. Treatment includes sustained cardiopulmonary resuscitation, repeated cardioversion, high doses of epinephrine, and use of bretylium to treat ventricular dysrhythmias. Intravenous intralipid has been used successfully in cases in which conventional resuscitation measures were unsuccessful. Suggested dose is initial bolus of 1.5-2.0 ml/kg of 20% intralipid solution, which can be repeated every 3 to 5 minutes up to a total maximum dose of 8 ml/kg.

17. **What is the risk of neurotoxicity with local anesthetics?**
    The overall risk of permanent neurologic injury due to neurotoxicity is extremely small. However, in recent years the following two complications have been described after spinal and epidural anesthesia:
    - Transient neurologic symptoms manifest in the form of moderate-to-severe pain in the lower back, buttocks, and posterior thighs. These symptoms appear within 24 hours of spinal anesthesia and generally resolve within 7 days. The delayed onset may reflect an inflammatory etiology for these symptoms. They are seen most commonly with lidocaine spinal anesthesia and are rare with bupivacaine. Patients having surgery in the lithotomy position appear to be at increased risk of neurologic symptoms following either spinal or epidural anesthesia.
    - Cauda equina syndrome: A few cases of diffuse injury to the lumbosacral plexus were initially reported in patients receiving continuous spinal anesthesia with 5% lidocaine dosed via microcatheters. The mechanism of neural injury is thought to be that nonhomogeneous distribution of spinally injected local anesthetic may expose sacral nerve roots to a high concentration of local anesthetic with consequent toxicity. Rare cases in the absence of microcatheters have also been described. Avoid injecting large amounts of local anesthetic in the subarachnoid space, especially if less than an anticipated response is obtained with the initial dose.

18. **Which local anesthetic is associated with the risk of methemoglobinemia?**
    Prilocaine and benzocaine are the two local anesthetics responsible for most cases of local anesthetic–related methemoglobinemia, although in rare instances other agents have been implicated. Prilocaine is metabolized in the liver to O-toluidine, which is capable of oxidizing hemoglobin to methemoglobin. Prilocaine in a dose greater than 600 mg can produce clinical methemoglobinemia, making the patient appear cyanotic. Benzocaine, used as a spray for topical anesthesia of mouth and throat, can result in methemoglobinemia if excessive amounts are used in the form of multiple sprays or if spraying the area for a longer duration than recommended. Methemoglobin is reduced through methemoglobin reductase, and this process is accelerated by intravenous methylene blue (1 to 2 mg/kg).

19. **Describe the role of lipid infusion in the treatment of local anesthetic toxicity.**
    Systemic local anesthetic toxicity is rare but can be fatal because of relative resistance of local anesthetic–induced cardiac arrest to standard resuscitative measures. Cardiotoxicity from bupivacaine has almost always been fatal, often requiring placement of the patient on cardiopulmonary bypass while the drug slowly clears from the cardiac muscle tissue. Animal studies have demonstrated that lipid infusion increases resistance to local anesthetic toxicity and improves success of resuscitation from local anesthetic overdose. In the past few years

there have been several case reports of successful use of lipid emulsion in the treatment of local anesthetic toxicity in humans. The mechanism of beneficial effect is thought to be a reduction in tissue binding of local anesthetic and a beneficial energetic-metabolic effect. The protocol for intralipid administration is as follows:

- Initially administer intralipid 20% at a dose of 1.5 to 2.0 ml/kg over 1 minute.
- Follow immediately with an infusion at a rate of 10 ml/minute.
- Continue chest compressions (lipid must circulate).
- Repeat bolus every 3 to 5 minutes up to 3 ml/kg total dosage until circulation is restored.
- Continue infusion until hemodynamic stability is restored.
- Increase the rate to 0.5 ml/kg/min if blood pressure declines.
- A maximum total dose of 8 ml/kg is recommended.

20. **What are some local anesthetics, and what are their potential applications?**
Ropivacaine is an amide local anesthetic that is structurally and behaviorally similar to bupivacaine. Like bupivacaine, it is highly protein bound and has a long duration of action. When compared to bupivacaine, it is less cardiotoxic and produces less motor block, thus allowing analgesia with less motor compromise (differential blockade). However, some of these benefits may be related to somewhat lower potency of ropivacaine and may not exist when equipotent doses are compared. Levobupivacaine is an S(−) isomer of the racemic bupivacaine and has a safer cardiac and CNS toxicity profile compared with that of bupivacaine. Local anesthetic effects are similar to those of bupivacaine. Because of their superior toxicity profile, both ropivacaine and levobupivacaine are suitable for situations requiring relatively large doses of local anesthetics.

WEBSITE

LipidRescue™ Resuscitation for Drug Toxicity: www.lipidrescue.org

SUGGESTED READINGS

Heavner JE: Local anesthetics, Curr Opin Anaesthesiol 20:336–342, 2007.

Litz RJ, Popp M, Stehr SN, et al: Successful resuscitation of a patient with ropivacaine-induced asystole after axillary plexus block using lipid infusion, Anaesthesia 61:800–801, 2006.

Mulroy ME: Systemic toxicity and cardiotoxicity from local anesthetics: incidence and preventive measures, Reg Anesth Pain Med 27:556–561, 2002.

Reinberg GL: Lipid emulsion infusion: resuscitation for local anesthetic and other drug overdose, Anesthesiology 117:180–187, 2012.

Rosenblatt MA, Abel M: Successful use of a 20% lipid emulsion to resuscitate a patient after a presumed bupivacaine-related cardiac arrest, Anesthesiology 105:217–218, 2006.

Strichartz GR, Berde CB: Local anesthetics. In Miller RD, editor: Anesthesia, ed 6, Philadelphia, 2005, Churchill Livingstone, pp 573–603.

CHAPTER 15

INOTROPES AND VASODILATOR DRUGS

Michael Kim, DO, and Nathaen Weitzel, MD

1. **What are the benefits of cardiovascular drugs?**

   All of the components of organ perfusion, including preload (end-diastolic volume), afterload, inotropy, heart rate, and myocardial oxygen supply and demand, can be pharmacologically modified. An underlying concept is the Frank–Starling principle, which states that increased myocardial fiber length, or preload, improves contractility up to a point of optimal contractile state. Further stretching results in declining performance. Furthermore, it should be remembered that the mean arterial pressure is the product of cardiac output and systemic vascular resistance, so that changes in the latter two may effect changes in the former (Figure 15-1).

2. **Discuss the limitations of drugs that alter vascular tone.**

   Preload can be altered with intravascular volume shifts as well as with drugs that change vascular tone and, most important, the venous capacitance vessels. In addition, arterial vasodilators may shift failing myocardium to a more effective contractile state due to afterload reduction and decreased impedance to ventricular ejection. However, the intrinsic contractile state is not improved by vasodilators, in contrast to the effect of positive inotropic agents, nor are they with pure vasoconstrictors such as phenylephrine. The salutary effects of arterial vasodilators are in most cases somewhat limited by their decreased but parallel impact on venous capacitance, which decreases preload and thus cardiac output. Vascular tone can also alter the ability of the intrinsic contractile state by increasing afterload, or increased vascular tone. This leads to increased impedance to ventricular ejection by making it more difficult on ventricular contraction. Although increasing systemic vascular resistance may be improved, actual ventricular ejection may be hampered and increase ventricular wall tension.

3. **What are the general goals of inotropic support and the characteristics of the ideal inotrope?**

   The general goal of inotropic support is increasing cardiac output by improving myocardial contractility to optimize end-organ perfusion. In addition, for enlarged hearts, a decrease in ventricular diameter, wall tension, and myocardial oxygen demand is desirable. Some inotropic agents may also serve to decrease pulmonary vascular resistance, improving right heart output and forward flow. The ideal inotrope increases contraction of cardiac muscle without changing preload or afterload, while improving pulmonary vascular resistance and myocardial oxygen demand, and has no propensity to cause arrhythmias. However, this agent does not currently exist.

4. **Discuss the hemodynamic profile of the phosphodiesterase (PDE) inhibitors amrinone and milrinone.**

   Amrinone and milrinone are approximately equipotent to dopamine and dobutamine in increasing cardiac output through increased inotropy and improved lusitropy (myocardial relaxation). In addition to direct myocardial effects, vasodilation typically occurs, making it difficult to separate the relative contributions of these effects on enhanced cardiac output. The observed dual hemodynamic effect has been coined *inodilation*. Right ventricular function can be favorably impacted as these agents decrease pulmonary vascular resistance (comparable to 20 ppm nitric oxide in cardiac surgery patients), thus improving forward flow. Coronary vessels become dilated, as well as arterial bypass grafts (internal mammary and gastroepiploic arteries and radial artery grafts); furthermore, in the presence of these

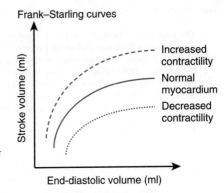

Figure 15.1. Frank–Starling curves illustrating functional assessment changes in stroke volume secondary to changes in end-diastolic volume under varying states of cardiac contractility (*Adapted from Hamilton M: Advanced cardiovascular monitoring. Surgery (Oxford) 31(2): 90-97, 2013.*)

drugs, they are less subject to the vasoconstrictive effects of concomitantly administered α-adrenergic agonists.

5. **What untoward effects can result from use of PDE inhibitors? How are these minimized?**
   Because the vasodilator effects may be profound, concurrent use of vasoconstrictors (e.g., epinephrine, norepinephrine, phenylephrine) is often necessary, particularly after cardiopulmonary bypass. Prolonged infusion of amrinone, but not milrinone, may cause significant thrombocytopenia, through non–immune-mediated peripheral platelet destruction.

6. **What are other advantages of the PDE inhibitors?**
   In addition to positive inotropy and lusitropy, vasodilation, and a relative lack of significant tachyarrhythmias, these inhibitors may transiently restore β-adrenergic function by decreasing cyclic adenosine monophosphate (cAMP) breakdown, which leads to increased calcium concentration, as well as potentiating the action of administered β-adrenergic agonists. These drugs dilate coronary arteries and conduits, improving collateral coronary circulation in addition to attenuating thromboxane activity and, in certain clinical situations, may help decrease myocardial oxygen consumption.

7. **What intracellular intermediary is involved in the actions of PDE III inhibitors and sympathomimetic amines?**
   Both drug classes increase intracellular cAMP concentrations, which in turn stimulates cardiac calcium channels but by different but similar mechanisms. Sympathomimetic β-adrenergic stimulation activates sarcolemmal adenyl cyclase, resulting in the generation of increased cAMP from adenosine triphosphate, whereas PDE III inhibitors decrease the breakdown of cAMP.

8. **How does increased intracellular cAMP affect the cardiac myocyte? What are the corresponding effects on myocardial function?**
   Increased intracellular cAMP activates protein kinases, which phosphorylate proteins in the sarcolemma, sarcoplasmic reticulum (SR), and tropomyosin complex. This causes elevated calcium (Ca^{2+}) influx via Ca^{2+} channels, amplifying the effects of Ca^{2+} on contractile elements. In addition, increased protein phosphorylation in the SR and tropomyosin complex improves diastolic relaxation (lusitropy) by stimulating reuptake of Ca^{2+} into the SR. The end result is a restoration of the myofilaments to their resting state. Therefore, both inotropy and lusitropy are improved.

9. **What is the result of combining adrenergic agonists with PDE III inhibitors?**
   An additive or synergistic effect results from the influence of PDE III inhibitors distal to the adrenergic receptor.

10. **Describe the hemodynamic profiles of epinephrine, norepinephrine, and dopamine.**

The effects of a low-dose infusion of epinephrine (<0.04 µg/kg/min) are primarily limited to stimulation of β_1- and α_2-adrenergic receptors in the heart and peripheral vasculature, resulting in positive chronotropy, dromotropy (conduction velocity), inotropy, increased automaticity, and vasodilation. Moderate-dose infusion (0.04–0.12 µg/kg/min) generates greater α-adrenergic effects and vasoconstriction, and high-dose infusion results in such prominent vasoconstriction that many of the β-adrenergic effects are blocked.

Hemodynamic dose-response relationship of epinephrine
- <0.04 µg/kg/min   Primarily beta stimulation
- 0.04–0.12 µg/kg/min   Mixed alpha and beta stimulation
- >0.12 µg/kg/min   Primarily alpha stimulation

The potency of norepinephrine in stimulating β-adrenergic receptors is similar to that of epinephrine, but it results in significant α-adrenergic stimulation at much lower doses. Typical dose ranges are 0.02–0.25 µg/kg/min.

Dopamine stimulates specific postjunctional dopaminergic receptors in renal, mesenteric, and coronary arterial beds to produce vasodilation. These dopaminergic effects occur at lower doses (0.5–1.0 µg/kg/min), becoming maximal at 2–3 µg/kg/min. At intermediate doses (2–6 µg/kg/min), β_1-adrenergic stimulation is evident. Beginning at doses of about 10 µg/kg/min (but as low as 5 µg/kg/min), α-adrenergic stimulation is seen, which at higher doses overcomes dopaminergic effects, producing vasoconstriction.

11. **Describe the hemodynamic profiles of isoproterenol and dobutamine.**

Isoproterenol is an extremely potent β_1 and β_2 agonist that possesses no alpha-stimulating properties. Therefore, isoproterenol increases heart rate, automaticity, and contractility and dilates both venous capacitance and arterial vessels. It may be a good choice for heart-rate maintenance in a denervated nonpaced transplanted heart. Dobutamine acts principally on β-adrenergic receptors, impacting β_1 receptors in a relatively selective fashion. In addition, it has a mild indirect β_1-stimulating effect that is secondary to prevention of norepinephrine reuptake but is offset by slightly more potent β_2 stimulation. Generally, at clinical doses, minimal increases in heart rate, positive inotropy, increased cardiac output, and minimal or modest decreases in systemic and pulmonary vascular resistance occur. Because of the indirect β_1-stimulating effect, patients concurrently receiving β blockers can exhibit marked increases in systemic vascular resistance without improvement in cardiac output. In addition, an occasional patient will display dose-related increases in heart rate.

12. **Which characteristics of β-adrenergic agonists limit their effectiveness?**
- Positive chronotropic and arrhythmogenic effects (dose-dependent effect with epinephrine, isoproterenol, and dobutamine), possibly resulting in increased myocardial oxygen consumption.
- Vasoconstriction secondary to α_1 activation (with norepinephrine, high-dose epinephrine, and high-dose dopamine), resulting in increased afterload and subsequent increased myocardial wall tension. Vasodilation due to stimulation of vascular β_2 receptors (with isoproterenol, and less so with dobutamine).

13. **How may the side effects and limitations of β-adrenergic agonists be minimized?**

Side effects may be decreased by appropriate dosage adjustments and use of combinations of agents. Currently, PDE III inhibitors have a prominent role in this regard. However, both vasopressin and nicardipine, at low doses, may prove beneficial in these circumstances as well.

14. **Is digitalis useful as an inotrope intraoperatively?**

Because of its narrow therapeutic ratio and adverse interactions with fluid and electrolyte shifts, digitalis is rarely used intraoperatively as an inotrope.

15. **What are the mechanism and sites of action of nitrovasodilators?**

Nitrates such as nitroglycerin and sodium nitroprusside are prodrugs that penetrate the vascular endothelium and become reduced to nitric oxide (NO). Nitroglycerin requires intact endothelial enzymatic activity, which is not present in the smallest or damaged vessels, while nitroprusside nonenzymatically degrades into NO and cyanide (a compound highly toxic to the mitochondrial respiratory chain). NO then stimulates production of cyclic guanosine monophosphate (cGMP), resulting in decreased cellular calcium levels and thus vascular smooth muscle relaxation.

Sodium nitroprusside acts primarily on the arterial vasculature while nitroglycerin has its most prominent effect on venous capacitance vessels (although this is less true with higher doses). NO can also be delivered directly to the pulmonary circulation by inhalation, thereby reaching the pulmonary vascular smooth muscle by diffusion across the alveolar-capillary membrane. Direct delivery to the pulmonary circulation reduces potentially undesirable systemic hypotension and causes specific pulmonary vasodilation.

16. **Describe the antianginal effects of nitrates.**
Beneficial effects of nitroglycerin and other nitrates in anginal therapy result from improved coronary perfusion, a reduction in myocardial oxygen consumption (MVO_2), and antiplatelet effects. Coronary artery spasm is ameliorated, and dilation of epicardial coronary arteries, coronary collaterals, and atherosclerotic stenotic coronary segments occurs. Venodilation reduces venous return, ventricular filling pressures, wall tension, and MVO_2 and improves subendocardial and collateral blood flow. Platelet aggregation is inhibited by release of NO and increased formation of cGMP.

17. **Describe the etiology of tachyphylaxis with nitrovasodilators.**
Therapy with nitroglycerin is often confounded by tachyphylaxis, especially with long-term use, due to changes in the enzymatic machinery responsible for its transformation into NO. Tachyphylaxis may also be due to adaptive changes in the vascular system itself in which nitroglycerin increases endogenous rates of O_2 production, which in turn inactivates NO released from nitroglycerin. Nitrates may also be of limited clinical effect in the presence of a preload-insensitive system as well as fixed pulmonary hypertension.

The presence of tachyphylaxis with administration of sodium nitroprusside suggests a therapeutic ceiling and ensuing cyanide toxicity and is usually associated with prolonged infusions of more than 2 µg/kg/min or when sulfur donors and methemoglobin stores are exhausted.

18. **Discuss the types and mechanisms of action of selective vasodilating agents available for clinical use.**
Hydralazine directly relaxes smooth muscle, dilating arterioles to a much greater extent than veins, decreasing diastolic more than systolic blood pressure. The response is slow, with onset of 15 to 20 minutes, and somewhat unpredictable, often causing prolonged hypotension.

Nicardipine is a short-acting selective calcium channel blocker (CCB), which acts on the arteriolar beds, providing easier titration and controlled reduction in systemic blood pressure. Nicardipine is becoming the arterial vasodilator of choice for cardiac surgery patients with hypertension as it has more selective coronary vasodilation than systemic vasodilation. The end result is a reduction in afterload, increased stroke volume, and increased coronary blood flow, which results in a favorable effect on myocardial oxygen balance. Onset is 5 to 15 minutes and duration of action is 4 to 6 hours.

Clevidipine is a new, third-generation CCB that is considered an ultra-short-acting arteriolar vasodilator. Metabolized by plasma esterases, the half-life of Clevidipine is approximately 2 minutes, with a context-sensitive half-time of 2 to 5 minutes regardless of duration of infusion. It acts much like nicardipine, in that it selectively dilates the arteriolar bed, reducing afterload without affecting cardiac filling pressures. It comes in an emulsion much like propofol and is currently available in the United States.

Fenoldopam is a unique parenteral vasodilator that acts via peripheral dopamine-1 receptors (DA-1). This causes a vasodilator effect that is selective for renal and splanchnic vasculature, as well as causing mild renal diuresis. Onset is 5 minutes and half-life is roughly 5 minutes with duration of action of 30 to 60 minutes with infusion. Fenoldopam was thought to provide some degree of renal protection against acute kidney injury, but trials in ICU patients and the operative setting have not shown clear benefit. Fenoldopam can cause significant hypotension, so if it is used as a renal protective agent, close monitoring of the blood pressure is needed to ensure adequate renal perfusion.

19. **Describe the mechanism of action of vasopressin.**

    Arginine vasopressin (AVP) is a polypeptide with a disulfide bond between the two cysteine amino acids. Vasopressin has action at three subtypes of receptors (V1, V2, V3). The V1 receptor stimulates vascular smooth muscle contraction, resulting in the vasopressor response of AVP. The V2 receptors act primarily in the renal collecting tubule of the kidney to produce water retention (antidiuretic hormone) by regulating osmolarity and blood volume, and the V3 receptors act in the CNS and modulate corticotropin secretion. The vasopressin system makes up one of the three vasopressor systems in the body; the sympathetic system and the renin-angiotensin system are the other two vasopressor systems. The plasma half-life of AVP is 4 to 20 minutes, so it must be delivered by infusion for prolonged effects.

20. **How may vasopressin aid in the management of cardiogenic or septic shock?**

    Vasopressin is becoming a mainstay in the treatment of shock states in combination with adrenergic inotropic agents. In the presence of a systemic inflammatory response, patients with septic shock tend to have low plasma vasopressin concentrations due to low vasopressin secretion. The verdict is out if these low secretions are due to low pituitary vasopressin or a defect in the baroreflex-mediated vasopressin secretion. The use of vasopressin has been shown to improve hemodynamics and reduce requirements of adrenergic agents. The dose range is still debated, with many studies showing effectiveness at doses of 0.01 to 0.04 U/min. There are published data supporting use of vasopressin following cardiopulmonary bypass, with doses up to 0.1 U/min. Bolus doses in situations of cardiac arrest are 20 to 40 U per advanced cardiovascular life support (ACLS) guidelines. Higher doses of vasopressin carry higher risk of intense vasoconstriction, bringing up concerns for splanchnic hypoperfusion; however, studies have not clearly defined the extent of this risk.

21. **How may β-type natriuretic peptide aid in the management of end-stage congestive heart failure?**

    Although large, prospective randomized trials with nesiritide (β-type natriuretic peptide) have not yet been conducted, some initial data indicate that nesiritide may be beneficial for the management of precardiac transplant patients with increased pulmonary vascular resistance and renal failure. Indeed, β-type natriuretic peptide improves the hemodynamic profile, increases renal sodium excretion, and suppresses the renin-angiotensin-aldosterone system, improving clinical symptomatology.

22. **What is diastolic heart failure, and what management options are available?**

    Congestive heart failure in the presence of preserved left ventricular systolic function (ejection fraction [EF] > 35%) and in the absence of ischemia and valvular pathology suggests diastolic heart failure. Chronic management with angiotensin-converting enzyme (ACE) inhibitors is being evaluated in several large clinical trials with the premise that decreased aldosterone and angiotensin levels ameliorate deleterious collagen remodeling of the cardiac structure. Acute management is directed at alleviating diastolic dysfunction in the following ways: tempered reduction in heart rate with beta blockade may benefit preload-sensitive diastolic dysfunction, low-dose PDE inhibitors and L-type CCBs (dihydropyridines) may improve cellular myocardial relaxation, and nitrates may improve symptomatology in certain volume-overloaded cases of diastolic dysfunction.

23. **What are the clinical indications and current evidence for using dopamine?**

    There is now scientific evidence that low-dose dopamine is ineffective for prevention and treatment of acute kidney injury and for protection of the gut. It may be apparent that low-dose dopamine, in addition to not achieving the preset goal of organ protection, may also be deleterious because it can induce renal failure in normovolemic and hypovolemic patients. Dopamine also suppresses the secretion and function of anterior pituitary hormones, thereby aggravating catabolism and cellular immune dysfunction and inducing central hypothyroidism. In addition, dopamine blunts the ventilatory drive, increasing the risk of respiratory failure in patients who are being weaned from mechanical ventilation. Recent observational trials seem to indicate an increased mortality in septic patients treated with dopamine, whereas similar patients treated with norepinephrine did not demonstrate this mortality risk. However, in patients with renal failure who require high-dose furosemide, low-dose dopamine could be useful in combination with low-dose furosemide. Based on current meta-analysis (lacking good, prospective randomized data), dopamine is now considered a fourth-line agent for cardiogenic, septic, or vasodilatory shock.

24. **Describe the new inotropic agent levosimendan, including its mechanism of action and its role in clinical therapy.**

Levosimendan is a pyridazinone-dinitrite drug, placed in a new class of pharmaceutical agents. The "calcium drug" acts to increase contractility without elevating intramyocardial calcium levels. This is achieved by stabilizing troponin C in an active form, thus providing inotropic support in similar fashion to other agents, but with much lower intracellular calcium requirements. It increases systolic force while maintaining coronary perfusion via coronary artery vasodilation, along with mild systemic and pulmonary vasodilation. It can be used synergistically with β-adrenergic agents and seems to have a low arrhythmogenic potential.

Numerous trials with this agent have shown success, but more randomized trials are needed. Infusion durations in current studies only reach 24 hours, limiting long-term use. Levosimendan performs as well, if not better, in patients with congestive heart failure when compared with dobutamine. In patients undergoing cardiac surgery, the combination of dobutamine and levosimendan resulted in better maintenance of stroke volume following bypass than dobutamine and milrinone combined. Based on current evidence, recommended dosing is to start with <36-µg/kg bolus followed by a 0.4-µg/kg/min infusion.

25. **What mechanism of action accounts for the inotropic effect of thyroid hormone?**

Thyroid hormone affects chronic changes in protein synthesis, such as alterations of nuclear synthetic machinery, structural changes of the myosin heavy chains while downregulating the B-isoform, and increasing expression of β-adrenergic receptors. In addition, more immediate augmentation of contractility occurs secondary to an increase in mitochondrial respiration and adenosine triphosphate (ATP) production. This enhances function of sarcolemmal Ca-ATPase through the inhibitory effect of phospholamban on sarcoplasmic reticulum, as well as augmented sodium entry into myocytes. Elevated intracellular sodium levels increase intracellular calcium concentration and activity. Thyroid hormone also acutely reduces peripheral vascular resistance by promoting relaxation in vascular smooth-muscle cells.

KEY POINTS: INOTROPES AND VASODILATOR DRUGS

1. Congestive heart failure with preserved left ventricular systolic function (EF > 35%) in the absence of ischemia and valvular pathology suggests diastolic heart failure.
2. Vasopressin has a role in blood pressure maintenance in septic shock, cardiogenic shock, and other shock states.
3. Beneficial effects of nitroglycerin and other nitrates in anginal therapy result from a reduction in MVO_2, improved coronary perfusion, and platelet effects.
4. Nicardipine and clevidipine are fast-acting CCB agents with a nearly ideal hemodynamic profile for many cardiac patients with hypertension. They act by reducing afterload, increasing coronary blood flow, and improving myocardial oxygen balance.
5. Because of its narrow therapeutic ratio and adverse interactions with fluid and electrolyte shifts, digitalis is rarely used intraoperatively as an inotrope.
6. There is now scientific evidence that low-dose dopamine is ineffective for prevention and treatment of acute renal failure and for protection of the gut, and that dopamine in general is not an effective treatment for septic shock.
7. Levosimendan is a newer agent that shows promise in the treatment of heart failure and cardiogenic shock following cardiac surgery.

SUGGESTED READINGS

Kikura M, Levy J: New cardiac drugs, Int Anesthisiol Clin 33:21–37, 1995.
Leone M, Martin C: Vasopressor use in septic shock: an update, Curr Opin Anaesthesiol 21:141–147, 2008.
McKinlay KH, Schinderle DB, Swaminathan M, et al: Predictors of inotrope use during separation from cardiopulmonary bypass, J Cardiothorac Vasc Anesth 18:404–408, 2004.

Merin RG: Positive inotropic drugs and ventricular function. In Warltier DC, editor: Ventricular function, Baltimore, 1995, Lippincott Williams & Wilkins, pp 181–212.

Ouzounian M, Lee DS, Liu PP: Diastolic heart failure: mechanisms and controversies, Nat Clin Pract Cardiovasc Med 5:375–386, 2008.

Raja SG, Rayen BS: Levosimendan in cardiac surgery: best available evidence, Ann Thorac Surg 81: 1536–1546, 2006.

Tobias JD: Nicardipine: applications in anesthesia practice, J Clin Anesth 7:525–533, 1995.

Treschan TA, Peters J: The vasopressin system, Anesthesiology 105:599–612, 2006.

Troncy E, Francoeur M, Blaise G: Inhaled nitric oxide: clinical applications, indications, and toxicology, Can J Anaesth 44:973–988, 1997.

Venkataraman R: Can we prevent acute kidney injury? Crit Care Med 36(4):S166–S171, 2008.

Warltier DC: Beta-adrenergic-blocking drugs, Anesthesiology 88:2–5, 1998.

Whitten CW, Latson TW, Klein KW, et al: Anesthetic management of a hypothyroid cardiac surgical patient, J Cardiothorac Anesth 5:156–159, 1991.

CHAPTER 16

PREOPERATIVE MEDICATION

James C. Duke, MD, MBA

1. **List the major goals of premedication.**

   Premedication needs to be tailored to the needs of the individual patient. Important goals include:
   - Sedation and anxiolysis
   - Analgesia and amnesia
   - Antisialagogue effect
   - To maintain hemodynamic stability, including decrease in autonomic response
   - To prevent and/or minimize the impact of aspiration
   - To decrease postoperative nausea and vomiting
   - Prophylaxis against allergic reaction

2. **List the most commonly used preoperative medications with the appropriate dose.**

   See Table 16-1.

3. **What factors should be considered in selecting premedication for a patient?**
   - Patient age and weight
   - Physical status
   - Levels of anxiety and pain
   - Previous history of drug use or abuse
   - History of postoperative nausea, vomiting, or motion sickness
   - Drug allergies
   - Elective or emergency surgery
   - Inpatient or outpatient status

4. **What factors limit the ability to give depressant medications preoperatively?**
   - Extremes of age
   - Head injuries or altered mental status
   - Limited cardiac or pulmonary reserve
   - Hypovolemia
   - Full stomach

5. **What is meant by psychological premedication?**

   Most patients are very anxious before surgery. An informative and comforting visit by an anesthesiologist may replace many milligrams of depressant medication and acts as psychological premedication. During this visit, a full description of the planned anesthetic events to anticipate in the perioperative period should be provided to the patient and family members, and all questions the patient or family may have should be answered. However, psychological preparation cannot accomplish everything and will not relieve all anxiety.

6. **Discuss the role of benzodiazepines in premedication.**

   Benzodiazepines are the most popular drugs used for premedication. They act on receptors for the inhibitory neurotransmitter, γ-aminobutyric acid, producing anxiolysis, amnesia, and sedation at doses that do not produce significant cardiovascular or ventilatory depression. These drugs are not analgesic and are not associated with nausea and vomiting. Side effects of benzodiazepines include excessive and prolonged sedation in occasional patients, especially with lorazepam. Sometimes paradoxical agitation, rather than anxiolysis, may result from taking these drugs. The most commonly used benzodiazepine in current practice is midazolam, administered intravenously in small incremental doses in the immediate preoperative period. Diazepam is associated with pain on intramuscular or intravenous injection and increased risk of phlebitis.

Table 16-1. Common Preoperative Medications, Route, Dose, and Purpose*

MEDICATION	ROUTE OF ADMINISTRATION	DOSE (MG)	PURPOSE
Diazepam	Oral, IV	5–10	Sedation
Midazolam	IV	1–2	Sedation
Morphine	IV	2–10	Analgesia
Meperidine	IM	25–100	Analgesia
Ranitidine	Oral, IV	150 and 50, respectively	Decrease gastric pH
Metoclopramide	Oral, IV	5–20	Gastrokinetic
Omeprazole	Oral	20	Proton pump inhibitor
Pantoprazole	IV	40	Proton pump inhibitor
Glycopyrrolate	IV	0.1–0.3	Weak sedative, antisialagogue
Scopolamine	IM, IV	0.3–0.6	Sedative, antisialagogue
Promethazine†	IM	25–50	Antiemetic
Ketamine	IM, oral	1–2 mg/kg and 6 mg/kg, respectively	Sedation

*Potent medications should always be titrated to effect.
†FDA black box warning against use in children younger than 2 years old.
FDA, Food and Drug Administration; IM, intramuscular; IV, intravenous.

7. List the most common side effects when opioids are used as premedication.

Pruritus   Histamine release
Nausea and vomiting   Delayed gastric emptying
Respiratory depression   Stiff chest syndrome
Orthostatic hypotension   Sphincter of Oddi spasm

8. Describe the reasons to include an anticholinergic agent in premedication.
   The main indications for these drugs include the following:
   • Drying of airway secretions. They are particularly useful for intraoral or airway surgery, before applying topical anesthesia to the airway, and for general anesthesia with endotracheal intubation.
   • Prevention of reflex bradycardia when vagal overactivity is anticipated, particularly during pediatric anesthetic induction and airway manipulation. Atropine or glycopyrrolate can best be given intravenously just before anticipated vagal stimulation.
   • Sedative and amnestic effect. Being tertiary amines, scopolamine and atropine can cross the blood-brain barrier and produce sedation and amnesia. In this regard, scopolamine is about 8 to 10 times as potent as atropine. Glycopyrrolate is a quaternary amine, does not cross the blood-brain barrier, and therefore is devoid of appreciable sedative effect.

9. Summarize the effects of commonly used anticholinergic agents.
   See Table 16-2.

10. List the common side effects of anticholinergic medications.
    • Drying and thickening of airway secretions
    • Decrease in lower esophageal sphincter tone
    • Mydriasis and cycloplegia
    • Central nervous system toxicity
    • Prevention of sweating
    • Hyperthermia

Table 16-2. Effects of Commonly Used Anticholinergic Agents

EFFECT	ATROPINE	SCOPOLAMINE	GLYCOPYRROLATE
Tachycardia	++	+	++
Antisialagogue effect	+	+++	++
Sedation, amnesia	+	+++	0
Central nervous system toxicity	+	++	0
Lower esophageal sphincter relaxation	++	++	++
Mydriasis and cycloplegia	+	+++	0

0, None; +, mild; ++, moderate; +++, marked.

11. A patient in the preoperative holding area is delirious after receiving only 0.4 mg of scopolamine as a premedication. What is the cause of the delirium? How is it managed?

   The most likely cause of the delirium is central anticholinergic syndrome produced by scopolamine. Central toxicity can follow the administration of tertiary amine scopolamine (and, less frequently, following atropine), which crosses the blood-brain barrier. The toxic symptoms are infrequent following the usual premedication dose. However, elderly patients are more prone to this side effect. Physostigmine is the only acetylcholinesterase inhibitor that crosses the blood-brain barrier and can be used to treat the central anticholinergic syndrome in a dose of 15 to 60 mcg/kg intravenously, administered slowly to prevent seizures.

12. How does the concern for aspiration pneumonitis influence the choice of premedication?

   Aspiration is discussed more fully in Chapter 13. The actual incidence of clinically significant aspiration pneumonitis is extremely rare in healthy patients having elective surgery. In the past, many anesthesiologists routinely administered pharmacologic agents such as H_2 antagonists, antacids, and gastrokinetics in an attempt to reduce the volume and increase the pH of the gastric contents of their patients in the preoperative period. In view of the extremely low incidence of clinically significant aspiration pneumonitis in healthy patients having elective surgery, *routine* and *indiscriminate* use of antacids, gastric acid secretion blockers, antiemetics, anticholinergics, and gastrokinetic medications is not warranted.

KEY POINTS: PREOPERATIVE MEDICATION

1. A preoperative visit by an informative and reassuring anesthesiologist provides useful psychological preparation and calms the patient's fears and anxiety before anesthesia.
2. The choice of premedication depends on the physical and mental status of the patient, whether the patient is an inpatient or outpatient, whether the surgery is elective or emergent, and whether the patient has a history of postoperative nausea and vomiting.
3. The risk of clinically significant aspiration pneumonitis in healthy patients having elective surgery is very low. Routine use of pharmacologic agents to alter the volume or pH of gastric contents is unnecessary.
4. In patients considered to be at increased risk of pulmonary aspiration, a 15- to 30-ml oral dose of nonparticulate acid given 15 to 30 minutes before induction of anesthesia is the most effective way to raise gastric pH above 2.5.
5. Many patients require little or no premedication.
6. Pediatric patients are especially prone to bradycardia during anesthesia and benefit from anticholinergic premedication.

13. **Is it safe to allow patients to drink some water to swallow preoperative medications?**

    Yes, it is acceptable to allow patients to take preoperative medications, including the patient's usual medications, with up to 150 ml of water in the hour preceding induction of anesthesia.

14. **What are the differences between premedication of pediatric versus adult patients?**

    Pediatric patients have the following special needs:
    - They are more difficult to prepare psychologically for surgery and anesthesia.
    - There is greater emphasis on the oral route of administration because most children fear needles.
    - Vagolytics are used more frequently because of a greater incidence of bradycardia on induction.

15. **How does the age of pediatric patients influence premedication?**

    Children up to 6 months of age do not appear to suffer anxiety when separated from parents. However, preschool children older than 6 months are at greatest risk of separation anxiety and may suffer long-term psychological trauma from a negative hospital experience. It is difficult to reassure and explain the expected events to this group. It is easier to communicate with patients older than 5 years, who can be reassured. Parental behavior is also important in the psychological preparation of pediatric patients. The needs of each patient must be assessed individually. Most children older than 1 year benefit from some sedative premedication. Oral midazolam (0.5 mg/kg dissolved in flavored syrup, to a maximum dosage of 20 mg) is commonly used. Atropine may be given intravenously once venous access has been obtained, just before airway manipulation, which can provoke vagal reflexes.

16. **Describe the preoperative management of a morbidly obese patient with a difficult airway. Assume that the patient is otherwise healthy.**

    A morbidly obese patient is considered at increased risk of pulmonary aspiration during induction of anesthesia because of delayed gastric emptying and the possibility of difficult airway management. Therefore H_2 blockers given the evening before (if possible) and the morning of surgery, preoperative metoclopramide, and oral nonparticulate antacids are in order. Glycopyrrolate is useful for planned fiberoptic intubation. It improves visualization by drying secretions, increases the effectiveness of the topical anesthesia, and decreases airway responsiveness. Opioids and benzodiazepines should be judiciously titrated, using supplemental oxygen and close observation to ensure an awake, appropriately responding patient who can protect his or her own airway.

SUGGESTED READINGS

Dotson R, Wiener-Kronish JP, Ajayi T: Preoperative evaluation and medication. In Stoelting RK, Miller RD, editors: Basics of anesthesia, ed 5, New York, 2007, Churchill Livingstone, pp 157–177.

Kararmaz A, Kaya S, Turhanoglu S, et al: Oral ketamine premedication can prevent emergence agitation in children after desflurane anaesthesia, Paediatr Anaesth 14:477–482, 2004.

3 PREPARING FOR ANESTHESIA

PREOPERATIVE EVALUATION

James C. Duke, MD, MBA, and Mark Chandler, MD

CHAPTER 17

1. What are the goals of the preoperative evaluation?

The preoperative evaluation consists of gathering information about the patient and formulating an anesthetic plan. The overall objective is a smooth anesthetic without perioperative morbidity and mortality.

2. Discuss the important features of the preoperative evaluation.

The anesthesiologist should review the surgical plan. Medical records review and focused physical examination are essential. Include allergies, medications, herbal supplements, drugs of abuse, review of systems, and prior anesthetic problems (e.g., difficult intubation, delayed emergence, malignant hyperthermia, prolonged neuromuscular blockade, or postoperative nausea and vomiting). There may be concerning features that warrant specialty consultation.

3. What is the physical status classification of the American Society of Anesthesiologist (ASA)?

The ASA classification was created in 1940 for the purposes of statistical studies and hospital records. It is useful both for outcome comparisons and as a means of communicating the physical status of a patient. Unfortunately it is imprecise and is a subject of disagreement. Finally, a higher ASA class only roughly predicts anesthetic risk. The six classes are:

- Class 1: A normal healthy patient
- Class 2: A patient with mild systemic disease
- Class 3: A patient with severe systemic disease
- Class 4: A patient with severe systemic disease that is a constant threat to life
- Class 5: A moribund patient who is not expected to survive without the operation
- Class 6: A declared brain-dead patient whose organs are being removed for donor purposes

Add an "E" for any unplanned or emergent procedure.

4. What are the features of informed consent?

The anesthetic must be conveyed, thorough, and in terms the patient understands. Often a translator is needed for a patient who speaks a foreign language. Include also cultural sensitivities.

5. Review appropriate pediatric fasting periods.

See Table 17-1. Current guidelines for pediatric patients include:

- Clear liquids up to 2 hours before surgery
- Breast milk up to 4 hours before surgery
- Solid foods, including nonhuman milk and formula, up to 6 hours before surgery

Guidelines may be modified if the child has gastrointestinal or airway concerns.

6. What are the appropriate preoperative laboratory tests?

No evidence supports the use of routine laboratory testing. Rather, there is support for the use of selected laboratory analysis based on the patient's circumstances (Table 17-2). Chest radiographs are rarely indicated. Chemistries should be drawn if electrolyte abnormalities are suspected. Patients with diabetes should have glucose checks. Hemoglobin and hematocrit values are reviewed if the patient appears anemic or if blood loss is anticipated. Coagulation studies are a function of history or bleeding stigmata.

Table 17-1. General Preoperative Fasting Recommendations

INGESTED MATERIAL	MINIMUM FASTING PERIOD (HOURS)
Clear liquids (e.g., water, fruit juices without pulp, carbonated beverages, clear tea and black coffee; clear liquids should not include alcohol)	2
Breast milk	4
Infant formula	6
Nonhuman milk	6
Light meal (a light meal typically consists of toast and clear liquids)	6
Full, heavy, fatty meal	8

Table 17-2. Appropriate Preoperative Laboratory Tests Based on Patient History and Physical Examination*

TEST	INDICATIONS
Electrocardiogram	Cardiac and circulatory disease, respiratory disease, advanced age[†]
Chest radiograph	Chronic lung disease, history of congestive heart disease
Pulmonary function tests	Reactive airway disease, chronic lung disease, restrictive lung disease
Hemoglobin/ hematocrit	Advanced age,[†] anemia, bleeding disorders, other hematologic disorders
Coagulation studies	Bleeding disorders, liver dysfunction, anticoagulants
Serum chemistries	Endocrine disorders, medications, renal dysfunction
Pregnancy test	Uncertain pregnancy history, history suggestive of current pregnancy

*At least 50% of the task force experts agreed that the listed tests were beneficial when used selectively. Because of a lack of solid evidence in the literature, these indications are somewhat broad and vague and limit the clinical use of the guidelines.

[†]The definition of advanced age is vague and should be considered in the context of that patient's overall health.

7. **What is the generally accepted minimum hemoglobin or hematocrit (H/H) for elective surgery?**
   It depends on the clinical setting. Surgeries without significant blood loss do not add any value. However, elderly anemic patients often have a poorer functional status, longer hospitalizations, and higher 1-year mortality.

8. **When are consultations indicated?**
   Specialty consultations are indicated when history, physical examination and other diagnostic data require specialty expertise to further risk stratify patients undergoing anesthesia. Cardiac consultations are probably most frequent, due in large part to the ambiguous nature of the symptoms of myocardial ischemia.

9. **What are the clinical risk factors for a major perioperative cardiac event?**
   The Revised Cardiac Risk Index (Box 17-1) has six components:
   • High-risk surgical procedures
   • History of ischemic heart disease

Box 17-1. Revised Cardiac Risk Index

Each of the following six risk factors is assigned one point.
1. **High-risk surgical procedures**
   Intraperitoneal
   Intrathoracic
   Suprainguinal vascular
2. **History of ischemic heart disease**
   History of myocardial infarction
   History of positive exercise test
   Current complaint of chest pain considered secondary to myocardial ischemia
   Use of nitrate therapy
   Electrocardiogram with pathologic Q waves
3. **History of congestive heart failure**
   Pulmonary edema
   Paroxysmal nocturnal dyspnea
   Bilateral rales or S3 gallop
   Chest radiograph showing pulmonary vascular redistribution
4. **History of cerebrovascular disease**
   History of transient ischemic attack or stroke
5. **Preoperative treatment with insulin**
6. **Preoperative serum creatinine >2 mg/dl**

Risk of Major Cardiac Event

Points	Class	Risk
0	I	0.4%
1	II	0.9%
2	III	6.6%
3 or more	IV	11%

Major cardiac events include myocardial infarction, pulmonary edema, ventricular fibrillation, primary cardiac arrest, and complete heart block.

- History of congestive heart failure
- History of cerebrovascular disease
- Preoperative treatment with insulin
- Elevated preoperative serum creatinine

The patient is assigned one point for each of these risk factors, which are then translated into percentage risks of perioperative major cardiac events such as myocardial infarction, pulmonary edema, ventricular fibrillation, primary cardiac arrest, and complete heart block.

10. What are active cardiac conditions?
Active cardiac conditions are serious cardiac conditions that warrant immediate evaluation and treatment before undergoing surgery. There are four active cardiac conditions:
- Unstable coronary syndromes, which include unstable or severe angina and recent myocardial infarction
- Decompensated heart failure
- Significant arrhythmias such as symptomatic ventricular arrhythmias, high-grade atrioventricular block, and symptomatic bradycardia
- Severe valvular disease such as symptomatic mitral stenosis or severe aortic stenosis

11. Are there ways of predicting postoperative pulmonary complications?
Among the most common risk factors for postoperative pulmonary complications (PPCs) are chronic obstructive pulmonary disease and advanced age. Observed PPC abnormalities rarely result in postoperative mortality; thus most surgeries may be performed even when these risk factors are present (Table 17-3).

Table 17-3. Risk Factors for Postoperative Pulmonary Complications

PREOPERATIVE RISK FACTORS	INTRAOPERATIVE RISK FACTORS
COPD	Site of surgery
Age	General anesthesia
Inhaled tobacco use	Pancuronium use
NYHA class II pulmonary hypertension	Duration of surgery
OSA	Emergency surgery
Nutrition status	

COPD, Chronic obstructive pulmonary disease; NYHA, New York Heart Association; OSA, obstructive sleep apnea.
From the New York Heart Association (NYHA).

Indications for pulmonary function testing are addressed in Chapter 9

KEY POINTS: PREOPERATIVE EVALUATION

1. Preoperative laboratory testing should be selective and individualized.
2. Current ACC/AHA guidelines for cardiac testing prior to noncardiac procedures are the gold standard for preoperative cardiac risk assessment.
3. The most important preanesthetic evaluation includes a thorough, accurate, and focused history and physical examination.
4. A patient's baseline hemoglobin tends to predict the need for transfusion when large blood loss occurs.
5. The four active cardiac conditions that will likely result in surgical cancellation to assess cardiac evaluation and treatment are unstable coronary syndrome, decompensated heart failure, significant cardiac arrhythmias, and severe valvular disease.
6. Before halting a patient's anticoagulation, one must consider the type and urgency of surgery, the possibility and consequences of intraoperative hemorrhage, and the reason why the patient is anticoagulated

12. **What benefits and risks are associated with preoperative cigarette cessation? How long before surgery must a patient quit smoking to realize any health benefits?**
   Patients randomized to receive an intervention to help them stop smoking 6 to 8 weeks before surgery saw a dramatic decrease in the overall complication rate in the smoking cessation group, mainly from diminished wound infections. The longer a patient can abstain from smoking before surgery, the greater the perioperative health benefit will be: bronchociliary function improves within 2 to 3 days of cessation, and sputum volume decreases to normal levels within about 2 weeks.

13. **For patients scheduled for noncardiac surgery, what are guidelines for perioperative cardiac evaluation?**
   An algorithmic approach to perioperative cardiac evaluation in patients who will undergo noncardiac surgery requires assessment of a patient's cardiac risks before surgery, taking into account the urgency of surgery, the presence of *active cardiac conditions*, the invasiveness of the planned surgery, the patient's functional status, and the presence of *clinical risk factors* for ischemic heart disease. Taken together, this algorithm underscores the importance of a history focused on cardiac issues for all surgical patients.

14. **What are the clinical risk factors for a major perioperative cardiac event?**
   The Revised Cardiac Risk Index (see Box 17-1) has six components: surgical risk, history of ischemic heart disease, history of congestive heart failure, history of cerebrovascular disease, preoperative treatment with insulin, and elevated preoperative serum creatinine. The

patient is assigned one point for each of these risk factors, which are then translated into percentage risks of perioperative major cardiac events such as myocardial infarction, pulmonary edema, ventricular fibrillation, primary cardiac arrest, and complete heart block.

15. **What constitutes the basic laboratory evaluation of coagulation status?**
The basic laboratory evaluation includes platelet count, prothrombin time (PT), partial thromboplastin time (PTT), and thrombin time. Thromboelastography is growing as a methodology. Thromboelastography measures the combined function of platelets and coagulation factors. The minimal number of normally functioning platelets to prevent surgical bleeding is 50,000/mm^3. Both the PT and PTT require about a 60% to 80% loss of coagulation activity before becoming abnormal, but patients with smaller decreases in function can still have significant surgical bleeding. Therefore the history is still very important.

16. **Are there special anesthetic considerations for surgical patients on warfarin?**
Warfarin is a vitamin K antagonist and is used to prevent thrombosis and emboli. A patient on warfarin is at high risk for intraoperative bleeding. Before stopping a patient's warfarin, it is important to know the indication for anticoagulation, the type and urgency of the surgery, and the consequences of intraoperative bleeding. Patients who are at very high risk of thromboembolism but nonetheless need to discontinue their anticoagulant (e.g., warfarin) in the perioperative setting are often bridged with low-molecular-weight heparin, another much shorter-acting anticoagulant. Because warfarin has such a long half-life (about 2.5 days) and heparin has such a short half-life (about 1.5 hours), a patient may be instructed to stop warfarin 4 days before surgery and then, often as an inpatient, undergo regular heparin injections up until a few hours before surgery. Once the surgery is completed (and depending on the postoperative bleeding risk), the warfarin can be restarted.

17. **What are considerations for patients with coronary stents?**
Coronary stents, small metal mesh tubes that maintain patency of stenosed coronary arteries, fall into two broad categories: bare metal stents and drug-eluting stents. The latter slowly release a chemical that helps prevent endothelialization. An ongoing debate among cardiologists is how long after stent placement a patient should remain anticoagulated. This anticoagulation issue adds considerably to the complexity of recommending cardiac workups for patients undergoing surgery. Patients with recent stent placement should not undergo surgery right away because delays in anticoagulants are known to precipitate acute myocardial infarctions.

18. **Why is it necessary to evaluate patients for obstructive sleep apnea (OSA) before surgery, and how should OSA be identified?**
Patients with OSA are known to have increased postoperative morbidity. Identifying those at risk remains a challenge despite an OSA diagnosis. Several screening tools (e.g., STOP-Bang, Berlin, and Flemons questionnaires) continue to challenge anesthesiologists regarding appropriate postoperative disposition.

SUGGESTED READINGS

Practice Advisory for Preanesthesia Evaluation: An Updated Report by the American Society of Anesthesiologists Task Force on Preanesthesia Evaluation, Anesthesiology 116(3):522–538, 2012.

Chung F, Yegneswaran B, Liao P, et al: Validation of the Berlin questionnaire and American Society of Anesthesiologists checklist as screening tools for OSA in surgical patients, Anesthesiology 108:822–830, 2008.

Eagle KA, Berger PB, Calkins H, et al: ACC/AHA Guideline update for perioperative cardiac evaluation for noncardiac surgery, Anesth Analg 94:1052–1064, 2002.

Gall B, Whalen FX, Schroder DR, et al: Identification of patients at risk for postoperative respiratory complications using a preoperative OSA screening tool and post-anesthesia care assessment, Anesthesiology 110:869–877, 2009.

Møller AM, Villebro N, Pedersen T, et al: 2002 Effect of preoperative smoking intervention on postoperative complications: a randomised clinical trial, Lancet 359:114–117, 2002.

Sweitzer BJ: Preoperative evaluation and medication. In Miller RD, Pardo MC, editors: Basics of anesthesia, ed 6, Philadelphia, 2011, Elsevier Saunders, pp 165–188.

Wijeysundera DM, Austin PC, Beattie WS, et al: Less is more. Outcomes and processes of care relate to preoperative consultation, Arch Intern Med 170:1365–1374, 2010.

CHAPTER 18

THE ANESTHESIA MACHINE AND VAPORIZERS, AND ANESTHESIA CIRCUITS AND VENTILATORS

James C. Duke MD, MBA

1. **What is an anesthesia machine?**

   A more modern and correct name for an anesthesia machine is an *anesthesia delivery system*. The job of the first anesthesia machines was to supply a mixture of anesthetizing and life-sustaining gases to the patient. A modern anesthesia delivery system performs these functions and also ventilates the patient and provides a number of monitoring functions. The most important purpose is to help the anesthesiologist keep the patient alive, safe, and adequately anesthetized. Anesthesia machines have become rather standardized. Currently there are two major manufacturers in the United States: Drager and Datex-Ohmeda.

2. **Describe the plumbing of an anesthesia machine to create an overview of its essential interconnections.**

   Leaving out the safety features and monitors, the anesthesia machine is divided into three sections:
   - A gas delivery system that supplies at its outlet a defined mixture of gases chosen by the anesthesiologist
   - The patient breathing system, which includes the patient breathing circuit, absorber head, ventilator, and often gas pressure and flow monitors
   - A scavenger system that collects excess gas and expels the gas outside the hospital, reducing the exposure of operating room personnel to anesthetic gases

3. **What gases are ordinarily available on all anesthesia machines, and what are their sources?**

   Oxygen (O_2) and nitrous oxide (N_2O) are available on almost every anesthesia machine. Most commonly, the third gas is air, but it can also be helium (He), heliox (a mixture of He and O_2), carbon dioxide (CO_2), or nitrogen (N_2). If the third gas does not contain O_2 (as do air and heliox), it is possible to deliver a (dangerous) hypoxic mixture to the patient.

   Usually the gas source for anesthesia machines in hospitals is from a centralized wall or pipeline supply. An emergency backup supply of gases is stored in tanks called E-cylinders attached to the rear of the anesthesia machine. These tanks should be checked daily to ensure that they contain an adequate backup supply in case of pipeline failure.

4. **Since the flow rates of N_2O and O_2 are controlled independently, can the machine be set to deliver a hypoxic mixture to the patient?**

   Different machine manufacturers have different ways of protecting the patient from hypoxic mixtures. The Drager's ORMC (oxygen ratio monitor and controller) senses the O_2 flow rate and controls N_2O flow pneumatically. Datex-Ohmeda's Link-25 system mechanically links the O_2 and N_2O flow knobs to ensure that the proportion of N_2O to O_2 remains in a safe range as the N_2O flow is increased.

5. **What is a *regulator*? How does it control the flow of gas?**

   O_2 and air in the E-cylinders are pressurized up to approximately 2200 psig, but the anesthesia machine needs to work with gas at an initial pressure of about 50 psig, slightly less than the pressure of the gas from the wall supply. A regulator performs this function. Each gas is regulated separately. Gas from both the cylinder and the wall supply encounters a check valve that selects the gas source with the highest pressure for use by the machine. Under normal circumstances, the wall supply is used preferentially, and the tank supply is spared for use if the wall supply fails.

6. **How does the hospital piped gas supply compare with the use of tank gas?**
   For practical purposes, wall gases are continuous in volume availability, as long as the central O_2 supply is refilled. Wall gas pressures are typically about 55 psig. Tank pressure is generally regulated by the first-stage regulator to 45 psig. The anesthesia machine preferentially chooses the source with the highest pressure. As long as everything is working correctly, the wall supply is used rather than the tank supply. Use of the wall supply oxygen is preferable because it is available in greater volume, is cheaper, and preserves the tank supply for use only in emergency situations.

7. **The hospital supply of oxygen is lost. The gauge on the O_2 tank reads 1000 psi. How long will you be able to deliver oxygen before the tanks are empty?**
   Contemporary anesthesia machines have two sources of gases: the wall outlet and E-cylinders attached to the machine itself. The cylinders are color coded and usually left shut off, being saved for use in an emergency, but a normally functioning anesthesia machine and normal wall outlet O_2 pressures will use the wall outlet preferentially.
   A full green E-cylinder of O_2 has a pressure of 2000 psi and contains about 625 L of O_2. Since the O_2 is a compressed gas, the volume in the tank correlates linearly with the pressure on the gauge. Therefore a pressure of 1000 psi means that the O_2 tank has about 312 L of gas left.
   In addition to providing for cellular respiration, oxygen is also used as the drive gas for powering the ventilator bellows. The amount of oxygen consumed during this function approximates the patient's minute ventilation. Thus, if a patient is receiving an O_2 flow of 2 L/min and a minute ventilation of 8 L/min, 10 L of O_2 will be drained from the oxygen tank every minute. A tank with 312 L remaining will last for 31 minutes at this rate. To reduce consumption of the tank oxygen, decrease the oxygen flow rate and hand-ventilate; also request that additional oxygen tanks be brought to the room.

8. **A new tank of N_2O is installed, and the pressure gauge reads only about 750 psig. Why is the pressure in the N_2O tank different from the pressures of other gases?**
   Air and O_2 are compressed gases and cannot be compressed to liquids in a room temperature environment because the critical temperature (the temperature at which a gas can be compressed into a liquid) is exceeded. However, at room temperature, N_2O condenses into a liquid at 747 psi. E-cylinders of N_2O contain the equivalent of about 1600 L of gas when full, whereas E-cylinders of O_2 and air hold only about 600 L. The pressure in the N_2O tank remains constant until the N_2O has been vaporized. About only a quarter of the initial volume of N_2O remains when the cylinder pressure drops, although accurate estimation would require weighing the cylinder, knowing the empty (tare) weight of the cylinder, and determining the moles of N_2O remaining.
   In contrast, because O_2 and air are compressed gases, the volume of gas remaining in an O_2 or air cylinder is directly proportional to the pressure. The pressure of a filled cylinder is 2200 psig. A pressure reading of 1100 would suggest that the tank is half-full or has about 300 L remaining.

9. **List the uses of O_2 in an anesthesia machine.**
   - Contributes to the fresh gas flow
   - Provides gas for the O_2 flush
   - Powers the low O_2 alarm
   - Controls the flow of N_2O
   - Powers the *fail-safe* valves
   - Is the driving gas for the ventilator

10. **Describe the safety systems used to prevent incorrect gas connections at the wall and cylinders.**
    - All wall supply gas connectors are keyed so only the O_2 supply hose can be plugged into the O_2 connector on the wall, the N_2O hose into the N_2O outlet, and so on. This is known as a Diameter Index Safety System (DISS).

- The gas cylinders are keyed using a Pin Index Safety System (PISS—no kidding) so that only the correct tank can be attached to the corresponding yolk on the anesthesia machine, *assuming that the pins have not been sheared off!*
- These safety systems should be backed up by a monitor that measures the delivered concentration of O_2 in a mixed gas. It is this monitor that is most critical in preventing delivery of a hypoxic gas mixture.

11. **In addition to the distinctions described previously, what other ways are gases distinguished to help prevent human error?**
   - First, the O_2 flow knob is distinctively fluted. Knobs for other gases are knurled.
   - Second, a color code exists such that each gas knob, flowmeter, tank, and wall attachment bears the corresponding color for its associated gas. In the United States O_2 is green, air is yellow, and N_2O is blue. International standards differ.

12. **There are two flowmeters for each gas on an anesthesia machine. Couldn't you safely get away with only one?**
   Two flowmeters are used to increase the range of flows over which an accurate measurement can be obtained. The flow tubes in anesthesia machines are always placed in series so all the gas flows sequentially through both tubes. To measure flows accurately in the ranges used for low flow or even closed-circuit anesthesia (200 to 1000 ml/min), two flow tubes are essential. Flowmeters, also known as *Thorpe tubes*, are also specific to the gas for which they have been designed and are not interchangeable with other gases.

13. **Why are the flowmeters for air, O_2, and N_2O arranged in a specific order?**
   Reasons include U.S. (National Institute for Occupational Safety and Health [NIOSH]) government standards, manufacturer's conventions, and safety. Requiring the O_2 knob to be in the same relative position on all anesthesia machines decreases the risk of the anesthesiologist turning the wrong knob. In the United States, the O_2 flowmeter must always be on the right, closest to the point of egress into the common gas manifold, just proximal to the anesthesia vaporizers. With the O_2 flowmeter in that position, most leaks tend to selectively lose gases other than O_2. This configuration is least likely to deliver a hypoxic gas mixture. Again, the best way to detect a hypoxic gas mixture is through use of an O_2 analyzer.

14. **What is meant by a fail-safe valve?**
   The fail-safe valve device is designed to cut off the flow of all gases except O_2 when the O_2 pressure falls below a set value, usually about 25 psig (Figure 18-1).

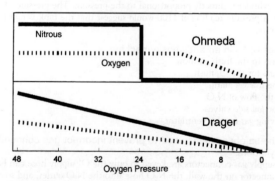

**Output when oxygen
pressure is lost**

Figure 18-1. Effect of fail-safe device and oxygen failure pressure device.

15. **Would it be safer to leave the tank O_2 supply on your machine turned on so, if the pipeline O_2 failed, the machine would automatically switch immediately to the backup tank supply?**

No. First, when all equipment is functioning properly, the disadvantage of leaving the tank on is that, if a failure in wall O_2 should occur, your machine will use gas from the tank, unknown to you. You may not recognize the problem until the machine (and tank) is totally out of O_2 and the low O_2 pressure alarm begins to sound. At this point you must scramble to find O_2 quickly.

The second reason allows for equipment failure, and there are two parts to the explanation:
1. When no gas is flowing, it is possible for pressure to be maintained in the gauge despite a leak where the tank is connected to the yolk. Thus it is possible to have a full indication on the pressure gauge and an empty tank. The pressure in the tank should be checked after the wall supply is disconnected and the system pressure bled down, and then the tank should be turned off.
2. If wall O_2 pressure drops too low, the tank could be drained, supplying the anesthesia machine rather than saving tank O_2 for emergencies. A second check valve prevents the tank O_2 from entering the wall supply plumbing if the wall supply fails. If this valve fails, the tank could, for the short period until the tank empties, backfill the hospital system, helping to supply O_2 to ward patients.

16. **How long can you continue to deliver O_2 when the wall supply fails?**

The E-cylinders that supply O_2 to most anesthesia machines hold 600 L when full. If the ventilator is not in use (remember that O_2 powers the ventilator), the O_2 flowmeter indicates how much O_2 is being used. With a flow of O_2 of 2 L/min, there is approximately 300 minutes (or 5 hours) of O_2 available. If the ventilator is in use, the additional gas required for this purpose is roughly equal to the ventilator minute volume, and the length of time the tank supply will last will be significantly decreased below the previously estimated 5 hours for a full tank. Manually ventilating the patient in this instance would preserve the oxygen supply. Reducing the oxygen flow would also extend the life of the tank.

17. **What physical principles are involved in the process of vaporization?**

The saturated vapor pressure of the volatile anesthetic, which varies with temperature, determines the concentration of vapor molecules above the liquid anesthetic. The heat of vaporization is the energy required to release molecules of a liquid into the gaseous phase. The liquid phase draws external heat during vaporization, or it will become cooler as molecules leave and enter the gaseous phase. To address this problem, vaporizers are constructed of metals with high thermal conductivity. High thermal conductivity ensures that there is a conduit of heat so the heat required for vaporization is constantly restored from the environment and the rate of vaporization of the volatile anesthetic is independent of changes in the temperature of the vaporizer.

18. **What does it mean when it is said that a vaporizer has variable bypass? What is the effect of having such a vaporizer turned on its side?**

The vaporizers are located downstream from the flowmeters. Fresh gas from the flowmeters enters the vaporizer and is divided into two streams. Most of the gas enters the bypass chamber and is not exposed to the volatile agent. The remaining gas enters the vaporizing chamber and becomes saturated with anesthetic. The concentration dial determines the proportion of gas flow that enters each of the two streams. These then reunite near the vaporizer outlet. The fresh gas leaving the vaporizer contains a concentration of vapor specified by the concentration dial.

If a variable bypass vaporizer is turned on its side, liquid anesthetic may spill from the vaporizing chamber to the bypass chamber, effectively creating two vaporizing chambers and increasing vaporizer output. This could create toxic levels of volatile anesthetic being delivered to the patient. However, most (but not all) modern vaporizers have mechanisms minimizing this effect.

19. **What does temperature compensation mean?**

During vaporization the liquid anesthetic will cool, drawing heat from the metal of the vaporizer, which draws heat from the operating room. As liquid anesthetic cools, the saturated vapor pressure decreases, as does vaporizer output. Temperature compensation means the vaporizer has mechanisms for adjusting the output to compensate for temperature.

20. **What is the pumping effect?**
Positive pressure can be transmitted back into the vaporizer during ventilation of the patient. The positive pressure can briefly cause gas to reverse flow within the vaporizer, allowing gas to periodically reenter the vaporizing chamber. The result of the pumping effect is increased vaporizer output beyond that indicated on the concentration dial. Modern vaporizers have mechanisms to reduce but not eliminate the pumping effect.

21. **How does altitude affect modern vaporizers?**
The effect of the change in barometric pressure on volume percent output can be calculated as follows: $x' = x (p/p')$, where x' is the output in volume percent at the new altitude (p'), and x is the concentration output in volume percent for the altitude (p), when the vaporizer is calibrated. Consider the following example: A vaporizer is calibrated at sea level ($p = 760$ mm Hg), taken to Denver, Colorado (5280 ft [~1609 m]) ($p' = 630$ mm Hg), and set to deliver 1% isoflurane vapor (x). The actual output (x') is 1% (760/630) = 1.2%. Remember that partial pressure of the vapor, and not the concentration in volume percent, is the important factor in depth of anesthesia. Note that 1% at sea level (760 mm Hg) is 7.6 mm Hg and that 1.2% in Denver (630 mm Hg) is 7.6 mm Hg; thus, regardless of altitude, the clinical effect is unchanged.

22. **What happens if you put the wrong agent in a vaporizer calibrated for another agent?**
The incorrect agent in an agent-specific vaporizer typically delivers either an overdose or underdose. The most important factor in determining the direction of error is the vapor pressure or the agent. If an agent with a high vapor pressure is put into a vaporizer meant for a less volatile agent, the output will be excessive. If an agent with a vapor pressure lower than the agent intended for the vaporizer is accidentally used, the anesthetic output will be lower than anticipated. Increasingly, vaporizers and bottles of volatile anesthetics are keyed to prevent incorrect addition of volatile anesthetics into vaporizers.

23. **What is different about the desflurane vaporizer?**
Desflurane has a vapor pressure of 664 mm Hg at 20° C. In other words, the boiling point of this agent is approximately at room temperature. Desflurane is also less potent than other common agents (minimum alveolar concentration [MAC] = 6%), and up to 18% volume percent may be delivered. Passively vaporizing this volume of agent will result in large temperature variations that require compensation. The desflurane vaporizer actively heats the liquid agent to 39° C. At this temperature the vapor pressure of the agent is approximately 2 atmospheres. This has proven a practical means of accurately delivering an anesthetic with such a high vapor pressure.

24. **What prevents turning on two vaporizers simultaneously?**
Modern anesthesia machines have an interlock system or an interlocking manifold that allows only one vaporizer to be turned on at a time. However, in anesthesia machines that allow for three vaporizers, the center spot must be occupied or the interlocking manifold will not be operational.

25. **At an altitude of 7000 feet, you have to set the vaporizer to deliver more desflurane than you would expect given the published MAC of that agent. Explain why this does not happen with vaporizers for other anesthetic agents.**
Conventional vaporizers (for halothane, isoflurane, and sevoflurane) are altitude compensated. The altitude compensation occurs because the diverting valve is functionally located at the outlet of the vaporizer, a variation in design that minimizes the pumping and pressurizing effects. The output of these vaporizers is a constant partial pressure of agent, not a constant volume percent. The desflurane vaporizer does not divert a portion of the fresh gas flow through a vaporizing chamber but rather adds vapor to the gas flow to produce a true volume percent output. Because it is the number of molecules of agent (the partial pressure) that anesthetizes the patient, conventional vaporizers provide the same anesthetizing power at any altitude. The desflurane vaporizer delivers the set volume percent regardless of altitude, which

represents a partial pressure (anesthetizing power) that is 24% less than the same concentration at sea level. Thus a correspondingly higher percentage of desflurane must be delivered to achieve MAC at 7000 feet.

26. **A patient with malignant hyperthermia needs to be anesthetized. Should the vaporizers be removed from the anesthesia machine?**

    Datex-Ohmeda vaporizers are easily removed simply by releasing a latch and lifting the vaporizer from the machine. On the Drager anesthesia machines, it is necessary to remove two Allen screws to release the vaporizers. Then, unless the vaporizer is being replaced by a second one, it is necessary to install a bypass block to the empty vaporizer slot. These tasks are easily accomplished by anyone capable of manipulating an Allen wrench, but Drager recommends that their vaporizers be changed only by authorized service personnel. However, flushing the machine with oxygen for several minutes should remove all of the agent (except from rubber parts in the absorber and circle). The anesthesia provider should ensure that the user of the machine cannot accidentally turn on a vaporizer.

KEY POINTS: THE ANESTHESIA MACHINE AND VAPORIZERS

1. Anesthesia machines are an integrated system that not only delivers anesthetic gases but also monitors both itself and the patient.
2. When compressed, some gases (N_2O and CO_2) condense into a liquid and some (O_2 and N_2) do not. These properties define the relationship between tank volume and pressure.
3. Anesthesia machines must have a backup supply of oxygen in case the wall oxygen fails.
4. Flowmeters accurately measure only the gas for which they are explicitly calibrated.
5. The output of traditional vaporizers depends on the proportion of fresh gas that bypasses the vaporizing chamber compared with the proportion that passes through the vaporizing chamber.
6. The desflurane vaporizer actively injects vapor into the fresh gas stream, whereas all traditional vaporizers use a passive variable bypass system.

---

27. **What is a scavenger?**

    Except in a close-circuit situation, gas is always entering and leaving the anesthesia breathing circuit. The exhaust gas is a mixture of expired gas from the patient and fresh gas that exceeded the patient's needs but contains anesthetic agent. To reduce exposure of operating room personnel to trace amounts of anesthetic agents, it is appropriate to capture and expel this anesthetic-laden gas from the operating room environment. The device used to transfer this gas safely from the breathing circuit into the hospital vacuum system is called a *scavenger*. Because of the periodicity of breathing, gas exits the breathing circuit in puffs. The scavenger provides a reservoir for the exhaust gas until the exhaust or vacuum system, which works at a constant flow rate, can dispose of the gas. The scavenger must also prevent excess suction or an occlusion from affecting the patient breathing circuit. It does this by providing both positive and negative relief valves. Thus, if the vacuum system fails or is adjusted to too low a rate, back pressure exits through a positive-pressure relief valve. (Granted it contaminates the operating room, but that problem is minimal compared to blowing the patient's lungs up like a balloon.) If the vacuum is adjusted too high, a negative-pressure relief valve allows room air to mix with the exhaust gas, preventing buildup of more than a 2.5 mm Hg suction at the breathing circuit.

28. **What are the different types of anesthesia breathing circuits?**

    Breathing circuits are usually classified as open, semiopen, semiclosed, or closed. They include various components configured to allow the patient to breathe (or be ventilated) with a gas mixture that differs from room air.

29. **Give an example of an open circuit.**

    An open circuit is the method by which the first true anesthetics were given 160 years ago. A bit of cloth saturated with ether or chloroform was held over the patient's face. The patient breathed the vapors and became anesthetized. The depth of anesthesia was controlled by the amount of liquid anesthetic on the cloth; thus it took a great deal of trial and error to become good at the technique.

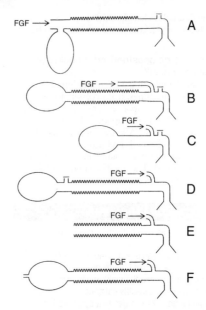

FGF

A

FGF

B

FGF

C

FGF

D

FGF

E

FGF

F

Figure 18-2. Mapleson A, B, C, D, E, and F circuits. *FGF*, Fresh gas flow. *(From Willis BA, Pender JW, Mapleson WW: Rebreathing in a T-piece.* Br J Anaesth *47:1239–1246, 1975, with permission.)*

30. Give an example of a semiopen circuit.

The various semiopen circuits were fully described by Mapleson and are commonly known as the Mapleson A, B, C, D, E, and F circuits (Figure 18-2). All have in common a source of fresh gas, corrugated tubing (more resistant to kinking), and a pop-off or adjustable pressure-limiting valve. Differences among the circuits include the locations of the pop-off valve, fresh gas input, and whether or not a gas reservoir bag is present. Advantages of the Mapleson series are simplicity of design, ability to change the depth of anesthesia rapidly, portability, and lack of rebreathing of exhaled gases (provided the fresh gas flow is adequate). Disadvantages include lack of conservation of heat and moisture, limited ability to scavenge waste gases, and high requirements for fresh gas flow. Semiopen circuits are rarely used today except for patient transport.

31. Give an example of a semiclosed circuit.

The prototypical semiclosed circuit is the circle system, which is found in most operating rooms in the United States (Figure 18-3). Every semiclosed system contains an inspiratory limb, expiratory limb, unidirectional valves, CO_2 absorber, gas reservoir bag, and a pop-off valve on the expiratory limb. Advantages of a circle system include conservation of heat and moisture, the ability to use low flows of fresh gas (thereby conserving volatile anesthetic and the ozone layer), and the ability to scavenge waste gases. A disadvantage is its complex design; it has approximately 10 connections, each of which has the potential for disconnection.

32. Give an example of a closed circuit.

Like the semiclosed circuit, the closed circuit is a circle system adjusted so the inflow of fresh gas just matches the patient's O_2 consumption and anesthetic agent uptake. The CO_2 is eliminated by the absorber.

33. Rank the Mapleson circuits in order of efficiency for controlled and spontaneous ventilation.

- Controlled: D > B > C > A (mnemonic: *D*og *B*ites *C*an *A*che)
- Spontaneous: A > D > C > B (mnemonic: *A*ll *D*ogs *C*an *B*ite)

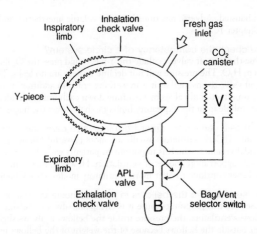

Figure 18-3. Circle system. APL, Adjustable pressure-limiting. *(From Andrews JJ: Inhaled anesthetic delivery system. In Miller RD, editor: Anesthesia, ed 4, New York, 1994, Churchill Livingstone, pp 185–228.*

34. What circuit is most commonly used in anesthesia delivery systems today?

Almost every anesthesia manufacturer supplies a circle system with its equipment. When compared with other available circuits, the circle system provides the most advantages.

35. How is a breathing circuit disconnection detected during delivery of an anesthetic?

Breath sounds are no longer detected with an esophageal or precordial stethoscope, and, if the parameters are properly set, the airway pressure monitor and tidal volume–minute volume monitor alarm will sound. The capnograph no longer detects CO_2, and soon thereafter the O_2 saturation begins to decline. Exhaled CO_2 is probably the best monitor to detect disconnections; a decrease or absence of CO_2 is sensitive although not specific for disconnection.

36. How is CO_2 eliminated from a circle system?

The exhaled gases pass through a canister containing a CO_2 absorbent such as soda lime or Baralyme. Soda lime consists of calcium hydroxide ($Ca[OH]_2$) with lesser quantities of sodium hydroxide (NaOH) and potassium hydroxide (KOH). Baralyme substitutes barium for calcium. Both soda lime and Baralyme react with CO_2 to form heat, water, and the corresponding carbonate. The soda lime reaction is as follows:

$$CO_2 + Ca(OH)_2 = CaCO_3 + H_2O + heat$$

37. How much CO_2 can the absorbent neutralize? What factors affect its efficiency?

Soda lime is the most common absorber and, at most, can absorb 23 L of CO_2 per 100 g of absorbent. However, the average absorber eliminates 10 to 15 L of CO_2 per 100 g absorbent in a single-chamber system and 18 to 20 L of CO_2 in a dual-chamber system. Factors affecting efficiency include the size of the absorber canister (the patient's tidal volume should be accommodated entirely within the void space of the canister), the size of the absorbent granule (optimal size is 2.5 mm or between 4 and 8 mesh), and the presence or absence of channeling (loose packing allowing exhaled gases to bypass absorber granules in the canister).

38. How do you know when the absorbent has been exhausted? What adverse reactions can occur between volatile anesthetic and CO_2 absorbents?

A pH-sensitive dye added to the granules changes color in the presence of carbonic acid, an intermediary in the CO_2 absorption chemical reaction. The most common dye in the United States is ethyl violet, which is white when fresh and turns violet when the absorbent is exhausted. Adverse reactions between volatile anesthetics and absorbents are discussed in Chapter 10.

39. **How can you check the competency of a circle system?**
You should close the pop-off valve, occlude the Y-piece, and press the O_2 flush valve until the pressure is 30 cm H_2O. The pressure will not decline if there are no leaks. Then you should open the pop-off valve to ensure that it is in working order. In addition, you should check the function of the unidirectional valves by breathing down each limb individually, making sure that you cannot inhale from the expiratory limb or exhale down the inspiratory limb.

40. **How do anesthesia ventilators differ from intensive care unit ventilators?**
Intensive care unit (ICU) ventilators usually are more powerful (allowing greater inspiratory pressures and tidal volumes, which is important in patients with decreased pulmonary compliance) and support more modes of ventilation. However, new generations of anesthesia machines continue to offer more ventilatory modes. (See Chapter 20.)

41. **What gas is used to drive the bellows in an anesthesia ventilator?**
O_2 is usually used for this purpose because it is cheap and always available. On modern ascending bellows ventilators, the pressure inside the bellows is always slightly higher than in the chamber outside the bellows because of the weight of the bellows itself and amounts to 1 to 2 cm H_2O. Where there is a bellows leak, any net gas flow would be out of (not into) the bellows and would not change the composition of the breathing mixture. When the bellows reaches the top of its ascent, an additional 1 to 2 cm H_2O pressure causes the exhaust valve to open.

42. **What is the status of the scavenger system when the bellows is below the top of its excursion?**
When the ventilator is engaged and the bellows is below the top of its excursion, the breathing circuit is completely closed. Excess gas can escape from the breathing circuit only when a special pneumatic value is activated by the bellows as it reaches the top of its range.

43. **What is the effect of the extra pressure required to open the exhaust valve on the patient?**
A patient being ventilated with an ascending bellows ventilator is usually subjected to 2.5 to 3 cm H_2O of positive end-expiratory pressure (PEEP). Most experts agree that this addition of PEEP is actually more physiologic than ventilating the patient with no PEEP.

44. **What parameters can be adjusted on an anesthesia ventilator?**
Most anesthesia ventilators allow adjustment of:
- Tidal volume (or minute volume)
- Respiratory rate
- Inspiratory-to-expiratory (I:E) ratio
- Sometimes inspiratory pause
- PEEP

Some newer anesthesia ventilators allow other adjustments, including the selection of different ventilation modes, such as pressure support and synchronized intermittent mandatory ventilation.

KEY POINTS: ANESTHESIA CIRCUITS AND VENTILATORS

1. Except for anesthesia machines in which there are flow compensators, fresh gas flow contributes to tidal volume.
2. Although the capabilities of anesthesia ventilators have improved greatly in recent years, they still are not as powerful as typical ICU ventilators.
3. Every patient ventilated with an ascending bellows anesthesia ventilator receives approximately 2.5 to 3 cm H_2O of PEEP because of the weight of the bellows.
4. The semiclosed circuit using a circle system is the most commonly used anesthesia circuit.
5. Advantages of a circle system include conservation of heat and moisture, the ability to use low flows of fresh gas, and the ability to scavenge waste gases. Disadvantages include multiple sites for disconnection and high compliance.

45. **Why have descending bellows been abandoned in favor of ascending bellows?**
Bellows are classified according to their movement during expiration (i.e., their position when the ventilator is not ventilating the patient). Hanging or descending bellows are considered unsafe for two reasons. First, if a circuit disconnection occurs, the bellows will fill with room air, and, although its movement may appear normal, the ventilator will be ventilating the room rather than the patient. Second, since the weight of the bellows creates a slight negative pressure in the circuit, this can cause negative end-expiratory pressure and can suck room air backward through the scavenger, interfering with the anesthesiologist's control of gas concentrations breathed by the patient.

46. **What would be the cause of bellows failing to rise completely between each breath?**
The most obvious reason for this is that a leak exists in the breathing circuit, a disconnect has occurred, or the patient has become extubated. If the fresh gas flow is too low, it is possible for the patient to use O_2 from the circuit faster than it is replenished.

47. **How does fresh gas flow rate contribute to tidal volume?**
The flow during the inspiration phase of the ventilatory cycle adds to the tidal volume. Let us assume that the respiratory rate is set at 10 breaths/min with an I:E ratio of 1:2 and a tidal volume of 1000 ml. Each breath cycle is then 6 seconds long: 2 seconds for inspiration and 4 seconds for expiration. If the fresh gas flow is 6 L/min, $2/60 \times 6000 = 200$ ml of fresh gas is added to each inspiration. Most modern anesthesia ventilators automatically compensate for this addition to tidal volume.

48. **How and where is tidal volume measured? Why are different measures frequently not equal?**
Tidal volume is measured using several techniques and at several sites in the breathing circuit. Common measures include the setting on the ventilator control panel, bellows excursion, and flow through the inspiratory or expiratory limbs of the circuit. These measures frequently differ because they may or may not include the contribution of the inspiratory flow, are measured at different pressures, and compensate differently for flow rates. Since each measure can, in theory, be an accurate measure of a different parameter, it is more important to record a consistent measure of tidal volume than to debate which measure is correct.

49. **When using very low flows of fresh gas, why is there sometimes a discrepancy between inspired O_2 concentration and fresh gas concentration?**
At low fresh gas flows, concentrations in the circuit are slow to change. However, this question refers to the fact that the patient will take up different gases (removing them from the circuit) at rates different from the rates at which the gases are added to the circuit. In the case of O_2, an average adult patient consumes (permanently removing from the circuit) approximately 200 to 300 ml/min of O_2. If N_2 or N_2O is supplied along with the O_2, the patient continues to consume O_2 while the N_2 or N_2O builds up in the circuit. It is possible for a hypoxic mixture to develop in the circuit, even though the fresh gas contains 50% or more O_2.

SUGGESTED READINGS

Brockwell RC, Andrews JJ: Inhaled anesthetic delivery systems. In Miller RD, editor: Miller's anesthesia, ed 6, Philadelphia, 2005, Elsevier Churchill Livingstone, pp 273–316.
Dorsch JA, Dorsch SE: Understanding anesthesia equipment, ed 5, Philadelphia, 2008, Lippincott Williams & Wilkins.

CHAPTER 19

PATIENT POSITIONING

James C. Duke, MD, MBA

1. **What is the goal of positioning a patient for surgery?**
   The goal of surgical positioning is to facilitate the surgeon's technical approach while balancing the risk to the patient. The anesthetized patient cannot make the clinician aware of compromised positions; therefore the positioning of a patient for surgery is critical for a safe outcome. Proper positioning requires that the patient be securely placed on the operating table; all potential pressure areas padded; the eyes protected; no muscles, tendons, or neurovascular bundles stretched; intravenous lines and catheters free flowing and accessible; the endotracheal tube in the proper position; ventilation and circulation uninterrupted; and general patient comfort and safety maintained for the duration of the surgery. It is always advisable to question a patient or ascertain if there is impaired mobility at any joint; never attempt to position patients beyond their limitations.

   Throughout the surgical procedure, it is also important to reassess the positioning, readjust as needed, and document any positioning actions and reassessments.

2. **Review the most common positions used in the operating room.**
   See Figure 19-1.

3. **What physiologic effects are related to change in body position?**
   An important consideration is the gravitational effects on the cardiovascular and respiratory systems. A change from an erect to a supine position increases cardiac output secondary to improved venous return to the heart, but there is minimal change in blood pressure secondary to reflex decreases in heart rate and contractility. Conditions that increase intraabdominal pressure in the supine position—including abdominal tumors, ascites, obesity, pregnancy, or carbon dioxide insufflation for laparoscopy—decrease venous return and cardiac output.

   The supine position results in decreased functional residual capacity and total lung capacity secondary to the abdominal contents impinging on the diaphragm. Anesthesia and muscular relaxation further diminish these lung volumes. Trendelenburg and lithotomy positions result in further compression of the lung bases, with a subsequent decrease in pulmonary compliance. Although some improvement is achieved with positive-pressure ventilation, the diaphragm is not restored to the awake position. In the supine position, spontaneous ventilation to the dependent lung areas increases. Matching of ventilation to perfusion improves because blood flow also increases to dependent areas.

4. **Describe the lithotomy position and its common complications.**
   The patient's hips and knees are flexed, and the patient's feet are placed in stirrups to gain ready access to the genitalia and perineum. The range of flexion may be modest (low lithotomy) or extreme (high lithotomy). The feet may be suspended on vertical structures known as candy canes or in boots, or the knees may be supported with crutches. With elevation of the legs, pressure is taken off the lower back, and blood is translocated from the lower extremities to the central compartments.

   Compression to lower extremity peripheral nerves is the most common injury, occurring in about 1% to 2% of patients placed in the lithotomy position. Neuropathies may be unilateral or bilateral and are a function of the time in this position (especially longer than 2 hours). They are noted soon after surgery, may present with paresthesias and/ or motor weakness, and usually resolve completely, although resolution may require a few months. Before these injuries are attributed to lithotomy positioning, consider if use of neuraxial needles, lower extremity tourniquets, or surgical trauma (e.g., use of retractors) may have contributed.

   To prevent dislocation of the hips, at case conclusion both feet should be released from the lithotomy stirrups and lowered simultaneously. When the leg section of the operating table is elevated, ensure that the fingers are clear to avoid crush or amputation injuries.

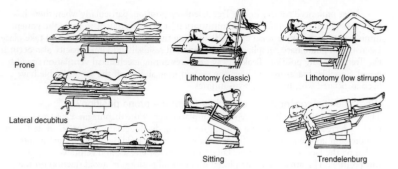

Figure 19-1. Patient positioning. *(From Martin JT: Positioning in anesthesia and surgery, ed 2, Philadelphia, 1987, WB Saunders.)*

5. **What nerves may be affected from lithotomy positioning?**
   - Femoral nerve: A reasonable practice is to avoid hip flexion >90 degrees, although it remains a matter of debate whether extreme flexion predisposes the patient to a femoral neuropathy. The femoral nerve is also at risk from pelvic retractors.
   - Common peroneal nerve: May be injured when the head of the fibula is insufficiently padded and compressed against the stirrup canes.
   - Sciatic nerve: Avoid stretching the hamstring muscle group by avoiding hip flexion >90 degrees.
   - Saphenous nerve: May become injured if the medial tibial condyle is compressed.
   - Obturator nerve: May be stretched as it exits the obturator foramen during thigh flexion.
   - Lateral femoral cutaneous nerve: Presents with only sensory findings.

6. **What are the special concerns for a patient positioned in the lateral decubitus position?**
   All patients in the lateral position should have an axillary roll positioned to distribute weight to the patient's rib cage and prevent compression of the neurovascular bundle of the dependent arm. Loss of pulse to the dependent arm suggests excessive compression, but the presence of a pulse does not ensure that the brachial plexus is protected. The arms are usually supported and padded in a position perpendicular to the shoulders. The dependent leg is usually flexed at the hip and knee, with padding between the legs and under the inferior fibular head to reduce pressure on the peroneal nerve. The head position should be in line with the vertebral column to prevent stretching of the brachial plexus of the nondependent arm. Horner's syndrome has been reported when the head was not supported in a neutral position. Facial structures, breasts, and genitalia should also be protected.
   Ventilation-perfusion mismatching is a risk in the lateral position. The dependent lung is underventilated and relatively overperfused. In contrast, the nondependent lung is overventilated because of the increase in compliance. Usually there is some physiologic compensation, and changes in ventilation and perfusion are usually well tolerated, although in a compromised patient they may prove problematic.

7. **What are the physiologic effects and risks associated with the Trendelenburg position?**
   Head down, or Trendelenburg position, further increases translocation of blood to the central compartment. Intracranial and intraocular pressure increases in the Trendelenburg position secondary to decreased cerebral venous drainage. Adverse outcomes in healthy patients have not been noted, although the Trendelenburg position is clearly contraindicated in patients with increased intracranial pressure. Lengthy procedures may result in significant facial and upper airway edema. The likelihood of postextubation airway obstruction should be considered, and the ability of the patient to breathe around the endotracheal tube with the cuff deflated is reassuring, although it does not completely ensure that postextubation airway obstruction will not occur.

After prolonged surgery in the Trendelenburg position, particularly when there has been substantial intravenous fluid administration, it may be prudent to leave the patient intubated with the upper torso elevated, allowing time for fluid redistribution to take place. Decreases in pulmonary compliance and functional residual and vital capacity also occur in the Trendelenburg position. Peak airway pressures during mechanical ventilation are also noted. Shoulder braces used to keep the patient from sliding off the surgical table have been associated with brachial plexus injuries.

8. **What specific concerns are associated with the prone position?**
The prone position results in a cephalad displacement of the diaphragm. Chest rolls are used to decrease abdominal compression, improving diaphragmatic excursion while limiting compression on the aorta and inferior vena cava. Proper padding of all pressure points, including the face, eyes, ears, arms, knees, hips, ankles, breasts, and genitalia, is necessary in this position. The arms should be placed in a neutral position to avoid traction on the brachial plexus, although modest abduction >90 degrees is acceptable. Electrocardiogram electrodes should not be placed so the patient is lying on them.

9. **What is the beach chair position?**
This position is used to improve access and mobility of the shoulder for surgery. When finally positioned, the anesthesiologist does not have easy access to the head or endotracheal tube; thus these structures must be well secured and in a neutral position before initiation of the surgery. Perfusion pressure must be closely monitored since the head is well above the level of the heart. Special care should also be taken to protect the eyes because the surgeon is working very close to the face and instruments and the like could place pressure on the eyes. Protective plastic eye shields are often used in this instance.

10. **When is a sitting position used?**
The sitting position is used to gain access to the posterior fossa of the cranium and perform cervical laminectomy. However, these procedures are now often performed with the patient in a prone position, and the use of the sitting position is decreasing.

11. **What are the advantages of the sitting position?**
   • Optimal positioning for surgical exposure with significantly less blood loss, improved surgical field, and perhaps improved resection of the lesion
   • Decreased facial swelling
   • Relatively easy access to the endotracheal tube
   • Less cranial nerve damage

12. **List the disadvantages of the sitting position.**
   • Hypotension. Because of decreased venous return, cardiac output may be reduced by as much as 20%, but it improves with fluid administration and pressors. Consider lower extremity compression hose to improve venous return. Intraarterial monitoring is essential. Place the transducer at the level of the external auditory meatus to monitor cerebral perfusion pressure.
   • Brainstem manipulations resulting in hemodynamic changes.
   • Risks of severe neck flexion include spinal cord ischemia and airway obstruction (caused by severe swelling of the tongue or kinking of the endotracheal tube). Two fingerbreadths of space should be allowed between the chin and sternum.
   • Venous air embolism (VAE).

13. **How does VAE occur? What are the sequelae?**
Because the surgical site is above the level of the heart, air entrainment into the venous circulation is a risk. VAE may result in pulmonary air embolism, hypotension, and paradoxic air embolism if an intracardiac shunt is present. Unless massive, VAE usually responds to fluid challenge and pressor therapy. The surgical site must also be flooded with fluid to prevent continued air entrainment.

14. **Review the sensitivity and limitations of monitors for detecting VAE.**
There are numerous monitors for detection of VAE. No single technique is totally reliable; thus the more monitors used, the greater the likelihood is for detecting VAE. In decreasing order of sensitivity, the monitors are transesophageal echocardiography and Doppler

ultrasound > increases in end-tidal nitrogen fraction > decreases in end-tidal carbon dioxide > increases in right atrial pressure > esophageal stethoscope.

A right atrial catheter has the advantage of being able to aspirate intracardiac air. Therefore, of all modalities mentioned, it is the only one capable of diagnosis and treatment. Multiorifice catheters are clearly preferable and should be placed high in the right atrium.

15. **What are the concerns for positioning a pregnant patient?**
The pregnant patient is susceptible to aortocaval compression secondary to the gravid uterus exerting pressure on these vascular structures, potentially decreasing the uteroplacental blood flow and venous return to the heart. Left uterine displacement decreases intraabdominal pressure and is achieved by placing a pillow or wedge under the right hip.

16. **What peripheral neuropathies are associated with cardiac surgery?**
The brachial plexus may be injured. Anatomic features of the plexus, including its superficial location, tethering between the intervertebral foramina and investing fascia, and the limited space in its course between the first rib and clavicle, render it vulnerable to injury. Sternal retraction and first rib fractures predispose to this injury. There does not appear to be a significant difference in brachial neuropathy when the arms are tucked against the body versus when the arms are abducted 90 degrees with elbows elevated and palms up. The best recommendations are to maintain the head in a neutral position, place the sternal retractor as far caudally as possible, and use asymmetric retractors cautiously.

17. **What is the most common perianesthetic neuropathy?**
The ulnar nerve is the most frequently injured peripheral nerve, although its incidence is still relatively infrequent. There is a distinct predilection for men older than 50 years of age, and it is not uncommon for there to be a few days' delay in presentation. Occasionally the neuropathy is bilateral. Of interest, the American Society of Anesthesiologists' (ASA's) Closed Claims Analysis found that 15% of ulnar neuropathies occurred in patients who were sedated and received spinal or epidural anesthesia or monitored anesthesia care. One would presume that, being awake, patients would readjust their arms if they felt numbness or paresthesias developing during the procedure. Ulnar neuropathies tend to be mild, mostly sensory in nature, and self-limited. Return of function within 6 weeks is reasonable advice for patients so affected, although deficits have been reported to last up to 2 years. There are numerous cases of ulnar neuropathy in which padding to protect the ulnar nerve was undertaken; thus perioperative ulnar neuropathies are clearly multifactorial in nature. Some patients may have even had a subclinical ulnar neuropathy present before surgery, only to have its initial recognition occur postoperatively.

18. **Review the incidence of brachial plexus injuries.**
Closed Claims Analysis found that brachial plexus injuries account for 20% of all anesthesia-related nerve injuries. Risk factors include use of shoulder braces in head-down positions, malposition of the arms, and sustained neck extension. Although not a matter of positioning, upper-extremity regional anesthetic techniques may also cause brachial plexus injuries. Of interest, eliciting paresthesias during needle placement or injection of local anesthetics was not a common finding.

19. **How might upper extremity neuropathies be prevented through careful positioning?**
Arm abduction should be limited to 90 degrees in supine patients. Protective padding is essential to avoid upper extremity neuropathies but using protective padding does not guarantee they won't occur. The ulnar groove should be padded and pronation avoided since this places the ulnar nerve in its most vulnerable position. When arms are tucked at the side, a neutral position is preferable. Flexion at the elbow may increase the risk of ulnar neuropathy. Pressure on the spiral groove of the humerus may result in radial neuropathy. Range limitation is not uncommon at the elbow, and overextension may place the median nerve at risk. Properly functioning automated blood pressure cuffs do not alter the risk of upper extremity neuropathy.

KEY POINTS: PATIENT POSITIONING

1. A conscientious attitude toward positioning is required to facilitate the surgical procedure, prevent physiologic embarrassment, and prevent injury to the patient.
2. Postoperative blindness is increasing in frequency, but it is unclear exactly which patients are at risk. Although not a guarantee to prevent this complication, during lengthy spine procedures in the prone position, maintain intravascular volume, hematocrit, and perfusion pressure.
3. The most common postoperative nerve injury is ulnar neuropathy. It is most commonly found in men older than 50 years, is delayed in presentation, is not invariably prevented by padding, and is multifactorial in origin.
4. In order of decreasing sensitivity, monitors for detection of VAE are transesophageal echocardiography and Doppler ultrasound > increases in end-tidal nitrogen fraction > decreases in end-tidal carbon dioxide > increases in right atrial pressure > esophageal stethoscope. It should be noted that, of all these monitors, only the right atrial catheter can treat a recognized air embolism.

---

20. **What injuries may occur to the eye?**

The most common injury is corneal abrasion, but patients may also develop conjunctivitis, chemical injury, direct trauma, blurred vision, and ischemic optic neuropathy (ION). Symptoms range from discomfort to pain to blindness. The relatively minor injuries are caused by direct pressure on the eye from facemasks, surgical drapes, chemicals that touch the eye, and failure to administer ocular protection. Positions other than supine are more commonly associated with eye injuries. Although in the past it was recommended that a corneal abrasion be treated with an eye patch, this appears to delay healing; use of nonsteroidal antiinflammatory ophthalmic ointments is now recommended by some. Repetitive use of local anesthetic or steroid drops is not recommended.

21. **Review the procedures that have been associated with postoperative visual loss (POVL).**

The incidence of blindness after cardiac surgery has been estimated at about 4%. The mechanisms are thought to be embolic, thrombotic, oncotic, and ischemic and related to the surgical procedures themselves. These patients may develop central retinal artery occlusion or ION.

Other surgical procedures that have been associated with POVL include neck dissections (including when there is ligation of the internal jugular veins), thyroidectomy, major vascular surgery, and craniotomy. It is of concern that the incidence of POVL associated with prone spine surgery seems to be on the increase.

22. **What factors may predispose a patient having spine surgery to POVL?**

The causative factors associated with POVL after spine surgery are not fully understood. The incidence appears to be about 0.2%. The ASA has developed a visual loss registry in an effort to identify predisposing factors and make recommendations to reduce the incidence of this tragic complication. It is thought that there is a subset of patients at high risk for this complication, although it is not always possible to identify before surgery which patients are at high risk. These patients may have a history of hypertension, diabetes mellitus, smoking, other vasculopathies, and morbid obesity.

Longer spine surgeries (lasting longer than 6 hours) with significant blood loss (1 to 2 L or more) are common features in patients who have sustained POVL. It does not appear to be a pressure effect on the globe since many of these patients were placed in Mayfield pins. Deliberate hypotensive anesthetic techniques do not appear to be a factor, although it may be argued that sustained hypotension in the setting of anemia requires therapy. It is interesting that, in this day when transfusion triggers are being pushed downward (to lower hematocrits), long spine cases may not be a subset in which profound anemia is acceptable. It may be that, in spine cases that require both anterior and posterior stabilization, staging the procedure might be advisable. Although the complication is devastating, its incidence remains small, and the patients at risk, the factors that contribute to POVL and recommendations for preventing it remain speculative.

23. **What patterns of blindness are noted?**

    ION is noted in about 90% of cases, and central retinal artery occlusion is noted in the remainder. Posterior ION is more common than anterior ION, and ION is more likely to be bilateral (approximately two thirds of the time), suggesting that the etiologies are different. Substantive recovery of vision is not frequent.

24. **How does the head position affect the position of the endotracheal tube with respect to the carina?**

    Flexion of the head may move the endotracheal tube toward the carina; extension moves it away from the carina. A general rule is that the tip of the endotracheal tube follows the direction of the tip of the patient's nose. The change in tube position is probably more problematic in a child than in an adult. Sudden increases in airway pressure or oxygen desaturation may be caused by mainstem bronchial intubation.

WEBSITE

American Society of Anesthesiologists: http://www.asahq.org

SUGGESTED READINGS

ASA Task Force on Perioperative Blindness: Practice advisory for perioperative visual loss associated with spine surgery, Anesthesiology 104:1319–1328, 2006.

Lee LA, Roth S, Posner KL, et al: The American Society of Anesthesiologists postoperative visual loss registry: analysis of 93 spine surgery cases with postoperative visual loss, Anesthesiology 105:652–659, 2006.

CHAPTER 20

MECHANICAL VENTILATION IN CRITICAL ILLNESS

James B. Haenel, RRT, and Jeffrey L. Johnson, MD

1. **Why might a patient require mechanical ventilation (MV)?**
   There are three conditions for which MV may be required:
   1. Inadequate respiratory drive
   2. Inability to maintain adequate alveolar ventilation
   3. Hypoxia

   The decision to provide MV should be based on clinical examination and assessment of gas exchange by arterial blood gas analysis. This decision must be individualized because arbitrary cutoff values for PO_2, PCO_2, or pH as indicators of respiratory failure may not be germane to all patients. Physiologic derangements necessitating the need for MV include primary parenchymal disorders such as pneumonia, pulmonary edema, or pulmonary contusion or systemic disease that indirectly compromises pulmonary function such as sepsis or central nervous system dysfunction. The principal goal of MV in the setting of respiratory failure is to minimize the potential for ventilator-induced injury and support gas exchange while the underlying disease process is reversed.

2. **Which is the most common mode of ventilation: volume or pressure control?**
   From a classification standpoint, neither is a true mode of ventilation. To be precise, conventional modes of MV control either volume or pressure. The mode of ventilation is a function of the types of breaths delivered (e.g., either mandatory and/or spontaneous breaths) and how the timing of each breath is determined. Volume control provides breaths that are volume constant and pressure variable. Pressure control provides breaths that are pressure constant and volume variable. It is the response of the ventilator to the patient's effort that determines the mode.

3. **What are the most commonly used modes of positive-pressure ventilation?**
   Currently there are nine modes that are based on using either volume or pressure as the control variable:
   - VC-CMV, volume control–continuous mandatory ventilation
   - VC-A-C, volume control–assist control (ventilation)
   - VC-IMV or VC-SIMV, volume-control intermittent or synchronized intermittent mandatory ventilation
   - PC-CMV, pressure control–continuous mandatory ventilation
   - PC-A-C, pressure control–assist control (ventilation)
   - PC-IMV or PC-SIMV, pressure control–intermittent mandatory ventilation or pressure control–synchronized intermittent ventilation
   - PSV, pressure support ventilation

4. **Does PC-CMV permit the patient to interact with the ventilator?**
   Use of an abbreviation such as PC-CMV frequently leaves the uninitiated confused. The term *controlled* MV implies that the patient is receiving a neuromuscular blocking agent and is prevented or locked out from triggering the ventilator. Therefore, when speaking of volume control or pressure control, more descriptive terms such as *volume-targeted* or *pressure-targeted ventilation* may minimize any misunderstanding.

5. **How does VC-A-C mode work?**
   The VC-A-C mode delivers a set minimum number of mandatory breaths and also allows the patient to trigger (or assist) additional breaths. Each breath (mandatory or assisted) is associated with a preset flow rate to deliver a preset tidal volume (V_T). AC-A-C may cause respiratory alkalosis more often and may promote auto-positive end-expiratory pressure

(auto-PEEP) because the patient receives a full set V_T with every breath, even when tachypneic.

6. **Do VC-A-C and VC-SIMV differ?**

   Both modes deliver mandatory breaths at a preset frequency, a preset V_T, and a preset inspiratory gas flow rate. Between machine-initiated breaths in the VC-A-C mode, the patient can trigger the ventilator and receive an assisted breath at the set V_T. In the VC-SIMV mode, the ventilator generates a timing window based on the set frequency of the mandatory breaths and attempts to *synchronize* the delivery of the breath in concert with the patient's spontaneous effort. In between the mandatory breaths, while in the SIMV mode, the patient is free to initiate a totally spontaneous effort and generate a V_T compatible with the patient's inspiratory muscular effort. Flow rates of gas vary during these spontaneous breaths and are based on the patient's efforts and demands.

7. **When initiating MV, how do you decide on VC-A-C over VC-SIMV?**

   If the intent of MV is to provide full ventilator support, provision of a sufficient level of alveolar ventilation is obligatory. The preference of VC-A-C over VC-SIMV, assuming that minute ventilation demands (set frequency and set V_T) are being met, is really a point of style or preference. However, once the patient has achieved cardiopulmonary stability and the goal is now to initiate partial ventilator support, the options for VC-A-C versus VC-SIMV are very different. A patient on a set respiratory frequency of 4 breaths/min in the VC-A-C mode with a total respiratory rate (RR) of 18 breaths/min is still receiving full ventilator support. In contrast, in the VC-SIMV mode, a patient with the same set frequency is considered to be in a partial mode of support and must be capable of supporting the bulk of his or her own gas exchange demands.

8. **What other variables are associated with conventional modes of MV?**

   Stated simplistically, ventilators are classified as either pressure, volume, or flow controllers. Current intensive care unit (ICU) ventilators can mix pressure control with flow control, all within a single breath. Next there are the phase variables, events that take place during a ventilator cycle. These phase variables control how the breath is
   - *Triggered* (i.e., patient or machine).
   - *Limited* (i.e., pressure or volume).
   - *Cycled* from inspiration to exhalation (i.e., pressure, volume, flow, or time).

9. **What is pressure support ventilation (PSV)?**

   PSV augments a patient's spontaneous inspiratory effort with a clinician-selected level of positive airway pressure. Inspiration is completed when the patient's spontaneously generated peak flow rate decreases below a minimum level or a percentage of the initial inspiratory flow, typically less than 25%. Therefore PSV is a purely patient-triggered, pressure-limited, and flow-cycled mode of ventilation. PSV allows patients to establish their own RR, vary their peak flow rate based on breath-to-breath demands, and enhance delivered V_T. Taken together, the RR, peak flow, and V_T determine the inspiratory to expiratory (I:E) ratio. It is much more physiologic and comfortable for the patient to control the I:E ratio than to impose a fixed I:E ratio that will not respond favorably to increased patient demands.

10. **How does pressure control ventilation differ from PSV?**

    PCV, unlike PSV, is a pressure-limited, time-cycled mode of ventilation. The V_T generated results from the clinician-determined inspiratory time and the applied airway pressure and are predominantly influenced by flow resistance and respiratory system compliance. Practically speaking, PCV is used as a mode of ventilation when full ventilatory support is necessary, whereas PSV is optimal for providing partial ventilatory support.

11. **What are trigger variables?**

    All modern ICU ventilators constantly measure one or more of the phase variables (i.e., pressure, volume, flow, or time) (Table 20-1). Inspiration occurs when one of these variables reaches a preset value. Clinically this is referred to as *triggering* the ventilator. The following conditions are necessary to initiate a breath under each individual variable:
    - Pressure triggering: requires patient-initiated effort to decrease circuit pressure below a preset value (e.g., 2 cm H_2O below baseline end-expiratory pressure, i.e. -2 cm H_2O, is common)

Table 20-1. Breath Types for Volume and Pressure Modes of Ventilator Operation

MODE (COMMON NAMES)	Mandatory			Assisted		
	TRIGGER	LIMIT	CYCLE	TRIGGER	LIMIT	CYCLE
VC-CMV	Time	Flow	Volume or Time	—	—	—
VC-A-C	Time	Flow	Volume or Time	Patient	Flow	Volume or Time
VC-SIMV	Time	Flow	Volume or Time	—	—	—
PC-CMV	Time	Pressure	Time	—	—	—
PC-A-C	Time	Pressure	Time	Patient	Pressure	Time
PC-SIMV	Time	Pressure	Time	—	—	—

- Flow or volume triggering: again requires patient effort that results in a drop in the flow rate or volume of gas that is continually present within the circuit
- Time triggering: does not require patient effort but occurs when the set RR on the ventilator becomes due
  Two potentially hazardous forms of triggering have also been identified:
- Auto-triggering: occurs when the ventilator is rapidly cycling without apparent patient effort. If the triggering system is overly sensitive (flow or pressure trigger) in the presence of leaks in the ventilator circuit or artificial airway cuff, cardiac oscillations, or excessive water condensation within the circuit tubing, then premature triggering of additional breaths may result. An extrinsic origin for auto-triggering may result from transmission of pleural suction in the face of a significant bronchopleural fistula that communicates with the tracheal airway. Generally increasing either the flow or pressure trigger will eliminate this phenomenon.
- Ineffective triggering: occurs when the ventilator doesn't recognize a patient's inspiratory effort. This is commonly seen during pressure triggering in the presence of auto-PEEP that may prevent the patient from achieving the necessary drop in circuit pressure.

12. **What are combined modes of ventilation?**
   Combined modes of ventilation take advantage of microprocessor technology and offer "hybrid modes" by combining aspects of volume-targeted and pressure-targeted ventilation, thereby circumventing both the high peak pressures of volume ventilation and the variable tidal volumes associated with pressure ventilation. Common examples are pressure-regulated volume control (PRVC), automatic tube compensation (ATC), and airway pressure-release ventilation (APRV). Although lacking strong evidence from large randomized prospective trials, many clinicians find that combined modes of ventilation offer potential advantages based on surrogate physiologic variables such as gas exchange and ventilator synchrony.

13. **What are the initial ventilator settings in acute respiratory failure?**
   Commonly one begins with the VC-A-C mode, which ensures delivery of a preset V_T. Pressure-cycled modes are acceptable but probably offer only theoretic advantage. The FiO_2 begins at 1 and is titrated downward as tolerated. High FiO_2 in the face of acute lung injury results in worsening of intrapulmonary shunting, probably as a result of absorption atelectasis. V_T is based on ideal body weight (IBW) and the pathophysiology of lung injury. Volumes of 6 to 10 ml/kg/IBW are acceptable as long as the plateau pressure is <30 cm H_2O. However, acute respiratory distress syndrome (ARDS) decreases the volume of the lung available for ventilation. Because large pressures or volumes may exacerbate the underlying lung injury, smaller volumes in the range of 6 to 8 ml/kg/IBW are chosen. A respiratory rate (f) is chosen, usually in the range of 10 to 20 breaths/min. Patients with high minute volume requirements or a low V_T (lung protective strategy) may require an f of 32 breaths/min. Carbon dioxide elimination does not improve significantly with rates

>25/min, and rates >30/min predispose to gas trapping secondary to abbreviated expiratory times.

14. **What is the role of positive end-expiratory pressure (PEEP)?**

PEEP has been a cornerstone in the management of respiratory failure for over 40 years. Specifically it is applied to the exhalation circuit of the mechanical ventilator. The main goals of PEEP are to:

- Increase functional residual capacity by preventing alveolar collapse and recruiting atelectatic alveoli.
- Decrease intrapulmonary shunting.
- Optimize pulmonary compliance, thus reducing the work of breathing.

PEEP adjustments should be considered in response to periods of desaturations (after common causes for hypoxemia, such as mucous plugging and barotrauma, have been ruled out) to assess recruitment potential.

15. **How is optimal PEEP identified?**

Although various methods for lung recruitment have been suggested, we use the following approach to identify the optimal PEEP:

Patients experiencing an acute desaturation event are placed in the pressure control mode, with RR set at 10 breaths/min, I:E ratio at 1:1, and peak pressure at 20 cm H_2O. The PEEP is increased to 25 to 40 cm H_2O for 1–2 minutes. The patient is continuously monitored for adverse effects. The PEEP is then returned to the baseline value. If the patient again desaturates, the trial is repeated, but the baseline PEEP is set 5 cm H_2O higher. This process is continued until the patient no longer desaturates. To enhance safety, identification of intravascular fluid deficits and optimization of the hemodynamic status should be addressed before application of high PEEP levels.

16. **What is intrinsic PEEP (PEEPi) or auto-PEEP?**

PEEPi is unrecognized positive alveolar pressure at end exhalation during MV. Patients with high minute ventilation requirements or patients with chronic obstructive pulmonary disease (COPD) or asthma are at risk for PEEPi. In healthy lungs during MV, if the RR is too rapid or the expiratory time too short, there is insufficient time for full exhalation, resulting in stacking of breaths and generation of positive airway pressure at end exhalation. Small-diameter endotracheal tubes may also limit exhalation and contribute to PEEPi. Patients with increased airway resistance and decreased pulmonary compliance are at high risk for PEEPi. Such patients have difficulty exhaling gas because of small airway obstruction/collapse and are prone to development of PEEPi during spontaneous ventilation and MV. PEEPi has the same side effects as extrinsic PEEP (PEEPe), but detecting it requires more vigilance.

Failure to recognize the presence of auto-PEEP can lead to inappropriate ventilator changes (Figure 20-1). The only way to detect and measure PEEPi is to occlude the expiratory port at end expiration while monitoring airway pressure. Decreasing rate or increasing inspiratory flow (to increase I:E ratio) may allow time for full exhalation. Administering a bronchodilator therapy in the setting of bronchospasm is usually beneficial.

17. **What are the side effects of PEEPe and PEEPi?**

- Barotrauma may result from overdistention of alveoli.
- Cardiac output may be decreased because of increased intrathoracic pressure, producing an increase in transmural right atrial pressure and a decrease in venous return. PEEP also increases pulmonary artery pressure, potentially decreasing right ventricular output. Dilation of the right ventricle may cause bowing of the interventricular septum into the left ventricle, thus impairing filling of the left ventricle, decreasing cardiac output, especially if the patient is hypovolemic.
- Incorrect interpretation of cardiac filling pressures. Pressure transmitted from the alveolus to the pulmonary vasculature may falsely elevate the readings.
- Overdistention of alveoli from excessive PEEP decreases blood flow to these areas, increasing dead space (V_D/V_T).
- Work of breathing may be increased with PEEPi because the patient is required to generate a larger negative pressure to trigger flow from the ventilator.
- Increase in intracranial pressure (ICP) and fluid retention.

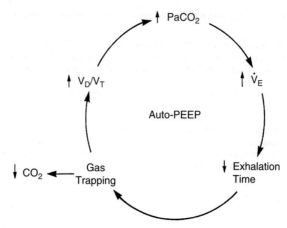

Figure 20-1. Failure to appreciate auto-PEEP can lead to a vicious cycle in which an increased minute ventilation (V_E) in response to a rise in $PaCO_2$ decreases exhalation time, augments gas trapping, increases dead space ventilation (V_D/V_T), and paradoxically decreases CO_2 elimination. A further increase in V_E repeats the cycle, allowing pleural pressure to increase so that the adverse effects of PEEP (e.g., decreased cardiac output) emerge.

18. **What is a ventilator bundle?**
    The ventilator bundle is a series of interventions related to ventilator care that have been identified to significantly reduce the incidence of ventilator-associated pneumonia. The key components of the ventilator bundle are:
    - Elevation of the head of the bed.
    - Daily *sedation vacations* and assessment for the readiness to extubate.
    - Stress ulcer prophylaxis.
    - Deep venous thrombosis.
      Additional interventions likely complementary to the ventilator bundle are implementation of a hand hygiene campaign, an oral care protocol, and endotracheal tube modifications such as implementation of subglottic secretion drainage cuffs and inhibition of biofilm formation.

19. **What is controlled hypoventilation with permissive hypercapnia?**
    Controlled hypoventilation (or permissive hypercapnia) is a pressure- or volume-limiting, lung-protective strategy whereby PCO_2 is allowed to rise, placing more importance on protecting the lung than on maintaining eucapnia. The set V_T is lowered to a range of approximately 4 to 6 ml/kg/IBW in an attempt to keep the peak airway pressure (Paw) below 35 to 40 cm H_2O and the static plateau pressure below 30 cm H_2O. Several studies of ARDS and status asthmaticus have shown decreases in barotrauma, number of days in the ICU, and mortality. The PCO_2 is allowed to rise slowly to a level of up to 80 to 100 mm Hg. If pH falls below 7.20, it may be treated with a buffer. Alternatively, one may wait for the normal kidney to retain bicarbonate in response to the hypercapnia. In contrast, the sick kidney may not be capable of retaining bicarbonate. Permissive hypercapnia is usually well tolerated. A potential adverse effect is cerebral vasodilation leading to increased ICP, and intracranial hypertension is the only absolute contraindication to permissive hypercapnia. Increased sympathetic activity, pulmonary vasoconstriction, and cardiac arrhythmias may occur but are rarely significant. Depression of cardiac contractility may be a problem in patients with underlying ventricular dysfunction.

20. **What is compliance? How is it determined?**
    Compliance is a measure of distensibility and is expressed as the change in volume for a given change in pressure. Determination of compliance involves the interrelationship

among pressure, volume, and resistance to airflow. The two relevant pressures that must be monitored during MV are peak and static pressures.

21. How is peak pressure measured?
Peak pressure is measured during the delivery of airflow at the end of inspiration. It is influenced by the inflation volume, airway resistance, level of PEEP, and elastic recoil of the lungs and chest wall and reflects the dynamic compliance of the total respiratory system.

22. How is static pressure measured?
Static or plateau pressure is measured during an end-inspiratory pause, during a no-flow condition, and reflects the static compliance of the respiratory system, including the lung parenchyma, chest wall, and abdomen.

23. How is compliance calculated?
Both dynamic and static compliance should be calculated. Dynamic compliance is calculated as $V_T/(Paw - \text{total PEEP})$, and plateau or static compliance is $V_T/(\text{plateau pressure} - \text{total PEEP})$. Normal values for both dynamic and static compliance are 60 to 100 ml/cm H_2O. A decrease in dynamic compliance without a change in the static compliance suggests an acute increase in airway resistance and can be assessed further by comparing peak pressure and plateau pressure. The normal gradient is approximately 10 cm H_2O. A gradient >10 cm H_2O may be secondary to endotracheal tube obstruction, mucous plugging, or bronchospasm. If volume is constant, acute changes in both dynamic and static compliance suggest a decrease in respiratory system compliance that may be caused by worsening pneumonia, ARDS, atelectasis, or increasing abdominal pressures.

Compliance is a global value and does not describe what is happening regionally in the lungs of patients with ARDS, in which diseased regions are interspersed with relatively healthy regions. Compliance values of 20 to 40 cm H_2O are common in advanced ARDS. Decreased lung compliance reflects the compliance of the lung that is participating in gas exchange, not the collapsed or fluid-filled alveoli.

24. Is ventilation in the prone position an option for patients who are difficult to oxygenate?
Absolutely! Studies have shown that the PaO_2 improves significantly in approximately two thirds of patients with ARDS when they are placed prone. The mechanisms include:
- Recruitment of collapsed dorsal lung fields by redistribution of lung edema to ventral regions.
- Reduction of overdistention, thus homogenizing the distribution of stress and strain within the lungs.
- Elimination of the compressive effects of the heart on the inferior lower lung fields, thus improving regional ventilation.
- Maintenance of dorsal lung perfusion in the face of improved dorsal ventilation, which leads to improved V/Q matching.

25. What are the indications for prone ventilation?
Timing for initiation of prone ventilation is not clearly established. We initiate a prone trial in any patient who remains hypoxemic or requires high FiO_2 concentrations after the performance of recruitment/PEEP maneuvers. A recent (2013) multicenter, prospective, randomized controlled trial in patients with severe ARDS showed that early (≤24 hours) proning sessions significantly decreased 28-day mortality versus the supine position (16% in the prone group and 32.8% in the supine group; p < 0.001).

26. How is the patient who is *fighting the ventilator* approached?
Initially the potential causes are separated into ventilator (machine, circuit, and airway) problems and patient-related problems. Patient-related causes include hypoxemia, secretions or mucous plugging, pneumothorax, bronchospasm, infection (pneumonia or sepsis), pulmonary embolus, myocardial ischemia, gastrointestinal bleeding, worsening PEEPi, and anxiety. The ventilator-related issues include system leak or disconnection; inadequate ventilator support or delivered FiO_2; airway-related problems such as extubation, obstructed endotracheal tube, cuff herniation, or rupture; and improper triggering sensitivity or flows. Until the problem is sorted out, the patient should be ventilated manually with 100%

oxygen. Breath sounds and vital signs should be checked immediately. Arterial blood gas analysis and a portable chest radiograph are valuable, but, if a tension pneumothorax is suspected, immediate decompression precedes the chest radiograph.

KEY POINTS: MECHANICAL VENTILATION IN CRITICAL ILLNESS

1. Three indications for MV are inadequate respiratory drive, inability to maintain alveolar ventilation, and hypoxia.
2. Two indications for noninvasive positive-pressure ventilation are hypercapnic respiratory failure and comfort in terminally ill patients.
3. Risk factors for auto-PEEP are high minute ventilation, small endotracheal tube, COPD, and asthma.
4. The normal airway gradient between peak and static pressure is approximately 10 cm H_2O.
5. The first step in the care of the hypoxic patient fighting the ventilator is to ventilate the patient manually with 100% oxygen.

---

27. **Should neuromuscular blockade be used to facilitate MV?**

Neuromuscular blocking agents (NMBAs) are commonly used to facilitate MV during ARDS, but, despite wide acceptance, there are few data and as yet no consensus available for when these agents should be used. Papazian et al (2010), in a multicenter, double-blind trial of early, severe ARDS, demonstrated that a 48-hour infusion of cisatracurium besylate resulted in improved 90-day survival (p = 0.04), less barotrauma, and increased time off the ventilator compared with the placebo group. Of interest, gas exchange measurements were essentially the same during neuromuscular blockade versus placebo. Although it remains to be elucidated why muscle paralysis may improve outcome, infusion of NMBAs in this study were theorized to lessen Ventilator Induced Lung Injury (VILI) by reducing atelectatrauma, barotrauma, and volutrauma. Muscle paralysis may also be of benefit in specific situations, such as intracranial hypertension or unconventional modes of ventilation (e.g., inverse ratio ventilation or extracorporeal techniques). Drawbacks to the use of these drugs include loss of neurologic examination, abolished cough, potential for an awake paralyzed patient, numerous medication and electrolyte interactions, potential for prolonged paralysis, and death associated with inadvertent ventilator disconnects. Use of NMBAs must not be taken lightly. Adequate sedation should be attempted first; if deemed absolutely necessary, use of NMBAs should be limited to 24 to 48 hours to prevent potential complications.

28. **Is split-lung ventilation ever useful?**

Split-lung ventilation (SLV) refers to ventilation of each lung independently, usually via a double-lumen endotracheal tube and two ventilators. Patients with severe unilateral lung disease may be candidates for SLV. SLV has been shown to improve oxygenation in patients with unilateral pneumonia, pulmonary edema, and contusion. Isolation of the lungs can save the life of patients with massive hemoptysis or lung abscess by protecting the good lung from spillage. Patients with a bronchopleural fistula also may benefit from SLV. Different modes of ventilation may be applied to each lung individually. The two ventilators need not be synchronized, and, in fact, hemodynamic stability is better maintained by using the two ventilators asynchronously.

WEBSITE

Institute for Healthcare Improvement: Implement the IHI ventilator bundle, http://www.ihi.org/resources/Pages/Changes/ImplementtheVentilatorBundle.aspx

SUGGESTED READINGS

Al-Hegelan M, MacIntyre NR: Novel modes of mechanical ventilation, Semin Respir Crit Care Med 34:499–507, 2013.

Futier E, Constantin JM, Paugam-Burtz C, et al: A trial of intraoperative low-tidal-volume ventilation in abdominal surgery, New Engl J Med 369:428–437, 2013.

Guérin CG, Reignier J, Richard JC, et al: Prone positioning in severe acute respiratory distress syndrome, N Engl J Med 368:2159–2168, 2013.

MacIntyre NR: Patient-ventilator interactions: optimizing conventional ventilation modes, Respir Care 56:73–84, 2011.

Neto AS, Cardoso SO, Manetta JA, et al: Association between use of lung-protective ventilation with lower tidal volumes and clinical outcomes among patients without acute respiratory distress syndrome, JAMA 308:1651–1659, 2012.

Papazian L, Forel JM, Gacouin A, et al: Neuromuscular blockers in early acute respiratory distress syndrome, N Engl J Med 363:1107–1116, 2010.

Pierson DJ: A primer on mechanical ventilation, Seattle, 2008, University of Washington. http://courses.washington.edu/med610/mechanicalventilation/mv_primer.html.

CHAPTER 21

PULSE OXIMETRY

Renee Koltes-Edwards, MD

1. Review pulse oximetry.

   Pulse oximetry is a noninvasive method by which arterial oxygenation can be approximated. It is based on the Beer-Lambert law and spectrophotometric analysis. When applied to pulse oximetry, the Beer-Lambert law essentially states that the intensity of transmitted light passing through a vascular bed decreases exponentially as a function of the concentration of the absorbing substances in that bed and the distance from the source of the light to the detector.

2. Is pulse oximetry an important monitor?

   Physiologic monitors provide the anesthesiologist information that must be integrated into the overall clinical picture. Every anesthesiologist should know the limits of the various physiologic monitors, and every monitor that is used in the operating room will, under the right conditions, give false readings. Pulse oximeters are no exception, and the clinician should have a good idea as to when the readings may be spurious.

3. How does a pulse oximeter work?

   A sensor is placed on either side of a pulsatile vascular bed such as the fingertip or earlobe. The light-emitting diodes (LEDs) on one side of the sensor send out two wavelengths of light: one red (600 to 750 nm wavelength) and one infrared (850 to 1000 nm wavelength). Most pulse oximeters use wavelengths of 660 nm (red) and 940 nm (infrared). The two wavelengths of light pass through the vascular bed to the other side of the sensor where a photodetector measures the amount of red and infrared light received.

4. How is oxygen saturation determined?

   A certain amount of the red and infrared light is absorbed by the tissues (including blood) that are situated between the emitters and detector. Therefore not all the light emitted by the LEDs makes it to the detector. Reduced hemoglobin absorbs much more of the red light (660 nm) than does oxyhemoglobin. Oxyhemoglobin absorbs more infrared light (940 nm) than does reduced hemoglobin. The detector measures the amount of light not absorbed at each wavelength, which in turn allows the microprocessor to determine a very specific number for the amount of hemoglobin and oxyhemoglobin present.

5. How does the pulse oximeter determine the degree of arterial hemoglobin saturation?

   In the vascular bed being monitored, the amount of blood is constantly changing because of the pulsation caused by each heartbeat. Thus the light beams pass not only through a relatively stable volume of bone, soft tissue, and venous blood but also through arterial blood, which is made up of a nonpulsatile portion and a variable, pulsatile portion. By measuring transmitted light several hundred times per second, the pulse oximeter is able to distinguish the changing, pulsatile component (AC) of the arterial blood from the unchanging, static component of the signal (DC) made up of the soft tissue, venous blood, and nonpulsatile arterial blood. The pulsatile component (AC), generally comprising 1% to 5% of the total signal, can then be isolated by canceling out the static components (DC) at each wavelength (Figure 21-1).

   The photodetector relays this information to the microprocessor. The microprocessor knows how much red and infrared light was emitted, how much red and infrared light has been detected, how much signal is static, and how much signal varies with pulsation. It then sets up what is known as the red/infrared (R/IR) ratio for the pulsatile (AC) portion of the blood. The R and IR of this ratio is the total of the absorbed light at each wavelength, respectively, for only the AC portion.

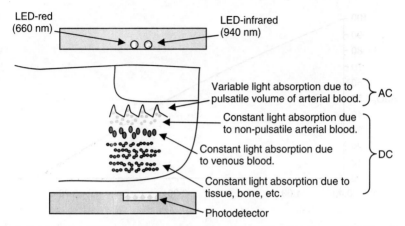

LED-red
(660 nm)

LED-infrared
(940 nm)

Variable light absorption due to pulsatile volume of arterial blood. } AC

Constant light absorption due to non-pulsatile arterial blood.

Constant light absorption due to venous blood.

Constant light absorption due to tissue, bone, etc.

} DC

Photodetector

Figure 21-1. Transmitted light passes through pulsatile arterial blood (AC) and other tissues (DC). The pulse oximeter can distinguish the AC from the DC portion by measuring transmitted light several hundred times per second.

6. **What is the normalization procedure?**
   Normalization involves dividing the pulsatile (AC) component of the red and infrared plethysmogram by the corresponding nonpulsatile (DC) component of the plethysmogram. This scaling process results in a normalized R/IR ratio, which is virtually independent of the incident light intensity.

$$R/IR \text{ ratio} = (AC_{red}/DC_{red})/(AC_{ir}/DC_{ir})$$

7. **How does the R/IR ratio relate to the oxygen saturation?**
   The normalized R/IR ratio is compared to a preset algorithm that gives the microprocessor the percentage of oxygenated hemoglobin in the arterial blood (the oxygen saturation percentage), and this percentage is displayed. This algorithm is derived from volunteers, usually healthy individuals who have been desaturated to a level of 75% to 80%; their arterial blood gas is drawn, and saturation is measured in a standard laboratory format. Manufacturers keep their algorithms secret, but in general an R/IR ratio of 0.4 corresponds to a saturation of 100%, an R/IR ratio of 1.0 corresponds to a saturation of about 87%, and an R/IR ratio of 3.4 corresponds to a saturation of 0% (Figure 21-2).

8. **Review the oxyhemoglobin dissociation curve.**
   It is a curve that describes the relationship between oxygen tension and binding (percentage oxygen saturation of hemoglobin) (Figure 21-3). Efficient oxygen transport relies on the ability of hemoglobin to reversibly load and unload oxygen. The sigmoid shape of the curve facilitates unloading of oxygen in the peripheral tissues, where the PaO_2 is low. At the capillary level, a large amount of oxygen is released from the hemoglobin, resulting in a relatively small drop in tension. This allows an adequate gradient for diffusion of oxygen into the cells and limits the degree of hemoglobin desaturation. The curve may be shifted to the left or right by many variables (Table 21-1).

9. **Why might the pulse oximeter give a false reading? Part 1—not R/IR related**
   • The algorithm the pulse oximeter uses to determine the saturation loses significant accuracy as saturation drops below 80%.
   • Saturation is averaged over a time period of anywhere from 5 to 20 seconds. As a patient is desaturating, the reading on the monitor screen will be higher than the actual saturation. This becomes critical as the patient enters the steep part of the oxyhemoglobin desaturation curve because the degree of desaturation increases dramatically and may exceed the ability of the monitor to change rapidly enough to

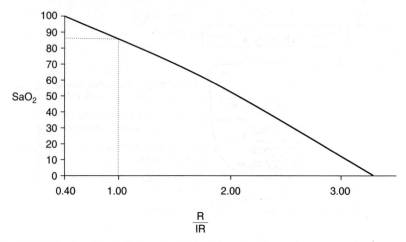

Figure 21-2. The ratio of absorbed red to infrared light corresponds to the appropriate percentage of oxygenated hemoglobin.

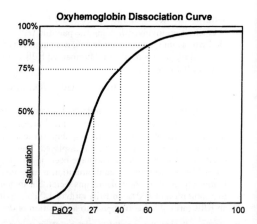

Figure 21-3. Oxyhemoglobin dissociation curve describes the nonlinear relationship between PaO_2 and percentage saturation of hemoglobin with oxygen (SaO_2). In the steep part of the curve (50% region), small changes in PaO_2 result in large changes in SaO_2.

Table 21-1. Left and Right Shifts of the Oxyhemoglobin Dissociation Curve

RIGHT SHIFT	LEFT SHIFT
Effects: Decreased affinity of Hb for O_2 (facilitates unloading of O_2 to tissues)	**Effects:** Increased affinity of Hb for O_2 (decreases unloading of O_2 from Hb)
Causes: Increased PCO_2 Hyperthermia Acidosis Increased altitude Increased 2,3-DPG Sickle cell anemia	**Causes:** Decreased PCO_2 Hypothermia Alkalosis Fetal hemoglobin Decreased 2,3-DPG Carboxyhemoglobin Methemoglobin

Hb, Hemoglobin; 2,3-DPG, 2,3-diphosphoglycerate.

show the true level of oxygen saturation. Likewise, as a person's saturation increases, the displayed reading on the screen will be lower than the actual saturation.

- Dark pigmentation of the skin may overestimate oxygen saturation.
- Response time to changes in saturation is related to probe location. Response time is less with ear probes and greater with finger probes.
- Anemia, hypotension; poor perfusion at the site of measurement; and nail polish, especially blue or black polish, also lead to false readings.

10. **Why might the pulse oximeter give a false reading? Part 2—R/IR related**

The R/IR ratio determines the displayed saturation. Any circumstance that erroneously drives the R/IR number toward 1.0 will result in a saturation reading approaching 87%. The overwhelming majority of times, these circumstances develop in well-oxygenated patients and result in a falsely low displayed saturation.

What can affect the R/IR number?

- Motion artifact causes a low signal-to-noise ratio, alters the absorption detection of both the red and infrared light by the photodetector, drives the R/IR ratio toward 1.0, and results in false saturation readings.
- Fluorescent lighting and operating room lights, because of their phased light production (and too fast for the human eye to detect), can cause false R/IR readings.
- Dyshemoglobinemias (carboxyhemoglobin [COHb] and methemoglobin [MetHb]) may create inaccurate oxygen saturation measurement. At 660 nm, COHb absorbs light, much like oxygenated hemoglobin, causing an overestimation of true saturation. The influence of methemoglobinemia on SpO_2 readings is more complicated. MetHb looks much like reduced Hb at 660 nm. However, more important, at 940 nm the absorbance of MetHb is markedly greater than that of either reduced or oxygenated Hb. Therefore the monitor reads it as absorption of both species, driving the R/IR number toward 1.0 and the saturation toward 87%. Therefore at a high SaO_2 level, the probe underestimates the true value; at a low SaO_2 level, the value is falsely elevated.

11. **What is methemoglobinemia?**

It is a blood disorder in which an abnormal amount of MetHb, greater than 1.5%, is found in the blood. MetHb is a form of hemoglobin that contains ferric (Fe^{3+}) instead of normal ferrous (Fe^{2+}) iron in the hemoglobin molecule. This abnormal hemoglobin species is unable to bind oxygen (O_2) and causes impaired release of oxygen from other O_2-binding sites. This prevents supplying oxygen to the body tissues and results in an O_2-Hb dissociation curve shift to the left.

12. **What are the causes of methemoglobinemia?**

Methemoglobinemia can be either inherited or acquired. The most common form is acquired from exposure to medications or chemicals. These agents include local anesthetics such as benzocaine, prilocaine, procaine, and lidocaine, vasodilators like nitroglycerin and nitroprusside, antibiotics like sulfonamides and benzene compounds and aniline dyes. A common feature of all these is the presence of nitrogen atoms. Nitrogen is capable of extracting electrons from iron, resulting in changes in Fe^{2+} to Fe^{3+}.

13. **How does methemoglobinemia affect the pulse oximeter reading?**

With increasing levels of methemoglobinemia in the blood, the pulse oximetry values decrease until the SpO_2 reads approximately 85%. At that point the SpO_2 reading does not decrease further even though the amount of MetHb may be increasing further and the true HbO_2 saturation is much lower. At this level of a pulse oximeter reading of 85%, the MetHb amount can be 35% or more. Conventional pulse oximetry uses two wavelengths of light and compares absorbance ratios to empirical data. Different Hb species have different absorption coefficients and in MetHb the ratios of absorbances approximate 1 at an SpO_2 of 85%.

14. **If one suspects methemoglobinemia, what test will establish it?**

If one suspects methemoglobinemia, then a direct measurement of oxyhemoglobin by a co-oximeter blood gas analysis is required. A conventional pulse oximeter can neither detect MetHb nor accurately determine SpO_2 when MetHb is present. A co-oximeter uses four different wavelengths of light and four species of hemoglobin are quantified; these four are oxygenated Hb, reduced Hb, MetHb, and COHb. The oxyhemoglobin saturation is then the percentage of HbO_2 of all the species determined to be present.

15. **How does methemoglobinemia affect the pulse oximeter reading?**
    With increasing levels of MetHb in the blood, the pulse oximetry values decrease until the SpO_2 reads approximately 85%. At that point the SpO_2 reading does not decrease further even though the amount of MetHb may be increasing further and the true HbO_2 saturation is much lower. At this level of a pulse oximeter reading of 85%, the MetHb amount can be 35% or more. Conventional pulse oximetry uses two wavelengths of light and compares absorbance ratios to empirical data. Different Hb species have different absorption coefficients and in MetHb the ratios of absorbances approximate 1 at an SpO_2 of 85%.

16. **What is the treatment for methemoglobinemia?**
    If the methemoglobinemia is severe, the treatment is intravenous methylene blue and increasing the O_2 to 100%, removing the offending agent, and providing hemodynamic support. Methylene blue acts as a cofactor to speed up the enzymatic reaction, thus reducing Fe_3^+ to Fe_2^+ (methemoglobin reductase.)
    Give 1 to 2 mg/kg over 5 min and the dose may be repeated in an hour to a maximum dose of 7 mg/kg. Methylene blue should not be used in patients with glucose-6-phosphate deficiency or a hemolytic anemia can be precipitated.

17. **The saturation plummets after injection of methylene blue. Is the patient desaturating?**
    No, methylene blue is sufficiently dark so as to deceive the actual hemoglobin saturation.

18. **Since the patient is oxygenated before anesthetic induction, if the pulse oximeter reaches 100%, does this indicate complete denitrogenation?**
    Replacing all alveolar nitrogen with oxygen provides a depot of oxygen that might be necessary if mask ventilation or intubation proves difficult. Hemoglobin may be completely saturated with oxygen before total pulmonary washout of nitrogen. Thus a reading of 100% in and of itself is not an accurate indication of denitrogenation.

19. **Is the pulse oximeter a good indicator of ventilation?**
    A pulse oximeter gives no indication of ventilation, only of oxygenation. For instance, a breathing patient may have an oxygen mask delivering 50% or more oxygen and an SpO_2 reading in the 90s, yet be hypoventilating and hypercapnic. In this situation, the oximeter reading gives a false sense of security. A better approach would be to administer less oxygen, and, as the pulse oximeter values decrease below 90, it would alert the nurse to tend to the patient. Arousing the patient from sleep, encouraging him or her to breathe deeply, and elevating the head of the patient's bed are better strategies than just increasing the delivered oxygen concentration. Always treat the cause, not the symptom; treat the patient, not the numbers.

20. **Are there complications associated with the use of pulse oximetry probes?**
    Pressure necrosis of the skin has been reported in both neonates and adults when the probe has been left on the same digit for prolonged periods of time. Digital burns from the LEDs have been reported in patients undergoing photodynamic therapy.

21. **How is the pulse oximeter waveform used to determine fluid responsiveness?**
    Arterial pulse volume will vary during the inspiratory and expiratory phases of the respiratory cycle, especially when preload is inadequate. Respiratory variations in the pulse oximetry waveform amplitude may give some indication of fluid resuscitation in selected patients.

KEY POINTS: PULSE OXIMETRY

1. Use of pulse oximetry has allowed anesthesiologists to rapidly detect and treat acute decreases in oxygen saturation.
2. As with all monitors, understanding both the methods of operation and the limitations of pulse oximeters is critical to the delivery of safe care. Pulse oximeters can give falsely high and low numbers; understand the reasons why that is so.
3. Treat the patient, not the symptom! Oxygenation and ventilation are separate processes, and pulse oximetry does not assess adequacy of ventilation.

WEBSITE

American Society of Anesthesiologists annual meeting abstract website: http://www.asa-abstracts.com

SUGGESTED READINGS

Barker S: Motion-resistant pulse oximetry: a comparison of new and old models, Anesth Analg 95:967–972, 2002.

Moyle J: Pulse oximetry, ed 2, London, 2002, BMJ Publishing Group.

Pedersen T, Moller AM, Pedersen BD: Pulse oximetry for perioperative monitoring: systematic review of randomized, controlled trials, Anesth Analg 96:426–431, 2003.

CHAPTER 22

CAPNOGRAPHY

James C. Duke, MD, MBA

1. **What is the difference between capnometry and capnography? Which is better?**
   Capnometry is defined as the numeric measurement and display of the level of CO_2. It is not nearly as valuable as capnography, in which the expired CO_2 level is graphically displayed as a function of time and concentration.

2. **Describe the most common method of gas sampling and the associated problems.**
   Sidestream devices aspirate gas (typically 50 to 250 ml/min), usually from the Y-piece of the circuit, and transport the gas via small-bore tubing to the analyzer. Sampling can also be performed by nasal cannulas; however, because of room air entrainment and dilution of the CO_2 concentration, the Y-piece provides qualitatively and quantitatively a better sample than nasal cannulas. Problems with sidestream measurement include a finite delay until the results of the gas sample are displayed and possible clogging of the tubing with condensed water vapor or mucus. Infrared absorption is the most common method of CO_2 analysis.

3. **What is the importance of measuring CO_2?**
   End-tidal carbon dioxide ($ETCO_2$) monitoring has been an important factor in reducing anesthesia-related mortality and morbidity. Short of bronchoscopy, carbon dioxide monitoring is considered the best method of verifying correct endotracheal tube (ETT) placement. In addition to its value as a safety monitor, evaluation of expiratory CO_2 provides valuable information about important physiologic factors, including ventilation, cardiac output, and metabolic activity, and proper ventilator functioning. $ETCO_2$ levels have also been used to predict outcome of resuscitation. A prospective observation study of 150 out-of-hospital cardiac arrests found that an $ETCO_2$ level less than 10 mm Hg after 20 minutes of standard advanced cardiac life support was 100% predictive of failure to resuscitate.

4. **Describe the capnographic waveform.**
   The important features include baseline level, the extent and rate of rise of CO_2, and the contour of the capnograph. Capnograms may be evaluated breath by breath, or trends may be assessed as valuable clues to a patient's physiologic status. There are four distinct phases to a capnogram (Figure 22-1). The first phase (A–B) is the initial stage of exhalation, in which the gas sampled is dead space gas, free of CO_2. At point B, there is mixing of alveolar gas with dead space gas, and the CO_2 level abruptly rises. The expiratory or alveolar plateau is represented by phase C–D, and the gas sampled is essentially alveolar. Point D is the maximal CO_2 level, the best reflection of alveolar CO_2, and is known as $ETCO_2$. Fresh gas is entrained as the patient inspires (phase D–E), and the trace returns to the baseline level of CO_2, approximately zero.

5. **What may cause elevation of the baseline of the capnogram?**
   The baseline of the capnogram may not return to zero at high respiratory rates. However, if the baseline is elevated more than approximately 2 mm Hg CO_2, the patient is receiving CO_2 during inspiration, and this is often termed *rebreathing* (Figure 22-2). Possible causes of rebreathing include the following:
   - An exhausted CO_2 absorber and unrecognized dye indicator
   - Channeling of the gas within the CO_2 absorber and unrecognized dye indicator
   - An incompetent unidirectional inspiratory or expiratory valve, often in circle systems
   - Accidental administration of CO_2 (perhaps from a CO_2 tank used for laparoscopy)
   - Bicarbonate administration
   - Tourniquet release
   - Inadequate fresh gas flow
   - Sepsis and other hypermetabolic event (fever, malignant hyperthermia)

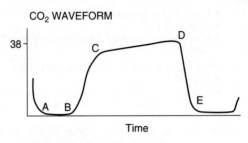

CO₂ WAVEFORM

Figure 22-1. The capnographic waveform. A–B, Exhalation of CO₂ free gas from dead space; B–C, combination of dead space and alveolar gas; C–D, exhalation of mostly alveolar gas; D, end-tidal point (alveolar plateau); D–E, inhalation of CO₂ free gas.

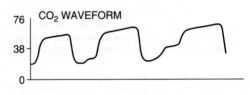

Figure 22-2. Rebreathing of CO₂ as demonstrated by failure of the waveform to return to a zero baseline.

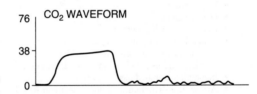

Figure 22-3. A sudden drop of ETCO₂ to near zero may indicate a loss of ventilation or catastrophic decreases in cardiac output.

6. **Does ETCO₂ correlate with PaCO₂?**
   CO₂ is easily diffusible across the endothelial-alveolar membrane; thus ETCO₂ should provide an estimate of alveolar CO₂ partial pressures and arterial carbon dioxide partial pressures (PaCO₂). Alveolar carbon dioxide partial pressures and PaCO₂ normally differ by about 5 mm Hg, the small difference caused mostly by alveolar dead space (nonperfused areas of the lung that are ventilated).
   As maldistribution between ventilation and perfusion increases, the correlation between ETCO₂ and PaCO₂ decreases, with ETCO₂ being lower. Increased dead space results in an increased gradient and may be associated with shock, air embolism or thromboembolism, cardiac arrest, chronic lung disease, reactive airway disease, or lateral decubitus positioning. Conversely, increases in cardiac output and pulmonary blood flow will decrease the gradient.
   When increases in dead space ventilation are suspected, the gradient between ETCO₂ and PaCO₂ can be determined by arterial blood gas analysis. With the gradient factored in, tracking of ETCO₂ is still a useful, indirect measure of arterial CO₂ content. Of note, shunt has minimal effect on arterial-alveolar CO₂ gradients.

7. **Is it possible to see exhaled CO₂ after accidental intubation of the esophagus?**
   Carbonated beverages or medications (e.g., Alka-Seltzer) return CO₂ after esophageal intubation. However, the usual CO₂ values and waveform would not be expected, and the CO₂ would likely exhaust quickly. Some CO₂ can also reach the stomach if mask ventilation is suboptimal.

8. **What might result in sudden loss of capnographic waveform?**
   A sudden loss of capnographic waveform (Figure 22-3) may be caused by the following:
   • Esophageal intubation
   • Ventilator disconnection or malfunction

- Capnographic disconnection or malfunction
- Obstructed ETT
- Catastrophic physiologic disturbance such as cardiac arrest or massive pulmonary embolus

9. **What else may result in increases in ETCO$_2$?**
   - Exhausted soda lime
   - Failure to recognize dye indicator and channeling of CO_2 through soda lime canister
   - Sepsis or other hypermetabolic events (fever, malignant hyperthermia)

KEY POINTS: CAPNOGRAPHY

1. Short of visualizing with bronchoscopy, CO_2 detection is the best method of verifying ETT location.
2. In the absence of ventilation-perfusion abnormalities, ETCO$_2$ roughly approximates PaCO$_2$.
3. Analysis of the capnographic waveform provides supportive evidence for numerous clinical conditions, including decreasing cardiac output; altered metabolic activity; acute and chronic pulmonary disease; and ventilator, circuit, and ETT malfunction.

---

10. **What process might lead to decreases in ETCO$_2$?**
    Rapid decreases in CO_2 waveforms may be associated with the following:
    - Hypotension
    - Hypovolemia
    - Decreased cardiac output
    - Lesser degrees of pulmonary embolism
    - Dislodgement of a correctly placed ETT
      Other, and usually less dramatic, decreases in ETCO$_2$ may be caused by the following:
    - Incomplete exhaled gas sampling
    - Airway leaks (including endotracheal cuff leaks)
    - Partial circuit disconnections
    - Partial airway obstruction
    - Hyperventilation
    - Hypothermia
    - Increasing dead space
    - Decreased metabolic activity (e.g., after neuromuscular blockade) (Figure 22-4)

11. **What processes may increase ETCO$_2$?**
    ETCO$_2$ values may rise gradually secondary to the following (Figure 22-5):
    - Hypoventilation
    - Increasing body temperature

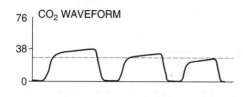

Figure 22-4. A gradual lowering of ETCO$_2$ indicates decreasing CO_2 production or decreasing pulmonary perfusion.

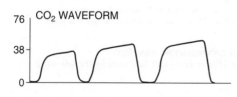

Figure 22-5. A rising ETCO$_2$ is associated with hypoventilation, increasing CO_2 production, and absorption of CO_2 from an exogenous source such as CO_2 laparoscopy.

Figure 22-6. A steep slope suggests obstructive lung disease.

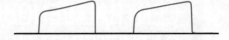

Figure 22-7. A cleft in the alveolar plateau usually indicates partial recovery from neuromuscular blockade. Surgical manipulation against the inferior surface of the diaphragm or weight on the chest may produce similar though usually other irregular waveforms as seen in Figure 22-8.

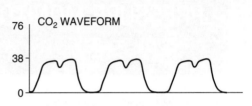

Figure 22-8. A sudden drop of $ETCO_2$ to a low but nonzero value is seen with incomplete sampling of patient exhalation, system leaks, or partial airway obstruction.

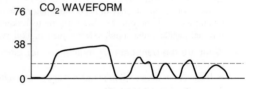

- Increased metabolic activity (e.g., fever, sepsis, malignant hyperthermia)
- Partial airway obstruction
- Bronchial intubation
- Rebreathing
- Exogenous CO_2 absorption (such as during laparoscopy) and venous CO_2 embolism
- Exhausted CO_2 absorber
- Inadequate fresh gas flow
- Faulty ventilator or anesthesia circuit valves
- Transient increases in $ETCO_2$ (may be noted after intravenous bicarbonate administration, release of extremity tourniquets, or removal of vascular cross-clamps)

12. **What processes can change the usual configuration of the waveform?**
    Asthma and chronic obstructive pulmonary diseases cause a delayed upslope and steep alveolar plateau (Figure 22-6).
    A commonly seen abnormal capnogram results when the patient makes spontaneous respiratory efforts and inhales before the next mechanical inspiration. This characteristic *cleft* in the alveolar plateau is a useful clinical sign indicating that the patient has started to breathe (Figure 22-7). Finally, a cuff leak may result in variable early decreases in the normal waveform configuration (Figure 22-8). Waveforms that are irregular and unlike neighboring waveforms may be caused by manipulation against the diaphragm by the surgeons, pressure of a surgeon against the chest wall, percussing against an abdomen distended by CO_2, or spontaneous breathing out of phase with mechanical ventilation.

WEBSITE

Capnography: www.capnography.com (Excellent and interactive)

SUGGESTED READINGS

Moon RE, Camporesi EM: Respiratory monitoring. In Miller RD, editor: Miller's anesthesia, ed 6, Philadelphia, 2005, Churchill Livingstone, pp 1437–1482.
Tautz TJ, Unwyler A, Antogini JF, et al: Case scenario: Increased end-tidal carbon dioxide: a diagnostic dilemma, Anesthesiology 112:440–4016, 2010.

CHAPTER 23

CENTRAL VENOUS CATHETERIZATION AND PRESSURE MONITORING

Daniel R. Beck, MD, MS, and Jacob Friedman, MD

1. **Define central venous catheterization.**

   Central venous catheterization involves inserting a catheter into the venous circulation and advancing it so its distal orifice is positioned immediately adjacent to or within the right atrium of the heart (Figure 23-1). Several access points can be chosen, and a patient's clinical condition, urgency of need, and anatomy may dictate the most successful approach. Operators should become familiar with the technique for cannulating the subclavian, internal jugular, antecubital, external jugular, axillary, and femoral veins.

2. **What are the perioperative indications for placement of a central venous catheter?**
   - Intravenous access when peripheral access is insufficient
   - Guiding fluid replacement
   - Evaluating cardiac function
   - Providing access for the following:
     - Aspiration of air emboli that can occur during neurosurgical procedures
     - Drug infusion
     - Blood and fluid infusion
     - Introducing a pulmonary artery catheter or transvenous pacemaker
     - Blood sampling

3. **What are the nonoperative indications for placement of a central venous catheter?**
   - Hyperalimentation
   - Temporary hemodialysis
   - Long-term chemotherapy
   - Frequent therapeutic plasmapheresis

4. **What are contraindications to central venous cannulation?**
   - Infection or obvious contamination of the site to be cannulated
   - Coagulopathy and choice of a non-compressible venous site (subclavian)
   - Presence, or concern for, thrombus in the vein to be cannulated
   - Patient intolerance

5. **How is a catheter introduced into the central venous circulation?**

   Before cannulation is attempted, Trendelenburg positioning will increase venous pressure at an upper body target vessel to avoid air embolism. As the needle is advanced toward a vessel, gentle, continuous aspiration is required. Occasionally during needle advancement, the vessel walls will collapse. Blood can be aspirated by slowly withdrawing the needle. Thorough knowledge of adjacent vital structures is important to avoid complications.

   Although a catheter can be inserted through a large-bore needle, the most common technique involves passing it over a guidewire, commonly referred to as the Seldinger technique. An 18- or 20-G needle is introduced into the vessel, and a guidewire is threaded through the needle and into the vein. The needle is removed, leaving the guidewire in place. The catheter is then passed over the guidewire and into the vessel. Finally the guidewire is removed. The obvious benefit of the Seldinger technique rests in the use of a smaller gauge introducer needle.

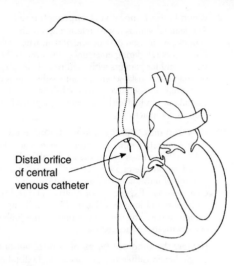

Distal orifice
of central
venous catheter

Figure 23-1. Placement of the central venous
catheter.

6. Describe the subclavian vein approach.
   The subclavian approach is commonly used because of the ease of access to the vessel.
   The vein is best cannulated from the infraclavicular approach with the patient in the
   Trendelenburg position. The subclavian vein runs parallel to and just below the middle
   third of the clavicle. The skin puncture is made just lateral to, and one finger-width below,
   the costoclavicular ligament. This structure can be identified by a notch two thirds of the
   length lateral to the sternal-clavicular junction. The needle is directed along the posterior
   border of the clavicle in the direction of the sternal notch until venous blood is aspirated.
   Care should be taken to approach with a flat trajectory just beneath the clavicle to avoid
   the dome of the lung.

7. Describe the internal jugular vein approach.
   There are several approaches to the internal jugular vein, three of which are briefly
   described here. The patient is first put in the Trendelenburg position.
   • **Low anterior:** Locate the point at which the sternal and clavicular heads of the
     sternocleidomastoid muscle join. Introduce the needle at this point and direct it at a
     30-degree angle to the skin. Advance the needle toward the ipsilateral nipple until
     venous blood is aspirated.
   • **High anterior:** Palpate the carotid artery at the level of the cricothyroid membrane.
     Introduce the needle just lateral to the carotid pulsation and advance it toward the
     ipsilateral nipple at a 30-degree angle until venous blood is aspirated. This approach
     frequently requires penetration of the sternocleidomastoid muscle by the introducer
     needle.
   • **Posterior:** Locate the junction of the posterior border of the sternocleidomastoid muscle
     and the external jugular vein. Introduce the needle just posterior to this point and
     advance it along the deep surface of the muscle toward the ipsilateral corner of the
     sternal notch until venous blood is aspirated.

8. Describe the external jugular vein approach.
   When the patient is in a Trendelenburg position, the external jugular vein frequently can
   be visualized where it crosses the sternocleidomastoid muscle. The needle is advanced
   in a direction paralleling the vessel and is introduced into the vein approximately two
   finger-widths below the inferior border of the mandible. Difficulty may arise in advancing
   the catheter or guidewire into the central circulation from the external jugular vein
   approach because the patient's anatomy frequently directs the catheter into the subclavian
   rather than the innominate vein. It is also frequently difficult to pass the guidewire or
   catheter past the clavicle.

9. **When is the femoral vein approach used?**
   The femoral vein is not a preferred approach because of the high risk of infection. Femoral venous cannulation may be undertaken when subclavian or internal jugular catheterization is unsuccessful, during emergency situations (CPR in progress or injury to upper extremity veins), and for patients with high risk of complications (coagulopathy, intolerance to pneumothorax risk) where a compressible site is desired. Alternatively, femoral lines may be desired perioperatively to establish access for emergency cardiopulmonary bypass cannulation in high-risk cardiothoracic procedures. Femoral lines should be removed as soon as it is practical.

10. **How can ultrasound guidance improve catheter placement?**
    Approximately 5 million central catheters are placed per year in the United States, with a 60% to 95% success rate using landmark techniques. This also leads to a mechanical complication rate of 5% to 19%, typically arterial puncture, hematoma, or pneumothorax. The use of ultrasound guidance drastically increases first pass success rates and limits complications. Experience with ultrasound technique, including visualizing structures in both short and long axis (Figure 23-2), will improve success rate and minimize complications. The use of ultrasound is not foolproof, and complications do still routinely occur with inexperienced users.

11. **Review the different types of central venous catheters.**
    Single-lumen catheters may have a single distal port or multiport tips. Triple-lumen catheters have three channels and lumens at slightly different positions on the distal cannula, providing ports for simultaneous drug infusion, blood drawing, and central venous pressure (CVP) monitoring. They are available in 7.5- and 9-Fr sizes. A percutaneous introducer sheath is designed for insertion of a pulmonary artery catheter into the central circulation. It is a large-bore catheter (9 Fr) and has a side port that can be used for CVP monitoring or for fluid infusion. Some catheters are heparin-coated, chlorhexidine or silver impregnated to help avoid thrombosis or infection.

12. **How do you verify venous puncture? Is blue blood enough?**
    Arterial blood may be dark because the patient is hypoxic, cardiac output is inadequate, or the patient may have methemoglobinemia, for example. Arterial flow of blood may be nonpulsatile in extreme cardiac failure. The best way to determine whether you are in a vein is to thread a short, small-gauge catheter (e.g., 18- or 20-G) over the wire, remove the wire, and transduce the small catheter. A short section of IV tubing connected to a catheter can be useful; venous cannulation will lead to a blood column height consistent with the CVP, and arterial cannulation will reveal pressure that overflows the tubing. Alternatively, ultrasound can visualize the guidewire in the vein (Figure 23-2), or bedside echocardiography can visualize the wire in the right atrium.

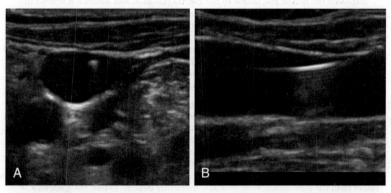

Figure 23-2. Ultrasound internal jugular guidewire in short (A) and long (B) axis views.

13. How is CVP measured?

The central venous catheter is typically attached to an electronic pressure transducer that converts the pressure transmitted via the catheter into an electrical signal that is displayed (in millimeters of mercury [mm Hg]) on a real-time display screen (1 mm Hg = 1.3 cm of H_2O of height above the reference point). When measuring CVP, it is crucial to place the pressure transducer or base of the manometer at the same (atrial) level each time because a variance of only a few centimeters from that level will result in a significant percentage measurement error given the typical CVP range of 0 to 13 cm of H_2O. For example, a 2.6-cm elevation of transducer will drop the CVP 2 mm Hg. For an actual CVP of 10, a 2–mm Hg error is 2/10 = 20% error. In contrast, variation in the transducer position during arterial or pulmonary artery pressure measurement will result in a much smaller error with the greater magnitude of pressures.

14. At what point on the body should CVP be measured?

The ideal point at which to measure CVP is at the level of the tricuspid valve. It is at this point that, in the healthy heart, hydrostatic pressures caused by changes in body position are almost zero. This phenomenon exists because, as the pressure at the tricuspid valve changes (e.g., if it increases from position change), the right ventricle will fill to a greater degree, right ventricular output will transiently increase, and the change in pressure at the tricuspid valve will be brought back toward zero. The opposite will occur if pressure at the tricuspid valve decreases.

An external landmark for the tricuspid is a point 2 inches behind the sternum, roughly the anterior axillary line, at the fourth intercostal space. Ongoing adjustment is necessary to ensure that the transducer or manometer is consistently at this level whenever the patient's position or bed height is changed (Figure 23-3).

15. Where should the distal orifice of the catheter be positioned?

When pressure measurements guide fluid management, the tip of the catheter can be positioned within either the atrium or the vena cava near the caval-atrial junction.

For monitoring the waveform of the CVP tracing, position the catheter within the atrium. By so positioning, the waveform will not be damped and will accurately reflect the pressure changes within the right atrium.

Placement of the catheter for aspiration of air emboli during neurosurgical cases requires positioning of the catheter (preferably multiport) tip in the right atrium near the superior vena cava–atrial junction. Embolized air flows past this point and accumulates in the superior aspect of the atrium. Positioning the catheter tip at the superior vena cava–atrial junction allows for optimal aspiration.

16. How can you judge the correct positioning of the distal orifice of the catheter?

- Before insertion, measure the distance from the point of insertion to the right atrium (external landmark—immediately to the right of the third costal cartilage), giving a rough estimate of the length of inserted catheter necessary.
- Advancing the catheter under fluoroscopy is the most accurate method for positioning the catheter tip but is time consuming and cumbersome.
- With a specialized central venous catheter, the tip can be used as an electrocardiogram (ECG) electrode. After insertion, the catheter is filled with electrolyte solution (normal

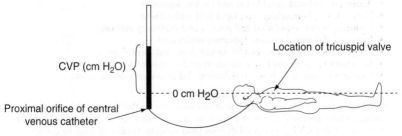

Figure 23-3. Positioning of the patient for central venous catheter measurement.

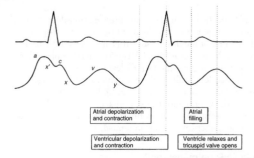

| Atrial depolarization and contraction | Atrial filling |
| Ventricular depolarization and contraction | Ventricle relaxes and tricuspid valve opens |

Figure 23-4. Normal central venous pressure waveform.

saline or 8.4% NaHCO$_3$), and the V lead of the ECG is attached to a proximal connection. The catheter is advanced toward the right atrium. The P-wave axis and voltage on the V lead tracing indicate the catheter tip position. As the catheter tip passes the area of the sinoatrial node, the P wave becomes equal in height to the R wave of the ECG. The catheter tip passing the mid-atrial position is demonstrated by a decreasing or biphasic P wave. Low atrial positioning is indicated by an inverted P wave or absence of the P wave.
- Surface transthoracic echocardiography or transesophageal echocardiography can also guide positioning, but training is required to obtain the appropriate views.

17. **Describe the normal CVP waveform, and relate its pattern to the cardiac cycle.**
The normal CVP waveform shows a pattern of three upstrokes and two descents that correspond to certain events in the cardiac cycle (Figure 23-4).
- The a wave represents the increase in atrial pressure that occurs during atrial contraction.
- The x' descent is the decrease in atrial pressure as the atrium begins to relax.
- Before total relaxation is completed, the c wave occurs, which is caused by the bulging of the tricuspid valve into the atrium during the early phases of right ventricular contraction.
- The x descent follows the c wave and is a continuation of the x' descent. The x descent is caused by a drop in pressure brought about by a downward movement of the ventricle and tricuspid valve during the later stages of ventricular contraction.
- The v wave represents the increase in atrial pressure that occurs while the atrium fills against a closed tricuspid valve.
- The y descent represents a drop in pressure as the ventricle relaxes, the tricuspid valve opens (because atrial pressure is higher than ventricular pressure at this point in time), and blood passively enters the ventricle.

18. **What influences CVP?**
CVP is directly related to returning blood volume, venomotor tone, and intrathoracic pressure and inversely related to cardiac function. The following perioperative events may change these variables:
- Anesthetic-induced vasodilation and cardiac depression
- Hypovolemia, hemorrhage, and rapid fluid replacement
- Positive-pressure ventilation and positive end-expiratory pressure
- Increased abdominal pressure (pneumoperitoneum)
- Sympathetic activation caused by agonist drugs and surgical stress
- Intraoperative ischemia may cause diastolic dysfunction or heart failure
- Patient positioning such as Trendelenburg, lithotomy, or seated position

19. **Is CVP an indicator of cardiac output?**
Cardiac output is primarily a function of venous return (in the absence of frank heart failure), along with modulation by heart rate, cardiac contractility, and peripheral vascular resistance. Since CVP does not solely reflect intravascular volume, it must be considered within the clinical context to be valuable. For instance, although a rising CVP suggests an

increased intravascular volume and improved venous return to the thorax, CVP will also increase in conditions such as right heart failure, cardiac tamponade, tension pneumothorax, pulmonary embolism, pulmonary hypertension, tricuspid regurgitation, and increasing intraabdominal pressure. These events are associated with decreasing cardiac output.

20. **How does CVP relate to right ventricular preload?**

CVP has long been thought to reflect right ventricular preload or, more specifically, right ventricular end-diastolic volume. End-diastolic volume is a key parameter in the Frank–Starling law of the heart. Recently it has been shown that CVP does not necessarily correlate with ventricular volume, cardiac performance, or the response of the heart to volume infusions in both normal and compromised patients. The likely reason for this is a large spread and nonlinearity in diastolic ventricular compliances among individuals and incomplete knowledge of transmural pressures.

Despite the previous findings, it is widely held that CVP measurement is useful to the clinician as a guide to intravenous fluid replacement, especially at the upper and lower ranges of CVP, or as a trend monitor. Thus a low (0 to 2 mm Hg) or decreasing CVP may indicate a need for fluid administration, whereas an increasing or elevated CVP (above 12 mm Hg) may indicate over-resuscitation or a patient with impaired cardiac performance. The response of CVP to a fluid bolus has also been shown to be useful in assessing fluid status. Figure 23-5 shows that a 200-ml fluid bolus in the hypovolemic patient will result in a small but transient increase in CVP, whereas the same bolus in the normovolemic patient will result in a larger but still transient increase. However, in the hypervolemic patient with right ventricular failure, the same bolus results in a sustained increase in CVP. The CVP is best used to monitor a trend; an isolated determination is of limited value.

KEY POINTS: CENTRAL VENOUS CATHETERIZATION AND PRESSURE MONITORING

1. Trends in CVPs are more valuable than isolated values and should always be evaluated in the context of the patient's scenario.
2. At best, CVP gives an estimate of cardiac preload, and there are many variables that influence its numeric value and interpretation.
3. Since complications of central venous catheterization are serious and include pneumothorax, arterial injury, hemothorax, thoracic duct laceration, air embolus, thromboembolism, and infection, with information obtained that is supportive rather than definitive, this procedure should not be performed casually. Ultrasound guidance may help mitigate risk of placement.
4. The CVP provides limited information about left heart function.

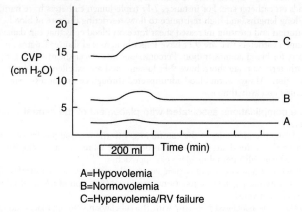

A=Hypovolemia
B=Normovolemia
C=Hypervolemia/RV failure

Figure 23-5. Central venous pressure (CVP) and fluid status. *RV,* Right ventricular.

21. **Does CVP relate to left ventricular preload?**
    CVP possibly reflects right ventricular preload only. In patients whose left and right ventricles are functioning normally, CVP often parallels the left atrial pressure, which may reflect the preload of the left ventricle. However, in patients with pulmonary hypertension, lung disease, right or left ventricular function abnormality, or valvular regurgitation, a pulmonary artery catheter provides better information with regard to the left side of the heart than does a central venous catheter. Echocardiography is slowly replacing pressure measurements as the gold standard for left ventricular filling status and biventricular function assessment in the operating room.

22. **Is there a single normal CVP reading?**
    No single CVP is normal for all patients. Resting CVP may range from 0 to 10 mm Hg in different individuals and varies little over time. The reason for this spread is not clear, although it is not necessarily related to blood volume. In the operating room there are frequent perturbations that can impact the CVP, and the correct interpretation of a changing CVP is often not obvious. Because of this, it becomes important to use all available clinical signs, including fluid resuscitation, urine output, blood pressure, and effects of anesthetic agents to determine an appropriate range of CVP for that patient.

23. **Are there noninvasive alternatives to CVP that better indicate volume status?**
    In recent years as it has become clear that CVP does not reliably correlate with preload and may be a useful indicator of the hemodynamic state only at the extremes, the more dynamic concept of *fluid responsiveness* has emerged for optimizing fluid therapy. Various techniques have been used to measure fluid responsiveness. For example, respiratory variation in systolic pressure during positive-pressure ventilation will decrease as volume is infused in a hypovolemic patient, or an esophageal Doppler or transesophageal echocardiogram can be used to measure increased descending aortic flow velocity (which mirrors cardiac output) as fluid is infused.

24. **How can an abnormal CVP waveform be used to diagnose abnormal cardiac events?**
    It may be used to assist in diagnosis of pathophysiologic events affecting right heart function. For example, atrial fibrillation is characterized by absence of the normal a wave component. Tricuspid regurgitation results in a *giant V wave* that replaces the normal c, x, and v waves. Other events that can change the normal shape of the CVP waveform include junctional rhythm with cannon A waves, atrioventricular dissociation, asynchronous atrial contraction during ventricular pacing, tricuspid stenosis, cardiac tamponade, increased ventricular afterload (from pulmonary hypertension or pulmonary embolus), and right ventricular ischemia and failure.

25. **Can you use the central venous catheter for blood transfusions?**
    It depends on catheter size. For instance, 7-Fr triple-lumen catheters have narrow lumens, long lengths, and high resistance to flow, restricting the rate of blood administration and creating increased shear force on blood cells that can damage them. Triple-lumen catheters that are 9 Fr have larger lumens and shorter lengths and are satisfactory for blood administration. Percutaneous introducer sheaths used for pulmonary artery catheterization are short, have 9-Fr lumens, and are excellent for blood administration. Always warm blood administered through central access to prevent hypothermia and arrhythmias.

26. **Describe complications associated with placement of the central venous catheter.**
    - Considering the proximity of the carotid artery to the internal jugular vein, it is not surprising that carotid artery puncture is one of the more common complications associated with all internal jugular vein approaches.
    - Pneumothorax may occur and is more commonly associated with a subclavian, low anterior (internal jugular), or junctional approach (junction of the internal jugular vein and subclavian vein).
    - Hemothorax is associated primarily with the subclavian vein approach and occurs secondary to subclavian artery puncture or laceration.

- The thoracic duct, as it wraps around the left internal jugular vein, can reach as high as 3 or 4 cm above the sternal end of the clavicle. This places the duct in a vulnerable position for puncture or laceration when a left internal jugular venipuncture is attempted.
- Shearing and embolization of a catheter tip may occur when a catheter is withdrawn through a needle. Likewise, a Seldinger guidewire can be sheared and embolized if attempts are made to withdraw it through an introducer needle. Therefore, if a catheter or wire cannot be advanced through an introducer needle, the parts should be removed in unison.
- Air embolism is a risk; to avoid this problem, the patient should be positioned head down (if entry is at a point superior to the heart) until the catheter is inserted and the hub of the catheter is occluded.
- Late complications include infection, vascular damage, hematoma formation, clot formation, dysrhythmia, and extravascular catheter migration.

27. Are any special precautions needed when removing a central venous catheter?

Before a subclavian or internal jugular catheter is removed, the patient should be placed in a head-down position to increase venous pressure at the point of removal and thereby prevent air aspiration into the vein. Following removal of the catheter, external pressure should be maintained on the area from which the catheter is withdrawn until clot formation has sealed the vessel.

SUGGESTED READINGS

Deflandre E, Bonhomme V, Hans P: Delta down compared with delta pulse pressure as an indicator of volaemia during intracranial surgery, Br J Anaesth 100:245–250, 2008.

Domino KB, Bowdle TA, Posner KL, et al: Injuries and liability related to central vascular catheters: a closed claims analysis, Anesthesiology 100:1411–1418, 2004.

Gelman S: Venous function and central venous pressure, Anesthesiology 108:735–748, 2008.

O'Leary R, Ahmed SM, McLure H, et al: Ultrasound guided infraclavicular axillary vein cannulation: a useful alternative to the internal jugular vein, Br J Anaesth 109(5):762–768, 2012.

Taylor RW, Palagiri AV: Central venous catheterization, Crit Care Med 35:1390–1396, 2007.

Troianos CA, Hartman GS, Glas KE, et al: Guidelines for performing ultrasound guided vascular cannulation, J Am Soc Echocardiogr 24:1291–1318, 2011.

CHAPTER 24

FLOW-DIRECTED THERAPY

Bethany Benish, MD

1. **Describe the role of transesophageal echocardiography (TEE) in cardiac surgery.**

   Since its introduction in 1976, the use of intraoperative TEE has steadily increased in popularity. Although TEE is traditionally used in cardiac surgery, the value of perioperative TEE for noncardiac surgery is becoming widely appreciated.

   In 1998, the American Society of Echocardiography and the Society of Cardiovascular Anesthesiologists (ASE/SCA) developed a standard comprehensive TEE examination, which includes the 20 views used for full cardiac evaluation and diagnosis of cardiac pathology.

   In 2013, ASE/SCA revisited this topic and developed the Basic Perioperative TEE exam for noncardiac surgery, which simplified the exam to 11 views focusing on intraoperative monitoring rather than diagnostics (Figure 24-1). Various cardiac chambers and vessels are apparent as well as the TEE probe diagrammed outside the cardiac image.

2. **What are the indications for TEE in noncardiac surgery?**

   See Box 24-1. TEE should be considered in cases where the nature of the procedure or the patient's underlying known or suspected cardiovascular pathology might result in hemodynamic, pulmonary, or neurologic instability or compromise. TEE should also be used to assist in diagnosis and management of unexplained life-threatening hemodynamic instability that persists despite initial corrective therapy. This is often referred to as a "rescue TEE."

3. **How are TEE images obtained?**

   TEE images result from transmission of ultrasound waves (2–10 mHz) from the TEE probe through target tissue (heart and great vessels). The time it requires for the wave to be reflected back determines the location of a structure. This can be combined with color flow Doppler to further examine dynamic structures. These high-resolution multiplane images and Doppler techniques provide real-time hemodynamic evaluation and assist in the diagnosis of cardiovascular pathology.

4. **How is TEE helpful for perioperative ischemia monitoring?**

   In the setting of myocardial ischemia, systolic wall motion abnormalities can often be detected before the ST segment changes on ECG. In addition, TEE can evaluate for complications of myocardial ischemia, including congestive heart failure, new septal defects or ventricular free wall rupture, valvular pathology, or new pericardial effusion.

5. **Are there complications to TEE?**

   Although complications of TEE are rare (0.2%), there have been serious and even fatal complications reported.

   Complications include:
   - Odynophagia
   - Dental injury
   - Oral/pharyngeal trauma
   - Upper gastrointestinal (GI) bleed
   - Esophageal laceration or perforation
   - Endotracheal tube displacement
   - Methemoglobinemia (related to topical benzocaine)

6. **What are the contraindications of TEE?**

   See Table 24-1.

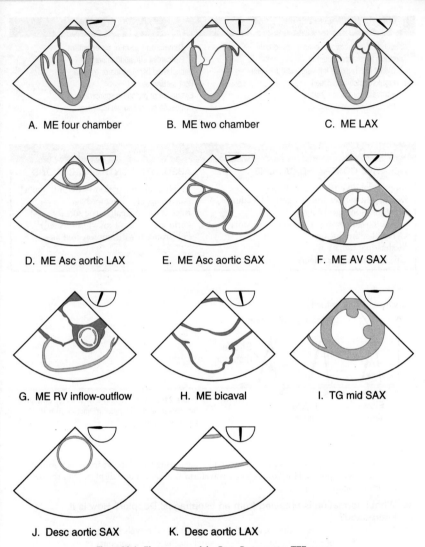

A. ME four chamber   B. ME two chamber   C. ME LAX

D. ME Asc aortic LAX   E. ME Asc aortic SAX   F. ME AV SAX

G. ME RV inflow-outflow   H. ME bicaval   I. TG mid SAX

J. Desc aortic SAX   K. Desc aortic LAX

Figure 24-1. Eleven views of the Basic Perioperative TEE exam.

7. **What is an esophageal Doppler monitor?**
   An esophageal Doppler monitor is a minimally invasive device that uses transesophageal ultrasonography to continuously monitor cardiac output and allow estimation of preload, afterload, and ventricular contractility in the perioperative or critical care setting.

8. **Describe how esophageal Doppler monitors work.**
   An esophageal Doppler monitor consists of a narrow flexible probe that is inserted into the esophagus via mouth or nose. It uses Doppler ultrasound to measure mainstream velocity of blood flow within the descending thoracic aorta. When combined with the cross-sectional area of the aorta, hemodynamic variables such as stroke volume and cardiac output can be calculated.

Box 24-1. Indications for TEE

Inadequate transthoracic echo image quality
Intraoperative assessment of:
   Global and regional left ventricular function
   Right ventricular function
   Intravascular volume status
   Basic valvular lesions

Thromboembolism or air embolism
Pericardial effusion/tamponade
Unexplained hypotension or hypoxia
Post cardiac arrest
Evaluation of preload responsiveness
Evaluation of myocardial ischemia

Table 24-1. TEE contraindications

RELATIVE CONTRAINDICATIONS	ABSOLUTE CONTRAINDICATIONS
Esophageal diverticulum or fistula	Esophageal obstruction (stricture, tumor)
Esophageal varices without active bleeding	Active upper GI hemorrhage
Previous esophageal surgery	Recent esophageal/gastric surgery
Severe coagulopathy or thrombocytopenia	Perforated viscus (known/suspected)
Cervical spine disease	Full stomach with unprotected airway
Mediastinal radiation	
Unexplained odynophagia	

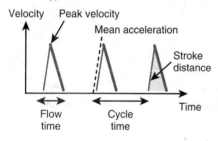

Figure 24-2. Aortic blood flow velocity estimated by measuring the Doppler frequency shift by the esophageal probe.

Aortic blood flow velocity is estimated by measuring the Doppler frequency shift by the esophageal probe. This flow velocity waveform is obtained and displayed on the device monitor (Figure 24-2).

9. **What information is obtained from an esophageal Doppler? How is it interpreted?**
   - Stroke distance (SD): distance (cm) a column of blood travels during systole
   - Stroke volume (SV): volume of blood ejected during systole (product of stroke distance and aortic cross-sectional area)
   - Flow time corrected (FTc): duration (ms) of flow during systole and corrected for heart rate
   - Peak velocity (PV): highest blood velocity during systole

   The esophageal Doppler waveform can be used both diagnostically and therapeutically, but interpretation requires clinical correlation.

   In general, FTc is inversely proportional to Systemic Vascular Resistance, therefore indicating preload and afterload. Measurements of peak velocity and mean acceleration are markers for left ventricular contractility (Figure 24-3 and Table 24-2).

10. **How can esophageal Doppler be used for goal-directed fluid therapy?**
    Fluid optimization using an esophageal Doppler involves intravenous administration of small boluses of fluid (200 ml) while monitoring stroke volume. If the SV/SD increases by >10%, the patient is "volume responsive" and repeat bolus should be considered to further

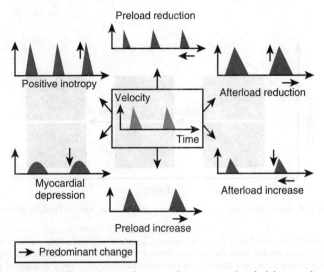

Preload reduction

Positive inotropy

Velocity

Afterload reduction

Time

Myocardial
depression

Afterload increase

Preload increase

→ Predominant change

Figure 24-3. Measurements of peak velocity and mean acceleration are markers for left ventricular contractility.

Table 24-2. Interpreting Esophageal Doppler

CLINICAL CONDITION	WAVEFORM CHARACTERISTICS	MANAGEMENT
Hypovolemia	Decreased SV or SD Shortened FTc Normal/slight reduced PV	Assess response to fluid challenge
Increased afterload	Shortened FTc Reduced PV	Consider vasodilator
Decreased afterload (sepsis or other vasodilatory state)	Widened FTc Reduced PV	Consider vasoconstrictors
Decreased contractility	Low PV Low mean acceleration	Consider inotrope

FTc, Flow time corrected; PV, peak velocity; SV, stroke volume; SD, stroke distance.

improve cardiac output. A decrease or an increase <10% following fluid bolus indicates that further volume expansion will likely be ineffective at improving cardiac output.

This concept of repeat fluid challenges to achieve the plateau on the patient's Frank–Starling curve is demonstrated in Figure 24-4.

11. **When should the use of esophageal Doppler be considered?**
Esophageal Doppler should be considered in any patient undergoing major or high-risk surgery in which the use of invasive cardiovascular monitoring would be considered.

12. **Does the use of intraoperative esophageal Doppler affect outcome?**
Intraoperative esophageal Doppler allows continuous monitoring of cardiac output to optimize intravascular volume and tissue perfusion. Although this is a relatively new technology, it has been serially tested in multiple prospective randomized controlled trials. When compared with conventional clinical parameters for fluid administration, in the setting of major abdominal surgery, the use of intraoperative esophageal Doppler has been

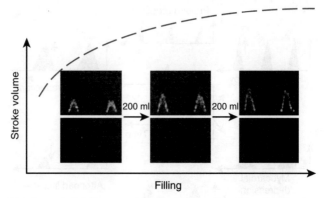

Figure 24-4. Repeat fluid challenges to achieve the plateau on the patient's Frank–Starling curve.

consistently associated with decreased hospital length of stay and improved outcome. In addition, some studies have shown fewer intensive care unit (ICU) admissions, decreased inotrope requirement, and earlier return of bowel function after major abdominal surgery.

13. **Has esophageal Doppler proven helpful in other types of surgeries?**
While the majority of studies have involved major bowel surgery, esophageal Doppler has also been shown to decrease hospital length of stay and perioperative complications in major orthopedic surgery, gynecologic/urologic procedures, multiple trauma, and even cardiac surgery when compared with standard practice either with or without the use of a central venous catheter.

14. **Describe the assumptions and limitations of esophageal Doppler monitoring.**
Using Doppler frequency shift to estimate stroke volume assumes that the proportion of blood flow in the ascending and descending aorta remains fixed despite hemodynamic changes. This proportion is in fact not constant. It is affected by acute illness, use of spinal/epidural anesthesia, and aortic cross-clamping, all of which can lead to redistribution of cardiac output. The aortic diameter is also assumed circular and to remain constant through the cardiac cycle.
    The main limitations of this technology are a requirement for procedural or deep sedation or general anesthesia so that the patient can tolerate probe placement, significant equipment costs, and the need for a skilled operator to accurately interpret the data.

15. **Are there any other new, minimally invasive cardiac output monitors available?**
Yes. Over the past decade, many new methods for estimating cardiac output (such as the Doppler) have regularly replaced the invasive insertion of PA catheters.

16. **Describe the main principles of these new minimally invasive cardiac output monitors.**
    • Pulse contour analysis
    • Lithium dilution
    • Gas rebreathing (applied Fick principle)
    • Electrical bioimpedance

PULSE CONTOUR ANALYSIS

Pulse contour analysis devices are based on the principle that cardiac output is proportional to arterial pulse pressure and that the contour of this arterial waveform is related to stroke volume and vascular resistance. These devices also provide information on respiratory-induced variation in stroke volume that can indicate ventricular preload dependence and be predictive of volume responsiveness. This technology depends on optimal arterial waveform signals. Arrhythmias, aortic regurgitation, and severe hemodynamic instability may affect the accuracy of these devices. In general, trends in cardiac output have been more useful than absolute values in these devices.

LITHIUM DILUTION

This technology requires both a venous and arterial line. A bolus of lithium chloride solution is injected into a venous line, and a concentration time curve is generated by a selective lithium electrode attached to the arterial pressure line. Cardiac output is then calculated from this measured lithium dose and the area under the concentration time curve. This method correlates well with PA catheter thermodilution but is less invasive. Accuracy in patients on lithium and on neuromuscular blockade has been questioned.

GAS REBREATHING (APPLIED FICK PRINCIPLE)

This system uses a mainstream infrared sensor to measure CO_2 in a disposable rebreathing loop attached to the ventilator circuit. Utilizing the applied Fick principle, the ratio between normal CO_2 and rebreathing CO_2 is used to calculate cardiac output. An obvious limitation to this device is that it requires mechanical ventilation. Additionally, changes in ventilation settings, mechanically assisted spontaneous breathing, severe chest trauma, presence of pulmonary shunting, and hemodynamic instability all affect the accuracy of this device and limit its clinical applicability. NiCO^{TM} uses this principle.

ELECTRICAL BIOIMPEDANCE

These devices use electric current stimulation to identify variations in thoracic or body impedance induced by cyclic changes in blood flow. These measurements are then used to estimate cardiac output. This technology is one of the least invasive methods for measuring cardiac output. Unfortunately, electrocautery, patient movement, and arrhythmias may interfere with the accuracy of these devices.

KEY POINTS: FLOW DIRECTED THERAPY

1. TEE should be considered in cases in which the nature of the procedure or the patient's underlying known or suspected cardiovascular pathology might result in hemodynamic, pulmonary, or neurologic instability or compromise.
2. Goal-directed individualized fluid therapy guided by esophageal Doppler monitoring reduces perioperative complications and hospital length of stay after major surgery and, therefore, should be considered for routine use in most types of high-risk surgeries. Accuracy of filling volume may limit unnecessary fluid infusions and reduce time to discharge.
3. In addition to TEE and esophageal Doppler, a variety of new, minimally invasive cardiac output monitoring devices are available and have, in many settings, replaced pulmonary artery catheters. Knowledge of how each of these devices estimates cardiac output and their clinical limitations is essential.

WEBSITES

National Board of Echocardiography: http://echoboards.org
Toronto General Hospital Department of Anesthesia: *Virtual transesophageal echocardiography.* http://pie.med.utoronto.ca/TEE

SUGGESTED READINGS

Reeves S, Finley AC, Skubas NJ, et al: Basic perioperative transesophageal echocardiography examination: a consensus statement of the American Society of Echocardiography and Society of Cardiovascular Anesthesiologists, Anesth Analg 117:543–558, 2013.
Singer M: Oesophageal Doppler, Curr Opin Crit Care 15:244–248, 2009.

CHAPTER 25

BLOOD PRESSURE DISTURBANCES, ARTERIAL CATHETERIZATION, AND BLOOD PRESSURE MONITORING

James C. Duke, MD, MBA

1. **What blood pressure value is considered hypertensive?**
   The numbers are somewhat arbitrary. Blood pressure (BP) changes throughout the day and can be affected by posture, exercise, medications, smoking, caffeine ingestion, and mood. Hypertension (HTN) cannot be diagnosed on the basis of one abnormal BP reading but requires sustained elevations over multiple measurements on different days. Systemic HTN is usually considered sustained elevations of diastolic BP greater than 90 to 95 mm Hg or a systolic BP greater than 140 to 160 mm Hg. Borderline HTN is defined as diastolic BP between 85 and 89 mm Hg or a systolic BP between 140 and 159 mm Hg. Diastolic pressures between 110 and 115 mm Hg define severe HTN, and malignant HTN is defined by BPs greater than 200/140 mm Hg. Malignant HTN is a medical emergency.

2. **What causes hypertension?**
   - Essential (or idiopathic) HTN: Unknown cause; >90% of all cases fall into this category.
   - Endocrine: Cushing's syndrome, hyperaldosteronism, pheochromocytoma, thyrotoxicosis, acromegaly, estrogen therapy
   - Renal: Chronic pyelonephritis, renovascular stenosis, glomerulonephritis, polycystic kidney disease
   - Neurogenic: Increased intracranial pressure, autonomic hyperreflexia
   - Miscellaneous: Obesity, hypercalcemia, preeclampsia, acute intermittent porphyria

3. **What are some of the physiologic processes that occur as a patient becomes hypertensive?**
   Often cardiac output temporarily increases, followed by sustained increases in systemic vascular resistance. Vascular smooth muscular hypertrophy is observed, and there is increased arteriolar tone. Extracellular fluid volume and renin activity have no consistent pattern, but usually intracellular sodium and calcium concentrations increase. Sustained HTN leads to concentric hypertrophy of the left ventricle and impaired ventricular relaxation, known as *diastolic dysfunction*. Diastolic dysfunction leads to increased end-diastolic pressures.

4. **What are the consequences of sustained HTN?**
   Untreated hypertensive patients develop end-organ disease, including left ventricular hypertrophy, coronary artery disease, congestive heart failure, cardiomyopathy, renal failure, and cerebrovascular accidents. Hypertensive patients also demonstrate labile BPs intraoperatively.

5. **Why should antihypertensives be taken up until the time of surgery?**
   A well-controlled hypertensive patient has less intraoperative lability in BP. Acute withdrawal of antihypertensives may precipitate rebound HTN or myocardial ischemia. In particular, β blockers and α_2 agonists are associated with rebound HTN. In general, antihypertensive therapy should be maintained until the time of surgery and restarted as soon as possible after surgery (Table 25-1).

Table 25-1. Commonly Prescribed Antihypertensive Medications

CLASS	EXAMPLES	SIDE EFFECTS
Thiazide diuretics	Hydrochlorothiazide	Hypokalemia, hyponatremia, hyperglycemia, hypomagnesemia, hypocalcemia
Loop diuretics	Furosemide	Hypokalemia, hypocalcemia, hyperglycemia, hypomagnesemia, metabolic alkalosis
β Blockers	Propranolol, metoprolol, atenolol	Bradycardia, bronchospasm, conduction blockade, myocardial depression, fatigue
α Blockers	Terazosin, prazosin	Postural hypotension, tachycardia, fluid retention
α_2 Agonists	Clonidine	Postural hypotension, sedation, rebound hypertension, decreases MAC
Calcium channel blockers	Verapamil, diltiazem, nifedipine	Cardiac depression, conduction blockade, bradycardia
ACE inhibitors	Captopril, enalapril, lisinopril, ramipril	Cough, angioedema, fluid retention, reflex tachycardia, renal dysfunction, hyperkalemia
Angiotensin receptor antagonists	Losartan, irbesartan, candesartan	Hypotension, renal failure, hyperkalemia
Vascular smooth muscle relaxants	Hydralazine, minoxidil	Reflex tachycardia, fluid retention

ACE, Angiotensin-converting enzyme; MAC, minimal alveolar concentration.

6. **Which antihypertensives should be held the day of surgery?**
   Although there is no universal agreement, many believe ACE inhibitors and angiotensin receptor antagonists should be held the day of surgery. Diuretics may be withheld when depletion of intravascular volume is a concern.

7. **Are hypertensive patients undergoing general anesthesia at increased risk for perioperative cardiac morbidity?**
   Although numerous studies have demonstrated that increased preoperative systolic BP is a significant predictor of postoperative morbidity, there are no data that establish definitively whether the preoperative treatment of hypertension reduces perioperative risk. However, poorly treated hypertensive patients have increased intraoperative BP lability, and hemodynamic fluctuations do have some relationship to postoperative complications. In addition, some patients with hypertension will have end-organ damage. It seems reasonable that for nonemergent surgical procedures, hypertension should be treated before surgery.

8. **Provide a differential diagnosis for intraoperative hypertension.**
   See Table 25-2.

9. **How is perioperative hypertension managed?**
   Pain is the most common cause of perioperative hypertension. Consider the usual hourly doses of common opioids and determine whether the maximum limit has been reached. The usual guidelines for opioid administration may not apply to patients receiving opioids chronically. If administration of volatile agents and opioids does not address HTN sufficiently, consider primary antihypertensive agents. After surgery, opioid therapy should be titrated to respiratory rate and the patient's interpretation of the severity of pain. Peripheral nerve blocks and analgesic adjuvants such as ketorolac should be considered. See Table 25-3.

Table 25-2. Differential Diagnosis of Intraoperative Hypertension

Related to preexisting disease	Chronic hypertension, increased intracranial pressure, autonomic hyperreflexia, aortic dissection, early acute myocardial infarction
Related to surgery	Prolonged tourniquet time, post cardiopulmonary bypass, aortic cross-clamping, post carotid endarterectomy
Related to anesthetic	Pain, inadequate depth of anesthesia, catecholamine release, malignant hyperthermia, shivering, hypoxia, hypercarbia, hypothermia, hypervolemia, improperly sized (too small) blood pressure cuff, intraarterial transducer positioned too low
Related to medication	Rebound hypertension (from discontinuation of clonidine, β blockers, or methyldopa), systemic absorption of vasoconstrictors, intravenous dye (e.g., indigo carmine)
Other	Bladder distention, hypoglycemia

Table 25-3. Antihypertensive Agents Used Perioperatively

DRUG	DOSE	ONSET
Labetalol	5–20 mg	1–2 minutes
Esmolol bolus	0.5 mg/kg over 1 minute	1–2 minutes
Esmolol infusion	50–300 mg/kg/min	1–2 minutes
Propranolol	1–3 mg	1–2 minutes
Hydralazine	5–20 mg	5–10 minutes
Sodium nitroprusside infusion	0.5–10 mg/kg/min	1 minute
Nitroglycerin	0.5–10 mg/kg/min	1 minute

10. **Broadly categorize the causes of perioperative hypotension.**
    - **Hypovolemia:** Dehydration, inadequate oral intake or preoperative intravenous fluid administration, bowel cathartics ("preps"), fever, diarrhea, vomiting
    - **Functional hypovolemia** (shock states):
      - Sepsis: decreased systemic vascular resistance, increased venous capacitance
      - Cardiac failure: ischemic heart disease, cardiomyopathy, pulmonary embolus, valvular disease, dysrhythmia
      - Hemorrhage: trauma, surgical blood loss, "third spacing"
      - Neurogenic: loss of systemic vascular resistance from spinal cord injury
      - Anaphylaxis: Acute loss of systemic vascular resistance
    - **Drugs:** Including anesthetic induction agents, volatile anesthetics, histamine-releasing medications, butyrophenones, medications used to induce hypotension (e.g., ganglionic blockers, vasodilators, α- and β-adrenergic blockers), regional anesthetics
    - **Positive-pressure ventilation**
    - **Cardiac tamponade, tension pneumothorax**
    - **Autonomic neuropathy:** Diabetes mellitus, spinal cord injuries, Guillain-Barré syndrome, familiar dysautonomia, Shy-Drager syndrome, human immunodeficiency virus, or acquired immunodeficiency syndrome. Orthostatic hypotension is discussed in Chapter 1.
    - **Medical and surgical disease:** Hematemesis, melena, diabetic ketoacidosis, diabetes insipidus, high-output renal failure, bowel disease, burns

11. **What is joint cement, and how does it cause hypotension?**
    Methylmethacrylate, cement used in joint replacement, undergoes an exothermic reaction that causes it to adhere to imperfections in the bony surface. Hypotension usually occurs 30 to 60 seconds after placement of the cement but can occur up to 10 minutes later.

Postulated mechanisms include tissue damage from the reaction, release of vasoactive substances when it is hydrolyzed to methacrylate acid, embolization, and vasodilation caused by absorption of the volatile monomer.

12. **Why does administration of renin-angiotensin system (RAS) antagonists result in hypotension in the peri-induction period? How might the hypotension be treated?**

The mechanism is believed to be loss of sympathetic tone superimposed on RAS blockade. The vasopressin system is the only intact system left to maintain BP, and vasopressin release is not a fast-response system compared with the sympathetic nervous system. Administration of intravenous fluids is a proper first response. The usual pressor agents used in the operating room (phenylephrine and ephedrine) may prove insufficient if administered because of the blockade of the RAS system and the loss of sympathetic tone associated with anesthetic induction. Preparations of vasopressin have been used to correct refractory hypotension.

13. **How does regional anesthesia create hypotension?**

Both spinal and epidural anesthesia produce hypotension through sympathetic blockade and vasodilation, although the effects of spinal anesthesia may be more precipitous. Hypovolemia exacerbates sympathetic blockade. Blocks lower than the fifth thoracic dermatome have less hypotension because of compensatory vasoconstriction of the upper extremities. Blocks higher than the fourth thoracic dermatome may affect cardioaccelerator nerves, resulting in bradycardia and diminished cardiac output.

14. **How is intraoperative hypotension evaluated and treated?**

Precipitous hypotension understandably requires quick treatment before all facts are at hand. Administration of adrenergic agonists and fluids is recommended. Decrease volatile or intravenous anesthetic levels. If hypotension is gradual and progressive, more facts can be taken into consideration as to the cause, but hypovolemia is the likely candidate. The effects of surgery, anesthesia, and coexisting disease are dynamic, and any single piece of information may be misleading. Thus always take into consideration as many variables as can be obtained. In addition, heart rate, BP, urine output, hematocrit, base deficit, serum lactate concentration, and response to fluid administration are valuable estimators of the cause of hypotension. Refractory hypotension requires invasive monitoring to obtain additional information about cardiac filling pressures and function.

15. **Review the standard adrenergic agonists used to manage hypotension during anesthesia. How should hypotension caused by cardiac ischemia be treated?**

The most common α-adrenergic agents are phenylephrine and ephedrine. Considerations to address ischemia include:
- Increasing delivered oxygen
- Decreasing heart rate
- Producing coronary vasodilation with nitroglycerin
- Reducing afterload (sodium nitroprusside is a useful arterial dilator)
- Increasing contractility, using inotropes such as dopamine, dobutamine, and amrinone

16. **What is the most commonly used noninvasive BP monitor and its limitations?**

Most frequently, BP is measured using an automated device (oscillometric method). Errors in measurement may be caused by inappropriate cuff size or positioning, atherosclerosis, or decreased blood flow (hypovolemia, vasopressors).

With the oscillometric method, a pneumatic cuff is inflated to occlude arterial blood flow. As the cuff is deflated, the arterial pulsations cause pressure changes in the cuff that are analyzed by a computer. The systolic pressure is taken at the point of rapidly increasing oscillations, the mean arterial pressure as the point of maximal oscillation, and the diastolic pressure as the point of rapidly decreasing oscillations. Errors in measurement with noninvasive BP monitoring include inappropriate cuff size, patient shivering, and prolonged use of the stat mode. Complications include ulnar nerve paresthesias, thrombophlebitis, or compartment syndrome.

17. **What are the indications for intraarterial BP monitoring?**
- BP changes may be rapid.
- Anticipated cardiovascular instability
- Moderate BP changes may cause end-organ damage.

- Clinical concerns such as massive fluid shifts, intracranial surgery, preexisting cardiovascular disease, valvular heart disease, diabetes mellitus, and massive obesity (where measuring cuff pressure is inaccurate)
- Frequent arterial blood gases may be needed to assess pulmonary function, acid-base status, blood loss, use of one lung ventilation, etc.
- Significant blood loss is likely.

18. What are the complications of invasive arterial monitoring?

Complications include distal ischemia, arterial thrombosis, hematoma formation, catheter site infection, systemic infection, necrosis of the overlying skin, pseudoaneurysms, and potential blood loss caused by disconnection. The incidence of infection increases with duration of catheterization. The incidence of arterial thrombosis increases with:

- Duration of catheterization
- Increased catheter size
- Catheter type (Teflon catheters cause more thrombosis than catheters made of polypropylene)
- Proximal emboli
- Prolonged shock
- Preexisting peripheral vascular disease

However, a closed claims liability analysis suggests complications of arterial catheterization are relatively uncommon.

19. How is radial artery catheterization performed?

The wrist is dorsiflexed and immobilized, the skin is cleaned with an antiseptic solution, the course of the radial artery is determined by palpation, and local anesthetic is infiltrated into the skin overlying the artery (if the patient is awake). A 20-G over-the-needle catheter apparatus is inserted at a 30- to 45-degree angle to the skin along the course of the radial artery. After arterial blood return, the angle is decreased, and the catheter is advanced slightly to ensure that both the catheter tip and the needle have advanced into the arterial lumen. The catheter is then threaded into the artery. Alternatively, the radial artery may be transfixed. After arterial blood return, the apparatus is advanced until both the catheter and the needle pass completely through the front and back walls of the artery. The needle is withdrawn into the catheter, and the catheter is pulled back slowly. When pulsatile blood flow is seen in the catheter, it is advanced into the lumen. If the catheter will not advance into the arterial lumen and blood return is good, a sterile guidewire may be placed into the lumen through the catheter and the catheter advanced over the wire.

Some arterial cannulation kits have a combined needle-guidewire-cannula system, in which the guidewire is advanced into the lumen after good blood flow is obtained and the catheter is then advanced over the guidewire. After cannulation low-compliance pressure tubing is fastened to the catheter, a sterile dressing is applied, and the catheter is fastened securely in place. Care must be taken to ensure that the pressure tubing is free from bubbles before connection. After the procedure, it is advisable to remove any devices that have dorsiflexed the wrist because of concerns for median nerve palsy.

20. Describe the normal blood supply to the hand.

The ulnar and radial arteries supply the hand. These arteries anastomose via four arches in the hand and wrist (the superficial and deep palmar arches and the anterior and posterior carpal arches). Because of the dual arterial blood supply, the hand usually has collateral flow, and either artery can supply the digits if the other is occluded. Both ulnar and radial arteries have been removed and used successfully as coronary artery bypass grafts without ischemic sequelae to the hand.

21. Describe the Allen test. Explain its purpose.

The Allen test is performed before radial artery cannulation to determine whether ulnar collateral circulation to the hand is adequate in case of radial artery thrombosis. Having the patient make a tight fist exsanguinates the hand. The radial and ulnar arteries are occluded by manual compression, the patient relaxes the hand, and the pressure over the ulnar artery is released. Measuring the time required for return of normal coloration assesses collateral flow. Return of color in less than 5 seconds indicates adequate collateral flow, return in 5 to 10 seconds suggests an equivocal test, and return in more than 10 seconds indicates inadequate collateral circulation. In 25% of the population, the collateral circulation to the hand is inadequate.

22. Is the Allen test an adequate predictor of ischemic sequelae?

Although some clinicians advocate use of the Allen test, others have demonstrated that the Allen test of radial artery patency has no relationship to distal blood flow. There are many reports of ischemic sequelae in patients with normal Allen tests; conversely, patients with abnormal Allen tests may have no ischemic sequelae. Apparently the Allen test alone does not reliably predict adverse outcome.

23. What alternative cannulation sites are available?

The ulnar, brachial, axillary, femoral, dorsalis pedis, and posterior tibial arteries are all acceptable cannulation sites. The ulnar artery may be cannulated if the radial artery provides adequate collateral flow. The brachial artery does not have the benefit of collateral flow, but many studies have demonstrated the relative safety of its cannulation. Cannulation of the axillary artery is also relatively safe, but the left side is preferred because of a lower incidence of embolization to the carotid artery. The femoral artery is an excellent site for cannulation because of the large size, the technical ease of cannulation, and the low risk of ischemic sequelae, but prolonged use is discouraged because of infection considerations. Cannulation is relatively difficult in patients with peripheral vascular disease and diabetes mellitus.

24. How does a central waveform differ from a peripheral waveform?

As the arterial pressure is transmitted from the central aorta to the peripheral arteries, the waveform is distorted (Figure 25-1). Transmission is delayed, high-frequency components such as the dicrotic notch are lost, the systolic peak increases, and the diastolic trough is decreased. The changes in systolic and diastolic pressures result from a decrease in the arterial wall compliance and from resonance (the addition of reflected waves to the arterial waveform as it travels distally in the arterial tree). The systolic BP in the radial artery may be as much as 20 to 50 mm Hg higher than the pressure in the central aorta.

25. What information can be obtained from an arterial waveform?

- The slope of the upstroke may be used to evaluate myocardial contractility.
- Large respiratory variations suggest hypovolemia.
- The waveform provides a visual estimate of the hemodynamic consequences of various arrhythmias.

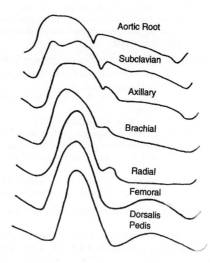

Figure 25-1. Configuration of the arterial waveform at various sites in the arterial tree. (*From Blitt CD, Hines RL: Monitoring in anesthesia and critical care medicine, ed 3, New York, 1995, Churchill Livingstone, with permission.*)

KEY POINTS: BLOOD PRESSURE DISTURBANCES, ARTERIAL CATHETERIZATION, AND PRESSURE MONITORING

1. Although numerous studies have demonstrated that increased preoperative systolic BP is a significant predictor of postoperative morbidity, no data have established definitively whether the preoperative treatment of hypertension reduces perioperative risk.
2. It seems rational that for nonemergent surgical procedures, hypertension should be treated before surgery.
3. With the exception of antagonists of the renin-angiotensin system and possibly diuretics, antihypertensive therapy should be taken up to, and including, the day of surgery.
4. Prolonged use of automated BP cuffs in the "stat" mode, in which the cuff reinflates immediately after each measurement is obtained, may lead to complications such as ulnar nerve paresthesia, thrombophlebitis, or compartment syndrome.
5. In 25% of the population, the collateral circulation to the hand is inadequate.
6. Ipsilateral ulnar arterial catheterization should not be attempted after multiple failed attempts at radial catheterization on the same side.
7. Peripherally measured arterial waveforms seem amplified and demonstrate higher systolic pressures, wider pulse pressures, and somewhat lower diastolic pressures. The mean arterial pressure is reduced only slightly.
8. The systolic BP in the radial artery may be as much as 20 to 50 mm Hg higher than the pressure in the central aorta.

26. **Define damping coefficient and natural frequency.**
Natural frequency, a property of the catheter-stopcock–transducer apparatus, is the frequency at which the monitoring system resonates and amplifies the signals it receives. The natural frequency is directly proportional to the diameter of the catheter lumen and an inverse function of the length of the tubing, the system compliance, and the density of the fluid contained in the system. Because the natural frequency of most monitoring systems is in the same range as the frequencies used to re-create the arterial waveform, significant amplification and distortion of the waveform may occur.

27. **What are the characteristics of overdamped and underdamped monitoring systems?**
The damping coefficient is estimated by evaluating the time for the system to settle to zero after a high-pressure flush (Figure 25-2). An underdamped system continues to oscillate for three or four cycles; it overestimates the systolic BP and underestimates the diastolic BP. An overdamped system settles to baseline slowly, without oscillating; it underestimates the systolic BP and overestimates the diastolic BP. However, in both cases the mean BP is relatively accurate.

28. **How can the incidence of artifacts in arterial monitoring systems be reduced?**
    • The connecting tubing should be rigid with an internal diameter of 1.5 to 3 mm and a maximal length of 120 cm.
    • The lines should be kept free of kinks, clots, and bubbles, which cause overdamping of the system.
    • Only one stopcock per line should be used to minimize possible introduction of air.
    • The mechanical coupling system should be flushed with saline to maintain the patency of the arterial line and minimize the risk of distal embolization and nosocomial infection.
    • The transducer should be placed at the level of the right atrium, the midaxillary line in the supine position.
    • The transducer should be electrically balanced or re-zeroed periodically because the zero point may drift if the room temperature changes.

29. **What are the risks and benefits of having heparin in the fluid of a transduction system?**
Heparinized infusions were used for over 25 years for the purposes of reducing the incidence of arterial catheter thrombosis. However, a recent comparison of the use of heparinized

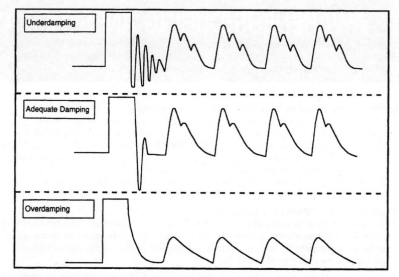

Figure 25-2. Underdamped, adequately damped, and overdamped arterial pressure tracings after a high-pressure flush.

versus nonheparinized solutions for arterial transducer systems found no increase in catheter thrombosis when a nonheparinized solution was used. The benefit of not using heparinized solutions would be decreased exposure to heparin and decreased possibility of heparin-induced thrombocytopenia.

30. **Are any risks associated with flushing the catheter system?**
On occasion, arterial catheter systems are flushed to improve the quality of the arterial waveform. Retrograde embolization of air or thrombus into the cerebral vasculature is a risk. Flush rates of greater than 1 ml/min have resulted in retrograde flow. It should be noted that adverse neurologic events associated with arterial cannulation are extremely rare events and remain anecdotal at this time.

SUGGESTED READINGS

Banakar SM, Liau DW, Kooner PK, et al: Liability related to peripheral venous and arterial catheterization: a closed claims analysis, Anesthesiology 109:124–129, 2009.

Brzezinski M, Luisetti T, London MJ: Radial artery cannulation: a comprehensive review of recent anatomic and physiologic investigations, Anesth Analg 109:1763–1781, 2009.

Donaldson AJ, Thompson HE, Harper NJ, et al: Bone cement implantation syndrome, Br J Anaesth 102:12–22, 2009.

Murphy GS, Szokol JW, Marymont JH, et al: Retrograde blood flow in the brachial and axillary arteries during routine radial arterial catheter flushing, Anesthesiology 105:492–497, 2006.

Truong AT, Thakar DR: Radial artery pseudoaneurysm. A rare complication with serious risk to life and limb, Anesthesiology 118:188, 2013.

Tuncali BE, Kuvaki B, Tuncali B, et al: A comparison of the efficacy of heparinized and nonheparinized solutions for maintenance of perioperative radial arterial catheter patency and subsequent occlusion, Anesth Analg 100:1117–1121, 2005.

CHAPTER 26

AWARENESS DURING ANESTHESIA

Aaron Murray, MD

1. **Review the classifications of memory and awareness.**

   Classifications of memory include both implicit (unconscious memory) and explicit (conscious memory). Explicit memory refers to conscious recollection of events such as intraoperative events. Awareness with recall (AWR) during general anesthesia is referred to as *anesthetic awareness*. Although patients may have "awareness" under general anesthesia, as shown by isolated forearm experiments, recall of events is what is key. The 2006 American Society of Anesthesiologists' (ASA's) practice advisory for intraoperative awareness excludes dreaming as anesthetic awareness.

2. **What is the incidence of awareness?**

   Incidence of AWR increases whenever "lighter" anesthesia is provided. An estimate of adult AWR in all risk populations combined is approximately 0.15%. Increased incidence occurs in higher risk populations such as obstetric, trauma, and cardiac surgery cases. Pediatric patients have a higher incidence of AWR.

3. **Are certain techniques and clinical situations more likely to result in awareness?**

   Recognized risk factors for AWR include:
   - Light levels of anesthesia (common in hypovolemic, obstetric, and trauma patients)
   - Prior history of intraoperative awareness
   - Cardiac surgery with cardiopulmonary bypass that has historically relied on narcotic-based anesthesia which, while minimizing myocardial depression, produces unreliable amnesia
   - Use of muscle relaxants is an independent risk factor
   - Machine malfunction (e.g., empty vaporizer), IV anesthetic pump malfunction, syringe swaps, etc.
   - Unrecognized increased anesthetic requirements such as in patients with chronic substance abuse and pediatric patients

4. **Describe the clinical signs and symptoms of insufficient anesthesia.**

   Motor responses and sympathetic activation can indicate light levels of anesthesia. Increased respiratory effort, accessory muscle use, swallowing, grimacing, and extremity motion are signs of insufficient anesthesia. Use of neuromuscular blockade eliminates the information that motor signs can provide regarding anesthetic depth. Sympathetic effects of light anesthesia include hypertension, tachycardia, mydriasis, tearing, and sweating. Such findings are nonspecific; thus their absence or presence may be unreliable indicators of AWR. Indeed, concomitant medications such as β blockers and sympathetic blockade may diminish changes in heart rate and blood pressure.

5. **What are the ramifications of AWR?**

   AWR is closely associated with patient dissatisfaction. The potential to hear operating personnel and experience weakness, paralysis, or pain can result in subsequent anxiety, sense of helplessness, and sleep disturbances. Posttraumatic stress disorder is a common sequela that may occur in 33% to 70% of patients who experience AWR.

6. **How should a patient who may have been aware during an anesthetic be approached?**

   Patients may volunteer information or seem angry or sad without clear reason. This should prompt a structured interview using general open-ended questions. An example would be "What is the last thing you remember?"

   Detailed documentation is appropriate once a case has been identified. Listen to and acknowledge the patient's recollections and explain the circumstances surrounding the situation (cardiovascular instability, trauma, etc.). Reassure the patient and offer psychological support. Notify the surgeons, nursing staff, and hospital legal counsel. The ASA Task Force on Intraoperative Awareness notes that not all patients need to be notified regarding the risk of AWR, but for high-risk patients, informed consent should include discussing the increased risk of AWR.

7. Are there strategies to decrease the incidence of AWR?

Premedication with amnestic drugs such as benzodiazepines or scopolamine can potentially reduce the likelihood of AWR, especially in higher risk patient populations or surgeries. Administer appropriate doses of induction agents and supplement with amnestic medications if airway management is difficult or prolonged. Avoid muscle relaxants unless necessary. Supplement nitrous-narcotic techniques with volatile anesthetics. Maintain anesthesia machines and ensure proper intravenous pump function. Consider neurophysiologic monitoring.

8. Are monitors available to assess depth of anesthesia?

Brain electrical activity monitoring can be used to assess depth of anesthesia and includes two commonly used modalities: processed electroencephalogram (pEEG), which is clinically easier to use compared with multichannel electroencephalogram (EEG) and evoked responses (e.g., auditory). No single monitor can provide a fail-safe answer to the question of anesthetic depth. pEEG technology has entered the operating room from a number of manufacturers and is the dominant technique of monitoring for awareness.

9. How does pEEG work? What are the target levels?

Raw EEG data, collected by electrodes placed on the forehead and temporal regions, are processed by the computer module to create a dimensionless numeric representation of the degree of cortical activity and thus the level of sedation. Lower numbers correspond to greater depths of hypnosis. One common format is the bispectral index (BIS). A BIS goal of 40 to 60 usually indicates adequate hypnosis. The ASA Task Force suggests that brain electrical activity monitoring is not routinely indicated but should be considered on an individualized basis for selected patients (high-risk patients, light general anesthesia).

10. Can end-tidal volatile agent monitoring be used instead of pEEG?

Targeting end-tidal anesthetic concentration (ETAC) of 0.7 to 1.3 minimal alveolar concentration (MAC) has been shown to be an appropriate goal. The BAG-Recall and MACS trials both compared large numbers of patients randomized to compare AWR with either a BIS pEEG protocol or an ETAC protocol. Neither was able to prove BIS superiority in reducing AWR in initial analysis.

11. Should pEEG or ETAC be used to monitor for patient awareness?

Several large studies have compared ETAC with pEEG for reducing AWR, and a trend has emerged. Most studies using volatile anesthesia have not shown any superiority for BIS monitoring. Contrary to this, secondary post hoc analysis of the MACS trial as well as the B-AWARE and Zhang et al. trials showed reduction of AWR in patients receiving total intravenous anesthesia (TIVA). These trials strongly suggest that when TIVA is used, pEEG monitoring can reduce the incidence of AWR, whereas an ETAC protocol is sufficient when volatile anesthetics are the primary anesthesia.

KEY POINTS: AWARENESS UNDER ANESTHESIA

1. Awareness is most likely in cases where minimal anesthetic is administered, such as cardiopulmonary bypass, hemodynamic instability, trauma, and obstetrics.
2. Symptoms of awareness can be nonspecific, and the use of neuromuscular blockade increases the risk of unrecognized awareness.
3. The small risk of awareness should be discussed during consent if patients are deemed at higher risk.
4. Processed EEG (e.g., BIS) can reduce awareness with recall during total intravenous anesthesia, while end-tidal anesthetic concentration monitoring is sufficient during cases predominated by volatile anesthesia.

WEBSITE

American Association of Nurse Anesthetists: Anesthetic awareness fact sheet and patient awareness brochure. www.aana.com/forpatients/pages/anesthetic-awareness.aspx

SUGGESTED READINGS

ASA Task Force on Intraoperative Awareness: Practice advisory for intraoperative awareness and brain function monitoring, Anesthesiology 104:847–864, 2006.

Avidan MS, Jacobson E, Glick D, et al: Prevention of intraoperative awareness in a high risk surgical population, N Engl J Med 365:591–600, 2011.

Avidan MS, Mashour GA: Prevention of intraoperative awareness with explicit recall: making sense of the evidence, Anesthesiology 118:449–456, 2013.

Mashour GA, Orser BA, Avidan MS: Intraoperative awareness: from neurobiology to clinical practice, Anesthesiology 114:1218–1233, 2011.

Osterman JE, Hopper J, Heran W, et al: Awareness under anesthesia and the development of post-traumatic stress disorder, Gen Hosp Psychiatry 23:198–204, 2001.

Rampersad SE, Mulroy MF: A case of awareness despite an "adequate depth of anesthesia" as indicated by a bispectral index monitor, Anesth Analg 100:1363–1364, 2005.

Zhang C, Xu L, Ma YQ, et al: Bispectral index monitoring prevents awareness during total intravenous anesthesia: a prospective, randomized, double blinded, multicenter controlled trial, Chin Med J 124:3664–3669, 2011.

CHAPTER 27

TEMPERATURE DISTURBANCES

James C. Duke, MD, MBA

1. **Describe the processes that contribute to thermoregulation.**

   There are three phases of thermoregulation: afferent sensing, central thermoregulatory integration, and efferent response. Distinct receptors are distributed about the body for sensing warmth and cold. Cold impulses travel centrally via myelinated A-delta fibers, warmth is transmitted by unmyelinated C fibers, and most ascending thermal information travels cephalad via the anterior spinothalamic tract. Thermal information is integrated within the spinal cord and centrally in the hypothalamus. Within a narrow range of temperatures (the interthreshold range), no efferent response is triggered by the hypothalamus. Above and below certain thresholds, efferent mechanisms activate in an attempt to decrease or increase body temperature, respectively. Warm responses include active vasodilation and sweating; cold responses include vasoconstriction, nonshivering thermogenesis, and shivering.

2. **Which patients are at risk for hypothermia?**

   All patients having either general or neuraxial anesthesia, or even just sedation, are at risk. Patients especially at risk include the elderly, who have reduced autonomic vascular control, and infants, who have a large surface area-to-mass ratio. Patients with burns, spinal cord injuries that involve autonomic dysfunction, and endocrine abnormalities are also at risk.

3. **Does hypothermia have an impact on patient outcome?**

   Mild hypothermia (1° to 3°C) has the following effects:
   - Increases incidence of surgical site infections (SSIs). Although this is a multifactorial problem, it has been noted that vasoconstriction secondary to hypothermia decreases blood flow to the wound and bacterial killing by neutrophils. Complications with bowel surgery have been related to hypothermia.
   - Increases the period of hospitalization by increasing the likelihood of SSIs and delayed healing
   - Reduces platelet function and impairs activation of the coagulation cascade, increasing blood loss and transfusion requirements (shown by some to also be a cause of increased SSIs)
   - Triples the incidence of ventricular tachycardia and morbid cardiac events
   - Prolongs the activity of muscle relaxants and anesthetic agents, increasing the likelihood of postoperative weakness and prolonged postoperative recovery.
   - The pathophysiologic effects of hypothermia are reviewed in Table 27-1.

4. **Characterize the different stages of hypothermia.**

   Hypothermia is a clinical state of subnormal body temperature in which the body is unable to generate enough heat to maintain a normal temperature.
   - **Mild hypothermia** (32° to 35°C [90° to 95°F]) is associated with mild central nervous system depression (dysarthria, amnesia, ataxia, and apathy), decreased basal metabolic rate, tachycardia, peripheral vasoconstriction, and shivering.
   - **Moderate hypothermia** (27° to 32°C [80° to 90°F]) results in further depression in consciousness, decreased motor activity, mild depression of vital signs, arrhythmias, and cold diuresis.
   - In **severe hypothermia** (<27°C [80°F]) the patient may be comatose and areflexic and have significantly depressed vital signs. Left untreated, such profound hypothermia leads to death.

Table 27-1. The Effects of Hypothermia on Organ Systems

SYSTEM	EFFECTS
Vascular	Increases systemic vascular resistance and peripheral hypoperfusion; plasma volume decreases because of cold diuresis
Cardiac	Decreases heart rate, contractility, and cardiac output and produces arrhythmias
Pulmonary	Increases pulmonary vascular resistance; decreases hypoxic pulmonary vasoconstriction; increases ventilation-perfusion mismatching; depresses ventilatory drive; decreases bronchial muscle tone, which increases anatomic dead space; oxyhemoglobin dissociation curve shifts to the left
Renal	Decreases renal blood flow and glomerular filtration rate; impaired sodium resorption and diuresis leading to hypovolemia
Hepatic	Decreases hepatic blood flow, metabolic and excretory functions
Central nervous system	Decreases cerebral blood flow; increases cerebral vascular resistance; decreases oxygen consumption by 7%/°C; increases evoked potential latencies; decreases MAC
Hematologic	Decreased platelet aggregation and clotting factor activity; increased blood viscosity, impaired immune response
Metabolic	Basal metabolic rate decreases; hyperglycemia and insulinopenia; decreased oxygen consumption and CO_2 production
Healing	Increased wound infections

MAC, Minimum alveolar concentration.

5. **Which perioperative events predispose a patient to hypothermia?**
   Heat loss is common in all patients during general anesthesia because of peripheral vasodilation, altered thermoregulation, and the inability to generate heat by shivering. General anesthesia widens the interthreshold range, and, because the thermoregulatory response is markedly less robust, body temperature changes passively with existing temperature gradients. Hypothermia is as common during neuraxial anesthesia as general anesthesia and is a result of sympathetic blockade, muscle relaxation, and a lack of afferent sensory input into central thermoregulatory centers.

6. **Which physical processes contribute to a patient's heat loss in the operating room?**
   • **Radiation:** The dissipation of heat to cooler surroundings, which accounts for about 60% of a patient's heat loss, depending on cutaneous blood flow and exposed body surface area
   • **Evaporation:** The energy required to vaporize liquid from any surface, be it skin, serosa, or mucous membranes; accounts for 20% of heat loss and is a function of the exposed surface area and the relative humidity
   • **Convection:** Is responsible for about 15% of heat loss and depends on the airflow over exposed surfaces
   • **Conduction:** Describes the transfer of heat between adjacent surfaces, accounts for about 5% of the total heat loss, and is a function of the temperature gradient and thermal conductivity
   • **Core temperature afterdrop** (a secondary decline in core temperature with rewarming): May result from the return of cold blood from the periphery

7. **As a practical matter, what is done to a patient in the operating room that increases heat loss?**
   Cool rooms, cold intravenous and sterile preparation solutions, and exposure of the patient to the environment contribute significantly to hypothermia. Cutaneous heat loss is

proportional to the exposed surface area and accounts for 90% of heat loss. One unit of refrigerated blood or 1 L of room-temperature crystalloid decreases the body temperature about 0.25°C. The effects of general anesthesia, regional anesthesia, and neuromuscular blockade have been discussed. Less than 10% of heat loss is through the respiratory tract.

8. **Should all patients receive temperature monitoring within the operating room? What are acceptable sites for temperature monitoring?**
The American Society of Anesthesiologists' Standards for Basic Anesthetic Monitoring state: "Every patient receiving anesthesia shall have temperature monitored when *clinically significant changes* in body temperature are intended, anticipated or suspected." Sites for monitoring temperature include skin, rectum, esophagus, external auditory canal, nasopharynx, bladder, and pulmonary artery catheter.

9. **Review shivering and nonshivering thermogenesis.**
Shivering is the spontaneous, asynchronous, random contraction of skeletal muscles in an effort to increase the basal metabolic rate. Shivering is modulated through the hypothalamus and can increase the body's production of heat by up to 300% in young, muscular individuals. It increases oxygen consumption and carbon dioxide production. This effect may be undesirable in a patient with coronary artery disease or pulmonary insufficiency.
Infants younger than 3 months of age cannot shiver and mount a caloric response by nonshivering thermogenesis, which increases metabolic heat production without producing mechanical work. Skeletal muscle and brown fat tissue are the major energy sources for this process.

10. **Describe the electrocardiographic manifestations of hypothermia.**
Mild hypothermia may be associated only with sinus bradycardia. Moderate hypothermia may result in prolonged PR intervals, widened QRS complexes, and a prolonged QT interval. Below 32°C, an elevation of the junction of the QRS and ST segments known as the hypothermic hump or Osborne or J wave may be seen. Its size increases with decreasing body temperature; it usually is seen in leads II and V6 and may spread to leads V3 and V4. Occasionally the J wave is identified in electrocardiograms. Nodal rhythms are common below 30°C. Below 28°C, premature ventricular contractions, atrioventricular blocks, and spontaneous atrial or ventricular fibrillation also occur. Ventricular fibrillation or asystole below 28°C is relatively unresponsive to atropine, countershock, or pacing. Resuscitative efforts should persist until the patient is rewarmed.

KEY POINTS: TEMPERATURE DISTURBANCES

1. Hypothermia is an extremely common event in the operating room because the environment and the effects of anesthetics increase heat loss. Anesthetics also decrease the ability to generate a response to hypothermia (shivering and vasoconstriction).
2. Even mild hypothermia has a negative influence on patient outcome, increasing wound infection rates, increasing nitrogen loss, delaying healing, increasing blood loss, and increasing hospitalization as well as cardiac morbidity.
3. The best method to treat hypothermia is use of forced-air warming blankets. Warm all fluids and blood products. Cover all body surfaces possible, including the head, to further reduce heat loss.

11. **How does hypothermia affect the actions and metabolism of drugs used in the operative environment?**
Drug effects are prolonged by decreased hepatic blood flow and metabolism and decreased renal blood flow and clearance. Protein binding increases as body temperature decreases. The minimum alveolar concentration of inhalational agents is decreased about 5% to 7% per degree centigrade decrease in core temperature. The effects of sedative agents are also decreased. Hypothermia may prolong the duration of neuromuscular blocking agents because of decreased metabolism. Hypothermia delays discharge from the postanesthetic care unit and may prolong the need for mechanical ventilation.

12. **Discuss methods of rewarming.**
    - **Passive rewarming** uses the body's ability to generate heat if continued heat loss is minimized by covering exposed areas.
    - **Active rewarming** is readily performed in the operating room and includes increasing the ambient temperature, administering warmed intravenous fluids, and warming with radiant heat. Forced-air warming devices are especially beneficial and superior to circulating water blankets. Their effect is maximal when a large surface area is exposed to active rewarming. A core temperature afterdrop (a secondary decline in core temperature with rewarming) may result from the return of cold blood from the periphery.
    - Warming inspired gases has no utility as the heat content of gases is minimal. The practice has been discontinued.

13. **Define hyperthermia.**
    Hyperthermia is a rise in body temperature of $2°C/hr$. Because it is uncommon in the operating room, its cause must be investigated. The usual cause is sepsis or overheating. Hypothalamic lesions and hyperthyroidism are less common causes. Malignant hyperthermia is a great concern because it is caused by volatile anesthetics or succinylcholine and can be fatal if left untreated.

14. **Describe the manifestations of hyperthermia.**
    Hyperthermia is a hypermetabolic state associated with increased oxygen consumption, increased minute ventilation, sweating, tachycardia, and vasodilation. An awake patient may experience general malaise, nausea, and light-headedness. With prolonged hyperthermia, the patient may develop heat exhaustion or heat stroke. In the anesthetized patient, signs and symptoms include tachycardia, hypertension, increased end-tidal carbon dioxide, increased drug metabolism, rhabdomyolysis, oliguria, and hypovolemia. Heart rate increases by 10 beats/min per degree centigrade increase in temperature.

15. **What conditions are associated with hyperthermia?**
    - Malignant hyperthermia, as discussed in Chapter 42
    - Hypermetabolic states, including sepsis, thyrotoxicosis, and pheochromocytoma
    - Hypothalamic lesions secondary to trauma, anoxia, or tumor
    - Neuroleptic malignant syndrome
    - Transfusion reaction
    - Medications

16. **What drugs increase the risk of hyperthermia?**
    Sympathomimetic drugs, monoamine oxidase inhibitors, cocaine, amphetamines, and tricyclic antidepressants increase the basal metabolic rate and heat production. Anticholinergic medications and antihistamines may elevate temperature by suppressing sweating.

17. **What are the pharmacologic effects of hyperthermia?**
    Increases in basal metabolic rate and hepatic metabolism decrease the half-life of anesthetic drugs. Anesthetic requirements may be increased.

18. **What is the treatment for the hyperthermic patient in the operating room?**
    Expose skin surfaces and use cooling blankets and cool intravenous fluids. Correctable causes of hyperpyrexia should be ruled out. Consider administering antipyretics, although it is always best to treat the cause, not the symptom.

WEBSITE

American Society of Anesthesiologists: Standards for basic anesthetic monitoring 2011. Available at http://www.asahq.org

SUGGESTED READINGS

Lemmens HJM, Brock-Utna JG: Heat and moisture exchange devices: are they doing what they are supposed to do? Anesth Analg 98:382–385, 2004.

Mauermann WJ, Nenergut EC: The anesthesiologist's role in the prevention of surgical site infections, Anesthesiology 105:413–421, 2006.

Rajagopalan S, Mascha E, Na J, et al: The effects of mild perioperative hypothermia on blood loss and the transfusion requirement, Anesthesiology 108:71–77, 2008.

Sessler DI: Temperature monitoring and perioperative thermoregulation, Anesthesiology 109:318–338, 2008.

CHAPTER 28

POSTANESTHETIC CARE

Michael M. Sawyer, MD

1. **Which patients should be cared for in the postanesthetic care unit (PACU)?**

   PACU care is traditionally divided into phase 1, during which monitoring and staffing ratios are equivalent to those in an intensive care unit, and phase 2, wherein transition is made from intensive observation to preparation for care on a surgical ward or at home.

   Fast-track recovery is emerging because of fast-offset anesthetic agents and adjunctive drugs. Most patients who have had monitoring plus sedation or extremity regional anesthesia should be appropriate for fast-track recovery, bypassing phase 1. Typically, however, after general or regional anesthesia, a period of phase 1 care is required. Coexisting disease, the surgical procedure, and pharmacologic implications of the anesthetic agents used ultimately determine the most appropriate sequence of postoperative care for each patient.

2. **Review important considerations for the immediate postanesthetic phase.**

   Transport from the operating room (OR) to the PACU can be a dangerous time for patients. Recent PACU designs have been developed to make this trip as short as possible. Many institutions still are burdened with PACUs remote from the ORs. Anesthetics conducted remote from the PACU (e.g., radiology, etc.) are also a site of potential instability. Before transport from remote locations, a patient should have oxygen administered, be able to maintain a patent airway with spontaneous respirations. The use of supplemental oxygen for transport is recommended. Patients with hemodynamic or respiratory instability will require the use of a transport monitor.

3. **Describe the process for PACU admission.**

   A report is given by the anesthesia caregiver to the PACU nurse, reviewing the patient's prior health status, surgical procedure, intraoperative events, agents used, and anesthetic course. The use of muscle relaxants and reversal of neuromuscular blockade, the intraoperative interventions for analgesia, and the intraoperative fluids and blood products received by the patient guide in planning PACU care. Initial assessment of the patient by the PACU nurse includes vital signs, baseline responsiveness, adequacy of ventilation, and adequacy of analgesia. Various scoring systems have been used to allow numeric scoring of subjective observations as an indicator of progress toward discharge. The Aldrete scoring system (Table 28-1) tracks five observations: activity, respiratory effort, circulation, consciousness, and oxygenation. Scales for each are 0 to 2, and a total score of 8 to 10 indicates readiness to move to the next phase of care. Regression of motor block in the case of regional anesthesia is also an important determinant of readiness for discharge, particularly when discharge home is planned and the patient has had lower extremity peripheral nerve blocks.

4. **What monitors should be used routinely in the PACU?**

   The level of care will depend on the clinical status of the patient. Pulse oximetry and periodic blood pressure monitoring should be used routinely on all patients. Interestingly, routine electrocardiogram (ECG) monitoring has not been found to be of value in patients without risk factors of coronary disease. Finally, temperature, urine output, and surgical drainage require monitoring as appropriate.

5. **What problems should be resolved during postanesthetic care?**
   - **Hypoventilation:** The patient should be breathing easily and able to cough on command and oxygenate to near preanesthetic levels.
   - **Hemodynamic stability:** Blood pressure should be within 20% of preanesthetic measurements with stable heart rate and rhythm.
   - **Attenuated sensorium:** The patient should be fully awake and voluntarily move all extremities.

Table 28-1. The Aldrete Scoring System

Activity	Able to move four extremities	2
	Able to move two extremities	1
	Not able to move extremities voluntarily or on command	0
Respiration	Able to breathe and cough	2
	Dyspnea or limited breathing	1
	Apneic	0
Circulation	BP ± 20% of preanesthetic level	2
	BP ± 21%–49% of preanesthetic level	1
	BP ± 50% of preanesthetic level	0
Consciousness	Fully awake	2
	Arousable on calling	1
	Not responding	0
O_2 saturation	Maintain O_2 saturation >92% in room air	2
	Needs O_2 to maintain O_2 saturation >90%	1
	O_2 saturation <90% with O_2 supplement	0

BP, Blood pressure.
Adapted from Aldrete AJ, Krovlik D: The postanesthetic recovery score. Anesth Analg 49:924–933, 1970.

Table 28-2. Ventilation Problems in the Postanesthetic Care Unit

PROBLEM	SYMPTOMS	TREATMENT
Residual neuromuscular blockade	Uncoordinated, ineffectual respiratory effort	Neostigmine, 0.05 mg/kg IV
Opioid narcosis	Slow ventilation, sedated and difficult to arouse	Respiratory support, naloxone, 0.04–0.4 mg IV
Residual inhalation anesthesia	Sleepy, shallow breathing	Encourage deep breathing

- **Postoperative pain:** Pain management should no longer require continuous nursing intervention.
- **Postoperative nausea and vomiting (PONV):** PONV should be treated aggressively since it is associated with prolonged length of stay in the PACU and decreased patient satisfaction with the perioperative experience.

6. **How is ventilation adversely affected by anesthesia?**
   Residual neuromuscular blockade, opioid effects, and lingering effects of inhalational anesthesia can result in postoperative hypoventilation (Table 28-2).

7. **Describe the appearance of a patient with residual neuromuscular blockade.**
   The patient appears *floppy*, with poorly coordinated and ineffective respiratory muscle activity. The patient may complain that breathing is restricted and efforts to deliver supplemental oxygen are suffocating. The patient is unable to sustain a head lift or hand grasp. In the worst case scenario, weakness of the pharyngeal muscles results in upper airway collapse and postextubation airway obstruction. Neither a good response to train-of-four testing in the OR nor spontaneous rhythmic ventilation before extubation rules out residual neuromuscular blockade.

8. **How do opioids and residual volatile anesthetics affect breathing?**
   Slow rhythmic breathing or apneic pauses in a patient who is hard to arouse suggest residual narcosis. In contrast to the patient with residual muscle relaxation, the narcotized patient is often unconcerned about ventilation despite obvious hypoxia. Surprising degrees of hypercapnia may be found, even with relatively normal pulse oximetry values when supplemental oxygen is delivered.

Table 28-3. Predicted FiO$_2$ with Supplemental Oxygen Delivery

SYSTEM	DELIVERY FLOW (L/MIN)	FIO$_2$ PREDICTED
Nasal cannula	2	0.28
Nasal cannula	4	0.36
Facemask	6	0.50
Partial rebreathing mask	6	0.6
Total rebreathing mask	8	0.8

FiO$_2$, Fractional inspired oxygen concentration.

9. **How should these causes of hypoventilation be treated?**
Hypoventilation resulting from residual neuromuscular blockade should be treated urgently and aggressively. Additional reversal agents may be given in divided doses up to the usual dose limitations. Treatment decisions for residual narcosis may prove to be more problematic. Indicated procedures include continuous stimulation until spontaneous ventilation improves or oral/nasal airways relieve an airway obstruction. Other supportive measures include increasing inspired oxygen concentrations (FiO$_2$). However, increasing FiO$_2$ does not reverse hypoventilation; it only masks it (Table 28-3).

10. **The patient has been delivered to the PACU. Oxygen saturations are noted to be in the upper 80s, and chest wall movement is inadequate. How should the patient be managed?**
Establish a patent airway (chin lift, jaw thrust) and administer oxygen. Suction the patient's airway if needed. Is the trachea in midline? Once the airway is patent, observe and auscultate the chest. Is the patient hypoventilating? Reversal of opioid effect may be necessary. Does the abdomen distend and the chest retract with inspiration (paradoxical respirations), suggesting airway obstruction or inadequate reversal of neuromuscular blockade?

Assess the patient's strength by hand grip and sustained head lift. Are there wheezes or rales, requiring inhaled β agonists? Is there diuresis? Palpate pulses and listen to the heart because circulatory depression causes oxygen desaturation. The patient may require assisted ventilation or reintubation.

Most hypoxia in the PACU is caused by atelectasis, which is treated by sitting the patient upright, asking him or her to breathe deeply or cough, and encouraging incentive spirometry.

11. **The patient develops stridorous breath sounds. Describe the likely cause and the appropriate management.**
A likely cause of stridorous breath sounds in the early postextubation period is laryngospasm, although other causes of upper airway obstruction (e.g., postextubation croup, expanding hematomas, soft-tissue swelling) should be excluded. Laryngospasm may be precipitated by extubation during light planes of anesthesia or secretions falling on the vocal cords. If laryngospasm is incomplete, the patient will have stridorous breath sounds. If laryngospasm is complete, little air movement is possible and breath sounds will be absent.

12. **How is laryngospasm treated?**
The treatment for laryngospasm is to support ventilation. Call for an assistant, provide a jaw thrust, and assist the patient's inspiratory efforts with positive-pressure ventilation, using 100% oxygen. If this proves unsatisfactory, administer succinylcholine, 0.15 to 0.30 mg/kg (about 10 to 20 mg in adults), to relax the vocal cords. (I have had success with even 5 mg of succinylcholine administered intravenously to an adult. In this setting, a little seems to go a long way. Another advantage is that the diaphragm and accessory muscles of respiration remain functional.) If the patient continues to experience difficulty with ventilation, reintubation after administering approximately 100 mg of succinylcholine may be necessary. Once intubation is completed and end-tidal CO$_2$ has been verified, the patient should receive assisted ventilation. Sedation may be appropriate. When re-extubation is

attempted, be prepared for a possible recurrence of laryngospasm. If stridorous breath sounds are caused by laryngeal edema, administration of nebulized racemic epinephrine and intravenous steroids may be indicated.

13. **The laryngospasm resolves. Chest auscultation reveals bilateral rales. What is the most likely cause?**
    Although congestive heart failure, fluid overload, adult respiratory distress syndrome, and aspiration of gastric contents need to be considered, negative-pressure pulmonary edema (NPPE) is the likely cause. NPPE results from generation of negative intrapleural pressures when the patient inspires against a closed or obstructed glottis. Whereas intrapleural pressures vary between −5 and −10 cm H_2O during a normal respiratory cycle, inspiration against a closed glottis may generate between approximately −50 and −100 cm H_2O pressure. Such increased pressures increase venous return to the thorax and pulmonary vasculature, increasing transcapillary hydrostatic pressure gradients, producing pulmonary edema. The onset of edema has been noted from 3 to 150 minutes after the inciting event. Some authorities refer to this syndrome as negative-pressure pulmonary injury (NPPI) because pink or frankly bloody pulmonary secretions suggest that some alveolar injury has taken place during attempts to breathe against a closed glottis.

14. **How is NPPE treated?**
    Once the airway obstruction is relieved, treatment is supportive. The pulmonary edema usually resolves between 12 and 24 hours. Continue oxygen therapy; continuous positive airway pressure and mechanical ventilation with positive end-respiratory pressure may occasionally be needed, depending on the severity of gas exchange impairment. Diuretics should be administered only if the patient has intravascular fluid overload or perhaps in the most severe cases.

15. **How are patients with undiagnosed with sleep apnea (SA) identified?**
    Postoperative SA is associated with increased mortality and morbidity. Patients with obstructed SA may never have been diagnosed. Hence, screening is indicated with undiagnosed though at-risk patients. Features suggesting a Sleep Apnea Clinical Score (SACS) can be assessed at the time of preoperative evaluation to identify those at risk. Characteristics include hypopnea, apnea, oxygen desaturation of pain-sedation mismatch and suggest the patient is likely to have oxygenation sedation events during routine floor care. These events may go undiagnosed and lead to increasing hypercarbia and cardiopulmonary arrest.

KEY POINTS: POSTANESTHETIC CARE AND COMPLICATIONS

1. Postanesthetic care is part of the continuum of perioperative care and the responsibility of the anesthesiologist.
2. Loss of normal respirations and airway obstruction are regular events that result in hypoxemia and require management.
3. Adequate oxygenation, controlled postoperative pain, and resolved PONV are common problems that allow PACU discharge.
4. Patients with suspected sleep apnea should be managed as sleep apnea patients should. Supplemental oxygen, regular checks, and oxygen saturations are the best standards for treatment.

16. **Describe an approach to the evaluation of postoperative hypertension and tachycardia.**
    A hyperdynamic postoperative phase is not an uncommon event. Frequently observed and readily treatable causes include pain, hypoventilation, hypercarbia, hypothermia with shivering, bladder distention, and essential hypertension. Also consider hypoxemia, hyperthermia and its causes, anemia, hypoglycemia, tachydysrhythmias, withdrawal (e.g., drug and alcohol), myocardial ischemia, prior medications administered, and coexisting disease. In rare cases, the hyperdynamic state may reflect hyperthyroidism, pheochromocytoma, or malignant hyperthermia.

17. **What might cause hypotension in the postoperative phase?**
   Prior or ongoing blood loss, third-space sequestration of fluid, and inadequate volume replacement manifest as hypotension. Myocardial ischemia or heart failure may present as hypotension, as can sepsis and anaphylaxis.

18. **How should hypotension be treated?**
   Consider the surgical procedure, intraoperative events, medications, and past medical history. Evaluate blood loss and urine output. Review the ECG rhythm strip and consider a 12-lead ECG. Volume expansion with balanced crystalloid solutions is first-line therapy. Elevation of legs and Trendelenburg positioning may help transiently. Circumstances may require administration of colloid or packed red blood cells. Should volume expansion prove unsatisfactory, vasopressors or inotropes may be necessary, but these suggest the need for further evaluation.

19. **Under what circumstances is a patient slow to awaken?**
   A reasonable initial assumption is that such patients are displaying residual drug effects. Should decreased awareness persist beyond a reasonable period of observation, ventilatory, metabolic, and central nervous system (CNS) etiologies must be considered. Does the patient have a seizure history and is the patient currently postictal? CNS ischemia caused by decreased perfusion or embolic phenomena should be considered. Has the patient had documented CNS ischemic events or strokes? Laboratory analysis should include arterial blood gases as well as measurements of serum sodium and glucose. If these levels are normal, perhaps a computed tomographic scan of the brain is needed.

20. **Discuss the issues surrounding PONV.**
   PONV remains a significant, troublesome postanesthetic problem. It results in delayed PACU discharge and occasional unplanned hospital admission and is a recurring cause of patient dissatisfaction. Both the surgical procedure and anesthetic agents administered may increase PONV risk. Procedural risks include laparoscopic surgery; surgery on genitalia; craniotomies; and shoulder, middle ear, or eye muscle procedures. Patient factors are female sex, nonsmokers, prior PONV or motion sickness history, and school-age children. Anesthetic agents with a high association with PONV include opioids, volatile inhalation agents, and nitrous oxide. Propofol has the lowest incidence of any of the induction agents and has been used effectively as a rescue medication. Risk assessment should be made on the basis of these factors, and prophylactic treatment or alteration of the anesthetic plan should be determined based on evidence of efficacy. PONV rescue (treatment once PONV has ensued) requires balancing drug benefits with side effects and cost.

21. **Should ambulatory patients be treated differently in the PACU?**
   The goal of postanesthetic care of the ambulatory patient is to render the patient *street ready*. Pain should be treated with short-acting agents such as fentanyl. Nonnarcotic analgesia and nerve blocks should be used whenever possible. Oral analgesics should be used in phase 2 recovery as prescribed for postoperative care. After regional anesthesia, extremities should be protected while the patient is mobilized, and ambulation should be assisted if transient segmental paresthesia makes movement unsteady. No ambulatory surgery patient should be discharged after receiving any sedating medication without a companion to ensure safe transportation to a place of residence.

22. **Should patients be required to tolerate oral intake before PACU discharge?**
   Taking clear liquids before discharge can increase length of stay in the PACU. It is unclear if the ability to tolerate clear liquids decreases adverse outcomes and at the present time is not recommended to be a requirement for PACU discharge. However, it may be helpful in selected patients.

23. **A patient has undergone a general anesthetic for an outpatient procedure. Recovery has been uneventful, yet the patient has no ride home. How should this be handled?**
   Patients should be required to have a responsible party accompany them home after anesthesia. It has been shown to decrease adverse events. The responsible party will be able to promptly report any adverse events that may arise. The patient in this case should be

kept at the health care facility, possibly under 23-hour observation, or until a responsible party is available.

24. **What is the reasonable minimal PACU stay?**

Although this time may be reasonable, the American Society of Anesthesiologists has no recommendation for the minimal length of stay in the PACU. Length of stay should be determined on a case-by-case basis. A discharge protocol should be designed that allows patients to reach postoperative goals that will direct them toward discharge.

WEBSITE

American Society of Anesthesiologists: http://www.asahq.org/

SUGGESTED READINGS

American Society of Anesthesiologists Task Force on Postanesthetic Care: Practice guidelines for postanesthetic care, Anesthesiology 96:742–752, 2002.

Gali B, Whalen FX, Schroeder DR, et al: Identification of patients at risk for postoperative respiratory complications using a preoperative obstructive sleep apnea screening tool and postanesthesia care assessment, Anesthesiology 110:869–877, 2009.

Gan TJ, Meyer T, Apfel CC, et al: Consensus guidelines for managing postoperative nausea and vomiting, Anesth Analg 96:62–71, 2003.

Gross JB, Bachenberg KL, Benumof J, et al: Practice guidelines for the perioperative management of patients with obstructive sleep apnea, Anesthesiology 104:1081–1093, 2006. Updated report available at http://www.ncbi.nlm.nih.gov/pubmed/24346178.

ISCHEMIC HEART DISEASE AND MYOCARDIAL INFARCTION

Tamas Seres, MD, PhD

1. **Name the known risk factors for the development of ischemic heart disease (IHD).**

   Age, male gender, and positive family history as risk factors are cannot be modified. Smoking, hypertension, diet, dyslipidemia, physical inactivity, obesity, and diabetes mellitus are modifiable and should be considered in all adults as risk factors for which interventions are likely to lower IHD risk.

2. **Describe the normal coronary blood flow (CBF).**

   The resting CBF averages about 225 ml/min, which is 4% to 5% of the total CO in normal adults. The CBF increases threefold to fourfold to supply the extra nutrients needed by the heart at maximum exercise level. The CBF is determined by the pressure gradient between the aorta and the ventricle. There are phasic changes in CBF during systole and diastole in the left ventricle. The blood flow falls to a low value during systole, especially in the subendocardial area because of the strong compression of the left ventricular muscle around the intramuscular vessels and the small pressure gradient between the aorta and the left ventricle (aortic systolic pressure–left ventricular systolic pressure). During diastole, the cardiac muscle relaxes and no longer obstructs the blood flow through the left ventricular capillaries. The pressure gradient is high during diastole (aortic diastolic pressure–left ventricular end-diastolic pressure).

   The phasic changes of the CBF are much less in the right ventricle because the force of contraction of the right ventricle is much weaker than that of the left ventricle and the pressure gradient is high between the aorta and the right ventricle during the entire cardiac cycle.

3. **Describe the coronary anatomy.**

   The right coronary artery system is dominant in 80% to 90% of people and supplies the sinoatrial node (60%), atrioventricular node (85%), and right ventricle. In 84% of people, it terminates as the posterior descending artery (PDA). Right-sided coronary artery occlusion can result in bradycardia, heart block, inferior or right ventricular myocardial infarction (MI).

   The left main coronary artery gives rise to the circumflex artery and left anterior descending (LAD) artery, which supply the majority of the interventricular septum (septal branches) and left ventricular wall (diagonal branches). When the circumflex gives rise to the PDA, the circulation is left dominant, and the left coronary circulation supplies the entire septum and the atrioventricular (AV) node. In 40% of patients, the circumflex supplies the sinoatrial (SA) node. Significant stenosis of the left main coronary artery (left main disease) or the proximal circumflex and LAD arteries (left main equivalent) may cause severely depressed myocardial function during ischemia.

4. **Explain the determinants of myocardial oxygen demand and delivery.**

   Myocardial oxygen demand is determined by wall tension and contractility. Wall tension (T) is the product of intraventricular pressure (P), radius (R), and wall thickness (h) (T = PR/2h). Increased ventricular volume (preload) and increased blood pressure (afterload) increase wall tension and O_2 demand. An increase in contractility in response to sympathetic stimulation or inotropic medications increases O_2 demand also.

   Increase in heart rate increases myocardial contractility but decreases the ventricular diameter and the wall tension. Thus, the increase in oxygen demand caused by enhanced contractility is in large part offset by the reduction in oxygen demand that accompanies the reduced wall tension. The oxygen demand is increasing because more contraction is performed per minute.

Myocardial oxygen delivery is determined by oxygen content and CBF. Oxygen content can be calculated by the following equation:

$$O_2 \text{ content} = [1.39 \text{ ml } O_2/g \text{ of hemoglobin} \times \text{hemoglobin (g/dl)} \times \text{saturation (decimal rate)}] + [0.003 \times PaO_2]$$

The oxygen content is decreased in anemia and hypoxemia.

CBF is determined by coronary perfusion pressure, the time available for perfusion, and the patency of coronary arteries. Coronary perfusion pressure is altered by diastolic hypotension, left ventricular hypertrophy, and increased left ventricular end-diastolic pressure. The diastolic time for perfusion is decreasing with tachycardia. The patency of the coronary arteries can be influenced by vasospasm or coronary occlusion caused by atherosclerosis.

5. **What is the clinical manifestation of myocardial ischemia?**
The clinical manifestations of myocardial ischemia are varied. Angina pectoris with or without signs of arrhythmias or heart failure is assumed to be the classic manifestation of myocardial ischemia. However, myocardial ischemia may present as ventricular failure or arrhythmias without angina or may remain clinically silent. The dynamic nature of coronary stenosis accounts for the changes in the caliber of a stenosis that may produce pain at rest at one time and angina with varying degrees of exercise at other times. Clinical manifestations are stable angina, unstable angina, Q or non-Q MI, MI with or without ST elevation. The different clinical entities need different management strategies.

6. **How can be the angina graded?**
The Canadian Cardiovascular Society introduced a grading system for angina:
Class I   Angina with strenuous or rapid prolonged exertion at work or recreation.
Class II   Angina with walking or climbing stairs rapidly, walking uphill. Walking more than two blocks on the level and climbing more than one flight of ordinary stairs at a normal pace.
Class III Angina with walking one to two blocks on the level and climbing one flight of stairs at a normal pace.
Class IV   Angina may be present at very low level of physical activity or at rest.

7. **Describe the pathogenesis of a perioperative MI.**
MI is usually caused by platelet aggregation, vasoconstriction, and thrombus formation at the site of an atheromatous plaque in a coronary artery. Sudden increases in myocardial O_2 demand (tachycardia, hypertension) or decreases in O_2 supply (hypotension, hypoxemia, anemia, tachycardia, coronary occlusion) can precipitate MI in patients with IHD. Recent studies have confirmed that most perioperative ischemic events are unrelated to hemodynamic perturbations, suggesting that intracoronary events may be important in the genesis of perioperative ischemia. Complications of MI include dysrhythmias, hypotension, congestive heart failure, acute mitral regurgitation, pericarditis, ventricular thrombus formation, ventricular rupture, and death.

8. **What clinical factors increase the risk of a perioperative MI following noncardiac surgery?**
There are active cardiac conditions, clinical risk factors, and minor clinical predictors based on an algorithm for risk stratification and appropriate use of diagnostic testing (ACC/AHA Task Force on Perioperative Evaluation of Cardiac Patients Undergoing Noncardiac Surgery, 2007). The guidelines integrate clinical risk factors, exercise capacity, and the surgical procedure in the decision-making process.
• Active cardiac conditions
  • Unstable angina
  • Severe angina (Canadian class III or IV)
  • Acute and recent MI

- Decompensated heart failure
- Significant arrhythmias
- Severe valvular disease
- Clinical risk factors
  - History of IHD
  - Compensated or prior heart failure
  - History of cerebrovascular disease
  - Diabetes mellitus
  - Renal insufficiency
- Minor clinical predictors
  - Advanced age (>70)
  - Abnormal ECG (LVH, LBBB, nonspecific ST-T abnormalities)
  - Rhythm other than sinus (AF)
  - Uncontrolled systemic hypertension

9. **How does the type of surgery influence the risk stratification for perioperative ischemia?**
   - High-risk surgery (risk of perioperative adverse cardiac events >5%) includes aortic and major vascular procedures as well as peripheral vascular surgeries.
   - Intermediate-risk procedures (risk of perioperative adverse cardiac events <5%) are carotid endarterectomy, head and neck surgery, intraperitoneal and intrathoracic surgery, orthopedic surgery, and prostate surgery.
   - Low-risk procedures (risk of perioperative adverse cardiac events <1%) are endoscopic procedures, superficial procedures, cataract surgery, and breast surgery.

10. **How can cardiac function be evaluated on history and physical examination?**
    If a patient's exercise capacity is excellent, even in the presence of IHD, the chances are good that the patient will be able to tolerate the stresses of the surgery. Poor exercise tolerance in the absence of pulmonary or other systemic disease indicates an inadequate cardiac reserve. All patients should be questioned about their ability to perform daily activities. The ability to climb two to three flights of stairs without significant symptoms (angina, dyspnea, syncope) is usually an indication of adequate cardiac reserve greater than 4 metabolic equivalents (METs) exercise capacity (1 MET equals 3.6 ml/kg/min oxygen uptake at rest).

    Signs and symptoms of congestive heart failure—including dyspnea, orthopnea, paroxysmal nocturnal dyspnea, peripheral edema, jugular venous distention, a third heart sound, rales, and hepatomegaly—must be recognized preoperatively.

11. **When would you consider noninvasive stress testing before noncardiac surgery?**
    The guidelines integrate clinical risk factors, exercise capacity, and the surgical procedure in the decision-making process. Noninvasive stress testing is considered if it will change the management of the following types of patients:
    - Patients with active cardiac conditions in whom noncardiac surgery is planned. These patients should be evaluated and treated according to the ACC/AHA guidelines before noncardiac elective surgery.
    - Patients with three or more clinical risk factors and poor functional capacity who require vascular surgery.
    - Patients with at least one or two clinical risk factors and poor functional capacity who require intermediate-risk noncardiac surgery.
    - Patients with at least one or two clinical risk factors and good functional capacity who are undergoing vascular surgery.

12. **What is the definition of recent MI and prior MI?**
    Recent developments in monitoring and therapy (including aggressive revascularization), combined with improved preparation of patients for surgery has significantly decreased the risk of perioperative re-infarction, even in patients with recent and prior MI. Based on the decreased risk for perioperative reinfarction, *recent MI* is defined as MI occurring 8 to 30 days before surgery, whereas *prior MI* is defined as MI that occurred more than 30 days before surgery.

13. **What tests performed by medical consultants can help further evaluate patients with known or suspected IHD?**

Exercise ECG is a noninvasive test that attempts to produce ischemic changes on ECG (ST depression = 1 mm from baseline) or symptoms by having the patient exercise to maximum capacity. Information obtained relates to the thresholds of heart rate and blood pressure that can be tolerated. Maximal heart rates, blood pressure response, and clinical symptoms guide interpretation of the results.

Exercise thallium scintigraphy increases the sensitivity and specificity of the exercise ECG. The isotope thallium is almost completely taken up from the coronary circulation by the myocardium and can then be visualized radiographically. Poorly perfused areas that later refill with contrast delineate areas of myocardium at risk for ischemia. Fixed perfusion defects indicate infarcted myocardium.

Dipyridamole thallium imaging is useful in patients who are unable to exercise. This testing is frequently required in patients with peripheral vascular disease who are at high risk for IHD and exercise test is limited by claudication. Dipyridamole is a potent coronary vasodilator that causes differential flow between normal and diseased coronary arteries detectable by thallium imaging.

Echocardiography can be used to evaluate left ventricular and valvular function and to measure ejection fraction. Stress echocardiography (dobutamine echo) can be used to evaluate new or worsened regional wall motion abnormalities in the pharmacologically stressed heart. Areas of wall motion abnormality are considered at risk for ischemia.

Coronary angiography is the gold standard for defining the coronary anatomy. Valvular and ventricular function can be evaluated and hemodynamic indices can be measured. Because angiography is invasive, it is reserved for patients who require further evaluation based on previous tests or who have a high probability of severe coronary disease.

14. **What are the main indications for coronary revascularization before noncardiac surgery?**

Consistent with the ACC/AHA 2004 Guideline Update for coronary artery bypass graft (CABG) surgery, the following patients need coronary revascularization before noncardiac surgery:
- Patients with stable angina who have significant left main coronary artery stenosis.
- Patients with stable angina who have three-vessel disease. Survival benefit is greater when left ventricular ejection fraction is less than 50%.
- Patients with stable angina who have two-vessel disease with significant proximal LAD stenosis and either ejection fraction less than 50% or demonstrable ischemia on noninvasive testing.
- Patients with high-risk unstable angina or non–ST-segment elevation MI.
- Patients with acute ST-elevation MI.

Coronary revascularization includes CABG or percutaneous coronary intervention (PCI).

15. **A patient who has undergone PCI is scheduled for surgery. What is your concern?**

After PCI, patients need to be on dual-antiplatelet therapy (aspirin and clopidogrel). Discontinuation of this therapy for surgical procedure poses a high risk for coronary artery thrombosis and myocardial events in the perioperative period. The appropriate timing of surgery is still under investigation, but the following guidelines are accepted:
- After balloon angioplasty, nonurgent surgery can be performed with aspirin after 14 days, but ideally these patients should be on dual-antiplatelet therapy for 4 to 6 weeks.
- After bare-metal or drug-eluting stent placement, nonurgent surgery can be performed with aspirin after 30 to 45 days or more than 365 days, respectively.

16. **Why do patients with drug-eluting stents need significantly longer dual-antiplatelet therapy?**

Drug-eluting stents in current clinical use were approved by the FDA after clinical trials showed they were statistically superior to bare-metal stents for treatment of coronary artery occlusions, having lower rates of major adverse cardiac events (usually defined as a composite clinical endpoint of death + MI + repeat intervention because of restenosis).

The drugs (sirolimus, paclitaxel) released from the stent inhibit endothelium surface formation inside the stent and require long-duration dual-antiplatelet therapy.

17. Should all cardiac medications be continued throughout the perioperative period?

Patients with a history of IHD are usually taking medications intended to decrease myocardial oxygen demand by decreasing the heart rate, preload, afterload, or contractile state (β blockers, calcium channel antagonists, nitrates) and to increase the oxygen supply by causing coronary vasodilation (nitrates). These drugs are generally continued throughout the perioperative period.

18. Should preoperative β-blocker therapy be continued into the perioperative period?

Yes, patients receiving preoperative β-blocker therapy should continue to receive their β blockers into the perioperative period.

19. Would you give prophylactic intraoperative nitroglycerin infusion?

The usefulness of intraoperative nitroglycerin as a prophylactic agent to prevent myocardial ischemia and cardiac morbidity is unclear for high-risk patients undergoing noncardiac surgery, particularly for those who have required nitrate therapy to control angina. The recommendation for prophylactic use of nitroglycerin must take into account the anesthetic plan and patient hemodynamics and must recognize that vasodilation and hypovolemia can readily occur during anesthesia and surgery.

20. What ECG findings support the diagnosis of IHD?

The resting 12-lead ECG remains a low-cost, effective screening tool in the detection of IHD. It should be evaluated for the presence of ST-segment depression or elevation, T-wave inversion, old MI as demonstrated by Q waves, disturbances in conduction and rhythm, and left ventricular hypertrophy. Ischemic changes in leads II, III, and aVF suggest right coronary artery disease, leads I and aVL monitor the circumflex artery distribution, and leads V_3, V_4, and V_5 look at the distribution of the LAD artery.

21. When is resting 12-lead ECG recommended?

- Patients with at least one clinical risk factor (history of IHD, history of compensated or prior heart failure, history of cerebrovascular disease, diabetes mellitus, and renal insufficiency) who are undergoing vascular surgical procedures
- Patients with known coronary heart disease, peripheral arterial disease, or cerebrovascular disease who are undergoing intermediate-risk surgical procedures
- It is reasonable in patients with no clinical risk factors who are undergoing vascular surgical procedures.

22. How long should a patient with a recent MI wait before undergoing elective noncardiac surgery?

The risk of reinfarction during surgery in a patient with recent MI has traditionally depended on the time interval between the MI and the procedure. The ACC/AHA Task Force eliminated the arbitrary 6-month time interval and suggested that elective surgery is associated with prohibitive risk only during the initial 4 to 6 weeks. The patient's functional status following rehabilitation from an MI is probably more important than the absolute time interval. Patients with ongoing symptoms are candidates for coronary revascularization prior to their noncardiac procedure.

23. Outline the hemodynamic goals of induction and maintenance of general anesthesia in patients with IHD.

The anesthesiologist's goal is to maintain the balance between myocardial O_2 demand and supply throughout the perioperative period. During induction, wide swings in heart rate and blood pressure should be avoided. Ketamine should be avoided because of the resultant tachycardia and hypertension. Prolonged laryngoscopy should be avoided, and the anesthesiologist may wish to blunt the stimulation of laryngoscopy and intubation by the addition of opiates, β blockers, or laryngotracheal or intravenous lidocaine. Maintenance drugs are chosen with knowledge of the patient's ventricular function. In patients with good left ventricular function, the cardiac depressant and vasodilator effects of inhaled

192 ANESTHESIA AND SYSTEMIC DISEASE

anesthetics may reduce myocardial O_2 demand. A narcotic-based technique may be chosen to avoid undue myocardial depression in patients with poor left ventricular function. Muscle relaxants with minimal cardiovascular effects are usually preferred. Blood pressure and heart rate should be maintained near baseline values. This can be accomplished by blunting sympathetic stimulation with adequate analgesia and aggressively treating hypertension (anesthetics, nitroglycerin, nitroprusside, β blockers), hypotension (fluids, phenylephrine, inotropic drugs), and tachycardia (fluids, anesthetics, β blockers).

24. **What monitors are useful for detecting ischemia intraoperatively?**
The V_5 precordial lead is the most sensitive single ECG lead for detecting ischemia and should be monitored routinely in patients at risk for IHD. Lead II can detect ischemia of the right coronary artery distribution and is the most useful lead for monitoring P waves and cardiac rhythm.

25. **Would you use TEE routinely in patients with high cardiac risk undergoing noncardiac surgery?**
Transesophageal echocardiography can provide continuous intraoperative monitoring of left ventricular function. In high-risk patients, detection of regional wall motion abnormalities with this technique is the most sensitive monitor for myocardial ischemia. However, a recent AHA/ACC recommendation suggests that it is reasonable to use intraoperative or perioperative transesophageal echocardiography to determine the cause of an acute, persistent, and life-threatening hemodynamic abnormality.

26. **Is a pulmonary artery catheter reasonable to use routinely for optimization of high-risk patients?**
The pulmonary artery occlusion (wedge) pressure gives an estimation of the left ventricular end-diastolic pressure, which is a useful guide for optimizing intravascular fluid therapy. Sudden increases in the wedge pressure may indicate acute left ventricular dysfunction due to ischemia. The use of pulmonary artery catheters in patients with IHD has not been shown to improve outcome; thus it should be restricted to a very small number of highly selected patients whose presentation is unstable and who have multiple comorbid conditions.

27. **A patient has high blood pressure (190/120 mm Hg) in the holding area. Would you cancel the surgery?**
Uncontrolled high blood pressure is a minor clinical predictor for outcome after surgery. If the patient does not have symptoms of acute organ failure because of the high blood pressure (such as headache, altered mentation, or chest pain) and does not have signs or symptoms of heart failure, the patient can undergo surgery. Preoperative blood pressure medications such as labetalol, hydralazine, β blockers, diuretics, Nipride or nicardipine infusions can be considered depending on the clinical conditions of the patient. General anesthesia, epidural anesthesia, and spinal anesthesia decrease the systemic blood pressure, so there is no need for anti-hypertensive medication during anesthesia in most of these cases. There should be a comprehensive plan for postoperative blood pressure control for these patients.

28. **Describe the stepwise evaluation of patients with cardiac disease who will have noncardiac surgery.**
   - Step 1: Determination of the urgency of the surgery: if the surgery is emergent, the patient should go to the operating room, and appropriate anesthesia and a monitoring plan should be established. Perioperative medical management and surveillance should be part of the plan.
   - Step 2: In cases when the surgery is not emergent, evaluate the patient for active heart condition (see Section 8). In patients being considered for elective noncardiac surgery, the presence of unstable coronary disease, decompensated heart failure, or severe arrhythmia or valvular heart disease usually leads to cancellation or delay of surgery until the cardiac problem has been clarified and treated appropriately.
   - Step 3: If the patient is not having active heart condition, evaluate the risk of surgery. If the surgery is low risk, the patient can go to the operating room.
   - Step 4: If the surgery is intermediate or high risk (see Section 9), evaluate functional capacity. In highly functional asymptomatic patients, management will rarely be changed

on the basis of results of any further cardiovascular testing. It is therefore appropriate to proceed with the planned surgery.
- Step 5: If the patient has poor functional capacity, evaluate for clinical risk factors.
  - No clinical risk factors: proceed with surgery.
  - One or two clinical risk factors:
    - Proceed with surgery.
    - Consider cardiovascular testing if it will change management.
  - Three or more clinical risk factors:
    - Consider heart rate control with β blocker if it is appropriate.
    - Consider cardiovascular testing if it will change management.

KEY POINTS: ISCHEMIC HEART DISEASE AND MYOCARDIAL INFARCTION

1. The clinical predictors, the surgical procedure, and exercise capacity should be integrated in the decision-making process to avoid adverse perioperative cardiac events.
2. Patients with active cardiac conditions (unstable or severe angina, recent MI) should be determined and treated before noncardiac elective surgery.
3. The risk of the surgical procedure also should be considered. Patients who are undergoing vascular surgery are at very high risk for perioperative ischemic events.
4. Patients with excellent exercise capacity, even in the presence of ischemic heart disease, will be able to tolerate the stresses of noncardiac surgery. The ability to climb two or three flights of stairs without significant symptoms (angina, dyspnea) is usually an indication of adequate cardiac reserve.
5. The type of acute revascularization should be carefully planned because patients with drug-eluting stent should be on dual-antiplatelet therapy for at least a year.

SUGGESTED READINGS

DiNardo JA: Anesthesia for cardiac surgery, ed 2, Philadelphia, 1998, Stamford, Appleton & Lange, pp 81–140.

Fleisher LA: Ischemic heart disease. In Sweitzer BJ, editor: Handbook of preoperative assessment and management, Philadelphia, 2000, Lippincott Williams & Wilkins, pp 39–62.

Fleisher L, Beckman JA, Brown KA, et al: Focused update on perioperative beta-blocker therapy, Anesth Analg 104:15–26, 2007.

Fleisher LA, Beckman JA, Kenneth A, et al: ACC/AHA 2007 Guidelines on perioperative cardiovascular evaluation and care for noncardiac surgery, Circulation 116:1971–1996, 2007.

Fleisher LA, Fleischmann KE, Auerbach AD, et al: 2014 ACC/AHA Guideline on Perioperative Cardiovascular Evaluation and Management of Patients Undergoing Noncardiac Surgery, J Am Coll Cardiol 64(22):e77–e137, 2014.

Guyton, AC, Hall JE: Textbook of medical physiology, ed 9, Philadelphia, 1996, Saunders, pp 253–264.

London M, Hur K, Schwartz GG, et al: Association of perioperative β-blockade with mortality and cardiovascular morbidity following major noncardiac surgery, JAMA 309:1704–1713, 2013.

Stoelting, RK: Anesthesia and co-existing disease, ed 4, New York, 2002, Churchill Livingstone, pp 1–24.

CHAPTER 30

HEART FAILURE

Tamas Seres, MD, PhD

1. **What is heart failure (HF)?**

   HF is a complex clinical syndrome that can result from any structural or functional cardiac disorder that impairs the ability of the ventricle to fill or eject blood. The cardinal manifestations of HF are dyspnea and fatigue, which may limit exercise tolerance and fluid retention and may lead to pulmonary congestion and peripheral edema. Some patients have exercise intolerance but little evidence of fluid retention, whereas others complain primarily of edema and report few symptoms of dyspnea or fatigue. Because not all patients have volume overload at the time of initial or subsequent evaluation, the term *heart failure* is preferred over the older term *congestive heart failure*.

2. **Name the causes of HF.**

   The most common causes of HF in the United States are coronary artery disease (CAD), systemic hypertension (HTN), dilated cardiomyopathy, and valvular heart disease (Box 30-1).

3. **Describe the staging of HF.**
   - **Stage A:** Patients with CAD, HTN, or diabetes mellitus who do not yet demonstrate impaired left ventricular (LV) function, LV hypertrophy, or geometric chamber distortion
   - **Stage B:** Patients who are asymptomatic but demonstrate LV hypertrophy, geometric chamber distortion, and/or impaired LV systolic or diastolic function
   - **Stage C:** Patients with current or past symptoms of HF associated with underlying structural heart disease
   - **Stage D:** Patients with HF refractory to medical therapy who might be eligible for specialized, advanced treatment strategies, such as mechanical circulatory support, procedures to facilitate fluid removal, continuous inotropic infusions, cardiac transplantation or end-of-life care, such as hospice

     This classification recognizes that there are established risk factors and structural prerequisites for the development of HF (stages A and B) and that therapeutic interventions introduced even before the appearance of LV dysfunction or symptoms can reduce the morbidity and mortality of HF.

4. **How is the severity of HF classified?**

   Typically, the status of patients with HF can be classified on the basis of symptoms, impairment of lifestyle, or severity of cardiac dysfunction. The New York Heart Association (NYHA) classification is used to assess symptomatic limitations of HF and response to therapy:
   - **Class I:** Ordinary physical activity does not cause symptoms. Dyspnea occurs with strenuous or rapid prolonged exertion at work or recreation.
   - **Class II:** Ordinary physical activity results in symptoms. Dyspnea occurs while walking or climbing stairs rapidly or walking uphill. Walking more than two blocks on the level and climbing more than one flight of ordinary stairs at a normal pace also result in symptoms.
   - **Class III:** Less than ordinary activity results in symptoms. Dyspnea occurs while walking one to two blocks on the level or climbing one flight of stairs at a normal pace.
   - **Class IV:** Dyspnea occurs at a low level of physical activity or at rest.

     The NYHA classification describes the functional status of patients with stage C or D HF. The severity of symptoms characteristically fluctuates even in the absence of changes in medications, and changes in medications can have either favorable or adverse effects on functional capacity in the absence of measurable changes in ventricular function. Some patients may demonstrate remarkable recovery associated with improvement in structural and functional abnormalities. Medical therapy associated with sustained improvement should be continued indefinitely.

Box 30-1. Causes of Heart Failure Conditions

Mechanical Abnormalities

    Pressure overload
        Aortic stenosis, systemic hypertension, and pulmonary hypertension
    Volume overload
        Valvular regurgitation, anemia, thyrotoxicosis, circulatory shunts
    Restriction of ventricular filling
        Mitral stenosis, constrictive pericarditis, left ventricular hypertrophy

Myocardial Disease

    Primary
        Cardiomyopathies, hypertrophic/restrictive/dilated cardiac disease
    Secondary
        Coronary artery disease, ischemic cardiomyopathy
        Metabolic: alcoholic cardiomyopathy, thyroid disorders, pheochromocytoma, uremic cardiomyopathy
        Drugs: doxorubicin, heroin, cocaine
        Metals: iron overload, lead poisoning, cobalt poisoning
        Myocarditis: bacterial/viral/parasitic/mycotic disease
        Connective tissue diseases: rheumatic arthritis, systemic lupus erythematosus, scleroderma
        Neurologic diseases: myotonic dystrophy, Duchenne muscular dystrophy
        Inherited diseases: glycogen storage diseases, mucopolysaccharidoses
        Other diseases: amyloidosis, leukemia, irradiation to heart

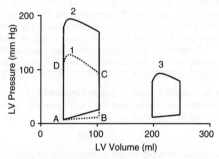

Figure 30-1. Left ventricular (LV) pressure-volume loops illustrating normal performance (*loop 1*), pressure overload (*loop 2*), and systolic dysfunction or volume overload (*loop 3*).
Loop 1: The phases of the heart cycle in normal heart. AB, diastolic filling; BC, isovolumic contraction; CD, ejection; DA, isovolumic relaxation.
Loop 2: This loop represents the pressure-volume relationship in chronic hypertension or aortic stenosis with concentric LV hypertrophy. The stroke volume and ejection fraction are normal. The high LV end-diastolic pressure suggests diastolic dysfunction based on decreased LV compliance.
Loop 3: In systolic dysfunction, the LV end-diastolic and end-systolic volumes are enlarged with normal or less than normal stroke volume. The end-diastolic pressure can be normal or higher than normal (secondary diastolic dysfunction), depending on the compliance of the LV. This loop may represent dilated cardiomyopathy or eccentric LV hypertrophy in volume overload.

5. **What major alterations in the heart occur in patients with HF?**

    Normal heart function can be characterized by pressure-volume curve showing the end-diastolic volume (B) and end-systolic volume (D) and pressure, stroke volume (CD), and ejection fraction (Figure 30-1, *loop 1*). It is also important to understand that the pressure for propelling the SV from the heart is generated mostly during isovolumetric contraction (BC) and the relaxation for diastole is happening mostly during isovolumetric relaxation (DA) (see Figure 30-1, *loop 1*). LV dysfunction begins with injury of the myocardium. The myocardial injury can be initiated by hypoxia, infiltration, or infection and is generally a progressive process causing systolic dysfunction with increasing end-systolic volume. The left ventricle dilates with increasing end-diastolic volume and becomes more spherical—a process called *cardiac remodeling* (see Figure 30-1, *loop 3*). Specific patterns of ventricular remodeling occur in response to augmentation in workload. In pressure overload the increased wall tension during systole initiates parallel addition of new myofibrils causing wall thickening and concentric hypertrophy (see Figure 30-1, *loop 2*). In volume overload the wall tension is increasing during diastole, which initiates new sarcomeres resulting in chamber enlargement and eccentric hypertrophy (see Figure 30-1, *loop 3*). Ventricular dilation allows the chamber to eject an adequate stroke volume (SV) with less muscle shortening, but wall stress is increased, as described by the Laplace relationship.

$$\text{Wall tension} = P \times R/2h$$

where P = intracavital pressure, R = the radius of the chamber, and h = the thickness of the chamber wall.

Increasing wall tension accompanies higher oxygen demand during similar performance. Myocardial hypertrophy with increasing wall thickness allows the heart to overcome pressure overload, with decreasing wall tension.

6. **What is the Frank–Starling law?**
The Frank-Starling law states that the force or tension developed in a muscle fiber depends on the extent to which the fiber is stretched. In a clinical situation, when increased quantities of blood flow into the heart (increasing preload), the tension will increase in the walls of the heart. The result of this increased stretch of the myocardium is that the cardiac muscle contracts with increased force and empties the expanded chambers with increasing SV. There is an optimal sarcomere length and thus an optimal fiber length from which the most forceful contraction occurs. The left ventricle normally operates at an LV end-diastolic volume, which is less than optimal fiber lengths. The clinical implication is that SV increases with increasing preload until the optimal fiber length of the myocardium is reached. In systolic HF, the myocardial contractility is decreased and the heart is working with higher end-diastolic and end-systolic volume. In this hemodynamic situation, relatively small changes in preload or afterload result in a decrease of SV and cardiac output.

7. **What is the role of cardiac output in patient evaluation?**
Cardiac output is the amount of blood that the heart can pump during 1 minute. The main determinants of the cardiac output are as follows:

$$CO = SV \times HR$$

where CO (cardiac output) = mean arterial pressure/total peripheral resistance, SV = stroke volume, and HR = heart rate.

Cardiac output varies widely with the level of physical activity. The average value for resting adults is about 5 liters/min. For women, this value is 10% to 20% less. Cardiac output increases in proportion to the surface area of the body. To compare the cardiac outputs of people of different sizes, the term of *cardiac index* (CI) was introduced, which is the cardiac output per square meter of body surface area. The normal CI for adults is more than 2.5 liters/min/m^2. The normal heart, functioning without any excess nervous stimulation, can pump an amount of venous return up to about 2.5 times the resting venous return, which is about 13 liters/min cardiac output. Nervous stimulation increases HR and contractility. These two effects can raise the cardiac output up to 25 liters/min. Patients with systolic HF are unable to generate appropriate cardiac output to the exercise level, and in patients with severe HF, the cardiac output decreases with exercise.

8. **What is the connection between exercise and cardiac output?**
Exercise increases the oxygen consumption of the body. This increased oxygen demand is matched by increasing oxygen delivery:

$$\text{Oxygen delivery} = CO \times \text{blood oxygen content}$$

Oxygen consumption and cardiac output increase in a parallel manner. HF results in a mismatch between tissue oxygen consumption and oxygen delivery based on the inappropriate cardiac output to the exercise level. The mismatch provokes tissue hypoxemia, acidosis, and inability to hold the exercise at the level where the mismatch occurs.

9. **What is systolic dysfunction?**
The symptoms and signs of HF can be caused by either an abnormality in systolic function that leads to diminished ejection fraction (EF) or an abnormality in diastolic function that leads to altered ventricular filling.

Systolic dysfunction leads to decreased ejection of blood from the left ventricle. The EF is diminished, the end-systolic and end-diastolic volume is enlarged, and the LV is dilated. The SV can be normal but is generated by a dilated ventricle with higher wall tension and oxygen consumption. In this pathologic condition, the LV has less reserve capacity to overcome pressure or volume load, which manifests in decreased exercise capacity (see Figure 30-1, *loop 3*).

10. **How can we diagnose systolic dysfunction and HF?**
The characteristic changes for systolic dysfunction are increased end-systolic and end-diastolic volume, decreased EF, decreased SV, wall motion abnormality, and secondary changes in diastolic function. These parameters can be obtained from an echocardiographic report and from evaluation of echocardiographic images. In general, the decreased SV with decreased cardiac output causes fatigue, and the secondary diastolic dysfunction with increased end-diastolic LV and left atrial (LA) pressure causes dyspnea. The functional status of the patient can be described by the NYHA functional classification. Patients with systolic dysfunction and clinical symptoms of HF have systolic HF.

11. **What is diastolic dysfunction?**
In normal condition the LV is filling up with blood at low (<12 mm Hg) LA pressure. The LA pressure stays low even with high cardiac output at strenuous exercise. This low pressure filling depends on the LV diastolic function. Early and late diastolic filling are the two phases of diastolic filling. Early diastolic filling starts with isovolumetric relaxation after the aortic valve closes until the mitral valve opens and continues during the early filling of the LV. It is energy-dependent and relies on reuptake of calcium from the cytosol into the sarcoplasmic reticulum of the myocytes. The LV generates negative pressure during this phase in normal condition, allowing the inflow of about 80% of the diastolic volume. Late diastolic filling (atrial contraction) depends on the LA contractility and LV compliance. Diastolic dysfunction can occur with normal or impaired systolic function. Impaired LV relaxation and/or decreased compliance are the major characteristic features of LV diastolic dysfunction. In diastolic dysfunction the size of the LV cavity can be normal, but ischemia, myocardial hypertrophy, pericardial constriction, fibrosis or myocardial diseases may alter the diastolic filling process. Systolic dysfunction with dilated left ventricle and high LV end-diastolic volume and pressure accompanies significant diastolic dysfunction because of decreased LV relaxation and compliance (see Figure 30-1, *loop 3*). Patients with normal EF but with the signs of diastolic dysfunction and clinical symptoms of HF have diastolic HF.

12. **How can we diagnose diastolic dysfunction?**
Evaluation of the echo data is important to diagnose the different type of diastolic dysfunction. Using intraoperative transesophageal echocardiography (TEE) helps make the diagnosis in the operating room. The diagnosis is made based on the Doppler study of the mitral valve inflow, pulmonary vein inflow, and tissue Doppler measurement of the velocity of the mitral valve annulus.
- **Mitral inflow:** The E wave represents the velocity curve of early diastolic filling, and the A wave is the velocity curve of late diastolic filling. E/A ratio is >0.8 in normal condition. The time from the peak to zero velocity of the E wave is the deceleration time of E (DecT), which is normally160 to 200 ms, and it represents effective early relaxation and normal LV compliance (Figure 30-2).
- **Pulmonary vein inflow:** During systole, blood is flowing from the pulmonary vein into the LA: S wave. During early diastole, the flow increases again from the pulmonary vein into the LA: D wave. During late diastole, during the atrial contraction there is a small back flow into the pulmonary vein: A reversal (Ar). In normal condition, the S/D ratio is close to 1 and the A reversal is <35 cm/s (Figure 30-3).

Mitral valve inflow

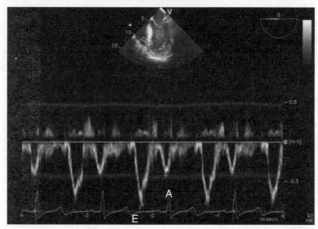

Figure 30-2. Pulsed-wave Doppler detection of mitral valve inflow. In the small segment of the upper part of the picture, the echo image of the four-chamber view can be seen. In this view, the Doppler probe detects the flow velocity through the mitral valve during the heart cycle. The Doppler probe is in the tip of the segment. The flow is going from the left atrium to the left ventricle away from the transducer during diastole; thus two negative velocity waves can be seen. The ECG helps to determine the phase of systole and diastole. The first wave is the E wave, which represents early diastolic filling, and the second wave is the A wave, which represents the atrial contraction.

Pulmonary vein inflow

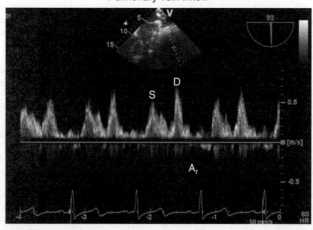

Figure 30-3. Pulsed-wave Doppler detection of pulmonary vein inflow. The small segment on the upper part of the figure represents the echo image of the two-chamber view. In this view the left upper pulmonary vein can be visualized just above the left atrial appendage. The flow is going from the pulmonary vein to the left atrium toward the transducer during systole and early diastole, and a small flow can be detected during the atrial kick back to the pulmonary vein. The first wave is the S wave, which represents the inflow during systole; the D wave represents the inflow during early diastole; and the small A_r (A reversal) is the flow back to the pulmonary wave during atrial contraction.

Tissue Doppler velocity

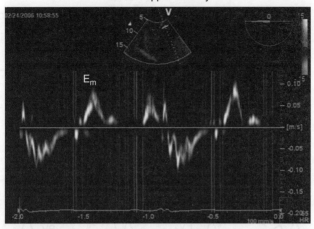

Figure 30-4. Tissue Doppler velocity measurement. The small segment of the upper part of the picture represents the echo image of the four-chamber view in tissue Doppler mode. The pulsed-wave Doppler probe is placed on the mitral valve annulus at the lateral wall and it shows the movement during systole and two waves during diastole. The ECG helps to differentiate between systole and diastole. The wave at early filling is the E_m velocity curve, which is a relatively volume-independent diastolic parameter.

- **Tissue Doppler:** The mitral valve and pulmonary vein inflow velocity curves are volume-dependent parameters that potentially change with the volume status of the patient. The mitral valve annulus velocities (E_m) during early diastole at the septum and the lateral wall are sensitive parameters of diastolic dysfunction and less sensitive to volume changes. In normal condition, the septal annulus velocity is >8 cm/s and the lateral annulus velocity is >10 cm/s (Figure 30-4).

13. **How can we characterize the different types of diastolic dysfunctions and their anesthetic management?**

    There are three types of diastolic dysfunctions:
    - **Grade 1 or relaxation abnormality:** The relaxation phase slows down, but the compliance of the LV is normal. In this situation the early diastolic filling is only 60% to 70% and the filling during late diastole increases. The LA pressure is normal in resting and during mild to moderate exercise. The LA pressure increases with tachycardia because the filling is shifting to late diastole and it needs high LA pressure to fill the LV without the suction effect of the early relaxation. In atrial fibrillation the SV and cardiac output decrease because of the lack of the atrial kick.
        - Clinical conditions include diseases with myocardial hypertrophy, such as HTN, aortic stenosis, and hypertrophic cardiomyopathy
        - Anesthetic management: These patients tolerate volume changes well because the LA pressure and LV compliance are normal. The goal is to keep the normal heart rate and avoid atrial fibrillation.
    - **Grade 2 or pseudonormal pattern:** This is a combination of relaxation abnormality and decreasing LV compliance. The decreasing LV compliance manifests in increasing LV end-diastolic and LA pressure. The increased LA pressure promotes bigger early diastolic filling with increasing E velocity resulting in normal E/A ratio. Pseudonormal pattern means that the E/A ratio is normal with higher than normal LA pressure. These patients have dyspnea at mild to moderate exercise.
        - Clinical conditions include ischemic and infiltrative heart disease or patients with LV hypertrophy have decreasing LV compliance.
        - Anesthetic management: These patients are sensitive for volume overload because of the elevated left atrial pressure (see Figure 30-5).

DIASTOLIC DYSFUNCTION

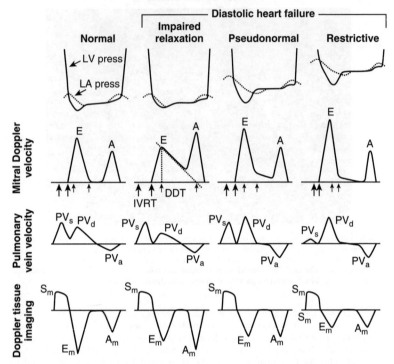

Figure 30-5. The evolution of diastolic dysfunction. The first row shows the left atrial (LA) and left ventricular (LV) pressure curve during diastole. The second row is the mitral valve inflow, the third row is the pulmonary vein inflow, and the fourth row is the tissue Doppler velocity curve. In normal condition, the pressure gradient in early diastole is generated by the suction effect of rapid LV relaxation (*column 1*). In impaired relaxation, the LA to LV pressure gradient is decreased because of the decreased suction effect of the LV resulting in decreased E, PV_d velocity, and E_m (*column 2*). In pseudonormal and restrictive pattern, the LV end-diastolic and LA pressure is increasing. The LA to LV pressure gradient is increasing in early diastole, generating normal E/A ratio in mitral valve inflow in pseudonormal (*column 3*) pattern or even bigger E/A ratio in restrictive pattern (*column 4*). The PV_s is decreasing and the PV_a (atrial contraction) is increased in pseudonormal and restrictive pattern with low tissue Doppler E_m. PV_s, S wave; PV_d, D wave; PV_a, A reversal.

- Grade 3 or restrictive pattern: The decreased LV compliance is the dominant diastolic abnormality with high LV end-diastolic and LA pressure. These patients might have dyspnea in rest and at mild exercise.
  - Clinical conditions include ischemic and infiltrative heart diseases. It often occurs in end stage heart failure.
  - Anesthetic management: These patients are volume overloaded and may react with flash pulmonary edema for fluid administration.
  - Higher than normal heart rate (tachycardia) is important to keep the cardiac output optimal because of the limited filling of the LV.

14. **What are the presenting symptoms of HF?**
    Exertional dyspnea and fatigue are most often the primary complaints. Paroxysmal nocturnal dyspnea, nocturia, coughing, wheezing, right upper quadrant pain, anorexia, nausea, and vomiting also may be complaints. Although HF is generally regarded as a

hemodynamic disorder, many studies have indicated that there is a poor relation between measures of cardiac performance and the symptoms produced by the disease. Patients with a very low EF may be asymptomatic (stage B), whereas patients with preserved EF may have severe disability (stage C). Patients with diastolic HF have the same symptoms, but they have normal EF. About 35% of patients with chronic HF have normal EF. The readmission and mortality rates of patients with diastolic HF might be similar to those observed in patients with systolic HF.

15. What physical signs suggest HF?

Cardiac palpation may reveal an expanded impulse area (ventricular dilation) or a forceful sustained impulse with LV hypertrophy. Auscultation reveals a gallop rhythm with S_3 or S_4 secondary to impaired LV filling or forceful atrial contraction, respectively. Murmurs of valvular diseases should be investigated. Severe failure may result in cyanosis.

Pulmonary examination often reveals rales located most prominently over the lung bases. Decreased breath sounds secondary to pleural effusions occur more often in patients with chronic HF.

Jugular venous distention >4 cm above the sternal angle with the patient recumbent at a 45-degree angle is considered abnormal.

16. What laboratory studies are useful in evaluating the patient with HF?

The posteroanterior and lateral chest radiograph may detect cardiomegaly or evidence of pulmonary vascular congestion, including perihilar engorgement of the pulmonary veins, cephalization of the pulmonary vascular markings, or pleural effusions.

The electrocardiogram (ECG) is often nonspecific, but ventricular or supraventricular dysrhythmias, conduction abnormalities, and signs of myocardial hypertrophy, ischemia, or infarction are present frequently.

Echocardiography characterizes chamber size, wall motion, valvular function, and LV wall thickness. SV can be measured using Doppler methods. EF can be calculated by measuring the end-diastolic and end-systolic volumes. Diastolic function can be evaluated by studying the flow pattern through the mitral valve and the left upper pulmonary vein using Doppler technique.

Radionuclide angiography provides a fairly reproducible and accurate assessment of left and right ventricular EF.

Serum electrolytes, arterial blood gases, liver function tests (LFTs), and blood cell counts are frequently evaluated. Many patients with HF are hyponatremic from activation of the vasopressin system or from the treatment with angiotensin-converting enzyme (ACE) inhibitors. Treatment with diuretics may lead to hypokalemia and hypomagnesemia. Some degree of prerenal azotemia, hypocalcemia, and hypophosphatemia is often present. Hepatic congestion may result in elevated bilirubin levels and elevated LFTs. Elevated brain natriuretic peptide (BNP) levels may help in suspected diagnosis of HF or trigger consideration of HF when the diagnosis is unknown but should not be used in isolation to confirm or exclude the presence of HF.

17. What treatment strategies are used in the different stages of HF?

- **Stage A: Patients at High Risk for Developing HF**

In patients with high risk for developing HF, systolic and diastolic HTN, lipid disorders, thyroid disorders, and diabetes mellitus should be controlled. Patients should be counseled to avoid smoking, excessive alcohol consumption, and illicit drug use that may increase the risk of HF. Patients who have known atherosclerotic vascular disease should be followed for secondary prevention. ACE inhibitors or angiotensin II receptor blockers can be useful to prevent HF in patients who have a history of atherosclerotic vascular disease, diabetes mellitus, or HTN.

- **Stage B: Patients with Cardiac Structural Abnormalities or Remodeling but Without Clinical Symptoms of HF**

All recommendations for stage A should apply to patients with cardiac structural abnormalities without clinical symptoms. β blockers and ACE inhibitors should be used in all patients with a recent or remote history of MI regardless of EF or presence of HF. β blockers and ACE inhibitors are indicated in all patients without a history of myocardial infarction who have a reduced EF with no HF symptoms.

- **Stage C: Patients with Current or Prior Symptoms of HF**
Patients with Reduced EF:
Measures listed as recommendations for patients in stages A and B are also appropriate for
patients in stage C. Diuretics and salt restriction are indicated in patients with current or
prior symptoms of HF and reduced EF who show evidence of fluid retention. ACE
inhibitors, angiotensin receptor blockers, and/or β blockers are recommended for all
patients with current or prior symptoms of HF and reduced EF, unless contraindicated.
Using one of the three β blockers proven to reduce mortality (i.e., bisoprolol, carvedilol,
and sustained-release metoprolol succinate) decreases mortality of these patients. Addition
of an aldosterone antagonist is reasonable in selected patients with moderately severe to
severe symptoms of HF and reduced EF. Automatic implantable cardioverter defibrillator
therapy and cardiac resynchronization therapy with dual-chamber pacemaker can be
instituted in high-risk patients.
Patients with Normal EF:
The goal is to reduce pulmonary congestion and correct precipitating factors such as HTN,
myocardial ischemia, and acute rhythm disturbances. Systolic and diastolic HTN should be
controlled in patients with HF and normal EF. Coronary revascularization is reasonable in
patients with CAD in whom symptomatic or demonstrable myocardial ischemia is judged to
be having an adverse effect on cardiac systolic and diastolic function. Ventricular rate
should be controlled in patients with atrial fibrillation. Diuretics should be used to control
pulmonary congestion and peripheral edema.
- **Stage D: Patients with Refractory End-Stage Heart Failure**
Such patients characteristically have symptoms at rest or on minimal exertion. They cannot
perform most activities of daily living, frequently have evidence of cardiac cachexia, and
typically require repeated and/or prolonged hospitalizations for intensive management. A
critical step in the successful management is the recognition and meticulous control of fluid
retention. These individuals represent the most advanced stage of HF and should be
considered for specialized treatment strategies, such as mechanical circulatory support,
continuous intravenous positive inotropic therapy, referral for cardiac transplantation, or
hospice care.

18. How would you plan anesthetic management of patients with HF?
    Patients with stage A or stage B HF have good functional status so they can go for surgery
    after routine preoperative evaluation.
       In stage C HF, the NYHA functional status should be evaluated and signs of
    decompensated HF should be checked. Patients with dyspnea, worsening dyspnea, or other
    change in clinical status are reasonable candidates to undergo preoperative noninvasive
    evaluation of LV function and postpone elective surgery until compensation.
       Stage D HF represents patients in NYHA class IV who are refractory to standard
    medical therapy. They can be on intravenous inotropic medications or assist device therapy
    and need special anesthetic management for noncardiac surgery.

19. How would you manage a patient with decompensated HF?
    In general, patients in decompensated HF are not candidates for elective procedures.
    Waiting a few days to optimize cardiac performance is indicated.
       In emergent circumstances, invasive monitoring (A-line, pulmonary artery catheter) is
    indicated to guide fluid therapy and assess response to anesthetic agents and inotropic or
    vasodilator therapy. Using TEE is extremely helpful to evaluate systolic and diastolic
    function, evaluate the effect of fluid therapy on the heart, and measure and monitor SV and
    cardiac output.
       If the patient needs optimization, continuous intravenous inotropic support or
    placement of a percutaneous LV assist device can be considered.

20. Which anesthetic agents can be used in decompensated HF?
    Avoidance of myocardial depression remains the goal of anesthetic management.
    Barbiturates and propofol generally produce the most profound depression of cardiac
    function and blood pressure when used for induction of general anesthesia. Etomidate
    produces only small aberrations in cardiovascular status, although hypotension may occur in
    the setting of hypovolemia. Ketamine administration may result in elevated cardiac output

and blood pressure secondary to increased sympathetic activity. However, in patients with increased sympathetic activation due to decompensated HF, ketamine acts as a negative inotropic agent and can cause severe hypotension and cardiac failure. All of the potent volatile anesthetic agents are myocardial depressants, but low doses are usually well tolerated. For patients with severely compromised myocardial function, narcotic-based anesthesia with or without low-dose volatile agent is useful. Remifentanil as a short-acting opioid can be well suited especially for short surgical procedures.

21. **Is regional anesthesia contraindicated in patients with HF?**
No. Regional anesthesia, when prudently administered, is an acceptable anesthetic technique. In fact, modest afterload reduction may enhance cardiac output. Continuous regional techniques (spinal or epidural) are preferable because they are associated with gradual loss of sympathetic tone, which may be treated with titration of fluids and vasoactive drugs. Invasive monitoring is necessary during regional anesthesia. An A-line is important to keep the blood pressure in an appropriate range, and pulmonary artery catheter can be helpful in selected cases.

22. **How would you support the heart in decompensated HF during anesthesia?**
Patients with HF often require circulatory support intraoperatively and postoperatively. After optimization of preload and afterload, inotropic drugs such as dopamine or dobutamine have been shown to be effective in low-output states. Phosphodiesterase III inhibitors, such as milrinone, possessing inotropic and vasodilating properties may improve hemodynamic performance. SV is inversely related to afterload in the failing ventricle, and the reduction of LV afterload with vasodilating drugs such as nitroprusside and nesiritide is also effective to increase cardiac output. Patients under anesthesia are vasodilated by most of the anesthetic agents. Epinephrine and dopamine have positive inotropic and vasoconstrictive properties and can be used alone. Dobutamine and milrinone cause vasodilation and should be combined with vasoconstrictive agents, such as vasopressin, epinephrine, or norepinephrine, in cases of low blood pressure.

23. **What are percutaneous LV assist devices?**
In patients with severe HF or in cardiogenic shock, percutaneous LV assist devices can be used to stabilize patients during recovery. They are available for short-term (several week) use only. It is important to understand the hemodynamic conditions in the presence of these devices to plan the anesthetic management and additional inotropic support. As a general concept, although these devices support the LV function, it is important to keep the RV function optimal to match the cardiac output generated by the devices.

24. **Why can't we use positive inotropic medications for long-term treatment of HF?**
Patients with HF are treated with β blockers, ACE inhibitors, and diuretics for long-term therapy. The effects of these medications are different compared with the effects of the β- and α-receptor agonist medications, which are used in the operating room to maintain hemodynamic stability during anesthesia and surgery. Outcome studies show that patients with HF have optimal long-term survival on β-blocker and ACE-inhibitor therapy and increasing mortality on medications with positive inotropic properties. This phenomenon can be explained by the protective effect of β blockers and ACE inhibitors on the heart against increased catecholamine, renin, and angiotensin levels in patients with HF.

KEY POINTS: HEART FAILURE

1. The symptoms and signs of heart failure (HF) can be caused by either an abnormality in systolic function that leads to a diminished ejection fraction (EF) or an abnormality in diastolic function that leads to a defect in ventricular filling.
2. Diastolic dysfunction can cause primary HF in the presence of normal EF, or it can be secondary in systolic HF with low EF with increased left atrial (LA) pressure. Different types of diastolic dysfunction need different types of fluid and hemodynamic management.
3. Patients in decompensated HF are not candidates for elective procedures and require a few days to optimize cardiac performance. However, in urgent cases, intravenous inotropic support and/or

percutaneous left ventricular (LV) assist device placement can be considered to perform anesthesia and surgery.
4. In emergent circumstances, invasive monitoring (arterial line, pulmonary artery catheter, and transesophageal echocardiography) is indicated to guide fluid therapy and assess response to anesthetic agents and inotropic or vasodilator therapy.
5. Patients with decreased myocardial reserve are more sensitive to the cardiovascular depressant effects caused by anesthetic agents, but careful administration with close monitoring of hemodynamic responses can be accomplished with most agents.
6. Noncardiac surgery for patients with an LV assist device requires an understanding of the hemodynamic effect of the device and of the monitoring options to maintain patient stability. As a general concept, the right ventricular function should be optimized to keep up with the cardiac output generated by the device.

WEBSITE

Systolic and diastolic dysfunction: www.uptodate.com

SUGGESTED READINGS

Braunwald E: Essential atlas of heart diseases, ed 2, Philadelphia, 2001, McGraw-Hill, pp 105–142.
Crawford MH: Current diagnosis and treatment in cardiology, ed 2, New York, 2003, McGraw-Hill, pp 217–249.
DiNardo JA: Anesthesia for cardiac surgery, ed 2, Stamford, 1998, Appleton & Lange, pp 81–140.
Falk S: Anesthetic considerations for the patient undergoing therapy for advanced heart failure, Curr Opin Anesthesiol 243:314–319, 2011.
Fleisher LA: Anesthesia and uncommon diseases, ed 5, Philadelphia, 2006, Saunders Elsevier, pp 29–38.
Fleisher LA, Beckman JA, Brown KA, et al: ACC/AHA 2007 Guidelines on perioperative cardiovascular evaluation and care for noncardiac surgery: executive summary, Circulation 116:1971–1996, 2007.
Hunt SA, Abraham WT, Chin MH, et al: ACC/AHA 2005 Guideline update for the diagnosis and management of chronic heart failure in the adult: a report of the American College of Cardiology/ American Heart Association Task Force on Practice Guidelines, Circulation 112:e154–e235, 2005.
Jessup M, Abraham WT, Casey DE, et al: 2009 Focused update: ACCF/AHA Guidelines for the diagnosis and management of heart failure in adults, Circulation 119:1977–2016, 2009.
Pirracchio R, Cholley B, De Hert S, et al: Diastolic heart failure in anesthesia and critical care, Br J Anesth 98:707–721, 2007.
Thomas Z, Rother AL, Collard CD: Anesthetic management for cardiac transplantation. In Hensley FA, Martin DE, Gravlee GP, editors: A practical approach to cardiac anesthesia, ed 4, Philadelphia, 2008, Lippincott Williams & Wilkins, pp 439–463.

CHAPTER 31

VALVULAR HEART DISEASE

Tamas Seres, MD, PhD

1. **Discuss the basic pathophysiology of valvular heart diseases.**

   Valvular heart diseases cause chronic volume or pressure overload, and each evokes a characteristic ventricular response called ventricular hypertrophy. *Ventricular hypertrophy* is defined as increased left ventricular (LV) mass. Pressure overload produces concentric ventricular hypertrophy with an increase in ventricular wall thickness with a cardiac chamber of normal size. Volume overload leads to eccentric hypertrophy with normal wall thickness and dilated cardiac chamber.

2. **Describe common findings of the history and physical exam in patients with valvular heart disease.**

   Most systolic heart murmurs do not signify cardiac disease, and many are related to physiologic increases in blood flow velocity. Diastolic murmurs virtually always represent pathologic conditions and require further cardiac evaluation, as do most continuous murmurs.

   A history of rheumatic fever, intravenous drug abuse, embolization in different organs, genetic diseases like Marfan syndrome, heart surgery in childhood, or heart murmur should alert the examiner to the possibility of valvular heart disease. Exercise tolerance is frequently decreased and patients may exhibit signs and symptoms of heart failure, including dyspnea, orthopnea, fatigue, pulmonary rales, jugular venous congestion, hepatic congestion, and dependent edema. Angina may occur in patients with a hypertrophied left ventricle, and atrial fibrillation frequently accompanies enlargement of the atria.

3. **Which tests are useful in the evaluation of valvular heart disease?**

   Echocardiography with Doppler technology is a fundamental diagnostic method in the evaluation of valvular heart diseases. The size and function of heart chambers, the pressure gradients at the valves, and the valve areas can be measured and the severity of the diseases determined.

   Echocardiography is recommended for:
   - Asymptomatic patients with diastolic murmurs, continuous murmurs, holosystolic murmurs, mid-peaking systolic murmurs, late systolic murmurs, murmurs associated with ejection clicks, or murmurs that radiate to the neck or back.
   - Patients with heart murmurs and symptoms or signs of heart failure, myocardial ischemia/ infarction, syncope, thromboembolism, infective endocarditis, or other clinical evidence of structural heart disease.

   An electrocardiogram (ECG) should be examined for evidence of ischemia, arrhythmias, atrial enlargement, and ventricular hypertrophy. Chest radiograph may show enlargement of cardiac chambers, suggest pulmonary hypertension, or reveal pulmonary edema and pleural effusions. Cardiac catheterization is used in the evaluation of such patients before surgery, mostly for diagnosing coronary artery disease. This method allows measurement pressures in various heart chambers and pressure gradients across different valves.

4. **How is echocardiography helpful in the anesthesia management?**

   Transesophageal echocardiography (TEE) can be used in the operating room during the surgical management of valvular diseases. The severity of the valvular disease and accompanying structural or functional changes can be reevaluated. Evaluation of valve repair or function of artificial valves is an important part of the patient management. Systolic and diastolic function of the left and right ventricles before and after cardiopulmonary bypass can be assessed and appropriate management can be planned and followed.

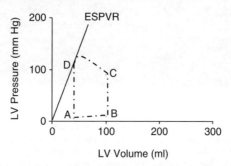

Figure 31-1. Pressure-volume loop in normal heart performance. *AB,* diastolic filling; *BC,* isovolumic contraction; *CD,* ejection; *DA,* isovolumic relaxation. *A,* mitral valve opening; *B,* mitral valve closing; *C,* aortic valve opening; *D,* aortic valve closing. The end-systolic pressure–volume relationship (ESPVR) curve is a load-independent index of myocardial contractility. If the contractility is increasing, the ESPVR curve is moving counterclockwise. The pressure-volume loop is an excellent tool to characterize the performance of the heart in different pathologic conditions. *LV,* Left ventricular.

5. **Which other monitors aid the anesthesiologist in the perioperative period?**
Besides standard American Society of Anesthesiologists (ASA) monitors, an arterial catheter provides beat-to-beat blood pressure measurement and continuous access to the bloodstream for sampling. Pulmonary artery catheters enable the anesthetist to measure cardiac output, mixed venous saturation, central venous and pulmonary artery pressures, and pulmonary capillary wedge pressure, which are important indexes of right and left ventricular function and filling and are useful for guiding intravenous fluid and inotropic therapy.

6. **What is a pressure-volume loop?**
A pressure-volume loop plots LV pressure against volume through one complete cardiac cycle. Each valvular lesion has a unique profile that suggests compensatory physiologic changes by the left ventricle.

7. **How does a normal pressure-volume loop appear?**
The AB segment is ventricular filling, BC is isovolumic contraction, CD is ejection, and DA is isovolumic relaxation. D point represents the aortic valve closing, A the mitral valve opening, B the mitral valve closing, and C the aortic valve opening (Figure 31-1). Stroke volume through the aortic valve is the distance between C and D points. End-systolic volume can be measured at the D point and end-diastolic volume can be measured at the B point. The end-systolic pressure–volume relationship (ESPVR) slope is a measure of contractility. A horizontal-clockwise shift of the slope represents a decrease in contractility.

8. **Discuss the pathophysiology of aortic stenosis (AS).**
AS is classified as valvular, subvalvular, or supravalvular obstruction of the LV outflow tract. Concentric hypertrophy (thickened ventricular wall with normal chamber size) develops in response to the increased intraventricular systolic pressure and wall tension necessary to maintain forward flow. Ventricular relaxation decreases, causing diastolic dysfunction. Decreasing LV compliance accompanies elevated LV end-diastolic pressure. Contractility and ejection fraction are usually maintained until late in the disease process. Atrial contraction may account for up to 40% of ventricular filling (normally 20%). In developing countries rheumatic valve disease is still the most common cause of AS. In North America and Europe, AS is primarily due to calcification of a native tri-leaflet or a congenital bicuspid valve. Patients often present with angina, syncope, or congestive heart failure. Angina with exertion can occur in the absence of coronary artery disease because the thickened myocardium is susceptible to ischemia and the elevated LV end-diastolic pressure reduces coronary perfusion pressure. Life expectancy with symptoms of angina is about 5 years. Once syncope appears, the average life expectancy is 3 to 4 years. Once congestive heart failure occurs, the average life expectancy is 1 to 2 years.

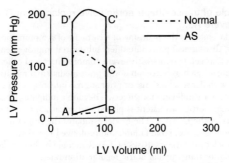

Figure 31-2. Pressure-volume loop in aortic stenosis *(AS)* compared with the normal loop. To generate normal stroke volume, the intraventricular pressure is high because of the pressure gradient at the aortic valve level. The end-diastolic pressure is higher than normal in cases when left ventricular *(LV)* hypertrophy alters LV compliance. Myocardial contractility is higher than normal.

9. **What is the indication for aortic valve replacement in AS?**
   According to the ACC/AHA guidelines, aortic valve replacement is indicated in the following patients:
   • Symptomatic patients with severe AS
   • Patients with severe AS undergoing coronary artery bypass graft surgery (CABG)
   • Patients with severe AS undergoing surgery on the aorta or other heart valves
   • Patients with severe AS and LV systolic dysfunction (ejection fraction less than 50%)
     In addition, aortic valve replacement is reasonable for patients with moderate AS undergoing CABG or surgery on the aorta or other heart valves.

10. **How are the compensatory changes in the left ventricle represented by a pressure-volume loop?**
    Because of AS, the left ventricle is working with higher intraventricular pressures to generate normal stroke volume. The higher systolic wall tension initiates myocardial thickening and LV hypertrophy. The hypertrophied left ventricle has increased contractility to accomplish the pressure work (Figure 31-2). As the AS is getting tighter, LV systolic pressure increases to the level where LV hypertrophy cannot normalize the wall tension. At this point, the heart starts dilating with the symptoms of systolic dysfunction and decreasing cardiac output.

11. **What are the hemodynamic goals in the anesthetic management of patients with AS?**
    Patients must have adequate intravascular volume to fill the noncompliant ventricle. Contractility should be maintained to overcome the high-pressure gradient through the aortic valve. Reduction in blood pressure or peripheral resistance does not decrease LV afterload, because of the fixed resistance against ejection of blood, but does decrease coronary perfusion with a great risk for development of subendocardial ischemia and sudden death. Extremes of heart rate should be avoided. Bradycardia leads to a decrease in cardiac output in patients with relatively fixed stroke volume. Tachycardia may produce ischemia with a limited diastolic time for coronary perfusion. Maintenance of sinus rhythm is imperative because of the importance of atrial contraction in LV filling. An emergent cardioversion is indicated if the patient suffers severe hemodynamic compromise due to arrhythmia.

12. **Discuss the management of the patients with AS after aortic valve replacement.**
    After the surgery, LV end-diastolic pressure decreases and stroke volume increases, but the hypertrophied left ventricle still may require an elevated preload to function adequately. Depressed myocardial function may suggest inadequate myocardial protection during the surgery due to the difficulty to perfuse the hypertrophied left ventricle. Inotropic agents (dopamine, dobutamine, epinephrine) can improve the LV performance in this situation.

13. **Describe the role of transcatheter aortic valve replacement (TAVR) in the treatment of severe AS.**

    Aortic valve replacement is the mainstay of treatment of symptomatic AS. In properly selected patients, this surgical procedure offers substantial improvements in symptoms and life expectancy. However, patients with severe comorbidities and others with technical limitations for surgery such as porcelain aorta, prior mediastinal radiation, previous pericardiectomy with dense adhesions, or prior sternal infection with complex reconstruction are not candidates for surgery. They are candidates for a relatively new procedure, where an aortic valve stent is placed with a catheter technique either through the femoral artery or the LV apex. The model estimates the risk of mortality and nonfatal complications such as stroke, renal failure, and prolonged ventilation. Survival after TAVR was improved in selected patients. Risks of TAVR include higher stroke and moderate or severe paravalvular or transvalvular aortic regurgitation rates.

14. **What is valve-in-valve procedure?**

    This is a catheter-based valve implantation inside an already implanted bioprosthetic valve. It can be performed not only at aortic but at any location of a bioprosthetic valve. This technique can be used to correct the valve function during the TAVR procedure or in the future when the stent valves start failing.

15. **Describe the special characteristics of anesthesia management for TAVR.**

    This procedure is performed in an elderly patient population with severe AS and significant comorbidities. Two large-bore intravenous lines, a central line with pulmonary artery catheter, and an intraarterial catheter are required. Standard monitors, invasive blood pressure, central venous pressure, pulmonary artery pressure, and cardiac output measurement are essential. TEE for evaluating right and left ventricular function during the case and evaluating the stenotic and the implanted valve are also a requirement. Anesthetic management is based on using medications with minimal effect on hemodynamics. Induction with fentanyl, etomidate, and rocuronium is working well. In case of hypertension during induction, inhalation of sevoflurane or a small dose of propofol blunts the hypertensive reaction well. Maintenance of anesthesia with anesthetic gases is sufficient. Awakening after sevoflurane anesthesia is smooth in most cases. The hemodynamic stability can be maintained with infusion of phenylephrine, vasopressin, norepinephrine, or epinephrine with cautious titration. The goal is to keep the blood pressure in a normal range to prepare for the rapid pacing period. During rapid pacing, a pacemaker is used to generate a heart rate of 160 to 180/min. At this heart rate the mean arterial pressure is low with minimal pulsation so the valvuloplasty and valve placement can be done without blowing away the dilating balloon. After the placement, the new valve is evaluated and if no further intervention needed, the cut at the groin or on the chest will be closed and the patient will be extubated.

16. **What complications can be expected during the TAVR procedure?**
    - Low cardiac output
    - Annular rupture: a rare life-threatening complication; needs aortic root replacement
    - Vascular complications: rupture or dissection of the arteries
    - Left bundle branch block can be transient or permanent during TAVR. Patient with right bundle branch block may develop third-degree atrioventricular block requiring pacemaker implantation.
    - Paravalvular regurgitation is a common complication. The presence of more than trace aortic regurgitation was associated with increased risk of late mortality.
    - Regurgitation: may indicate improper valve sizing and deployment. Severe leak is an indication for valve-in-valve deployment.
    - Brain infarction: The reported 30-day risk of stroke following TAVR is 2% to 5%. The rate of stroke is higher in TAVR compared with medical or surgical treatment.
    - Aortic insufficiency

17. **Discuss the pathophysiology of aortic insufficiency (AI).**

    In the developing world, the most common cause of AI is rheumatic heart disease. In developed countries, AI is most often due to aortic root dilation, congenital bicuspid aortic

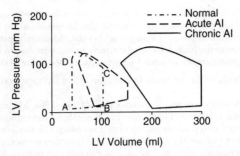

Figure 31-3. Pressure-volume loops in aortic regurgitation compared to the normal loop. In acute aortic insufficiency (*AI*), the end-diastolic and end-systolic volume is increasing. The stroke volume can be increased, normal, or decreased depending on the severity of AI. The left ventricular (*LV*) volume is increasing during the isovolumic relaxation period (*DA segment*). The end-diastolic pressure (*AB segment*, B point) is high. Contractility is decreased because the myocardium is overstretched. In chronic AI, the end-diastolic, end-systolic, and stroke volumes are enlarged. Cardiac output is normal and the contractility is decreased. The LV volume is increasing during the isovolumic relaxation period also (*DA segment*) but the end-diastolic pressure (*AB segment*, B point) is normal so the heart has diastolic reserve to accommodate to limited volume or pressure load.

valve, or infective endocarditis. Causes of acute AI are infective endocarditis, aortic dissection (Marfan syndrome), and AI after aortic balloon valvotomy or a failed surgical valve repair.

In chronic AI, there is LV diastolic volume overload because part of the stroke volume regurgitates across the incompetent aortic valve in diastole. Patients have large end-diastolic volumes and stroke volumes. The volume load generates high wall tension in diastole, initiating eccentric hypertrophy (dilated left ventricle with normal or thickened wall). Increasing regurgitant orifice area, slow heart rate (relatively more time spent in diastole), and increased systemic vascular resistance increase the amount of regurgitant flow. Compliance and stroke volume may be markedly increased in chronic aortic insufficiency, whereas contractility gradually diminishes (Figure 31-3). Aortic insufficiency can be due to a disease of the valve leaflets or to enlargement of the aortic root.

Ideally, patients with chronic AI should have valve replacement surgery before the onset of irreversible myocardial damage. In acute AI, the left ventricle is subjected to rapid, massive volume overload with elevated end-diastolic pressure. Hypotension and pulmonary edema may necessitate emergent valvular replacement.

18. **What is the indication for aortic valve replacement in AI?**
    - Symptomatic patients with severe AI irrespective of LV systolic function
    - Asymptomatic patients with chronic severe AI and LV systolic dysfunction (ejection fraction 50% or less) at rest
    - Asymptomatic patients with chronic severe AI while undergoing CABG or surgery on the aorta or other heart valves
    - It is reasonable for asymptomatic patients with severe AI with normal LV systolic function (ejection fraction greater than 50%) but with severe LV dilation (end-diastolic dimension greater than 75 mm or end-systolic dimension greater than 55 mm).

19. **What does the pressure-volume loop look like in acute AI and chronic AI?**
    In acute AI, the end-diastolic and end-systolic volume is increasing. The stroke volume can be increased, normal, or decreased depending on the severity of AI. The LV volume is increasing during the isovolumic relaxation period (DA segment). The end-diastolic pressure (AB segment, B point) is high. End-diastolic pressure higher than 25 to 30 mm Hg manifests in pulmonary edema. Contractility is decreased because the myocardium is overstretched. There is no diastolic reserve so the heart cannot increase the stroke volume with increasing systemic pressure (see Figure 31-3).

In chronic AI the end-diastolic, end-systolic and stroke volumes are enlarged. Cardiac output is normal and the contractility decreased. The LV volume is also increasing during the isovolumic relaxation period (DA segment) but the end-diastolic pressure (AB segment, B point) is normal so the heart has diastolic reserve to accommodate to limited volume or pressure load determining the patient's exercise capacity (see Figure 31-3).

20. **What are the hemodynamic goals in the anesthetic management of patients with AI?**
Appropriate preload is necessary for maintenance of forward flow. Modest tachycardia reduces ventricular volumes and limits the time available for regurgitation. Contractility must be maintained with β-adrenergic agonists if necessary. Dobutamine can be ideal because it does not increase the afterload. Afterload reduction augments forward flow, but additional intravascular volume may be necessary to maintain preload. Increases in afterload result in increasing LV end-diastolic pressure and pulmonary hypertension. In acute AI, the goal is to achieve the lowest tolerable systemic blood pressure to increase the stroke volume and cardiac output.

21. **Discuss the hemodynamic changes in patients with AI after aortic valve replacement.**
After the surgery, LV end-diastolic volume and pressure decrease. Preload should be increased by volume administration to maintain filling of the dilated left ventricle. The decreased myocardial contractility may necessitate inotropic or intraaortic balloon pump support.

22. **What is the pathophysiology of mitral stenosis (MS)?**
MS is usually secondary to rheumatic disease (80%-90%), infective endocarditis (3.3%), and mitral annular calcification (2.7%). Symptoms (fatigue, dyspnea on exertion, hemoptysis) may be worsened when increased cardiac output is needed, as with pregnancy, illness, anemia, and exercise. Blood stasis in the left atrium is a risk for thrombus formation and systemic embolization. Critical stenosis of the valve occurs 10 to 20 years after the initial rheumatic disease. As the orifice of the mitral valve narrows, the left atrium experiences pressure overload. In contrast to other valvular lesions, the left ventricle in patients with MS shows relative volume underload due to the obstruction of forward blood flow from the atrium. The elevated atrial pressure may be transmitted to the pulmonary circuit and thus lead to pulmonary hypertension and right-sided heart failure. The overdistended atrium is susceptible to fibrillation with resultant loss of atrial systole, leading to reduced ventricular filling and cardiac output.

23. **What are the indications for mitral valve replacement in MS?**
Mitral valve (MV) surgery (repair if possible) is indicated in patients with symptomatic (NYHA functional class III–IV) moderate or severe MS when:
• Percutaneous mitral balloon valvotomy is unavailable, percutaneous mitral balloon valvotomy is contraindicated because of left atrial thrombus despite anticoagulation or because concomitant moderate to severe mitral regurgitation (MR) is present and the valve morphology is not favorable for percutaneous mitral balloon valvotomy in a patient with acceptable operative risk.
• Symptomatic patients with moderate to severe MS who also have moderate to severe MR should receive MV replacement, unless valve repair is possible at the time of surgery.
• MV replacement is reasonable for patients with severe MS and severe pulmonary hypertension (pulmonary artery systolic pressure greater than 60 mm Hg) with NYHA functional class I–II symptoms who are not considered candidates for percutaneous mitral balloon valvotomy or surgical MV repair.

24. **What are the indications for percutaneous mitral balloon valvotomy?**
More and more patients are undergoing percutaneous balloon valvotomy. The indications for this procedure include:
• It is effective for symptomatic patients (NYHA II–IV) with moderate or severe MS and valve morphology favorable for percutaneous mitral balloon valvotomy in the absence of left atrial thrombus or moderate or severe MR.

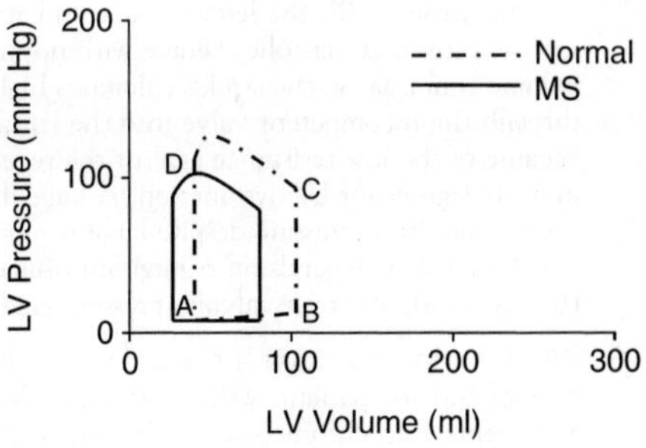

Figure 31-4. Pressure-volume loop in mitral stenosis (MS) compared with the normal loop. In mitral stenosis, the end-diastolic, end-systolic, and stroke volume is small. The left ventricle generates low blood pressure. The contractility is decreasing due to the chronic underfilling of the left ventricle. *LV,* Left ventricular.

- It is effective for asymptomatic patients with moderate or severe MS who have pulmonary hypertension (systolic pressure >50 mm Hg at rest or >60 mm Hg with exercise).
- It is reasonable for symptomatic (NYHA III–IV) patients with moderate or severe MS who have a nonpliable calcified valve and either are not candidates for surgery or are at high risk for surgery.

25. **How is the pressure-volume loop changed from normal in MS?**
    The end-diastolic, end-systolic, and stroke volume are small because of the limited flow into the left ventricle. The left ventricle generates low blood pressure. The contractility is decreased because of chronic underfilling of the left ventricle (Figure 31-4).

26. **What are the anesthetic considerations in MS?**
    The intravascular volume must be adequate to maintain flow across the stenotic valve. A slower heart rate is beneficial to allow more time for the blood to flow across the valve and to increase ventricular filling. Sinus rhythm should be maintained for adequate filling of the left ventricle as atrial contraction contributes about 30% of the stroke volume. Afterload should be kept in the normal range for these patients because of the fixed resistance of the blood flow between the left atrium and left ventricle. Chronic underfilling of the left ventricle leads to depressed ventricular contractility even after the restoration of normal filling. Negative inotropic agents should be avoided. Increases in pulmonary vascular resistance may exacerbate right ventricular failure so hypoxemia, hypercarbia, and acidosis should be avoided. For this reason, the respiratory depressant effects of preoperative medications may be particularly deleterious.

27. **Discuss the postoperative management of patients with MS after mitral valve replacement or balloon valvotomy.**
    Decline of left atrial pressure decreases pulmonary artery resistance and pulmonary artery pressure, increasing cardiac output. However, the LV performance can be depressed because of the chronic underfilling of the left ventricle, especially after cardiopulmonary bypass. Preload augmentation and afterload reduction should be applied to improve forward blood flow. Inotropic or intraaortic balloon pump support may be necessary to improve the systolic performance of the left ventricle.
    After balloon valvotomy, the gradient through the mitral valve and mitral regurgitation will be evaluated. Severe acute mitral regurgitation is an indication for immediate surgical management. A mean arterial pressure of about 60 mm Hg is desirable. Cautious administration of epinephrine also may achieve this goal.

28. **Describe the pathophysiology of mitral regurgitation (MR).**
    The causes of primary valve disease and chronic mitral regurgitation include mitral valve prolapse, infective endocarditis, trauma, rheumatic heart disease, drugs (ergotamine, pergolide), and congenital valve cleft. Acute MR may occur in the setting of flail leaflet due to mitral valve prolapse, infective endocarditis, or trauma. The secondary causes of MR include ischemic heart disease, LV systolic dysfunction, or hypertrophic cardiomyopathy.
    In acute MR, end-diastolic volume and pressure increase, the pulmonary circuit and right side of the heart are subject to sudden increases in pressure and volume, and may precipitate acute pulmonary hypertension, pulmonary edema, and right-sided heart failure.

In chronic MR, the left ventricle and atrium show volume overload, leading to increased LV end-diastolic volume with normal end-diastolic pressure. LV end-systolic volume is normal so the stroke volume is high, but part of the stroke volume escapes through the incompetent valve into the left atrium. Ejection fraction is usually high because of the low resistance against the regurgitation. An ejection fraction of 50% may indicate significant LV dysfunction. A large distensible left atrium can maintain near-normal left atrial pressure despite large regurgitant volumes. As in AI, in chronic MR regurgitant flow depends on regurgitant orifice size, time available for regurgitant flow (bradycardia), and transvalvular pressure gradient.

29. **What is the indication for mitral valve replacement in MR?**
    • Symptomatic patients with acute severe MR
    • Patients with chronic severe MR and NYHA functional class II, III, or IV symptoms in the absence of severe LV dysfunction (severe LV dysfunction is defined as ejection fraction less than 30%) and/or end-systolic dimension greater than 55 mm
    • Asymptomatic patients with chronic severe MR and mild to moderate LV dysfunction, ejection fraction 30% to 60%, and/or end-systolic dimension greater than or equal to 40 mm
    • MV repair is recommended over MV replacement in the majority of patients with severe chronic MR who require surgery, and patients should be referred to surgical centers experienced in MV repair.

30. **How is the pressure-volume loop in MR changed from normal?**
    In acute MR, the end-diastolic volume increases with high end-diastolic pressure. End-systolic volume is normal or decreased, stroke volume is increased, but the ejected volume into the aorta is relatively small depending on the regurgitant volume (Figure 31-5).
    In chronic MR, the end-diastolic volume is increased with normal end-diastolic pressure due to the chronic myocardial remodeling process. The end-systolic volume is normal or increased. The markedly increased stroke volume preserves the forward cardiac output despite the significant regurgitation. The contractility is normal or decreased (see Figure 31-5).

31. **What are the hemodynamic goals in anesthetic management of MR?**
    The intravascular volume should supply the dilated left ventricle. The best level of preload augmentation for a patient must be based on the clinical response to a fluid load. Bradycardia increases the regurgitant volume, decreasing the ejected volume into the aorta. Normal or slightly elevated heart rate helps to decrease the regurgitant flow volume.

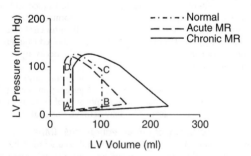

Figure 31-5. Pressure-volume loop in mitral regurgitation *(MR)* compared with the normal loop. In acute MR, the end-diastolic volume is increasing with higher end-diastolic pressure. The end-systolic volume is either normal or less than normal because part of the stroke volume is flowing back the low-pressure left atrium during the isovolumic contraction period *(BC segment)*. In chronic MR, the end-diastolic volume is high with normal or slightly elevated end-diastolic pressure. The end-systolic volume is normal or bigger than normal, depending on the severity of the MR and the systolic function of the left ventricle. The ejected stroke volume is sufficient to maintain adequate cardiac output. The contractility is decreased. *LV*, Left ventricular.

Contractility should be maintained and afterload reduced with an inotropic agent such as dobutamine or milrinone. Afterload reduction augments forward flow and decreases regurgitation. As in MS, drugs and maneuvers that increase pulmonary vascular resistance must be avoided.

32. **Discuss the hemodynamic management after mitral valve repair or replacement in patients with MR.**
    Once the valve is in place, the left ventricle has to eject the full stroke volume into the aorta. This immediate pressure load increases LV tension and may compromise the ejection fraction. Therefore, inotropic or intraaortic balloon pump support may be necessary until the left ventricle can adjust to the new hemodynamic condition. Preload should be augmented to fill up the dilated left ventricle.

KEY POINTS: VALVULAR HEART DISEASE

1. Hemodynamic goals in aortic stenosis include maintaining intravascular volume, contractility, peripheral vascular resistance, and sinus rhythm while avoiding extremes in heart rate. Arrhythmias associated with hypotension require emergent cardioversion.
2. Hemodynamic goals in the patient with aortic insufficiency include augmenting preload, maintaining contractility, maintaining normal or elevated heart rate, and reducing afterload.
3. Hemodynamic goals in the patient with mitral stenosis include maintaining intravascular volume, afterload, sinus rhythm, and a slower heart rate. Avoid hypoxemia, hypercarbia, and acidosis because they may increase pulmonary vascular resistance. Sedative medications should be given with great care.
4. Hemodynamic goals in the patient with mitral regurgitation include maintaining intravascular volume, contractility, and elevated heart rate while reducing afterload. As in mitral stenosis, avoid situations that will increase pulmonary vascular resistance.
5. Anesthetic management in patients undergoing transcatheter aortic valve replacement is similar to that of patients having aortic valve surgery. A unique part of the procedure is the rapid pacing, which generates a low output state for the valvuloplasty or valve placement. Maintaining normal blood pressure before rapid pacing is the key element for quickly getting back to normal output state and blood pressure.

WEBSITE
Online STS risk calculator: http://riskcalc.sts.org

SUGGESTED READINGS

Bonow RO, Carabello BA, Chatterjee K, et al: ACC/AHA 2006 guidelines for the management of patients with valvular heart disease, Circulation 114:450–527, 2006.

Braunwald E: Essential atlas of heart diseases, ed 2, Philadelphia, 2001, McGraw-Hill, pp 254–279.

Crawford MH: Current diagnosis and treatment in cardiology, ed 2, Philadelphia, 2003, McGraw-Hill, pp 108–150.

DiNardo JA: Anesthesia for cardiac surgery, ed 2, Stamford, 1998, Appleton & Lange, pp 109–140.

Gaasch WH, Brecker SJD, Aldea GS: Transcatheter aortic valve replacement. Available from the UpToDate website: http://www.uptodate.com/contents/transcatheter-aortic-valve-replacement.

Sukernik M, Martin DE: Anesthetic management for the treatment of valvular heart diseases. In Hensley FA, Martin DE, Gravlee GP, editors: A practical approach to cardiac anesthesia, ed 4, Philadelphia, 2008, Lippincott Williams & Wilkins, pp 316–347.

CHAPTER 32

AORTO-OCCLUSIVE DISEASES

Gurdev S. Rai, MD

1. **Define aorto-occlusive disease.**

   Aorto-occlusive disease is characterized by atherosclerotic changes within the aorta (usually abdominal) that extend into the iliac and femoral arteries and result in hypoperfusion of vital organs and the lower extremities. Involvement at the iliac bifurcation and renal arteries is common; aneurysmal changes may be found as well. Seventy percent of aortic aneurysms are infrarenal and many include renal arteries as well.

2. **What risk factors and coexisting diseases are common in patients with aorto-occlusive disease?**

   Risk factors include smoking, family history, obesity, atherosclerotic disease elsewhere, advanced age, and male sex. Common diseases include hypertension, ischemic heart disease, heart failure, chronic obstructive pulmonary disease (COPD), diabetes mellitus, chronic renal disease, and carotid artery disease.

3. **What is the natural progression of aorto-occlusive disease?**

   The natural history of aneurysmal disease is one of continuing enlargement. Operative or endovascular repair should be undertaken when the aneurysm is 6 cm or larger. The incidence of rupture increases with size (9.4% chance of rupture within 1 year for aneurysms 5.5 to 5.9 cm, increasing to 32.5% for aneurysms 7 cm and larger).

   National mortality from elective open abdominal aneurysm repair is <5%. For repair of an acutely ruptured aneurysm, perioperative mortality remains high, about 50%. Mortality with open thoracic aneurysm repair ranges from 5% to 14%. Endovascular repair results in decreased mortality. The survival rate is 92% at 1 year and 67% at 5 years.

   Aorto-occlusive disease results in hypoperfusion distal to the occlusion. Unlike surgery for aneurysmal disease, surgery for occlusive disease should be undertaken when the patient becomes symptomatic and fails medical therapy.

4. **Describe preoperative preparation of such patients in the presence of concurrent disease.**

   The goal of preoperative evaluation is to optimize any significant organ dysfunction.
   - **Coronary artery disease:** This is the major cause of perioperative mortality and morbidity. Myocardial infarction occurs in 4% to 15% of patients, and heart failure is noted in 30% of postoperative aneurysm repairs. If the patient has an acute coronary syndrome, decompensated heart failure, severe valvular disease, or significant arrhythmias, he or she should undergo preoperative cardiac testing, including echocardiography, stress testing, and coronary angiography. Similarly, coronary artery evaluation may be strongly indicated in the presence of renal insufficiency, history of heart failure or cerebrovascular disease, or if the patient has diabetes mellitus or cannot achieve a metabolic equivalent (MET) level of 4.
   - **Pulmonary:** It has been mentioned that COPD is common. Physical examination, pulmonary function testing, arterial blood gas analysis, and chest radiography may suggest the need for preoperative incentive spirometry and bronchodilator and antibiotic therapy.
   - **Renal:** The incidence of postoperative renal dysfunction in elective infrarenal aorta repair is 3% and up to 30% in thoracic aorta repair. The primary cause of postoperative renal failure is preexisting kidney disease. The degree of renal dysfunction should be characterized and the patient adequately hydrated. Poorly controlled hypertension should be optimized. If the patient requires a contrast study before surgery, he or she should be well hydrated before dye administration and exposed to a minimum amount of contrast; repeated studies should be avoided.

- **Cerebrovascular disease:** Signs and symptoms of cerebrovascular insufficiency should be elucidated. Cerebral hypoperfusion during surgery could result in stroke. If carotid stenosis is found, endarterectomy may need to precede aortic repair. Chronically hypertensive patients also have shifts in cerebral autoregulation, and this is a second justification for preoperative management of hypertension.
- **Diabetes mellitus:** This should be well controlled.

5. List the appropriate intraoperative monitors for aortic surgery.
    - Standard monitors include pulse oximetry and noninvasive blood pressure and temperature monitoring. Continuous cardiac rhythm monitoring for rhythm (lead II) and ischemia (lead V_5) is essential.
    - Also essential are the usual anesthesia machine monitors, including capnography and delivered oxygen concentration.
    - Intraarterial monitoring rapidly detects swings in blood pressure and facilitates laboratory analysis.
    - Monitoring of urine output with a Foley catheter and urometer is essential.
    - Use of central venous pressures, pulmonary artery catheters, and/or transesophageal echocardiography is appropriate when myocardial dysfunction and valvular disease are present.
    - Somatosensory and motor-evoked potential can be useful if spinal cord ischemia is considered a risk.

6. Discuss the physiologic implications of aortic clamping and unclamping.
    Aortic cross-clamping increases left ventricular afterload. Preparation for this cross-clamping includes increasing depth of anesthesia, vasodilator therapy with nitroglycerin or sodium nitroprusside, and possibly administration of α blockers or calcium channel blockers. A decrease in renal blood flow occurs in about 90% of patients having thoracic aortic cross-clamping and in about 40% of patients having infrarenal cross-clamping. There is redistribution of renal blood flow to the renal cortex and a decrease in glomerular filtration. These changes persist to some degree even after cross-clamp removal. The potential for a clinically profound decrease in anterior spinal artery blood flow is more likely in thoracic aortic repair, making spinal cord an ischemic risk; in certain cases lumbar drainage of spinal fluid has been instituted to mitigate decreases in spinal cord perfusion pressure.

    Hypotension and a decrease in systemic vascular resistance are noted after unclamping. Ischemic metabolites, lactic acid, and potassium returning to the central circulation depress contractility and potentiate the hypotension.

7. Review the anesthetic goals for these surgical patients.
    - Typically a general anesthetic provides anesthesia, analgesia, amnesia, and muscle relaxation. (These are classic principles.)
    - Maintain cardiac output and coronary perfusion and limit myocardial workload by controlling heart rate and afterload, especially during aortic cross-clamping.
    - Aggressively replace blood loss with crystalloids, colloids, and blood and blood products when necessary. Massive blood loss will likely result in a coagulopathy that will require anticoagulants associated with the massive blood transfusion.
    - Maintain oxygenation and ventilation, guided by blood gas analysis. Excessive ventilatory pressures may compromise preload.
    - The best way to preserve renal function is to maintain normal intravascular volume, cardiac output, and oxygenation.
    - Especially in patients with diabetes, blood glucose should be monitored and controlled. Insulin therapy not only controls hyperglycemia but also prevents ketoacidosis and may improve wound healing and long-term outcome.
    - Hypoperfusion of the anterior spinal artery during aortic cross-clamping or extended hypoperfusion places the patient at risk for paraplegia, especially during thoracic aorta surgery.
    - Before unclamping, an intravenous bolus of fluid is wise. It may be necessary to reclamp the aorta or provide some minor degree of occlusion to allow the patient time to equilibrate and stabilize.

8. **What can be done intraoperatively to preserve renal function?**

The incidence of acute kidney injury after elective repair of infrarenal aneurysms is about 3%. Of these patients the mortality is 40%, and this incidence has not changed in decades.

The biggest predictor of postoperative renal dysfunction is preexisting renal disease. The adequacy of renal perfusion cannot be assumed by the amount of urine output since it does not correlate with postoperative renal function. Urine output stimulated by diuretics (furosemide, mannitol) and dopamine does not ensure that renal function will be preserved postoperatively.

Major factors that affect postoperative renal function include preoperative renal function, the degree of aortic disease, and the duration of cross-clamping. Therefore optimizing renal function before surgery, maintaining euvolemia and renal perfusion, and minimizing cross-clamp time are paramount. Nephrotoxic medications (e.g., gentamicin) or medications that decrease renal blood flow (nonsteroidal antiinflammatory drugs) should be eliminated from the perioperative period as well. Intravenous radiocontrast is also nephrotoxic if administered immediately before surgery.

Dopamine, furosemide, mannitol, and fenoldopam (a selective dopamine type 1 receptor agonist) have all been used to prevent renal failure, but evidence is either lacking or controversial as to the efficacy of these treatments. Evidence that low-dose dopamine (2 mcg/kg/min) has a positive effect is equivocal at best. In addition, dopamine has the harmful property of increasing tachycardia and cardiac workload in patients predisposed to myocardial disease. Furosemide may cause renal hypoperfusion in hypovolemic states and induce electrolyte imbalances. Evidence of renal protection with mannitol is inconclusive, but it is still widely used to encourage preclamping diuresis. Many clinicians believe that this osmotic diuretic benefits the kidneys by increasing cortical blood flow and reducing endothelial edema and vascular congestion. Fenoldopam is an antihypertensive agent that dilates renal and splanchnic vessels. This increase in renal blood flow may be advantageous, but more prospective studies are required.

9. **What are the potential advantages to postoperative epidural analgesia?**

Epidural anesthesia may suppress sympathetic tone and the stress response while providing excellent analgesia. This limits myocardial work by attenuating tachycardia and hypertensive swings in a patients predisposed to cardiac ischemia. It also provides titratable postoperative pain relief without excessive sedation. However, a concern with neuraxial analgesia is hematoma formation in the setting of anticoagulation. Use of these techniques is considered safe practice as long as there is at least 1 hour from epidural placement to heparinization of the patient.

10. **What specific concerns exist for endovascular repair of the aorta?**

Endovascular repair of the aorta uses stents passed through an artery (usually femoral) and guided to the aorta via fluoroscopy. The patient must be motionless during the procedure, but general, neuraxial, or local anesthesia is appropriate. Local anesthesia has the advantage of requiring less fluid and vasopressor support, although the same degree of pulmonary and cardiac complications occur when compared with general anesthesia. Usually only an arterial line and standard monitors are necessary, but conversion to an open procedure is possible, and aggressive intravenous access is justified. Overall endovascular techniques require less fluid and hemodynamic support, and the 30-day mortality for abdominal aortic aneurysms is less than that for open repairs (3% vs. 4%). The cardiac, pulmonary, renal, and bleeding complications are fewer as well.

11. **Describe the primary management aspects when a patient presents with an acute abdominal aortic rupture.**

The primary determinants of morbidity and mortality are extent, size, and location. Rupture of the intimal and medial aortic layers is less ominous in the short term when a pseudoaneurysm forms. Although hemorrhage is minimal, proximal increases in afterload and distal ischemia are risks. A larger aortic tear results in rapid and significant blood loss. A retroperitoneal rupture may be temporarily more stable than the almost always fatal intraabdominal rupture.

Resuscitation should be done in the operating room since rapid surgical intervention is necessary to prevent death. Rapid airway control must be obtained to optimize ventilation and oxygenation. The initial goal is to maintain perfusion and oxygenation to the heart and brain. Efforts are directed toward intravascular volume restoration. Multiple large-bore intravenous lines are necessary, as is intraarterial monitoring and probably central venous pressure monitoring as well. Transesophageal echocardiography or pulmonary artery catheterization may be valuable when preexisting myocardial dysfunction is present, but vigorous intravascular restoration and treatment of the inevitable coagulopathy should take precedence. The patient should have 10 units of blood available, universal donor blood if necessary, and the laboratory should be made aware that this case will probably require massive transfusion, with requirements for fresh frozen plasma, platelets, and cryoprecipitate. Disturbances in coagulation are best followed with thromboelastography. Blood pressure may require inotropic or chronotropic support, although volume resuscitation is the mainstay of treatment. A systolic blood pressure of 80 to 100 mm Hg is an ideal goal, although communication about hemodynamic goals should involve the surgeons.

KEY POINTS: AORTO-OCCLUSIVE DISEASE

1. Coexisting diseases are extremely common and include coronary artery disease, hypertension, COPD, chronic renal disease, and diabetes mellitus. These comorbidities have a very important impact on outcome.
2. Preoperative assessment is made as guided by the 2007 ACC/AHA Guidelines if the need for testing and evaluation is necessary.
3. The most common cause of perioperative mortality is cardiac disease. Postoperative renal failure also has an important impact on outcome.
4. Goals of anesthesia are to maintain intravascular volume and attenuate the acute and severe hemodynamic changes that occur with vascular cross- and uncross-clamping.

12. Discuss the important elements of postoperative care.
   - Intensive care unit admission is absolutely essential.
   - **Cardiac:** Patients should be monitored for ischemia and hypotension. The incidence of myocardial ischemia is greatest on about the third postoperative day.
   - **Pulmonary:** Many patients remain intubated after surgery if poor baseline pulmonary function exists, if they have left ventricular dysfunction, or if massive fluid shifts have occurred. Epidural analgesia may be of benefit in weaning the patient from mechanical ventilation.
   - **Renal:** Monitoring electrolytes, renal markers, and urine output is important for assessing kidney failure and fluid status.
   - Other complications include bleeding, graft dysfunction, bowel ischemia, stroke, embolic events, and extremity hypoperfusion.

SUGGESTED READINGS

Greenberg RK, Lytle B: Endovascular repair of thoracoabdominal aneurysms, Circulation 117:2288–2296, 2008.

Jones DR, Lee HT: Perioperative renal protection: best practice and research, Clin Anaesthesiol 22:193–215, 2008.

Kee ST, Dake MD: Endovascular stent grafting. In Jaffe RA, Samuels SI, editors: Anesthesiologist's manual of surgical procedures, ed 3, Philadelphia, 2004, Lippincott Williams & Wilkins, pp 313–316.

Oliver WC Jr, Nuttall GA, Cherry KJ, et al: A comparison of fenoldopam with dopamine and sodium nitroprusside in patients undergoing cross-clamping of the abdominal aorta, Anesth Analg 103:833–840, 2006.

CHAPTER 33

INTRACRANIAL AND CEREBROVASCULAR DISEASE

Gurdev S. Rai, MD

1. **What is cerebrovascular insufficiency?**
   Cerebrovascular insufficiency results from an inadequate supply of blood flow, oxygen, and/or glucose to the brain. Cerebral ischemia develops, and neurologic damage will ensue if the underlying process is not corrected within 3 to 8 minutes.

2. **Compare global ischemia with focal ischemia.**
   Global ischemia refers to global hypoxia (respiratory failure, asphyxia) or circulatory arrest wherein the brain is not perfused. Focal ischemia may result from vasospasm, traumatic, hemorrhagic, embolic, or atherosclerotic events. If the underlying cause is reversed rapidly and perfusion and oxygenation are restored, neurologic damage can be avoided.

3. **How does cerebrovascular insufficiency manifest itself?**
   Manifestations include transient ischemic attacks (TIAs) and cerebrovascular accidents (CVAs).
   - TIAs are acute in onset, involve neurologic dysfunction for minutes to hours (<24 hours), resolve spontaneously, and are associated with a normal computed tomography (CT) and magnetic resonance scan.
   - CVAs may develop acutely or chronically progress over time (minutes to days). Strokes can be classified as minor, with an eventual full recovery, or major, with severe and permanent disability or death. In addition to cerebrovascular abnormalities, CVAs are associated with other comorbidities, including hypertension, diabetes, coagulopathies, atrial fibrillation, mitral valve disease, endocarditis, and substance abuse.
   - A third group of patients experience neurologic dysfunction for longer than 24 hours, with spontaneous and complete recovery within 1 to 2 weeks. This phenomenon is termed *reversible ischemic neurologic deficit* and should be pathophysiologically grouped with TIAs.

4. **What is the etiology of CVAs and TIAs?**
   Atherosclerosis at the bifurcation of the common carotid artery is the source of most cerebral ischemic events. The thrombus itself or, more likely, embolic plaques and debris can dislodge to the brain, resulting in neurologic injury. Resolution of TIAs within 24 hours is the result of the inherent mechanisms of the body for breaking down such emboli. Ischemia of the brainstem and the temporal and occipital lobes is thought to be caused by a transient decrease in blood flow or blood pressure in the vertebrobasilar system. Hypoperfusion to the brain secondary to the atherosclerotic stenosis itself accounts for less than 10% of ischemic events.

5. **Are other factors involved in neurologic outcome following an episode of cerebrovascular insufficiency?**
   The type and size of plaque or embolus, the site of ischemia, the extent of collateral circulation, the duration of inadequate perfusion, and the inherent response of the brain to the insult all contribute to the neurologic sequelae.

6. **List the risk factors for cerebral ischemic events.**
   Hypertension and cigarette smoking are the strongest risk factors. Cardiac diseases (e.g., left ventricular hypertrophy, atrial fibrillation, cardiomyopathy, endocarditis, valvular disease, coronary artery disease) are major risk factors. Other risk factors include age, diabetes, hyperlipidemia, coagulopathies, vascular disease elsewhere, and a maternal history of stroke. The 5-year risk of stroke in a patient who has had a TIA is nearly 35%.

7. **Who is a candidate for carotid endarterectomy (CEA)?**

Asymptomatic bruits are heard in 5% to 10% of the adult population. A 1989 prospective study of 566 patients with asymptomatic carotid bruits revealed a 1-year stroke or TIA rate of 2.5% compared with a rate of 0.7% in patients without carotid bruits. The European Carotid Surgery Trial (ECST) demonstrated that CEA is not indicated for most patients with moderate (30% to 69%) stenosis, even if they are symptomatic. However, the rate of stroke or TIA increases dramatically with increasing stenosis, reaching a 1-year stroke or TIA rate of 46% for stenosis greater than 80%. It is well accepted that symptomatic patients and asymptomatic patients with a stenosis greater than 70% are candidates for CEA.

Carotid stenting is now available for patients who fit these criteria but are high-risk surgical candidates. Stenting is an alternative to CEA in this select patient population and involves only local anesthesia and a small femoral incision.

8. **Define cerebral autoregulation. How is it affected in cerebrovascular disease, and what are the anesthetic implications?**

Cerebral autoregulation is the ability of the brain to maintain cerebral blood flow relatively constant (40 to 60 ml/100 g/min) over a wide range (50 to 150 mm Hg) of arterial pressures. Stenosis or obstruction in the internal carotid artery causes a pressure drop beyond the obstruction. In an effort to maintain cerebral blood flow, the cerebral vasculature dilates. As the degree of carotid obstruction progresses, the cerebral vasculature distal to the obstruction maximally dilates. At this point the cerebral vasculature loses its autoregulatory ability. Cerebral blood flow becomes passive and depends on systemic blood pressure. It thus becomes critically important to maintain the blood pressure of patients with carotid stenosis because they have minimal or no autoregulatory reserve to counter anesthetic-induced reductions in blood pressure.

9. **How are the cerebral responses to hypercapnia and hypocapnia altered in cerebrovascular disease? What are the anesthetic implications?**

Normal cerebral vessels are highly sensitive to arterial carbon dioxide partial pressure ($PaCO_2$), dilating in response to hypercapnia and constricting in response to hypocapnia. However, in ischemic and already maximally vasodilated areas of the brain, this relationship breaks down, and responses to hypercapnia and hypocapnia may be paradoxical. Because cerebral vessels in an area of ischemia are already maximally dilated, hypercapnia may result in dilation of only normally responsive vessels outside the area of ischemia. This phenomenon, termed *steal*, may divert blood flow away from the ischemic area, further compromising perfusion. On the other hand, hypocapnia may cause vessels in normal areas to undergo constriction, diverting blood to marginally perfused areas. This phenomenon is termed the *Robin Hood* or *inverse steal* effect. Therefore it is generally recommended that normocapnia be maintained in patients undergoing endarterectomy.

10. **What is normal cerebral blood flow? At what level is cerebral blood flow considered ischemic?**

Normal cerebral blood flow in humans is 40 to 60 ml/100 g/min (15% of cardiac output). The cerebral metabolic rate for oxygen in adults is 3 to 4 ml/100 g/min (20% of whole-body oxygen consumption). The cerebral blood flow at which ischemia becomes apparent on electroencephalogram (EEG), termed the *critical regional cerebral blood flow*, is 18 to 20 ml/100 g/min.

11. **How do inhalational anesthetics affect cerebral perfusion and cerebral metabolic rate?**

In the normal brain, cerebral blood flow varies directly with the cerebral metabolic rate for oxygen. Inhalational agents are said to *uncouple* this relationship. They decrease the cerebral metabolic rate for oxygen but concurrently cause dilation of cerebral blood vessels, thus increasing cerebral blood flow.

12. **How should patients having CEA be monitored?**

In addition to standard monitoring, intraarterial blood pressure monitoring is indicated to continuously monitor blood pressure. Carotid surgery does not involve large fluid shifts, and monitoring central venous or pulmonary artery pressures is rarely necessary. Since the potential for uncontrolled carotid arterial bleeding always exists, large-bore intravenous access is recommended. Additional intravenous lines dedicated for the use of vasoactive and anesthetic agents are also recommended.

13. **Is regional or general anesthesia preferred for the endarterectomy patient?**
No controlled, randomized, prospective study exists that demonstrates a long-term benefit of one technique over the other. Ultimately the choice between regional and general anesthesia is based on patient suitability and preference, surgeon and anesthesiologist experience and expertise, and the availability of cerebral perfusion monitoring.

14. **What are the advantages of regional anesthesia for CEA?**
The main advantage of regional anesthesia is the ability to perform continuous neurologic assessment of the awake, cooperative patient and thus evaluate the adequacy of cerebral perfusion. However, this can become a disadvantage if the patient develops cerebral ischemia. Cerebral ischemia in this setting may lead to disorientation, inadequate ventilation and oxygenation, and a disrupted surgical field. Providing maximal cerebral protection often requires conversion to a general anesthetic, but endotracheal intubation in this setting may prove difficult. Sedation may impair the value of the awake neurologic assessment and must be titrated carefully. There is some evidence that 30-day mortality and postoperative hemorrhage are reduced with regional anesthesia.

15. **What are the advantages and disadvantages of general anesthesia for patients undergoing CEA?**
Advantages of general anesthesia include control of the airway, a quiet operative field, and the ability to maximize cerebral perfusion if ischemia develops. The main disadvantage of general anesthesia is loss of the continuous neurologic evaluation that is possible in the awake patient.

16. **What methods of monitoring cerebral perfusion during general anesthesia are available?**
Available techniques include stump pressure monitoring, intraoperative EEG, monitoring of somatosensory-evoked potentials, monitoring of jugular venous or transconjunctival oxygen saturation, transcranial Doppler, and tracer wash-out techniques. Newer methods include transcutaneous cerebral oximetry. None of the methods has been demonstrated to improve outcome, and none has gained widespread acceptance as the monitor of choice.

17. **Do stump pressures provide reliable cerebral perfusion information?**
No. The stump pressure is the pressure in the portion of the internal carotid artery immediately cephalad to the carotid cross-clamp. This pressure is presumed to represent pressure transmitted from the contralateral carotid and vertebral arteries via the circle of Willis. Stump pressures have no correlation with flow. Some patients with stump pressures less than 50 mm Hg are adequately perfused, whereas some patients with "adequate" stump pressures have suffered ischemic injury.

18. **Does intraoperative EEG provide clinically useful information during CEA?**
No data show that EEG during CEA results in improved patient outcomes. Although the EEG is a highly sensitive and an early indicator of global cortical ischemia, it is not highly specific and results in many false-positive (although few false-negative) warnings. Other concerns include the time of ischemia needed before detecting EEG changes. The issue is that, once EEG changes occur, irreversible damage might have already taken place.

19. **What are the common postoperative complications of CEA?**
   • **Hypotension:** A common complication due to an intact carotid sinus responding to higher arterial pressures after removal of the atheromatous plaque. Such hypotension responds well to fluid administration and vasopressors.
   • **Hypertension:** Also common but less understood. Obviously the high incidence of preoperative hypertension, particularly when it is poorly controlled, may result in labile postoperative hypertension. It may also be the result of denervation or trauma to the carotid sinus. Given the high association of postoperative hypertension with onset of new neurologic deficit, postoperative hypertension must be monitored and treated with some consideration given to the patient's baseline blood pressures.

- **Cerebral hyperperfusion:** After correction of the stenosis, blood flow may increase by as much as 200%. Poorly controlled hypertension contributes to this complication. Symptoms and side effects of hyperperfusion are headache, face and eye pain, cerebral edema, nausea and vomiting, seizure, and intracerebral hemorrhage. The blood pressure of such patients should be very carefully controlled, preferably without the use of cerebral vasodilators.
- **Airway obstruction:** This could result from hematomas and tissue edema. Treatment involves reestablishing an airway, possibly requiring intubation, opening the incision, and draining the hematoma. Respiratory problems also may result from vocal cord paralysis caused by damage to recurrent laryngeal nerves and from phrenic nerve paresis after cervical plexus block. The chemoreceptor function of the carotid bodies is predictably lost in most patients after CEA, as evidenced by a complete loss of the respiratory response to hypoxia and an average increase in the resting $PaCO_2$ of 6 mm Hg.
- Most **strokes** associated with CEA occur after surgery as a result of surgical factors involving carotid thrombosis and emboli from the surgical site. Immediate and progressive postoperative strokes are a surgical emergency and require prompt exploration.
- **Myocardial ischemia:** Due to the comorbidities common in these patients, CEA carries a risk of myocardial ischemia. This risk might be mitigated by performing carotid artery stenting rather than CEA.

20. **What are the major causes and presentations of spontaneous subarachnoid hemorrhage (SAH)?**
Intracranial aneurysm rupture is the most common cause of SAH (75% to 80%). Risk factors are smoking and systemic hypertension. Rupture depends on the size, with a 6% chance per year if the aneurysm is 25 mm or larger. Arteriovenous malformation (AVM, ≈5%), idiopathic (≈14%), hemorrhagic tumors, and vasculitides are other causes. SAH often presents as a severe frontal or occipital headache, often with associated neurologic deficits, photophobia, stiff neck, and nausea/vomiting. SAH may also manifest as temporary loss of consciousness or even death. Changes in the electrocardiogram (T-wave and ST-segment changes) and signs of pulmonary edema within 2 days of the bleed are the result of catecholamine release. Establishing the diagnosis and implementing quick intervention decrease the patient's morbidity and mortality.

21. **List the Hunt-Hess classification of neurologic status following spontaneous SAH.**
- **Grade I:** Asymptomatic, minimal headache and/or nuchal rigidity
- **Grade II:** Moderate to severe headache/nuchal rigidity, cranial nerve palsy (often cranial nerve III)
- **Grade III:** Confusion, drowsiness, or mild focal deficit
- **Grade IV:** Stupor, hemiparesis, early decerebrate rigidity, vegetative disturbances
- **Grade V:** Moribund, deep coma, decerebrate rigidity

22. **Describe the management of intracranial aneurysms following spontaneous SAH.**
Early surgical intervention (aneurysm clipping) within the first 72 hours of the initial bleed improves neurologic outcome, but early treatment may be technically difficult secondary to cerebral edema and unstable concomitant medical conditions. Surgery is often delayed until the risk of maximal vasospasm has decreased. Initial treatment includes close hemodynamic monitoring and stabilization. Anticoagulation, if present, should be reversed. If a patient does not have any neurologic deficits, is alert and appropriate, and has appropriate cerebral perfusion pressure (CPP), antihypertensive therapy may be used, but most hypertensive patients are left untreated so as to maintain CPP.
  When blood pressure control is necessary, usually nitroprusside or nitroglycerin is avoided because it increases cerebral blood flow; labetalol is an acceptable alternative. The use of fibrinolytics is controversial and discouraged. Glucocorticoids confer neither a benefit nor a risk. If the patient is stuporous, has decerebrate posturing, or is in a coma, interventional radiologic procedures, ventriculostomy, or burr holes may be indicated. Patients chosen for aneurysmal coiling often have a number of uncontrolled comorbidities. Interventional radiologic procedures have become the treatment of choice for selected

patient groups after cerebral aneurysm rupture. Complete obliteration of the aneurysm is encouraged with postoperative imaging to confirm success.

23. **Why is early surgical clipping so critical in the management of spontaneous SAH resulting from aneurysm rupture?**
Rebleeding and vasospasm are two devastating early complications of SAH. Rebleeding, the principal cause of death in patients after SAH, can be seen years after the initial bleed. Yet 20% of aneurysms rebleed in the first 2 weeks, with the highest risk posed on postbleed day 1. Surgical intervention prevents rebleeding, thus the reason for early clipping. Vasospasm causes delayed cerebral ischemia following SAH. It can present on a neurologic continuum from drowsiness to stroke. The etiology is believed to be subarachnoid blood around the circle of Willis in the basal cisterns. Such blood can be removed at the time of surgical clipping to decrease the incidence of vasospasm. Signs/symptoms of vasospasm are seen in roughly 30% of patients 4 to 14 days following aneurysm rupture.

24. **How is vasospasm diagnosed? Who is at risk?**
Patients at risk for vasospasm include those with hypertension on admission, age older than 60, decreased level of consciousness, large amount of blood in subarachnoid space on CT scan, hydrocephalus, and overall poor health. Intravascular volume depletion, hydrocephalus, sepsis, and electrolyte abnormalities must be considered as alternative causes of acute neurologic deterioration. Vasospasm is most clearly demonstrated by angiography and involves the middle cerebral artery 75% of the time. The pathophysiology of vasospasm is complex and not well understood, but it is thought to be related to products released by the breakdown of erythrocytes in the subarachnoid space. Autoregulation is lost in the vasospastic vessels. Surgery is often delayed if vasospasm is suspected.

25. **Describe the treatment options if vasospasm is suspected following a spontaneous SAH.**
Traditionally vasospasm has been treated with hypertension, hypervolemia, and hemodilution. Hypervolemia is achieved with colloid administration, with a goal of central venous pressure of 8 to12 mm Hg or pulmonary artery wedge pressure of 18 to 20 mm Hg. The desired level is a hematocrit of 27 to 30, thereby reducing viscosity and improving microcirculation. If the aneurysm is clipped, vasopressors (dopamine, phenylephrine) can be used to induce hypertension, with the goal being a mean arterial pressure approximately 20 to 30 mm Hg greater than baseline systolic pressure. Increased perfusion pressure will attenuate any cerebral ischemia and promote blood flow to transitional areas of injury (known as the *penumbra*). Calcium channel blockers (CCBs) are usually started empirically following SAH. CCBs have not been found to be consistent in decreasing the incidence of vasospasm (either angiographically or clinically). The CCB nimodipine has been shown to improve outcomes in SAH and should be used with appropriate monitoring. The overall mechanism of action in this setting is unknown, but decreased platelet aggregation, dilation of small arterioles, and reduction of calcium-mediated excitotoxicity are considered possible etiologies. Angioplasty can be performed and papaverine infused if segmental vasospasm is present on angiogram.

KEY POINTS: INTRACRANIAL AND CEREBROVASCULAR DISEASE

1. Atherosclerosis at the bifurcation of the common carotid artery is the source of most cerebral ischemic events.
2. Cerebral autoregulation usually maintains cerebral blood flow relatively constant over a wide range of arterial pressures. It is critically important to maintain the blood pressure of patients having carotid endarterectomy (CEA) because they have minimal or no autoregulatory reserve to counter anesthetic-induced reductions in blood pressure.
3. Normal cerebral vessels are highly sensitive to $PaCO_2$, dilating in response to hypercapnia and constricting in response to hypocapnia. However, in ischemic and already maximally vasodilated areas of the brain, this relationship breaks down, and responses to hypercapnia and hypocapnia may be paradoxical.

4. In the normal brain, cerebral blood flow varies directly with the cerebral metabolic rate. Inhalational agents are said to *uncouple* this relationship in that they decrease the cerebral metabolic rate while concurrently dilating cerebral blood vessels and increasing cerebral blood flow.
5. No particular anesthetic technique for CEA has been shown to improve outcome.
6. None of the methods of monitoring cerebral blood flow during CEA has been demonstrated to improve outcome, and none has gained widespread acceptance as the monitor of choice.
7. The key to SAH management is early diagnosis and surgical treatment within 72 hours. Vasospasm should be treated with hypertension, hypervolemia, and hemodilution.

26. **How can surgical exposure be improved and the brain be protected during aneurysm surgery?**
Hypocapnia can be used to relax the brain, but cerebral ischemia to marginally perfused regions is a concern and usually is best avoided. Mannitol is usually given after the dura is opened to facilitate exposure and relax the brain. Lumbar cerebrospinal fluid (CSF) drains can be placed, and CSF can be drained off after the dura has been opened. Glucose must be maintained between 80 and 120 mg/dl to prevent further neurologic insult. Neurosurgeons commonly place temporary occlusion clips on the parent artery that feeds the aneurysm before clipping it. Most studies have shown that this is tolerated for 10 to 14 minutes. The risk of ischemic injury increases up until 31 minutes of temporary clipping, at which time the chance of ischemic insult is nearly 100%. Induced hypertension, mild hypothermia, and burst suppression with high-dose barbiturates should be considered during temporary occlusion to protect against cerebral ischemia. EEG should be used to monitor the effects of occlusion and/or burst suppression. Overall, maintaining CPP and minimizing the time of vessel occlusion best protect the brain.

27. **What is a cerebral arteriovenous malformation (AVM)?**
AVMs are congenital vascular abnormalities that usually arise during the fetal stage of development as capillary beds are formed. The development of capillary beds is arrested, and direct communications between arteries and veins are formed. As the brain develops, the AVM acquires increased arterial blood flow and becomes a shunt system of high flow and low resistance. AVMs increase in size as they acquire further blood supply.

28. **How do AVMs typically present?**
Most AVMs are symptomatic by the age of 40, usually with the presentation of hemorrhage (nearly 50%), seizure (17% to 50%), or headache (7% to 45%). Less commonly focal neurologic deficits, increased intracranial pressure, and high-output heart failure are the presenting features. Hemorrhage, epilepsy, and neurologic deficits are the traditional indications for surgery, but newer techniques (endovascular and microsurgical/radiation) have allowed for more aggressive surgical intervention in nonruptured aneurysms. Age is also an important factor in the decision to operate.

29. **What are the common treatment modalities for AVMs?**
Conservative treatment is reserved for inoperable AVMs. Inoperable AVMs (e.g., because of size, location) can now be treated with radiosurgery or endovascular embolization. Radiosurgery directs radiation to the AVM to induce fibrosis and obliteration of the communicating vessels. Embolization is often used to decrease the size of an AVM before surgery, decreasing the risks of intraoperative bleeding and postoperative hyperemia. Surgical resection remains the definitive treatment for AVMs, virtually eliminating the risk of hemorrhage following excision.

30. **Describe the anesthetic management for surgical excision of an AVM.**
Most important, acute hypertensive episodes must be avoided. Intraarterial blood pressure monitoring and large-bore intravenous access are imperative because of the potential for rapid and massive blood loss. Such blood loss can be decreased by preoperative embolization. Some surgeons still advocate high-dose barbiturates, hypocapnia, hypothermia, and deliberate hypotension for cerebral protection.

31. What is normal perfusion pressure breakthrough?

This phenomenon of cerebral edema is also called *autoregulation breakthrough*. It is commonly seen following AVM resection or embolization. With large AVMs, the high-flow, low-resistance shunt can lead to underperfusion of adjacent brain tissue so the vessels supplying the underperfused region of brain lose the ability to autoregulate. Once the shunt is excised, all of the blood flow is diverted to the previously marginally perfused tissues, and the maximally dilated vessels are unable to vasoconstrict. This leads to the potential of cerebral edema, hyperperfusion, and hemorrhage into surrounding areas. The precise mechanism of how and why this occurs is not clear. Neurologic dysfunction following such episodes is a major cause of morbidity and mortality following AVM surgery. Treatment modalities of hyperperfusion include hyperventilation, osmotic diuresis (mannitol), head-up positioning, cautious use of deliberate hypotension, barbiturate coma, and moderate hypothermia.

SUGGESTED READINGS

Connolly ES, Rabinstein AA, Carhuapoma JR, et al: Guidelines for the management of aneurysmal subarachnoid hemorrhage: a guideline for healthcare professionals from the American Heart Association/American Stroke Association, Stroke 43:1711–1737, 2012.

Goldstein LB, Bushnell CD, Adams RJ, et al: Guidelines for the primary prevention of stroke: a guideline for healthcare professionals from the American Heart Association/American Stroke Association Council on Stroke, Stroke 42:517–584, 2011.

Gupta PK, Ramanan B, Mactaggart JN, et al: Risk index for predicting perioperative stroke, myocardial infarction, or death risk in asymptomatic patients undergoing carotid endarterectomy, J Vasc Surg 57:318–326, 2013.

Suarez JI, Tarr RW, Selman WR: Aneurysmal subarachnoid hemorrhage, N Engl J Med 354:387–396, 2006.

van Gijn J, Kerr RS, Rinkel GJ: Subarachnoid haemorrhage, Lancet 369:306–318, 2007.

CHAPTER 34

REACTIVE AIRWAY DISEASE

Malcolm Packer, MD

1. **Define reactive airway disease, in particular, asthma.**

   The term *reactive airway disease (RAD)* is used to describe a family of diseases that share the characteristic of airway sensitivity to physical, chemical, or pharmacologic stimuli. This sensitivity results in a bronchoconstrictor response and is seen in patients with asthma, chronic obstructive pulmonary disease (COPD), emphysema, viral upper respiratory illness, and other disorders.

   Asthma is defined by the American Thoracic Society as "a disease characterized by an increased responsiveness of the trachea and bronchi to various stimuli manifested by a widespread narrowing of the airways that changes in severity either spontaneously or as a result of therapy." Asthma is manifested by episodes of dyspnea, cough, and wheezing. These symptoms are related to the increased resistance to airflow in the patient's airways.

2. **What are the different types of asthma?**

   Although the common denominator lies in airway hyperreactivity, patients may fit into two subgroups: allergic (extrinsic) and idiosyncratic (intrinsic). Many believe that the terms *extrinsic* and *intrinsic* should be discarded. Underlying all types of asthma are airway hyperreactivity, inflammation, and an interaction between allergic and nonallergic stimuli.

   Allergic asthma is thought to result from an immunoglobulin E–mediated response to antigens such as dust and pollen. Among the mediators released are histamine, leukotrienes, prostaglandins, bradykinin, thromboxane, and eosinophilic chemotactic factor. Their release leads to inflammation, capillary leakage in the airways, increased mucus secretion, and bronchial smooth muscle contraction.

   Idiosyncratic asthma is mediated by nonantigenic stimuli, including exercise, cold, pollution, and infection. Bronchospasm is caused by increased parasympathetic (vagal) tone. Although the primary stimulus differs, the same mediators as those in allergic asthma are released (and some patients with allergic asthma have enhanced vagal tone).

3. **What diseases mimic asthma?**
   - COPD
   - Upper and lower airway obstruction from tumor, aspirated foreign bodies, or stenosis
   - Left ventricular failure (cardiac asthma) and pulmonary embolism
   - Gastroesophageal reflux and aspiration
   - Viral respiratory illnesses (e.g., respiratory syncytial virus)
   - Allergic reactions and anaphylaxis

   A careful history and physical examination will differentiate these diseases from primary reactive disease.

4. **What are the important historical features of an asthmatic patient?**
   - Duration of disease
   - Frequency, initiating factors, and duration of attacks
   - Has the patient ever required inpatient therapy? Did the patient require intensive care admission or intubation?
   - What are the patient's medications, including daily and as-needed usage, over-the-counter medications, and steroids?

5. **What symptoms and physical findings are associated with asthma?**

   Common symptoms include coughing, shortness of breath, and tightness of the chest. The most common physical finding is expiratory wheezing. Wheezing is a sign of obstructed airflow and is often associated with a prolonged expiratory phase. As asthma progressively worsens, patients use accessory respiratory muscles. A significantly symptomatic patient with quiet auscultatory findings may signal impending respiratory failure because not enough air is moving to elicit a wheeze. Patients also may be tachypneic and probably are dehydrated; they prefer an upright posture and demonstrate pursed-lip breathing. Cyanosis is a late and ominous sign.

6. What preoperative tests should be ordered?

The patient's history guides the judicious ordering of preoperative tests. A mild asthmatic patient maintained on as-needed medication and currently healthy will not benefit from preoperative testing. Symptomatic patients with no recent evaluation may deserve closer attention.

The most common test is a pulmonary function test, which allows simple and quick evaluation of the degree of obstruction and its reversibility (see Chapter 9). A comparison of values obtained from the patient with predicted values aids the assessment of the degree of obstruction. Severe exacerbation correlates with a peak expiratory flow rate (PEFR) or forced expiratory volume in 1 second (FEV_1) of less than 30% to 50% of predicted, which for most adults is a PEFR of less than 120 L/min and an FEV_1 of less than 1 L. Tests should be repeated after a trial of bronchodilator therapy to assess reversibility and response to treatment.

Arterial blood gases are usually not helpful. Electrocardiograms, chest radiographs, and blood counts are rarely indicated for evaluation of asthma unless particular features of the patient's presentation suggest alternative diagnoses (e.g., fever and rales, suggesting pneumonia).

7. Describe the mainstay of therapy in asthma.

The mainstay of therapy remains inhaled β-adrenergic agonists. Selective short-acting β_2 agonists such as albuterol and terbutaline offer greater β_2-mediated bronchodilation and fewer side effects (e.g., β_1-associated tachydysrhythmias and tremors). Albuterol can be nebulized or administered orally or by metered-dose inhaler (MDI). Terbutaline is effective via nebulizer, subcutaneously, or as a continuous intravenous infusion. But they may produce hypokalemia, lactic acidosis, and cardiac tachydysrhythmias, particularly with intravenous use. Epinephrine is available for subcutaneous use in severely asthmatic patients. Patients with coronary artery disease have difficulty with tachycardia and need the β_2-specific agents. Routinely the inhaled route is preferred.

Long-acting β_2 agonists such as salmeterol and formoterol are used for chronic dosing and are sometimes paired with a steroid.

8. What other medications and routes of delivery are used in asthma?

- **Corticosteroids:** Reverse airway inflammation, decrease mucus production, and potentiate β-agonist–induced smooth muscle relaxation. Steroids are strongly recommended in patients with moderate to severe asthma or patients who have required steroids in the past 6 months. Onset of action is 1 to 2 hours after administration. Methylprednisolone is popular because of its strong antiinflammatory powers but weak mineralocorticoid effect. Side effects include hyperglycemia, hypertension, hypokalemia, and mood alterations, including psychosis. Long-term steroid use or prolonged use with muscle relaxants is associated with myopathy. Steroids may be given orally, via MDI, or intravenously.
- **Anticholinergic agents:** Cause bronchodilation by blocking muscarinic cholinergic receptors in the airways, therefore attenuating bronchoconstriction caused by inhaled irritants and associated with β-blocker therapy. They are invaluable in patients with COPD or with severe airway obstruction (predicted $FEV_1 < 25\%$). Ipratropium, glycopyrrolate, and atropine may be given via nebulizer, and ipratropium is available in an MDI.
- **Leukotriene receptor antagonist:** Relative newcomers in the treatment of mild to moderate asthma. They act by inhibition of the 5-lipoxygenase pathway or antagonism of the cysteinyl-leukotriene type 1 receptors. They are commonly prescribed and may be used in conjunction with inhaled steroids.
- **Theophylline:** The use in asthma is controversial. Theophylline has some bronchodilatory effects and improves diaphragmatic action. Such benefits must be weighed against a long list of side effects: tremor, nausea and vomiting, palpitations, tachydysrhythmias, and seizures. Until definite proof is available, many investigators

Table 34-1. Useful Medications for Patients with Reactive Airway Disease

MEDICATION	DOSE	COMMENTS
Albuterol	2.5 mg in 3 ml of normal saline for nebulization or 2 puffs by MDI	May need repeat treatments
Terbutaline	0.3–0.4 mg subcutaneously	May repeat as required every 20 minutes for three doses IV dosing of terbutaline has several protocols available through literature search
Epinephrine	0.3 mg subcutaneously	May repeat as required every 20 minutes for three doses
Corticosteroids	Methylprednisolone, 60-125 mg intravenously every 6 hours, or prednisone, 30-50 mg orally daily	Steroids are usually tapered at the first opportunity
Anticholinergics	Ipratropium, 0.5 mg by nebulization or 4-6 puffs by MDI; atropine, 1-2 mg per nebulization	Useful with severe RAD and COPD
Theophylline	5 mg/kg intravenously over 30 minutes (loading dose in patients not previously taking theophylline)	After the loading dose, start continuous infusion at the appropriate rate according to age and disease state of the patient, being watchful for any drug interactions

COPD, Chronic obstructive pulmonary disease; *MDI,* metered-dose inhaler; *RAD,* reactive airway disease.

suggest that theophylline therapy should be initiated only in patients with acute asthma who do not improve with maximal β-agonist and corticosteroid therapy. Careful monitoring of serum levels is mandatory. Theophylline is the oral preparation, whereas aminophylline, its water-soluble form, is for intravenous use.
- **Cromolyn sodium:** A mast cell stabilizer useful for long-term maintenance therapy. Patients younger than 17 years of age and with moderate to severe exercise-induced asthma appear to benefit the most. Side effects include some minimal local irritation on delivery. Cromolyn sodium may be administered via MDI or as a powder in a turboinhaler. Cromolyn sodium is not effective in acute asthmatic attacks and in fact is contraindicated.
- **Methotrexate or gold salts:** Patients with severe asthma may require one of these medications. Both have undesirable side-effect profiles and are reserved for patients who have major difficulties with corticosteroids (Table 34-1).

9. **What is the best approach to preoperative management of the patient with RAD?**
   Patients should be classified according to the urgency of the operation required and their particular history of reactive airways.
   - Patients who are scheduled for elective procedures but are actively wheezing are probably best cancelled, administered therapy, and rescheduled.
   - Asymptomatic patients on no medications currently and with no recent bouts of asthma and no history of serious illness may require no therapy or, at most, inhaled β agonists.
   - Mild asthmatics ($FEV_1 > 80\%$) with ongoing or recent symptoms should definitely have β-adrenergic therapy before surgery.
   - Moderate asthmatics (FEV_1 65% to 80%) should continue their β-adrenergic therapy and either double their inhaled steroid dose for a week before surgery or start oral steroids 2

days before surgery. When symptomatic, these patients should start β-adrenergic and oral steroid therapy. Important factors to consider before beginning steroids include the following:
- Have the patients had intensive care admissions or mechanical ventilation related to their asthma?
- Have steroids been administered in the past 6 months?
- Are the patients at risk for adrenal insufficiency?
- Severe asthmatics (FEV < 65%) should be on β-adrenergic therapy and be given 2 days of oral steroids before surgery. Patients with FEV_1 < 70% have improvements in pulmonary function with either inhaled β-adrenergic therapy or oral steroids with only 1 day of therapy. Combining β-adrenergic and oral steroid therapy also significantly decreases postintubation wheezing when compared with β-adrenergic therapy alone. Finally, patients having upper abdominal or thoracic surgery and emergency cases are at particular risk and deserve aggressive therapy.

10. **Review the pros and cons of induction agents in asthmatic patients.**
Intravenous induction agents used in asthmatic patients include propofol and ketamine. Ketamine has well-known bronchodilatory effects secondary to the release of endogenous catecholamines with $β_2$-agonist effects. Ketamine also has a small, direct relaxant effect on smooth muscles. Propofol decreases both airway resistance and airway reflexes after administration. Intravenous lidocaine is a useful adjunct for blunting the response to laryngoscopy and intubation.

Mask induction with halothane or sevoflurane is an excellent method to block airway reflexes and to relax airway smooth muscles directly. These agents are much more palatable to the airway than isoflurane or desflurane.

Atracurium and mivacurium are commonly used muscle relaxants that have demonstrated histamine release and may cause bronchoconstriction. Vecuronium, rocuronium, and pancuronium are not associated with histamine release. Cisatracurium is associated with less histamine release relative to atracurium.

11. **What agents may be used for maintenance anesthesia?**
Sevoflurane, halothane, and isoflurane are effective in blocking airway reflexes and bronchoconstriction. Inhaled anesthetics have been used in the intensive care unit to provide bronchodilation in intubated patients with severe asthma, improving indices of respiratory resistance (inspiratory and expiratory flows), decreasing hyperinflation, and lowering intrinsic positive end-expiratory pressure (PEEP).

Opioids at higher doses block airway reflexes but do not provide direct bronchodilation. Morphine remains controversial because of its histamine-releasing activity. Anesthetics relying primarily on opioids may cause problems with respiratory depression at emergence (particularly in patients with COPD with an asthmatic component).

Neuromuscular blocking agents with a benzylisoquinolinium nucleus such as d-tubocurarine, atracurium, and mivacurium release histamine from mast cells on injection. They also may bind directly to muscarinic receptors on ganglia, nerve endings, and airway smooth muscle. Both mechanisms theoretically may increase airway resistance. Relaxants with an aminosteroid nucleus such as pancuronium and vecuronium continue to be used safely in asthmatic patients. In patients with bronchospasm, neuromuscular blocking agents improve chest wall compliance, but smooth muscle airway tone and lung compliance remain the same. Prolonged use of muscle relaxants in ventilated asthmatic patients is associated with increases in creatine kinase and clinically significant myopathy.

12. **What are the complications of intubation and mechanical ventilation in asthmatic patients?**
The stimulus of intubation causes significant increases in airway resistance. Lung hyperinflation occurs when diminished expiratory flow prevents complete emptying of the alveolar and small airway gas. Significant gas trapping may cause hypotension by increasing intrathoracic pressure and reducing venous return. Pneumomediastinum and pneumothorax are also potential causes of acute respiratory decompensation.

Several measurements of ventilator function may give some insight into a patient's improving or worsening status. Plateau pressures (the pressure measured at end inspiration and before expiration starts, averaged over a 0.4-second pause) correlate loosely with complications at pressures greater than 30 cm H_2O. Auto-PEEP is the measurement of end-expiratory pressure (taken at end expiration while the expiratory port is momentarily occluded) and may correlate with alveolar pressures in the bronchospastic patient. However, auto-PEEP does not specifically correlate with complications. Plateau pressure and auto-PEEP measurements require a relaxed patient.

Patients on prolonged high-dose corticosteroids and muscle relaxants are at risk for severe myopathy. Pancuronium and vecuronium are the worst offenders, but all muscle relaxants are suspect.

Several strategies for mechanically ventilating bronchospastic patients have been developed:

- Pressure-support ventilation allows for spontaneous ventilation in the sedated patient with less work of breathing and less risk of barotrauma and if mandatory breaths are required.
- Increase expiratory time by decreasing ventilator rate, increasing inspiratory flow rates to decrease inspiratory time, and directly increasing the inspiratory-to-expiratory ratio.
- Be careful of ventilator-applied PEEP.
- Decrease minute volume, allowing controlled hypoventilation and permissive hypercapnia.

13. What are the causes of intraoperative wheezing and the correct responses to asthmatic patients with acute bronchospasm?

Causes include airway secretions, foreign body partial obstruction, pulmonary edema (cardiac asthma), partially obstructed endotracheal tube, endotracheal tube at the carina or down a mainstem bronchus, allergic or anaphylactic response to drugs, and asthma. A number of medications cause wheezing in asthmatic patients, including β blockers, muscle relaxants, and aspirin.

After carefully checking the endotracheal tube, assessing airway pressures, and listening for bilateral breath sounds, increase the inspired oxygen to 100% and deepen the anesthetic if hemodynamically tolerated by the patient. Provoking factors such as medication infusions, misplaced endotracheal tubes, or other causes of airway stimulation should be corrected. Administration of medications suggested in Questions 7 and 8 may help.

14. Describe the emergence techniques for asthmatic patients under general endotracheal anesthesia.

Awake and deep extubations are alternatives in patients under general endotracheal anesthesia. The endotracheal tube is a common cause of significant bronchospasm, and its removal under deep-inhaled anesthetic in a spontaneously ventilating patient often leads to a smooth emergence. Deep extubations should be avoided in patients with difficult airways, morbidly obese patients, and patients with full stomachs.

15. What new therapies are available to anesthesiologists treating asthmatic patients in bronchospasm?

- **Magnesium sulfate:** Has been administered to patients in status asthmaticus. Hypothetically, magnesium interferes with calcium-mediated smooth muscle contraction and decreases acetylcholine release at the neuromuscular junction. Magnesium reduces histamine- and methacholine-induced bronchospasm in controlled studies.
- **Heliox:** A blend of helium and oxygen that decreases airway resistance, peak airway pressures, and $PaCO_2$ levels when administered to spontaneously and mechanically ventilated patients. The mixture contains 60% to 80% helium and 20% to 40% oxygen and is less dense than air. The decrease in density allows less turbulent flow and significant declines in resistance to flow. The device for heliox administration in intubated patients is cumbersome unless the anesthesia machine is already equipped.
- **LITA tube:** This endotracheal tube allows intraoperative instillation of lidocaine at and below the cords of the intubated patient. This technique decreases airway stimulation from the endotracheal tube and may prevent reflex bronchospasm.
- **Extracorporeal oxygenation:** Using veno-venous oxygenation and CO_2 removal allows for minimal ventilatory support (lung rest) and the removal of dangerously high CO_2

with resulting improvement in pH. This should be considered if ventilation is becoming increasingly difficult and/or air leaks require ventilatory rest.

KEY POINTS: REACTIVE AIRWAY DISEASE

1. The patient with reactive airway disease (RAD) is at increased risk for intraoperative bronchoconstriction as manifested by increased peak airway pressures, difficulty in ventilation, and hypoxemia.
2. Most, if not all, patients with RAD will benefit from preoperative bronchodilator therapy.
3. Actively wheezing patients scheduled for elective surgery should be delayed until the reactive component of their pulmonary disease and other contributing factors have been treated and have come under satisfactory control.

WEBSITES

American Academy of Allergy, Asthma, and Immunology: http://www.aaai.org
Asthma and Allergy Foundation of America: http://www.aafa.org

SUGGESTED READINGS

Applegate R, Lauer R, Gatling J, et al: The perioperative management of asthma, J Aller Ther S11:007, 2013.
Apter AJ: Advances in the care of adults with asthma and allergy in 2007, J Allergy Clin Immunol 121:839–844, 2008.
Bishop MJ: Preoperative corticosteroids for reactive airway? Anesthesiology 100:1047–1048, 2004.
Chonghaile M, Higgins B, Laffey J: Permissive hypercapnia: role in protective lung ventilatory strategy, Curr Opin Crit Care 11:56–62, 2005.
Doherty G, Chisakuta A, Crean P: Anesthesia and the child with asthma, Pediatr Anesth 15:446–454, 2005.
Jean L, Brown RH: Should patients with asthma be given preoperative medications including steroids? In Fleisher LA, editor: Evidence-based practice of anesthesiology, Philadelphia, 2004, Saunders, pp 77–81.
Reddel H, Taylor DR, Bateman ED, et al: An official American Thoracic Society/European Respiratory Society statement: asthma control and exacerbations, Am J Respir Crit Care Med 180:59–99, 2009.
Szelfler S: Advances in pediatric asthma, J Allergy Clin Immunol 121:614–619, 2008.
Watanabe K, Mizutani T, Yamashita S: Prolonged sevoflurane therapy for status asthmaticus, Pediatr Anesth 18:543–545, 2008.

ASPIRATION

Malcolm Packer, MD

CHAPTER 35

1. **What is aspiration, and what differentiates aspiration pneumonitis from aspiration pneumonia?**

   Aspiration is the passage of material from the pharynx into the trachea. Aspirated material can originate from the stomach, esophagus, mouth, or nose. The materials involved can be particulate (e.g., food), a foreign body, fluid (e.g., blood, saliva), or gastrointestinal contents. Aspiration of gastric contents may occur by vomiting or by passive regurgitation.

   Aspiration pneumonitis describes the initial inflammatory response after aspiration, and aspiration pneumonia describes the consolidation along with the inflammation.

2. **How often does aspiration occur, and what is the morbidity and mortality rate?**

   The incidence of significant aspiration is 1 per 10,000 anesthetics. Studies of children's anesthetics demonstrate about twice that occurrence. The average hospital stay after aspiration is 21 days, much of which is in intensive care. Complications range from bronchospasm, pneumonia, and acute respiratory distress syndrome, lung abscess, and empyema. The average mortality rate is 5%.

3. **What are risk factors for aspiration?**
   - Extremes of age
   - Emergency cases
   - Type of surgery (most common in cases of esophageal, upper abdominal, or emergency laparotomy surgery)
   - Recent meal (Preoperative fasting guidelines for elective surgery are discussed in Chapter 17.)
   - Delayed gastric emptying and/or decreased lower esophageal sphincter tone (diabetes, gastric outlet obstruction, hiatal hernia)
   - Medications (e.g., narcotics, anticholinergics)
   - Trauma
   - Pregnancy
   - Pain and stress
   - Depressed level of consciousness
   - Morbid obesity (even bariatric surgery and the resulting weight loss)
   - Difficult airway
   - Neuromuscular disease (impaired ability to protect the trachea)
   - Esophageal disease (e.g., scleroderma, achalasia, diverticulum, Zenker diverticulum)

4. **What precautions before anesthetic induction are required to prevent aspiration or mollify its sequelae?**

   The main precaution is to recognize which patients are at risk. Patients should have an adequate fasting period to improve the chances of an empty stomach. Gastrokinetic medications such as metoclopramide have been thought to be of benefit because they enhance gastric emptying, but no good data support this belief. It is helpful to increase gastric pH by either nonparticulate antacids such as sodium citrate and histamine-2 (H_2) receptor antagonists, either of which decreases acid production. The market now includes several H_2 antagonists, giving anesthesiologists a choice (e.g., cimetidine, ranitidine, and famotidine). Although cimetidine increases gastric pH, it also has a significant side-effect profile, including hypotension, heart block, central nervous system dysfunction, decreased hepatic blood flow, and significant retardation of the metabolism of many drugs. Ranitidine, a newer H_2 antagonist, is much less likely to cause side effects; only a few cases of central nervous system dysfunction and heart block have been reported. Famotidine is equally as potent as cimetidine and ranitidine and has no significant side effects. To be effective at induction, H_2 blockers must be administered 2 to 3 hours before the procedure, although medications given near the time of induction may have some benefit after extubation. The use of proton pump inhibitors in place of, or in concert with, H_2 antagonists has not proven to be more efficacious. The use of orogastric or nasogastric drainage before induction is most effective in patients with intestinal obstruction.

5. **How might a patient with a difficult airway and at risk for aspiration be managed?**
   A regional anesthetic is a desirable alternative when appropriate for the surgery and has been shown to be of value in the setting of cesarean section, where the patient population is definitely at aspiration risk. A rapid sequence induction with cricoid pressure is preferred when a general anesthetic is needed. Discussions on the efficacy and potential hazards of cricoid pressure continue, but to date it is usually recommended for rapid sequence intubations.

   Patients with difficult airways may require awake placement of an endotracheal tube to allow protection of the airway from aspiration. Patient comfort is aided by the judicious use of sedation and topical local anesthetic. Oversedation and topicalization of the airway may make the patient less able to protect the airway. Therefore keeping the patient conscious and applying topical local anesthetic only to the airway above the glottis may increase safety. Endotracheal intubation does not guarantee that no aspiration will occur. Material may still slip past a deflated or partially deflated cuff.

6. **Describe the different clinical pictures caused by the three broad types of aspirates.**
   - **Acidic aspirates** with a pH less than 2.5 and volumes of more than 0.4 ml/kg immediately cause alveolar-capillary breakdown, resulting in interstitial edema, intraalveolar hemorrhage, atelectasis, and increased airway resistance. Hypoxia is common. Although such changes usually start within minutes of the initiating event, they may worsen over a period of hours. The first phase of the response is direct reaction of the lung to acid—hence the name *chemical pneumonitis*. The second phase, which occurs hours later, is caused by a leukocyte or inflammatory response to the original damage and may lead to respiratory failure.
   - Aspiration of **nonacidic fluid** destroys surfactant, causing alveolar collapse and atelectasis. Hypoxia is common. The destruction of lung architecture and the late inflammatory response are not as great as in acid aspiration.
   - Aspiration of **particulate food matter** causes both physical obstruction of the airway and a later inflammatory response. Alternating areas of atelectasis and hyperexpansion may occur. Patients may have hypoxia and hypercapnia caused by physical obstruction of airflow. If acid is mixed with the particulate matter, damage is often greater and the clinical picture worse.

7. **Review the clinical signs and symptoms after aspiration.**
   Fever occurs in over 90% of aspiration cases, with tachypnea and rales in at least 70%. Cough, cyanosis, and wheezing occur in 30% to 40% of cases. Aspiration may occur *silently*—without the anesthesiologist's knowledge—during anesthesia. Any of the previous clinical deviations from the expected course may signal an aspiration event. Radiographic changes may take hours to occur and may be negative, especially if radiographic images are taken soon after an event.

8. **When is a patient suspected of aspiration believed to be out of danger?**
   The patient who shows none of the previously mentioned signs or symptoms and has no increased oxygen requirement at the end of 2 hours should recover completely.

9. **Describe the treatment for aspiration.**
   Any patient who is thought to have aspirated should receive a chest radiograph and, at a minimum, many hours of observation. Supportive care remains the mainstay. Immediate suctioning should be instituted. Supplemental oxygen and ventilatory support should be initiated if respiratory failure is a problem. Patients with respiratory failure often demonstrate atelectasis with alveolar collapse and may respond to positive end-expiratory pressure. Patients with particulate aspirate may need bronchoscopy to remove large obstructing pieces. Antibiotics should not be administered unless there is a high likelihood that gram-negative or anaerobic organisms (i.e., bowel obstruction) have been aspirated. However, a worsening

clinical course over the next few days suggests that a broad-spectrum antibiotic may be indicated. Corticosteroids have not been shown to be helpful in human studies. Lavaging the trachea with normal saline or sodium bicarbonate after aspiration has not been shown to be helpful and may actually worsen the patient's status.

More aggressive treatments of severe aspiration usually occur in the critical care setting. Surfactant installation, high-frequency oscillatory ventilation, and prone positioning have all shown some promise for certain patients with severe aspirations.

KEY POINTS: ASPIRATION

1. Numerous patient subgroups are at increased risk of aspiration, including patients presenting for emergency surgery, those having had a recent meal, those with bowel obstruction or delayed gastric emptying, the obese, patients who are in trauma or are pregnant, those having pain or being treated with opioids, and those who cannot protect the airway (e.g., patients with a depressed level of consciousness or neuromuscular disease).
2. Such patients may require prophylaxis to decrease the severity of aspiration should it occur, and medications valuable for decreasing the acidity of gastric secretions include nonparticulate antacids, H_2 blockers, and proton pump inhibitors. Patients with bowel obstruction should receive gastric decompression before anesthetic induction.
3. Regional anesthetics are ideal for patients at risk for aspiration if appropriate. A rapid-sequence induction with cricoid pressure is the technique of choice when general anesthesia is required in patients with manageable airways. Awake intubation may be necessary in patients with difficult airways.
4. Should aspiration occur, the treatment is mostly supportive.

SUGGESTED READINGS

Apfelbaum JL, Caplan RA, Connis RT, et al: Practice guidelines for preoperative fasting and the use of pharmacologic agents to reduce the risk of pulmonary aspiration, Anesthesiology 114:495–511, 2011.
Cohen NH: Is there an optimal treatment for aspiration? In Fleisher LA, editor: Evidence-based practice of anesthesiology, ed 2, Philadelphia, 2009, Saunders, pp 327–335.
Jean J, Compère V, Fourdrinier V: The risk of pulmonary aspiration after weight loss due to bariatric surgery, Anesth Analg 107:1257–1259, 2008.
Kluger M, Visvanathan T, Myburgh J, et al: Crisis management during anesthesia: regurgitation, vomiting and aspiration, Qual Saf Health Care 14:4–9, 2005.
Marrano G, Marco L: Selected medicated (saline vs. surfactant) bronchoalveolar lavage in severe aspiration syndrome in children, Pediatr Crit Care Med 8:476–481, 2007.
Neelakanta G: Chikyarapra A: A review of patients with pulmonary aspiration of gastric contents during anesthesia reported to the Departmental Quality Assurance Committee, J Clin Anesth 18:102–107, 2006.
Tasch M: What reduces the risk of aspiration? In Fleisher LA, editor: Evidence-based practice of anesthesiology, Philadelphia, 2004, Saunders, pp 118–124.

CHAPTER 36

CHRONIC OBSTRUCTIVE PULMONARY DISEASE

Howard J. Miller, MD

1. **Define chronic obstructive pulmonary disease (COPD).**
   COPD is a spectrum of diseases that includes emphysema, chronic bronchitis, and asthmatic bronchitis. It is characterized by progressive increased resistance to breathing. Airflow limitation may be caused by loss of elastic recoil or obstruction of small or large (or both) conducting airways. The increased resistance may have some degree of reversibility. Cardinal symptoms are cough, dyspnea, and wheezing.

2. **What are the features of asthma and asthmatic bronchitis?**
   Asthma
   - This heterogeneous disorder is characterized by reversible airway obstruction.
   - Precipitating factors include exercise, dander, pollen, and intubation.
   - Symptoms improve with bronchodilator and immunosuppressive therapy.
   Asthmatic bronchitis
   - It consists of airway obstruction, chronic productive cough, and episodic bronchospasm.
   - It can result from progression of asthma or chronic bronchitis.
   - There is less improvement with bronchodilator therapy; some degree of airway obstruction at all times.

3. **Describe chronic bronchitis and emphysema.**
   - **Chronic bronchitis:** Characterized by cough, sputum production, recurrent infection, and airway obstruction for many months to several years. Patients with chronic bronchitis have mucous gland hyperplasia, mucus plugging, inflammation and edema, peribronchiolar fibrosis, airway narrowing, and bronchoconstriction. Decreased airway lumina caused by mucus and inflammation increase resistance to flow of gases.
   - **Emphysema:** Characterized by progressive dyspnea and variable cough. Destruction of the elastic and collagen network of alveolar walls without resultant fibrosis leads to abnormal enlargement of air spaces. In addition, the loss of airway support leads to airway narrowing and collapse during expiration (air trapping).

4. **List contributory factors associated with the development of COPD.**
   - **Smoking:** Smoking impairs ciliary function, depresses alveolar macrophages; leads to increased mucous gland proliferation and mucus production, increases the inflammatory response in the lung, leads increased proteolytic enzyme release, reduces surfactant integrity, and causes increased airway reactivity.
   - **Occupational and environmental exposure:** Animal dander, toluene and other chemicals, various grains, cotton, and sulfur dioxide and nitrogen dioxide in air pollution.
   - **Recurrent infection:** Bacterial, atypical organisms (mycoplasma), and viral (including human immunodeficiency virus, which can produce an emphysema-like picture).
   - **Familial and genetic factors:** A predisposition to COPD exists and is more common in men than women. α_1-Antitrypsin deficiency is a genetic disorder resulting in autodigestion of pulmonary tissue by proteases and should be suspected in younger patients with basilar bullae on chest x-ray film. Smoking accelerates its presentation and progression.

5. **What historical information should be obtained before surgery?**
   - Smoking history: number of packs per day and duration in years
   - Dyspnea, wheezing, productive cough, and exercise tolerance
   - Hospitalizations for COPD, including the need for intubation and mechanical ventilation

- Medications, including home oxygen therapy and steroid use, either systemic or inhaled
- Recent pulmonary infections, exacerbations, or change in character of sputum
- Weight loss that may be caused by end-stage pulmonary disease or lung cancer
- Symptoms of right-sided heart failure, including peripheral edema, hepatomegaly, jaundice, and anorexia secondary to liver and splanchnic congestion

6. **What features distinguish *pink puffers* from *blue bloaters*?**

Pink puffers (emphysema)	Blue bloaters (chronic bronchitis)
Usually older (>60 years)	Relatively young
Pink in color	Cyanotic
Thin	Heavier in weight
Minimal cough	Chronic productive cough; frequent wheeze

7. **List abnormal physical findings in patients with COPD.**
   - Tachypnea and use of accessory muscles
   - Distant or focally diminished breath sounds, wheezing, or rhonchi
   - Jugular venous distention, hepatojugular reflux, and peripheral edema suggest right-sided heart failure
   - Palpation of peripheral pulses is an indirect measure of stroke volume

8. **What laboratory examinations are useful?**
   - White cell count and hematocrit: Elevation suggests infection and chronic hypoxemia, respectively.
   - Electrolytes: Bicarbonate levels are elevated to buffer a chronic respiratory acidosis if the patient retains carbon dioxide. Hypokalemia can occur with repeated use of β-adrenergic agonists.
   - Chest x-ray film: Look for lung hyperinflation, bullae or blebs, flattened diaphragm, increased retrosternal air space, atelectasis, cardiac enlargement, infiltrate, effusion, masses, or pneumothorax.
   - Electrocardiogram: Look for decreased amplitude, signs of right atrial (peaked P waves in leads II and V_1) or ventricular enlargement (right axis deviation, R/S ratio in $V_6 \leq 1$, increased R wave in V_1 and V_2, right bundle-branch block), and arrhythmias. Atrial arrhythmias are common, especially multifocal atrial tachycardia and atrial fibrillation.
   - Arterial blood gas: Hypoxemia, hypercarbia, and acid-base status, including compensation, can be evaluated.
   - Spirometry is discussed in Chapter 9.

9. **How does a chronically elevated arterial carbon dioxide partial pressure ($PaCO_2$) affect the respiratory drive in a person with COPD?**
   Persons with COPD have a reduced ventilatory drive in response to levels of carbon dioxide (CO_2). Chronically elevated $PaCO_2$ produces increased cerebrospinal fluid bicarbonate concentrations. The respiratory chemoreceptors at the medulla become "reset" to a higher concentration of CO_2. Thus diminished ventilatory drive secondary to CO_2 exists. In these patients, ventilatory drive may be more dependent on partial pressure of oxygen (PO_2).

10. **What are the deleterious effects of oxygen administration in these patients?**
    Inhalation of 100% oxygen may increase ventilation-perfusion mismatch by inhibiting hypoxic pulmonary vasoconstriction (HPV). HPV is an autoregulatory mechanism in the pulmonary vasculature that decreases blood flow to poorly ventilated areas of the lung, ensuring that more blood flow is available for gas exchange in better ventilated areas of the lung. Inhibition of HPV results in increased perfusion of poorly ventilated areas of lung, contributing to hypoxemia and/or hypercarbia. It is prudent to always administer the minimum oxygen necessary to achieve the desired goal, perhaps a pulse oximetry value between 90% and 95%.

11. **How do general anesthesia and surgery affect pulmonary mechanics?**
    Vital capacity is reduced by 25% to 50%, and residual volume increases by 13% following many general anesthetics and surgical procedures. Upper abdominal incisions and thoracotomy affect pulmonary mechanics the greatest, followed by lower abdominal

Table 36-1. Pulmonary Function Values Associated with Increased Perioperative Mortality/Morbidity*

PFT	ABDOMINAL SURGERY	THORACOTOMY	LOBECTOMY/ PNEUMONECTOMY
FVC	<70%	<70%	<50% or <2 L
FEV_1	<70%	<1 L	<1 L
FEV_1/FVC	<50%	<50%	<50%
FEF_{25-75}	<50%	<50%	
RV/TLC	40%		
$PaCO_2$	>45–55 mm Hg	>45–50 mm Hg	

*Percentages are of predicted values.
FEF_{25-75}, Forced expiratory flow in the midexpiratory phase; FEV_1, forced expiratory volume in 1 second; FVC, forced vital capacity; PFT, pulmonary function test; RV, residual volume; TLC, total lung capacity.

incisions and sternotomy. Expiratory reserve volume decreases by 25% after lower abdominal surgery and 60% after upper abdominal and thoracic surgery. Tidal volume decreases 20%, and pulmonary compliance and functional residual capacity decrease 33%. Atelectasis, hypoventilation, hypoxemia, and pulmonary infection may result. Many of these changes require a minimum of 1 to 2 weeks to resolve.

12. **What factors are associated with an increased perioperative morbidity or mortality?**
Increased morbidity results from hypoxemia, hypoventilation resulting in acute hypercarbia, pulmonary infection, prolonged intubation, and mechanical ventilation. The number of intensive care days is increased, overall hospitalization is prolonged, and rate of mortality is increased.
    Patients presenting for lobectomy or pneumonectomy must have pulmonary function and arterial blood gas values that are superior to the values in Table 36-1. If any of the aforementioned criteria are not satisfied, further preoperative testing is indicated to determine the risk-benefit ratio for lung resection. Further tests include split-lung function, regional perfusion, regional ventilation, regional bronchial balloon occlusion, and pulmonary artery balloon occlusion studies. A forced expiratory volume in 1 second (FEV_1) less than 800 ml in a 70-kg person is probably incompatible with life and is an absolute contraindication to lung resection because of the high incidence for extended mechanical ventilation.

13. **List the common pharmacologic agents used to treat COPD and their mechanisms of action.**
See Table 36-2.

14. **What therapies are available to reduce perioperative pulmonary risk?**
    • Stop smoking.
        • Cessation for 48 hours before surgery decreases carboxyhemoglobin levels. The oxyhemoglobin dissociation curve shifts to the right, allowing increased tissue oxygen availability.
        • Cessation for 4 to 6 weeks before surgery has been shown to decrease the incidence of postoperative pulmonary complications.
        • Cessation for 2 to 3 months before surgery results in all of the previous benefits plus improved ciliary function, improved pulmonary mechanics, and reduced sputum production.
    • Optimize pharmacologic therapy. Continue medications even on the day of surgery.
    • Recognize and treat underlying pulmonary infection.
    • Maximize nutritional support, hydration, and chest physiotherapy.

Table 36-2. Agents Used to Treat Chronic Obstructive Pulmonary Disease

CLASS AND EXAMPLES	ACTIONS
β-Adrenergic agonists: albuterol, metaproterenol, fenoterol, terbutaline, epinephrine	Increases adenylate cyclase, increasing cAMP and decreasing smooth muscle tone (bronchodilation); short-acting β-adrenergic agonists (e.g., albuterol, terbutaline, and epinephrine) are the agents of choice for acute exacerbations
Methylxanthines: aminophylline, theophylline	Phosphodiesterase inhibition increases cAMP; potentiates endogenous catecholamines; improves diaphragmatic contractility; central respiratory stimulant
Corticosteroids: methylprednisolone, dexamethasone, prednisone, cortisol	Antiinflammatory and membrane stabilizing; inhibits histamine release; potentiates β agonists
Anticholinergics: atropine, glycopyrrolate, ipratropium	Blocks acetylcholine at postganglionic receptors, decreasing cGMP, relaxing airway smooth muscle
Cromolyn sodium	Also a membrane stabilizer, preventing mast cell degranulation, but must be given prophylactically
Antileukotrienes: zileuton, montelukast	Inhibition of leukotriene production and/or zafirlukast, leukotriene antagonism; antiinflammatory; used in addition to corticosteroids; however, may be considered first-line antiinflammatory therapy for patients who cannot or will not use corticosteroids

cAMP, Cyclic adenosine monophosphate; cGMP, cyclic guanosine monophosphate.

- Institute effective postoperative analgesia, allowing the patient to cough effectively, take large tidal volumes, and ambulate early after surgery.

15. **Do advantages exist with regional anesthesia techniques in patients with COPD?**
Regional anesthesia, including extremity and neuraxial blockade, avoids the need for endotracheal intubation. However, spinal or epidural blockade above the T10 dermatome may reduce effective coughing secondary to abdominal muscle dysfunction, leading to decreased sputum clearance and atelectasis. Concerning brachial plexus anesthesia, pneumothorax or blockade of the phrenic nerve, causing hemidiaphragmatic paralysis, is a risk. Sedation administered during or after these procedures may depress respiratory drive and should be titrated to effect.
Local anesthetics infused through catheters placed into the brachial plexus sheath or the lumbar and thoracic epidural space provide superior postoperative analgesia. Neuraxial techniques improve pulmonary mechanics, and opioids can be administered at much lower doses and with less sedation when compared to other parenteral routes.

16. **What agents can be used for induction and maintenance of general anesthesia?**
All of the standard induction agents can be used safely. Ketamine produces bronchodilation secondary to its sympathomimetic effects by direct antagonism of bronchoconstricting mediators, but secretions increase remarkably. Anecdotal evidence exists of bronchodilating properties from propofol. Intravenous lidocaine given before intubation can help blunt airway reflexes.
All volatile anesthetics are bronchodilators. Desflurane is an airway irritant, although once the patient is intubated this is rarely a problem; it has the advantage of rapid clearance once discontinued.
Nitrous oxide increases the volume and pressure of blebs or bullae, thereby increasing the risk of barotrauma and pneumothorax. In addition, it may increase pulmonary vascular resistance and pulmonary artery pressures. This would be especially deleterious in patients

with coexisting pulmonary hypertension or cor pulmonale. Therefore nitrous oxide should be avoided in patients with COPD.

17. **Discuss the particular concerns regarding muscle relaxation (and reversal) in patients with COPD.**

Atracurium and *d*-tubocurarine produce histamine release and might best be avoided. Succinylcholine also produces histamine release, and the benefits and risks of rapid paralysis and endotracheal intubation must be evaluated when considering its use.

Anticholinesterases (neostigmine and edrophonium) reverse the effects of nondepolarizing relaxants. Theoretically they may precipitate bronchospasm and bronchorrhea secondary to stimulation of postganglionic muscarinic receptors. However, clinically bronchospasm is rarely seen after administration of these agents, possibly because anticholinergic agents (atropine or glycopyrrolate) are concurrently administered.

18. **Discuss the choice of opioids in patients with COPD.**

Opioids blunt airway reflexes and deepen anesthesia. Morphine produces histamine release and should be used with caution. Hydromorphone, fentanyl, sufentanil, and remifentanil do not cause histamine release. Always consider the residual respiratory depressant effects of opioids at the end of surgery.

19. **Define auto-PEEP.**

Air trapping is known as auto-PEEP (positive end-expiratory pressure) and results from "stacking" of breaths when full exhalation is not allowed to occur. Auto-PEEP results in impairment of oxygenation and ventilation and hemodynamic compromise by decreasing preload and increasing pulmonary vascular resistance. Increasing expiratory time reduces the likelihood of auto-PEEP. Increasing the expiratory phase of ventilation and decreasing the respiratory rate can accomplish this.

KEY POINTS: CHRONIC OBSTRUCTIVE PULMONARY DISEASE

1. Patients with a significant reactive (and reversible) component to their lung disease require thorough preoperative preparation, including inhaled β-agonist therapy and possibly steroids.
2. Consider alternatives to general anesthesia in patients with a significant reactive component. An actively wheezing patient is not a good candidate for an elective surgical procedure.
3. *All that wheezes is not asthma.* Also consider mechanical airway obstruction, congestive failure, allergic reaction, pulmonary embolus, pneumothorax, aspiration, and endobronchial intubation.
4. Patients with chronic bronchitis may require antibiotic therapy, inhaled β agonists, and measures to mobilize and reduce sputum before surgery to improve outcome. Smoking cessation is very beneficial in the long term.
5. Patients for planned pulmonary resections absolutely require pulmonary function tests to ensure that more lung is not resected than is compatible with life. Injudicious resections may create a ventilator-dependent patient.

---

20. **Form a differential diagnosis for intraoperative wheezing.**
    - Bronchoconstriction (remember, *all that wheezes is not asthma*)
    - Mechanical obstruction of the endotracheal tube by secretions or kinking
    - Aspiration of gastric contents or of a foreign body (e.g., a dislodged tooth)
    - Endobronchial intubation (most commonly right mainstem intubation)
    - Inadequate anesthesia
    - Pulmonary edema (cardiogenic and noncardiogenic)
    - Pneumothorax
    - Pulmonary embolus

21. **How would you treat intraoperative bronchospasm?**
    - Administer 100% oxygen and manually ventilate, allowing sufficient expiratory time. Identify and correct the underlying conditions as discussed in Question 20.

- Administer therapy:
  - Relieve mechanical obstructions.
  - Increase the volatile anesthetic agents and/or administer intravenous lidocaine, ketamine, or propofol.
  - Administer β-adrenergic agonists: aerosolized via the endotracheal tube (e.g., albuterol), subcutaneously (e.g., terbutaline), or intravenously (e.g., epinephrine or terbutaline).
  - Administer anticholinergic bronchodilators: aerosolized via the endotracheal tube (e.g., ipratropium) or intravenously (e.g., atropine or glycopyrrolate).
  - Intravenous aminophylline and corticosteroids are also suggested therapies.
  - Although controversial, extubation may be beneficial because the endotracheal tube may be a stimulus for bronchoconstriction.

22. **What factors may determine the need for postoperative mechanical ventilation?**
Patients who exhibit a resting $PaCO_2 > 45$ to 50, $FEV_1 < 1$ L, forced vital capacity (FVC) < 50% to 70% of predicted, or $FEV_1/FVC < 50\%$ may require postoperative ventilation, especially for upper abdominal and thoracic surgeries. Consider how well the patient was prepared before surgery, the respiratory rate and work of breathing, the tidal volume and negative inspiratory force generated by the patient, arterial blood gas parameters, and body temperature. Is there residual neuromuscular blockade or effects of anesthetic agents? Is analgesia satisfactory?

23. **Should H_2-receptor antagonists be avoided in patients with COPD?**
H_1-receptor stimulation results in bronchoconstriction, and H_2-receptor stimulation results in bronchodilation. Theoretically H_2-receptor antagonists would result in unopposed H_1-receptor stimulation, causing bronchoconstriction. Many patients with COPD take corticosteroids, have symptoms of gastritis or peptic ulcers, and receive H_2 antagonists. Use of H_2-receptor antagonists should be individualized and the patients observed for adverse side effects.

24. **At the conclusion of surgery, should a patient with COPD be extubated when deeply anesthetized or emerging?**
Perhaps the better question is can the surgical procedure be performed under regional anesthesia, avoiding endotracheal anesthesia altogether? If general anesthesia is required, perhaps a mask anesthetic or use of the laryngeal mask airway would limit the stimulation inherent in endotracheal intubation.

   In an intubated patient with reactive airway disease, airway reflexes may be blunted through use of lidocaine (intravenous or intratracheal) and aerosolized β-adrenergic agonists. Selected patients may be candidates for deep extubation. Patients at risk for aspiration and those with difficult airways are not candidates for deep extubation. Typically deep extubation is accomplished with the patient breathing spontaneously, deeply anesthetized with a volatile agent, with airway reflexes suppressed. Deep extubation is not a 100% guarantee against bronchospasm as the patient awakens further.

SUGGESTED READINGS

Qaseem S, Snow V: Risk assessment for and strategies to reduce perioperative pulmonary complications for patients undergoing noncardiothoracic surgery: a guideline from the American College of Physicians, Ann Intern Med 144:575–580, 2006.

Rabe KF, Wedzicha JA: Controversies in treatment of chronic obstructive pulmonary disease, Lancet 378:1038–1047, 2011.

Stoller JK: Clinical practice. Acute exacerbations of chronic obstructive pulmonary disease, N Engl J Med 346:988–994, 2002.

Sutherland ER, Cherniack RM: Management of chronic obstructive pulmonary disease, N Engl J Med 350:2689–2697, 2004.

Wedzicha JA, Seemungal TA: COPD exacerbations: defining their cause and prevention, Lancet 370:786–796, 2007.

CHAPTER 37

ACUTE RESPIRATORY DISTRESS SYNDROME (ARDS)

James B. Haenel, RRT, and Jeffrey L. Johnson, MD

1. **Is there a difference between acute lung injury (ALI) and acute respiratory distress syndrome (ARDS)?**

   Not really. Historically, these two syndromes were officially classified separately. The North American-European Consensus Committee (NAECC, 1992) on ARDS convened with the goal of providing a clearer and more uniform definition of ALI/ARDS. Two years later, ALI, like ARDS, was defined as an acute inflammatory condition resulting in increased lung permeability. At the time, however, the clinical presentation of ALI and ARDS in terms of timing, etiologies, physiology, and radiographic appearance were considered equivalent. ALI/ARDS is the same syndrome, but the degree of hypoxemia is worse in ARDS; this is reflected in the newer "Berlin" definition (see Box 37-1). Of importance, the degree of the hypoxemia is reflective of disease severity only; it does not predict mortality.

2. **How would you define ARDS?**

   Three clinical definitions are commonly used: the NAECC definition, the Murray Lung Injury Score, and the Berlin definition (Box 37-1). The NAECC definition of ALI/ARDS served as an important benchmark and offers some advantages. For example, it is simple enough for those with limited experience to readily apply. One significant drawback is the NAECC has no reference to the set positive end-expiratory pressure (PEEP) level. This absence of a minimum level of PEEP and other ventilator settings maintains the simplicity of the NAECC definition but makes it too nonspecific. For example, a patient on 5 cm H_2O of PEEP could have a PaO_2/FiO_2 ratio of <200; however, after a recruitment maneuver (RM) using a higher level of PEEP, 5 minutes later that same patient may have a PaO_2/FiO_2 level of >300. The Berlin definition factors this in, by stating that PaO_2/FiO_2 should be measured on ≥5 cm of PEEP, though this is a modest requirement. Additionally, the Berlin definition allows for coexistence of ARDS and high filling pressures, and dispatches the term ALI by describing ARDS as a continuum from moderate to severe.

3. **What are the risk factors for ARDS?**

   Historically, ARDS has been described as being a diffuse inflammatory reaction of the pulmonary parenchyma to a variety of insults. Most classifications of risk factors for ARDS are based on whether the inciting event is either a direct or indirect insult to the lung parenchyma (Table 37-1).

   Stratification of risk factors based on whether ARDS is caused by a pulmonary or extrapulmonary etiology has important implications beyond establishing its epidemiology and incidence. There are identified important mechanical differences in the lungs and chest wall compliance of patients based on whether there is a pulmonary or extrapulmonary cause for the ARDS. ARDS resulting from direct pulmonary disease is associated predominantly with lung tissue consolidation; therefore the response of a stiff lung to an RM with PEEP may be modest at best and carry the risk of overdistention of normal alveoli. In contrast, the lung suffering from an indirect insult demonstrates increased interstitial edema and diffuse alveolar collapse. Application of an RM with PEEP in this situation often results in a salient improvement in lung compliance and oxygenation.

4. **What is the most common cause of ARDS, and what is the mortality rate for ARDS?**

   Severe sepsis is a common risk factor for the development of ARDS. In the 1980s three prospective studies evaluated the risk factors for ARDS, and sepsis was identified as a risk in 43% of the cases. The most common diagnosis associated with ARDS, reported in the

Box 37-1. Definitions of Acute Lung Injury and Acute Respiratory Distress Syndrome (American-European Consensus Conference)

Acute Lung Injury Criteria

Timing: acute

Oxygenation: $PaO_2/FiO_2 \leq 300$ mm Hg (regardless of PEEP)

Chest radiograph bilateral infiltrates on anteroposterior film

Pulmonary artery occlusion pressure: <8 mm Hg or no clinical evidence of left arterial hypertension

ARDS Criteria

Same as acute lung injury except:

Oxygenation: $PaO_2/FiO_2 \leq 200$ mg Hg regardless of PEEP)

Murray Lung Injury Score

Chest Radiograph Score

No alveolar consolidation	0
Alveolar consolidation: 1 quadrant	1
Alveolar consolidation: 2 quadrants	2
Alveolar consolidation: 3 quadrants	3
Alveolar consolidation: 4 quadrants	4

Hypoxemia Score

$PaO_2/FiO_2 \geq 300$	0
PaO_2/FiO_2 225–299	1
PaO_2/FiO_2 175–224	2
PaO_2/FiO_2 100–174	3
PaO_2/FiO_2 100	4

PEEP Score (when ventilated)

PEEP ≥ 5 cm H_2O	0
PEEP 6–8 cm H_2O	1
PEEP 9–11 cm H_2O	2
PEEP 12–14 cm H_2O	3
PEEP ≥ 15 cm H_2O	4

Respiratory System Compliance Score

Compliance ≥ 80 ml/cm H_2O	0
Compliance 60–79 ml/cm H_2O	1
Compliance 40–59 ml/cm H_2O	2
Compliance 20–39 ml/cm H_2O	3
Compliance ≤ 19 ml/cm H_2O	4

The final value is obtained by dividing the aggregate sum by the number of components that were used: no lung injury, 0; mild-to-moderate injury, 1–2.5; severe lung injury (ARDS), 2.5.

Summary of the "Berlin" Definition of ARDS

Factor Description:

Onset: within 1 week of known risk factor

Imaging: bilateral opacities not explained by effusion, collapse, or nodules

Type of pulmonary edema not explained by cardiac failure or fluid overload. If no clinical risk factor identified, objective assessment required

Severity (with PEEP ≥ 5)

Mild: P/F ≤ 300

Moderate: P/F ≤ 200

Severe: P/F ≤ 100

ARDS, Acute respiratory distress syndrome; *FiO₂*, fraction of inspired oxygen; *PaO₂*, arterial oxygen partial pressure; *PEEP*, positive end-expiratory pressure.

Table 37-1. Classification of Inciting Events Associated with ALI/ARDS

DIRECT LUNG INJURY	INDIRECT LUNG INJURY
Aspiration of gastric contents	Sepsis
Pulmonary contusion	Multisystem trauma associated with shock
Diffuse pulmonary infections	Massive transfusion >6 units PRBCs in ≤12 hours
Bacterial	Drug overdose
Fungal	Acute pancreatitis
Viral	Cardiopulmonary bypass (rare)
Pneumocystis	Fat emboli syndrome
Inhalational injury	
Near drowning	

ALI, Acute lung injury; *ARDS*, acute respiratory distress syndrome; *PRBCs*, packed red blood cells.

National Institutes of Health (NIH) Acute Respiratory Distress Syndrome Network (ARDS NET) study, was pneumonia (incidence = approximately 35%); sepsis as an etiology had an incidence of 27%.

A single mortality figure for the broad definition of ARDS might not be appropriate to offer; the definition for this syndrome has varied, and the ARDS-specific mortality varies widely depending on etiology. That being said, three large randomized trials involving over 2000 patients provided consistent mortality data of between 33.9% and 36.3%.

5. **What is the pathogenesis of ARDS?**
Common to all inciting risk factors is an intense inflammatory pulmonary reaction initially targeted at the interstitial and alveolar-capillary membrane. As a result of injury to the alveolar epithelial and endothelial membranes, flooding of the alveolar space with proteinaceous exudate containing vast numbers of neutrophils occurs. This results in severe shunting and altered gas exchange. Attraction of polymorphonuclear leukocytes (PMNs) to the injured lung has been linked to the presence of proinflammatory cytokines, endotoxins, thrombin, complement, and vascular endothelial growth factor. Lung injury and other organ dysfunction may be exacerbated and perpetuated by inappropriate mechanical ventilation, suggesting that a combined biochemical and biophysical injury from alveolar overdistension and shear injury related to repeated opening and closing of distal airways exacerbates parenchymal damage.

6. **Describe the stages of ARDS.**
Regardless of the specific etiology, clinical, radiographic, and histopathologic abnormalities generally progress through three overlapping phases: an acute or exudative phase, a proliferative phase, and finally a fibrotic phase, also referred to as late ARDS. Identifying each phase in a particular patient is complicated and may be influenced by other confounding variables such as episodes of ventilator-associated pneumonia and the harmful effects of mechanical ventilation.
   1. The exudative phase persists for about a week and is characterized clinically by symptoms of respiratory distress (dyspnea and tachypnea), refractory hypoxemia, and patchy bilateral radiographic infiltrates and pathologically by sequestration of neutrophils.
   2. The proliferative phase manifests early in the second week. Clinically lung compliance remains low because of edema and replacement of fibrin and cell debris with collagen within the intraalveolar space. There is persistent hypoxemia and increased alveolar dead space hampering CO_2 elimination. Pulmonary hypertension progressively worsens as the capillary network is destroyed, and intimal proliferation leads to a reduction of the luminal cross-sectional area. Radiographically there are diffuse alveolar infiltrates and air bronchograms on the chest x-ray film. Histologically, there are increased amounts of inflammatory exudate consistent with PMNs and the beginning of fibroblast proliferation within the interstitium and alveoli.
   3. Some time after 10 days, the fibrotic or late phase of ARDS occurs. Clinically, lung compliance is markedly decreased, with static compliance values as low as 10 to 20 cm

Box 37-2. Causes of Acute Noninfectious Lung Diseases

Acute interstitial pneumonia
Acute eosinophilic pneumonia
Acute bronchiolitis obliterans organizing pneumonia
Diffuse alveolar hemorrhage
Acute hypersensitivity pneumonia

H_2O, resulting in increased work of breathing and ventilator dependence. Radiographically the chest x-ray film reveals linear opacities consistent with fibrosis. The histopathologic correlate is progressive scarring of the lungs caused by dramatic increases in collagen levels. Many investigators have used steroids during this late phase of ARDS to attenuate host inflammatory responses.

7. **How do patients who develop ARDS typically present?**
Within 24 hours of an identified risk factor, 80% of patients present with respiratory dysfunction, and within 72 hours the remaining patients progress to signs of respiratory compromise. Most patients will be receiving mechanical ventilation based on physiologic instability from their injury. The extent of hypoxemia (refractory to supplemental O_2) cannot be predicted but may be exacerbated by the patient's baseline pulmonary function, intravascular volume status, adequacy of cardiac output, and severity of the inciting risk factor. Concurrent with worsening of intrapulmonary shunting, the lung compliance is reduced, as evidenced by rising peak alveolar pressures (static plateau pressure). This reflects that the volume of aerated lung is diminished from persistent edema, atelectasis, and consolidation of the diseased lung. It is important to emphasize that the decreased compliance reflects the poor compliance of the lung tissue that is participating in ventilation and not the fluid-filled, consolidated lung. In the nonsedated patient, tachypnea and air hunger with elevated minute ventilation are common. Auscultation of the lungs is surprisingly normal, and, as a rule, volume of secretions aspirated from the artificial airway is minimal.

8. **Do any pulmonary diseases mimic ARDS?**
Based on the current definitions, a number of diffuse noninfectious parenchymal lung diseases can fulfill the criteria for ALI/ARDS (Box 37-2). Most of the patients who meet these criteria are initially diagnosed with ALI/ARDS secondary to pneumonia. Although pneumonia is one of the most prevalent causes for ARDS, an infectious etiology can be found in about 50% of the cases. Patients who present without an obvious risk factor for pneumonia should undergo a sampling of the distal airways, and may even require an open lung biopsy to fully exclude a noninfectious etiology for their lung disease. The misdiagnosis of a patient having a noninfectious cause for the onset of acute pulmonary dysfunction may exclude him or her from receiving appropriate therapy.

9. **Are any drug therapies available to treat ARDS?**
Despite the establishment of an NIH network (ARDS NET) of interactive critical-care treatment groups involved in performing prospective, randomized, controlled, multicenter trials, no effective drug therapy has been identified. Thromboxane synthetase inhibitors, nitric oxide (NO), corticosteroids, surfactant, N-acetylcysteine, inhaled prostacyclin, liquid ventilation, activated protein C, and other agents have also been trialed but with unconvincing success. The only proven therapy for ARDS involves low tidal volume (and low plateau pressure) ventilation. It can be argued that a minimal fluid strategy has also been proven effective, though this produced a modest decrease in intensive care unit (ICU) length of stay with no difference in mortality.

10. **Does that mean that medical therapy has no role in patients with refractory ARDS?**
Because no pharmacologic agent has demonstrated a reduction in mortality rates doesn't mean that an individual patient may not respond favorably to a targeted drug therapy. For example, inhaled NO, once considered a promising therapy because of its ability to provide

selective pulmonary vasodilation and improve ventilation-perfusion mismatch, has not demonstrated improved mortality outcomes. However, if a patient is dying from refractory hypoxemia, trials of inhaled NO have consistently resulted in improved oxygenation and pulmonary hemodynamics in 60% of patients. These benefits are short lived, diminishing over a 24- to 48-hour period, but this bought time may allow for other therapies such as antibiotics to become effective. Similarly, a recent study from ARDS NET pertaining to the safety and efficacy of corticosteroids in persistent ARDS concluded that the routine use of methylprednisolone was not warranted. Nonetheless, to date there have been five trials consisting of 518 patients who have received corticosteroids as part of an ARDS protocol and have demonstrated significant improvements in gas exchange, reduction in markers of inflammation, decreased duration of mechanical ventilation, and decreased number of days spent in the ICU. There is nothing routine about refractory ARDS; therefore decisions regarding advanced pharmacologic therapies must be evaluated in light of the patient's physiologic status.

11. **Is there an optimal fluid strategy in ARDS?**
    Recently the ARDS NET study demonstrated that a conservative fluid management approach that resulted in a negative fluid balance at day 7 (-136 ± 491 ml) versus a liberal fluid strategy (6992 ± 502 ml) resulted in fewer ventilator days, fewer ICU days, and no increase in nonpulmonary organ failures. As an aside, the use of a pulmonary artery catheter when compared to a central venous catheter demonstrated no differences in outcome.

12. **Does mechanical ventilation produce a uniform effect on the lung affected by ARDS?**
    No. While described as a diffuse process, at a regional and microscopic level, the syndrome of ARDS is actually an inhomogeneous pattern of lung consolidation. There are likely to be regions of the lung that are very different. Some zones consist of normal lung; others are partially flooded/potentially recruitable lung regions; others are consolidated, gravity-dependent lung; and areas of hyperinflated lung tissue; finally, some regions may be relatively overdistended with the application of positive pressure. As a consequence of the ongoing structural changes occurring within the lung parenchyma, a ventilator-associated lung injury (VILI) may result from maldistribution of tidal volumes (V_Ts) and high airway pressures exacerbating overdistention of remaining aerated lung.

13. **Can mechanical ventilation hurt the lung affected by ARDS?**
    Yes. Conceptually, there are two types of injuries caused by positive-pressure ventilation: stress and strain. Stress can be thought of as tension on the lung skeleton related to static distention (transpulmonary pressures); higher pressures produce injury by overdistending normally compliant units. Strain can be thought of deformation of lung units through the respiratory cycle, including the potential for repetitive "opening" and "closing" of alveoli. This is related to tidal volumes used and the end-expiratory volume. Of note, since lung units share walls, and one unit may not have the same compliance as its neighbor, strain can result from the interaction of two or more adjacent units. Both stress and strain are thought to potentiate ongoing lung inflammation. Undoubtedly there needs to be a balance between providing a sufficient inspiratory plateau pressure (peak alveolar pressure) while at the same time avoiding insufficient amounts of end-expiratory pressures.

14. **So how should patients with ARDS be ventilated?**
    As a result of mounting evidence for increased morbidity and mortality associated with VILI, clinicians have focused on providing lung protective strategies in patients with ALI/ARDS. Numerous trials have compared the efficacy of a low V_T approach to more traditional V_T. The largest trial was the ARDS NET study involving 861 patients that compared a V_T of 6 ml/kg of predicated body weight to a V_T of 12 ml/kg. Further reduction in V as low as 4 ml/kg was permitted in the low group if end-inspiratory plateau pressures remained >30 cm H_2O, whereas V_T reduction could not occur in the traditional group unless plateau pressures were >50 cm H_2O. Mortality was 39.8% in the traditional V_T group and 31% in the low V_T patients, resulting in an approximately 20% reduction in mortality. In other words, for every 10 patients ventilated with a lung protective approach, one life will be saved.

Table 37-2. Techniques for Performance of Recruitment Maneuvers

CONVENTIONAL VENTILATION	UNCONVENTIONAL MODES	POSITIONING
Sustained inflation/CPAP CPAP of 30–40 cm H_2O PEEP 1. Incremental increases by 2.5–5 cm H_2O until increase in P/F ratio 2. PCV mode: RR 10/min, I:E 1: PIP 20 cm H_2O, increase PEEP to 30–40 cm H_2O for 2 minutes Addition of sighs Consider spontaneous breathing	High-frequency ventilation High-frequency oscillation Airway pressure release ventilation Pressure-control inverse ratio ventilation	Prone ventilation Use reverse Trendelenburg position; maintain for PEEP 12–24 hours Supine position Maintain head of bed at 30 to 45 degrees with frequent turning

CPAP, Continuous positive airway pressure; I:E, inspiratory-to-expiratory ratio; PCV, pressure-control ventilation; PEEP, positive end-expiratory pressure; PIP, peak inspiratory pressure; RR, respiratory rate.

15. **Since low tidal volumes are good, isn't high-frequency oscillation the best bet?**
   While conceptually attractive as a lung protective mode, high-frequency oscillation has proved disappointing in adults. Two trials were reported in 2013: one was stopped early for potential harm in the oscillation group, and the other was completed with no benefit in 30-day mortality.

16. **What is a lung recruitment maneuver? How is it done?**
   Lung recruitment is defined as the application of a prolonged increase in airway pressure, with the goal being reversal of atelectasis; this is followed by the application of sufficient amounts of PEEP to ensure that the lung stays open. Various techniques are available to accomplish recruitment maneuvers (RMs) (Table 37-2). Most RMs are performed on an intermittent basis through manipulation of the mechanical ventilator, whereas some other techniques are continuous.
   Although RMs are commonly accepted as part of a lung protective strategy for ALI/ARDS, there is still much to be learned about their use: which patients will benefit, direct versus indirect lung injury, optimal duration for RM, whether RMs should be applied routinely or only during acute hypoxic events, and whether the baseline PEEP makes a difference in terms of response.

17. **How does prone ventilation improve oxygenation?**
   The primary pulmonary defect based on computed tomographic scans of supine patients with ARDS is the opacification of the gravity-dependent areas of the lung as a result of atelectasis and consolidation. It is clear that alveolar flooding from formation of edema fluid is partially responsible for the atelectasis, but mechanical imbalances caused by cephalic displacement of the diaphragm with positive-pressure ventilation, decreased thoracic and abdominal compliance, increased pleural pressure in dorsal lung regions, and the weight of the heart causing compression of the lower lung regions all act in concert to worsen atelectasis and promote ventilation-perfusion mismatching. Gravity plays only a minor role in perfusion heterogeneity in the lung; therefore the dorsal regions of the lung, regardless of positioning, always receive preferential perfusion. Improvements in oxygenation by using the prone position probably result from:
   - Recruitment of collapsed dorsal lung fields by a redistribution of lung edema to ventral regions.
   - Increased diaphragm motion enhancing ventilation.
   - Elimination of the compressive effects of the heart on the inferior lower lung fields, thus improving regional ventilation.
   - Maintenance of dorsal lung perfusion in the face of improved dorsal ventilation leads to improved ventilation-perfusion matching.

18. Does prone ventilation offer a survival benefit in patients with ARDS?

Since 2001 there have been more than nine randomized prospective trials of prone ventilation in critically ill patients. In 2008 alone, there were four meta-analyses of prone ventilation reporting on approximately 1562 patients. All but two of these trials used some form of lung-protective ventilation strategy. The unwavering findings from all of these reports is that prone ventilation results in a consistent improvement in oxygenation. Whether this translates into improved outcomes remains something of a debate. A recent (2013) large randomized study of the early application of prone ventilation in patients with severe ARDS (defined as P/F < 150) demonstrated a hazard ratio of 0.44 in the prone ventilation group and is likely to increase the enthusiasm for this approach.

KEY POINTS: ADULT RESPIRATORY DISTRESS SYNDROME

1. Historically, sepsis has been identified as the most common risk factor for ARDS.
2. VILI is thought to be caused by two mechanisms:
   - Stress: overdistention of normal aerated lung by using high tidal volumes/pressures
   - Strain: repetitive alveolar collapse that occurs as a result of ventilating the lungs with low end-expiratory volumes and pressures
3. Mechanical ventilation settings for patients with ARDS or ALI include tidal volume at 6 to 8 ml/kg of ideal body weight and limiting plateau pressures to <30 cm H_2O.
4. PEEP should be adjusted to prevent end-expiratory collapse.
5. High-frequency oscillation appears ineffective in adults.

SUGGESTED READINGS

Calfee CS, Matthay MA: Nonventilatory treatments for acute lung injury and ARDS, Chest 131:913–920, 2007.

Ferguson NA, Frutos-Vivar F, Esteban A, et al: Acute respiratory distress syndrome: underrecognition by clinicians and diagnostic accuracy of three clinical definitions, Crit Care Med 33:2228–2234, 2005.

Ferguson ND, Fan E, Camporata L, et al: The Berlin definition of ARDS: an expanded rationale, justification and supplementary material, Intensive Care Med 38:1573–1582, 2012.

Ferguson ND, Cook DJ, Guyatt GH, et al: High-frequency oscillation in early acute respiratory distress syndrome, N Engl J Med 368:795–805, 2013.

Guerin C, Reignier J, Richard J-C, et al: Prone positioning in severe acute respiratory distress syndrome, N Engl J Med 368:2159–2168, 2013.

Matthay MA, Ware L, Zimmerman G: The acute respiratory distress syndrome, J Clin Invest 122:2731–2740, 2012.

Meduri GM, Marik PE, Chrousos GP, et al: Steroid treatment in ARDS: a critical appraisal of the ARDS network trial and the recent literature, Intensive Care Med 34:61–69, 2008.

Shuster KM, Alouidor R, Barquist ES: Nonventilatory interventions in the acute respiratory distress syndrome, J Intensive Care Med 23:19–33, 2008.

CHAPTER 38

PULMONARY HYPERTENSION

Benjamin Atwood, MD, and Nathaen Weitzel, MD

1. **Define pulmonary hypertension and pulmonary artery hypertension.**
   - Pulmonary hypertension (PH) refers to a mean pulmonary arterial pressure (>25 mm Hg) from any cause.
   - Pulmonary artery hypertension (World Health Organization (WHO) Group 1) was previously referred to as primary pulmonary hypertension. Pulmonary artery hypertension (PAH) is defined by mean pulmonary artery pressure (PAP) >25 mm Hg at rest with a pulmonary capillary wedge pressure (PCWP), left atrial pressure or left ventricular end-diastolic pressure less than or equal to 15 mm Hg, and pulmonary vascular resistance (PVR) greater than 3 Wood units.[1]

2. **List the WHO classifications of pulmonary hypertension.**
   WHO Group Number:
   1. Pulmonary arterial hypertension (PAH)
      a. Idiopathic (IPAH): formally called "primary pulmonary hypertension"
      b. Familial (FPAH)
      c. Associated (APAH): APAH is secondary or associated with connective tissue disorders, congenital systemic to pulmonary shunts, portal hypertension, HIV infection, drugs, toxins, metabolic disorders including thyroid disorders, glycogen storage disease, Gaucher disease, hereditary hemorrhagic telangiectasia, hemoglobinopathies, chronic myeloproliferative disorders, splenectomy, chronic hemolytic anemia
      d. Associated with significant venous or capillary involvement
      e. Persistent PH of the newborn
   2. PH with left-sided heart disease (left atrial, ventricular systolic or diastolic dysfunction, aortic or mitral valvular disease, restrictive cardiomyopathy, constrictive pericarditis, left atrial myxoma)
   3. PH associated with lung diseases (chronic obstructive pulmonary disease [COPD], interstitial lung disease, obstructive sleep apnea, alveolar hypoventilation disorders, chronic high altitude disease)
   4. PH due to chronic thromboembolism disease: thrombotic pulmonary embolism, tumor, infection
   5. Miscellaneous: myeloproliferative disorders, sarcoidosis, histiocytosis X, lymphangiomatosis, exterior compression of pulmonary, sickle cell disease[1]

3. **How is pulmonary vascular resistance calculated, and what are normal values?**

$$PVR \, (dyne \times sec/cm^5) = (80 \times (PAP - PCW)/CO)$$

   Pulmonary capillary wedge (PCW) is equal to the left atrial pressure. Cardiac output (CO) is often substituted for pulmonary blood flow, although intracardiac and other shunts make these unequal, and thus need to be accounted for if present. Normal PVR is 1.1 to 1.4 Woods units, or about 90 to 120 dynes/sec/cm⁻⁵. (A Woods unit is 240 dynes/sec/cm⁻⁵.) A PVR greater than 300 dynes/sec/cm⁻⁵ is indicative of PH.

4. **What is cor pulmonale?**
   Cor pulmonale is right ventricular (RV) failure as a result of elevated PAP.

5. **What is Eisenmenger syndrome?**
   Eisenmenger syndrome is chronic left-to-right shunt that induces PAH from remodeling and eventually reverse of shunt flow. Also, it is seen in arterial or ventricular septal defects, patent ductus arteriosus, or truncus arteriosis. Eisenmenger syndrome implies a fixed PVR.

6. **What is hypoxic pulmonary vasoconstriction?**

    Hypoxic pulmonary vasoconstriction (HPV) is when a segment of the lung is not well oxygenated, leading to vasoconstriction of affected pulmonary vessels. HPV serves to optimize ventilation-perfusion (V/Q) matching by shunting blood flow to more oxygenated areas of the lung. This is the opposite of what happens in tissue elsewhere in the body, which is vasodilated if hypoxic. HPV reduces intrapulmonary shunt and resulting hypoxemia of blood exiting the lung into the right atrium. PAP increases when many lung segments vasoconstrict because of HPV.

7. **Discuss the pathophysiology and natural history of pulmonary hypertension.**

    Endothelial cell injury leads to imbalances between vasodilator and vasopressor molecules. Reductions in the endogenous vasodilators nitric oxide (NO) and prostacyclin (PGI_2) are noted, whereas the vasoconstrictors thromboxane and endothelin are increased. But vasoconstriction appears to be only part of the answer because thrombosis, inflammation, free radical generation, and smooth muscle hyperplasia are also common features noted in PH. Vascular remodeling is a prominent feature of PH.

    The pulmonary circulation has high flow and low resistance. Changes in CO, airway pressure, and gravity affect the pulmonary circulation more than the systemic circulation. The right ventricle is thin walled and accommodates changes in volume better than changes in pressure. To accommodate increases in flow such as during exercise, unopened vessels are recruited, patent vessels distended, and PVR may decrease. Normal adaptive mechanisms can accommodate a threefold to fivefold increase in flow without significant increases in PAPs.

    Early in the evolution of PH, the pressure overload results in hypertrophy of the right ventricle without significant changes in CO or RV filling pressures, either at rest or during exercise. As the disease progresses, the vessel walls thicken and smooth muscle cells proliferate. Vessels become less distensible, and the actual cross-sectional area of the pulmonary circulation decreases. CO eventually declines despite modest increases in right ventricular end-diastolic pressure (RVEDP). Mechanisms for enhancing contractility are few for the right ventricle. RV failure (RV ejection fraction below 45%) worsens and patients become symptomatic even at rest. RV myocardial blood flow becomes compromised. Tricuspid regurgitation develops secondary to right ventricle distention and worsening failure. In addition, LV filling may be compromised by excessive septal incursion into the left ventricle, with a resultant decrease in CO.

    Survival rates of 1, 3, and 5 years for patients with idiopathic pulmonary hypertension are 68%, 48%, and 34%, respectively.[2]

8. **What symptoms suggest pulmonary hypertension?**
    - Dyspnea
    - Angina (50% of patients)
    - Fatigue (20% of patients)
    - Weakness
    - Syncope

9. **What signs suggest pulmonary hypertension?**

    Cyanosis, clubbing, peripheral venous insufficiency, edema, rales, hepatomegaly, ascites, increase in the pulmonic component of S2 (pulmonic valve closure), RV S3 or S4 heart sound (RV hypertrophy), holosystolic murmur louder with inspiration (tricuspid regurgitation), RV heave, jugular V waves (tricuspid regurgitation), jugular A waves (decreased right ventricle compliance).

10. **What are some electrocardiographic and radiologic features of the disease?**

    The electrocardiogram commonly shows right axis deviation, RV hypertrophy (tall R waves in V1-V3), RV strain (T-wave inversion in V1-V3), S wave in V6, and enlarged P waves in II, III, and aVF. Arrhythmias, such as atrial fibrillation, are problematic because the right ventricle loses atrial kick.

    Abnormalities on chest radiographs include prominence of the right ventricle, right atrium, increased right-sided heart border and the hilar pulmonary artery trunk, rapid tapering of vascular markings, a hyperlucent lung periphery, peripheral hypovascularity, and decrease in the retrosternal air space.

11. **What additional diagnostic tests are available for evaluating pulmonary hypertension? What results may be expected?**
    Lung perfusion scans are important in patients when thromboembolic disease is suspected, and typically demonstrate segmental defects in patients with thromboemboli.
    Right-sided heart catheterization is the gold standard for confirming the diagnosis of PH because it directly measures the pressure. It is usually reserved until advanced therapy is needed. An elevated wedge pressure is an indication for further testing to rule out left-sided heart pathology as a cause of PH. Vasoreactivity tests can be performed during right-sided heart catheterization to determine which drug therapies are effective.

12. **What are transesophageal echo signs of pulmonary hypertension?**
    Echocardiographic features of PH include RV dilation and/or hypokinesis, small LV dimension, abnormal septal motion, thickened interventricular septum, RV pressure overload (paradoxical bulging/flattening of septum into LV, RV hypertrophy), RA dilation, and tricuspid regurgitation (TR) secondary to RV dilation (not intrinsic tricuspid velocity [TV] abnormality).

13. **How do you calculate PAP with transesophageal echocardiography?**
    See Figure 38-1 and Figure 38-2.
    - PASP = $(4 \times [TRV]^2) + RA$ (derived from the Bernoulli equation: $P = 4[V^2] + R$)
    - PASP (pulmonary artery systolic pressure) is the same as RVSP (right ventricular systolic pressure). PASP > 50 means PH is likely.
    - TRV = tricuspid regurgitant jet velocity
    - RAP = right atrial pressure (either estimated or taken from direct hemodynamic measurements)
    - This method cannot be used if there is no regurgitant jet detected.

14. **What are possible treatments for PH (WHO Group 1–5)?**
    Treatment depends on the cause of PH. Treatment for PAH (WHO Group 1) is different from treatment of PH with an underlying cause. Below are examples of treatments considered for all WHO groups.

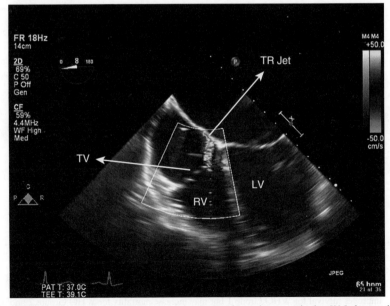

Figure 38-1. Mid-esophageal four-chamber view with color Doppler on the tricuspid valve. *LV*, Left ventricle; *RV*, right ventricle; *TR Jet*, tricuspid regurgitant jet; *TV*, tricuspid valve.

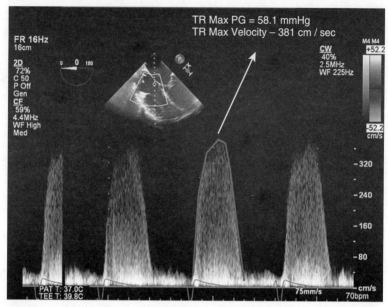

Figure 38-2. Continuous wave Doppler tracing of tricuspid regurgitant (TR) jet. To calculate the systolic pulmonary artery pressure (PAP), use the Bernoulli equation $(PAP = (4 \times [TRV]^2) + RAP)$. In this example, convert the 381 cm/s to 3.81 m/s and use this value for the velocity. Assuming a normal right atrial pressure (RAP) of 10 mm Hg, the calculated PAP would be 68 mm Hg.

Anticoagulation is controversial for PH. There are several retrospective studies showing some survival benefit. Anticoagulation is also used more commonly used in patients with drug-induced PH or thromboembolic PH (WHO Group 4).[3,4]

Diuretics are considered for symptomatic control of RV failure, hepatic congestion, and peripheral edema in patients with PH (WHO Groups 1–5). However, excessive diuresis may decrease RV preload and CO.

Cardiac glycosides (digoxin) are used when there are signs of RV failure and in patients who have developed atrial arrhythmias (e.g., multifocal atrial tachycardia, atrial fibrillation, or atrial flutter). Serum electrolytes must be closely followed when digoxin is administered to a patient on diuretics.

15. **Discuss therapies for patients suffering from PAH (WHO Group 1).**
    There is no treatment for the underlying cause of PAH (WHO Group 1) so therapies are focused on dilating the pulmonary artery. Patients often undergo right-sided heart catheter vasoreactivity tests to assess for responsiveness of potential treatments. Therapies tested include calcium channel blockers, epoprostenol, and NO. If patients do not respond to those, then they may be given a trial of endothelin receptor antagonists (bosentan or ambrisentan) or phosphodiesterase-5 inhibitors (sildenafil, tadalafil, or vardenafil).

16. **Discuss therapies for patients suffering from pulmonary hypertension in WHO Groups 2 through 5.**
    In pulmonary hypertension (WHO Groups 2–5), therapy is first directed at the underlying cause to prevent progression of PH. Therapies studied that improve PAH (WHO Group 1) are not always beneficial for PH from other known causes. For example, epoprostenol improves survival for WHO Group 1 but may increase mortality for WHO Groups 2 and 3 by causing V/Q mismatch, worsening left-sided heart failure, increased hypoxemia, or pulmonary edema.[5]

- WHO Group 2—Medical and surgical treatment of underlying left-sided heart disease is helpful to prevent worsening PH (e.g., mitral valve repair).
- WHO Group 3—In patients with severe COPD causing PH, oxygen therapy to raise PaO_2 is correlated with improved survival. It is administered to maintain oxygen saturation greater than 90%.[6]
- WHO Group 4—Treatment includes anticoagulation and surgical thromboendarterectomy from thromboembolic occlusion of pulmonary vasculature.
- WHO Group 5—Treat underlying causes.

17. What are some surgical therapies for patients suffering from pulmonary hypertension?

- Thromboendarterectomy
- Atrial septostomy: Creation of right-to-left interatrial shunt that relieves right-sided heart filling pressures. Creating a shunt decreases systemic arterial saturation but improves CO and oxygen delivery. It is reserved for treating critically ill PAH patients and is often a bridge to transplant. However, it is associated with high morbidity and mortality.[7]
- Right ventricular assist device: Various models of assist devices can be used in RV failure and should be considered a bridge to transplant. There are no mechanical support devices approved for destination therapy in right-sided heart failure as of early 2014.
- Extracorporeal membrane oxygenation (ECMO): A bridge to transplant[8]
- Bilateral lung or heart-lung transplantation is the final treatment option for selected patients with PH. Three-year survival is approximately 50%.[9]

18. Describe calcium channel blocker (CCB) use in PAH.

Examples of CCBs include nifedipine, diltiazem, and amlodipine. Some patients with PAH respond with PA vasodilation in response to CCB in right-sided heart catheterization vasoreactivity tests. Those patients tend to have long-term functional improvement and survival in observational studies, but no randomized trials have compared outcomes. Some potential side effects include systemic hypotension and worsening hypoxemia from blunting of HPV and worsening V/Q mismatch.[10]

19. What are endothelin receptor antagonists?

ET-1 is a vasoconstrictor and causes pulmonary artery vasoconstriction. Common endothelin receptor antagonists include bosentan and ambrisentan. Endothelin receptor antagonists have been shown to improve symptoms of PH but have not been proven to decrease mortality. Adverse effects include hepatotoxicity and peripheral edema.[11,12]

20. What are prostanoids and their therapeutic counterparts?

Patients with PAH have low levels of prostacyclin synthase and prostacyclin. Prostacyclin is a strong vasodilator, and decreased levels cause decreased vasodilation. Prostacyclin also has antiproliferative effects.

A prostanoid (synthetic prostacyclin analog) acts like prostacyclin and causes vasodilation in the pulmonary artery and prevents platelet aggregation. Examples of prostanoids include epoprostenol, treprostinil, beraprost, and iloprost. They have been shown to decrease PAP and increase CO. Prostanoids can be inhaled or administered intravenously, subcutaneously, or enterally. Intravenous administration causes more systemic vasodilation and V/Q mismatch than does the inhalational route. For this reason, the inhalational route is generally preferred in the operating room and the intensive care unit.

Epoprostenol is the most studied and commonly used prostanoid. When administered by continuous intravenous infusion, epoprostenol (PGI_2) has a half-life of 2 to 3 minutes. Intravenous prostanoids lack pulmonary selectivity. It can cause systemic hypotension and decreased RV coronary perfusion. Epoprostenol has been shown to prolong survival and improve functional status in patients with PAH (WHO Group 1).[13] Epoprostenol may cause increased mortality in PH WHO Groups 2 and 3. It can cause increased pulmonary venous hypertension, inhibit HPV, and cause V/Q mismatch.[14]

21. What are phosphodiesterase-5 inhibitors?

NO activates guanylate cyclase to make cGMP in smooth muscle. Next, cGMP causes vasodilation. The enzyme PDE-5 degrades cGMP, which causes vasoconstriction. The

PDE-5 inhibitors are orally administered vasodilators that potentiate the effect of NO. Currently available PDE inhibitors include sildenafil, tadalafil, and vardenafil. They are synergistic when used in conjunction with NO or prostanoids. PDE-5 inhibitors have not been shown to affect mortality but do improve the functional status of patients with PAH.[12]

22. **How should a patient with pulmonary hypertension be monitored intraoperatively?**
Intraarterial pressure monitoring is commonly used for patients with moderate to severe PH. It allows beat-to-beat assessment of blood pressure and allows frequent blood gas analysis. Arterial pulse pressure variation (also know as "delta down") can assess volume status, although it has not been validated in PH.[15]

Pulmonary artery catheters directly monitor PAP and right atrial pressure. They allow indirect assessment of the LV by measuring wedge pressures. PA catheters help in differentiating causes of systemic hypotension when PH is present. Patients with PH are at increased risk for PA rupture from PA catheters, and Eisenmenger patients are at even higher risk of rupture. Many consider PAC use in patients with Eisenmenger syndrome to be contraindicated.

Transesophageal echocardiography (TEE) is useful in assessing volume status, LV and RV performance, valvular regurgitation, and early detection of segmental wall motion abnormalities secondary to myocardial ischemia. This should be considered the monitor of choice when using a general anesthetic.

23. **How do you manage systemic hypotension with pulmonary hypertension using a PA catheter?**
   - Decreased SVR (increased CO, normal CVP, normal or decreased PCWP, normal or increased PAP): Treat the cause of decreased SVR, vasopressors, volume.
   - Decrease RV preload (decreased CO, decreased CVP, decreased PCWP, decreased PAP, normal or increased SVR): Treatment is volume.
   - Increased PVR (decreased CO, increased CVP, decreased PCWP, normal or increased PAP): Treat cause of increased PVR (e.g., acidosis, hypercarbia, hypoxia) and pulmonary vasodilators.
   - Decreased RV contractility (decreased CO, increased CVP, normal PCWP, increased SVR): Reverse cause of decreased contractility and inotropes.

24. **Why does the difference between right and left ventricular (LV) pressure matter?**
High RV pressure can cause shifting of the intraventricular septum into the LV and decrease CO. Unlike the left ventricle, coronary perfusion to the right ventricle occurs during systole and diastole under normal conditions. As RVEDP increases, perfusion from coronary arteries during diastole decreases, causing further RV failure and increasing pressure. Thus, too much preload could be detrimental in PH.[16]

25. **What is the potential morbidity and mortality for noncardiac surgery on patients with PH?**
   - Mortality (1%-10%)
   - Morbidity (15%-42%)
   - Postoperative respiratory failure (7%-28%)
   - Heart failure (10%-13%)
   - Hemodynamic instability (8%)
   - Dysrhythmias (12%)
   - Renal insufficiency (7%)
   - Sepsis (7%-10%)
   - Ischemia/myocardial infarction (4%)
   - Delayed tracheal extubation (8%-21%)
   - Longer ICU/hospital stay[17]

26. **What risk factors predict major complication?**
   - Elevated right atrial pressure >7 mm Hg
   - History of PE
   - NYHA/WHO functional capacity ≥2

- ECHO: RVH, RVMPI > 0.75 (right ventricular myocardial performance index)
- RVSP/SBP ratio > 0.66
- 6-min walking distance <399 m at the last preoperative assessment
- Perioperative use of vasopressors
- Need for emergency surgery
- History of CAD
- PASP > 70 mm Hg
- >3 hr general anesthesia[18,19]

27. **What intraoperative measures may decrease pulmonary hypertension?**
- Patients on chronic PH medication should take their PH medication up to and including the day of surgery. Prostaglandin infusions must be continued intraoperatively.
- Avoid hypoxia, hypercarbia, and acidosis. In contrast to systemic vessels, pulmonary vessels constrict with hypoxia, hypercarbia, and acidosis. Hypoxic pulmonary vasoconstriction (HPV) optimizes ventilation and flow in the lungs but increases PAP.
- Assess myocardial performance; increasing PA pressures may be secondary to a failing LV. In the setting of a failing LV, supportive measures for optimizing myocardial oxygen supply and demand should be employed, such as reducing heart rate, increasing the diastolic pressure, and providing coronary vasodilation if ischemia is suspected.
- Inotropic drugs such as milrinone or dobutamine can improve contractility, provide moderate pulmonary vasodilation, and improve CO. The effects of acidosis are worse in the presence of hypoxemia. Moderate hyperventilation (a $PaCO_2$ of about 30 mm Hg) is suggested.
- Ensure adequate preload. Patients with PAH have a fixed afterload and are more preload dependent. However, RV volume overload can shift the intraventricular septum into the left ventricle and decrease CO.
- Avoid spinal anesthesia because it can cause a sudden decrease in SVR and preload.
- Catecholamine release will increase PA pressure, so adequate depth of anesthesia is needed.
- If systemic hypotension and coronary perfusion are problematic, consider vasopressin because it does not increase PVR like phenylephrine. Norepinephrine increases SVR more than PVR so it promotes RV coronary perfusion.
- Consider the use of direct-acting pulmonary vasodilators such as NO and epoprostenol for PAH.

28. **What effect does positive end-expiratory pressure (PEEP) have in PH?**
Recruitment maneuvers decrease atelectasis and improve V/Q matching. However, high levels of PEEP may constrict blood vessels in well-ventilated areas of the lungs, causing increased shunting and decreased PaO_2. Increasing PEEP causes increased intrathoracic pressure and decreases RV preload by decreasing venous return. It also increases RV afterload, which can exacerbate PH. Increasing FiO_2 may be better than high PEEP to improve PaO_2 in patients with PAH.

29. **Discuss the effect of volatile anesthetics and NO on the pulmonary pressure.**
Volatile anesthetics (isoflurane, desflurane, sevoflurane) cause vasodilation and decreased PAP. High concentrations of volatiles can cause V/Q mismatch by blunting HPV and can lead to hypoxemia. Volatile anesthetics should be titrated carefully since impaired RV function is a risk with higher concentrations. NO can increase PVR because of worsening hypoxemia.[20]

30. **What patient and surgical factors should be considered preoperatively?**
- General: risks and benefits of surgery, anesthetic technique, potential for fluid shifts, potential for hypoxia, hypercarbia, acidosis
- Severity of PH: history and physical exam, ECG, 6-min walk test (6MWT), echocardiography, right-sided heart catheterization (the "gold standard")
- Medication management: Discontinue PH anticoagulation if indicated. Bridge anticoagulation if taking for history of DVT, atrial fibrillation, artificial valves, etc. Continue home medical therapy for PH up to time of surgery. Consider NO or epoprostenol for intraoperative management.

31. **What are the effects of intravenous anesthetics on PAP?**
    - Etomidate does not change SVR, PVR, or contractility, so it is often used for patients with PH. Etomidate is associated with adrenal suppression and must be used with caution.
    - Propofol infusions have been shown to decrease PVR, SVR, and contractility.
    - Opioids do not have a direct vasodilator effect but may attenuate the vasoconstrictor effect of noxious pain stimuli, preventing increased PAP. Respiratory depression can lead to hypercapnia and cause increased PAP in spontaneously breathing patients.
    - Ketamine increases PVR and is not ideal for PH. In children with intracardiac shunts, ketamine may prevent reversal of left-to-right shunts because it increases systemic vascular resistance to a greater extent than PVR.[21]

32. **Is neuraxial anesthesia an option?**
    Epidural anesthesia has been used safely in patients with PH. Acute changes in SVR associated with spinal anesthesia suggest that epidural anesthesia is preferred. Invasive monitoring is still suggested. Loss of cardioaccelerator fibers from T1-T4 may result in undesirable bradycardia. Ensure adequate preload prior to neuraxial anesthesia and have medications to treat acute decreases in SVR or heart rate.
    Many PH patients take anticoagulation medications so this must be taken into account when performing regional anesthesia. Regional anesthesia is also useful as an adjunct for postoperative pain control and avoids use of narcotics.

33. **Discuss the advantages and disadvantages of the intravenous nitrovasodilators.**
    Commonly used nitrovasodilators include nitroglycerin and sodium nitroprusside. Nitroglycerin has the advantage of providing coronary vasodilation. Nitroglycerin may excessively decrease preload because it is primarily a venodilator. Nitroglycerin infusions are started at 1 mcg/kg/min. Venodilation may become excessive above 3 mcg/kg/min, causing decreased preload and requiring intravenous fluid augmentation.
    Sodium nitroprusside (SNP) is principally an arterial vasodilator. Infusions begin at 0.5 to 1 mcg/kg/min and are carefully adjusted upward to effect. SNP is extremely effective at afterload reduction. Despite its potency and potential for creating excessive hypotension, SNP is safe for short-term use. Long-term use is associated with tachyphylaxis and the potential for cyanide toxicity.
    Nitroglycerin and nitroprusside are nonselective and also decrease SVR. They nonselectively dilate pulmonary blood vessels and cause V/Q mismatch. Avoid nitroprusside and nitroglycerine on patients taking sildenafil as it can cause severe hypotension.

34. **Discuss the properties of nitric oxide (NO).**
    NO is a small molecule produced by vascular endothelium. Formed from the action of NO synthetase on arginine, NO crosses into vascular smooth muscle and stimulates guanylate cyclase. Subsequently cGMP produces smooth muscle relaxation and vasodilation.
    NO is administered by inhalation and crosses the alveolar membrane to the vascular endothelium, producing smooth muscle relaxation. But when it crosses into the circulation, it is rapidly bound to hemoglobin (with an affinity 1500 times greater than carbon monoxide) and deactivated; thus it has no systemic vasodilator effect. Since it is only delivered to ventilated alveoli, it increases blood to those areas and improves V/Q matching. Dosage ranges can be quite wide, but 20 to 40 parts per million is not an atypical dose.
    Deactivation on entering the circulation also limits the effectiveness of NO to the period in which it is administered by inhalation. Because storage in oxygen produces toxic higher oxides of nitrogen, especially nitrogen dioxide (NO_2), NO is stored in nitrogen and blended with ventilator gases immediately before administration. The potential for increased methemoglobin levels during NO administration should also be recognized. It has proinflammatory and antiinflammatory effects, and the significance of this is not fully understood. It also impairs platelet aggregation and adhesion.

35. **Discuss the therapeutic usefulness and limitations of NO in pulmonary artery hypertension.**
    Cardiopulmonary bypass (CPB) induces pulmonary endothelial injury, probably caused by ischemia-reperfusion injury, although other factors are probably involved as well. Levels of

the vasoconstrictors thromboxane and endothelin are increased, whereas levels of the vasodilators PGI_2 and endogenous NO are decreased. PH coming off of CPB is a predictor of increased mortality and postoperative myocardial infarction. NO has been tested for the treatment of PAH after valve replacement, correction of congenital cardiac defects, and cardiac transplantation. It has also been used as a bridge to lung transplantation.

Numerous neonatal conditions are associated with PAH, including congenital diaphragmatic hernias, congenital heart disease, and persistent PAH of the neonate. NO is used in infants with respiratory distress syndrome.

36. **List potential surgeries that pose the risk of increasing pulmonary hypertension.**
    - Liver transplantation: microembolization and large volume infusion may overwhelm the right side of the heart and cause increased PH.
    - Hip replacement: bone cement implantation syndrome occurs when many small pulmonary embolisms of cement, bone, and air occur during placement of prosthesis.
    - Laparoscopic procedures: inflation of CO_2 can cause hypercapnia, leading to increased PH.

37. **What effect do vasopressors and inotropes have on pulmonary hypertension?**
    The goal is to maintain systemic pressures above pulmonary pressures to ensure coronary artery perfusion to the right ventricle. The right coronary artery supplying the right ventricle occurs during systole and diastole. Loss of the pressure gradient can cause ischemia to the right ventricle and increased RVEDP in a downward spiral.
    Norepinephrine—β_1 and α_1 agonist. An effective vasopressor in acute RV failure, it increases SVR > PVR, and so favors RV perfusion while supporting cardiac output. Causes more pronounced increase in PVR at higher doses >0.5 mcg/kg/min in animal studies.
    Phenylephrine—α_1 agonist. Increases PVR causing increased RV afterload.
    Vasopressin—vasopressinergic V1 receptor agonist. Increases SVR with no change in PVR decreasing PVR/SVR ratio. Vasopressin is useful in vasodilatory shock with PH.
    Dopamine—increases CO without increasing PVR. Side effects include tachycardia and arrhythmias that prevent its use in cardiogenic shock.
    Dobutamine—increases contractility and CO while decreasing PVR and SVR. It has less chronotropic effect than dopamine.
    Milrinone—decreases PVR and SVR and increases CO.
    Epinephrine—increases CO. Decreases PVR/SVR ratio.
    Isoproterenol—used as chronotrope after cardiac transplant. It is also associated with arrhythmias.[22]

38. **Why is it recommended to avoid pregnancy in pulmonary hypertension?**
    The mortality rate during pregnancy with PH is 30% to 50%. Avoiding pregnancy is commonly recommended to patients with PH. Pregnancy causes increased circulating volume and CO that is poorly tolerated with PH, especially during the peripartum period up to several months after delivery.[23,24]

KEY POINTS: PULMONARY HYPERTENSION

1. Milrinone is an effective drug in decreasing PAP and increasing CO.
2. Epoprostenol and nitric oxide are effective intraoperative medications to decrease PAP.
3. Hypoxia, hypercarbia, and acidosis all worsen PAP.
4. Vasopressin increases SVR without increasing PAP. Norepinephrine increases SVR > PVR so is also useful in PAH.
5. Nonselective vasodilators (e.g., calcium channel blockers, nitroglycerine, nitroprusside, volatile anesthetics) can cause hypoxemia by blunting HPV.
6. Treatment for PH depends on the underlying cause. Effective treatments for PAH (WHO Group 1) such as epoprostenol may worsen the condition of other WHO groups of PH.
7. Unlike the left ventricle, coronary perfusion to the right ventricle occurs during both systole and diastole. As RVEDP increases, perfusion from coronary arteries during diastole decreases, causing further RV failure.

REFERENCES

1. McLaughlin VV, Archer SL, Badesch DB, et al: ACCF/AHA 2009 expert consensus document on pulmonary hypertension, J Am Coll Cardiol 53:1573–1619, 2009.
2. McLaughlin VV, Presberg KW, Doyle RL, et al: Prognosis of pulmonary arterial hypertension: ACCP evidence-based clinical practice guidelines, Chest 126:78S–92S, 2004.
3. Johnson SR, Mehta S, Granton JT: Anticoagulation in pulmonary arterial hypertension: a qualitative systemic review, Eur Respir J 28:999–1004, 2006.
4. Raja SG, Raja SM: Treating pulmonary arterial hypertension: current treatments and future prospects, Ther Adv Chronic Dis 2:359–370, 2011.
5. Hoeper MM, Barbera JA, Channick RN, et al: Diagnosis, assessment, and treatment of non-pulmonary arterial hypertension pulmonary hypertension, J Am Coll Cardiol 54:S85–S96, 2009.
6. Ashutosh K, Dunsky M: Noninvasive tests for responsiveness of pulmonary hypertension to oxygen. Prediction of survival in patients with chronic obstructive lung disease and cor pulmonale, Chest 92:393–399, 1987.
7. Reichenberger F, Pepke-Zaba J, McNeil K, et al: Atrial septostomy in the treatment of severe pulmonary arterial hypertension, Thorax 58:797–800, 2003.
8. Keogh AM, Mayer E, Benza RL, et al: Interventional and surgical modalities of treatment in pulmonary hypertension, J Am Coll Cardiol 54(1 Suppl):S67–S77, 2009.
9. Yusen RD, Christie JD, Edwards LB, et al: The registry of the International Society for Heart and Lung Transplantation: thirtieth adult lung and heart-lung transplant report—2013, J Heart Lung Transplant 32:965–978, 2013.
10. Sitbon O, Humbert M, Jaïs X, et al: Long-term response to calcium channel blockers in idiopathic pulmonary arterial hypertension, Circulation 111:3105–3111, 2005.
11. Galiè N, Olschewski H, Oudiz RJ, et al: Ambrisentan for the treatment of pulmonary arterial hypertension, Circulation 117:3010–3019, 2008.
12. Ryerson CJ, Nayar S, Swiston JR, et al: Pharmacotherapy in pulmonary arterial hypertension: a systematic review and meta-analysis, Respir Res 11:12, 2010.
13. McLaughlin VV, Shillington A, Rich S: Survival in primary pulmonary hypertension: the impact of epoprostenol therapy, Circulation 106:1477–1482, 2002.
14. Califf RM, Adams KF, McKenna WJ, et al: A randomized controlled trial of epoprostenol therapy for severe congestive heart failure, Am Heart J 134:44–54, 1997.
15. Marik PE, Cavallazzi R, Vasu T, et al: Dynamic changes in arterial waveform derived variables and fluid responsiveness in mechanically ventilated patients, Crit Care Med 37(9):2642–2647, 2009.
16. Minai OA, Yared JP, Kaw R, et al: Perioperative risk and management in patients with pulmonary hypertension, Chest 144(1):329–340, 2013.
17. McGlothlin D, Ivascu N, Heerdt PM: Anesthesia and pulmonary hypertension, Prog Cardiovasc Dis 55(2):199–217, 2012.
18. Meyer S, McLaughlin VV, Seyfarth HJ, et al: Outcomes of noncardiac, nonobstetric surgery in patients with PAH: an international prospective survey, Eur Respir J 41(6):1302–1307, 2013.
19. Ramakrishna G, Sprung J, Ravi BS, et al: Impact of pulmonary hypertension on the outcomes of noncardiac surgery: predictors of perioperative morbidity and mortality, J Am Coll Cardiol 45(10):1691–1699, 2005.
20. Gille J, Seyfarth HJ, Gerlach S, et al: Perioperative anesthesiological management of patients with pulmonary hypertension, Anesthesiol Res Pract 2012:356982, 2012.
21. Williams GD, Maan H, Ramamoorthy C, et al: Perioperative complications in children with pulmonary hypertension undergoing general anesthesia with ketamine, Paediatr Anaesth 20(1):28–37, 2010.
22. Price LC, Wort SJ, Finney SJ, et al: Pulmonary vascular and right ventricular dysfunction in adult critical care: current and emerging options for management, Crit Care 14:R169, 2010.
23. Bédard E, Dimopoulos K, Gatzoulis MA: Has there been any progress made on pregnancy outcomes among women with pulmonary arterial hypertension? Eur Heart J 3:256–265, 2009.
24. Bassily-Marcus AM, Yuan C, Oropello J, et al: Pulmonary hypertension in pregnancy: critical care management, Pulm Med 2012:709407, 2012.

PERIOPERATIVE HEPATIC DYSFUNCTION AND LIVER TRANSPLANTATION

Matthew J. Fiegel, MD

CHAPTER 39

1. What is the normal physiologic function of the liver?

The human liver consists of four anatomic lobes (left, right, caudate, quadrate) and eight surgical lobes (I–VIII). The liver receives approximately 20% to 25% of the cardiac output and contains 10% to 15% of the total blood volume. The portal vein supplies 75% of the blood flow of the liver and 50% of its oxygen requirements.

Almost all plasma proteins are synthesized in the liver. These include albumin, α_1-acid glycoprotein, pseudocholinesterase, and all coagulation factors except factors III, IV, and VIII. The liver is also involved in carbohydrate, lipid, and cholesterol metabolism and bile synthesis. The liver produces 20% of the body's heme. The liver possesses an immune function in that hepatic Kupffer cells filter splanchnic venous blood of bacteria. Last, the liver serves as the main organ of drug metabolism and detoxification. Through three hepatic reactions (phases I, II, and III), drugs are metabolized to a more water-soluble form and excreted in the urine or bile. Phase I reactions use the cytochrome P-450 family of proteins and consist of oxidation, reduction, or hydrolysis. Phase II reactions undergo conjugation with substances such as glucuronic acid and amino acids. In phase III reactions, endogenous hepatic proteins use adenosine triphosphate to excrete various substances. Within the liver, nitrogen-containing compounds are degraded to urea.

2. Review the most common cause of acute parenchymal liver disease.

Viral infection is responsible for the majority of cases of acute hepatitis. Traditionally hepatitis B (HBV) was the most common form of acute viral hepatitis. However, with the advent of the HBV vaccine, hepatitis A and C now account for the majority of viral hepatitis cases worldwide. Epstein-Barr virus and cytomegalovirus also cause acute hepatitis, as do drugs and toxins. Drug-induced liver injury (DILI) can mimic acute viral hepatitis and is most commonly caused by alcohol, antibiotics, and nonsteroidal antiinflammatory drugs. Because it causes an elevation in bilirubin, DILI carries a 10% mortality rate.

3. What is cirrhosis?

Cirrhosis, the most serious sequela of chronic hepatitis, is characterized by diffuse hepatocyte death, causing fibrosis and nodular hepatocellular regeneration. Distortion of hepatic circulation further propagates cellular damage and results in progressive reduction of hepatocytes, eventually manifesting as impaired hepatic function. Hepatic synthetic failure, indicated by a prolonged prothrombin time (PT)/international normalized ratio (INR), hypoalbuminemia, and impaired detoxification mechanisms resulting in encephalopathy, is often termed *end-stage liver disease* (ESLD).

4. Describe the neurologic derangements in patients with cirrhosis.

Central nervous system dysfunction presents as hepatic encephalopathy, ranging from confusion to coma, and may be secondary to increased dietary protein consumption or gastrointestinal (GI) bleeding. Increased ammonia levels do not correlate with the degree of encephalopathy. Treatment consists of a low-protein diet, lactulose, and rifaximin. Fulminant liver failure may present with cerebral edema and increased intracranial pressure, necessitating a stay in the intensive care unit as well as intracranial pressure monitoring.

5. **Review pulmonary changes occur in patients with cirrhosis.**

   Arterial hypoxemia with compensatory hyperventilation may be secondary to atelectasis from ascites/hydrothorax or hepatopulmonary syndrome (HPS). HPS is caused by intrapulmonary arteriovenous (AV) shunting. Portal hypertension and neovascularization are responsible for these AV shunts. The clinical features of HPS include platypnea (shortness of breath while standing) and orthodeoxia (decreased saturation when upright). They are indicative of the ventilation/perfusion mismatching.

   Portal pulmonary hypertension (PPH), defined as a mean pulmonary artery pressure (PAP) greater than 25 mm Hg, is seen in 2% to 4% of patients with cirrhosis. Its etiology is unclear. It is unclear which PPH patients should undergo transplantation because the outcome is unpredictable. Severe PPH (mean PAP > 45) is a contraindication to liver transplantation.

   Vasodilators reduce PAP and prolong survival in some PPH patients. The prostaglandin epoprostenol (Flolan) can reduce PAP when given as a chronic infusion and has been used to bridge patients to transplantation. Nitric oxide inhaled in doses up to 80 ppm acutely reduces PAP in a small number of PPH patients and has been used in the operating room to reduce PAP.

6. **Describe cardiovascular changes in patients with cirrhosis.**

   As liver disease progresses, most patients develop a hyperdynamic circulatory state, characterized by a fall in total peripheral resistance and a compensatory rise in cardiac output. The circulating plasma volume increases in response to vasodilation, and peripheral blood flow is enhanced. Although total body volume is increased, cirrhotic patients possess decreased effective arterial blood volume. The AV oxygen gradient narrows as a result of increased peripheral shunting. Consequently the mixed venous oxygen saturation is higher than normal. The response to vasopressors is decreased. Pulmonary blood flow is increased and can result in increased PAP; pulmonary vascular resistance usually remains normal.

   Coronary artery disease (CAD) with resulting impaired myocardial function (previously thought uncommon in patients with liver disease) may be present, especially when the patient has diabetes. CAD in liver transplant patients older than 50 years occurs in the range of 5% to 27%. Abnormalities in both systolic and diastolic function (cirrhotic cardiomyopathy) may be present and result in an inadequate cardiac output for the degree of vasodilation. This is especially true in patients with a history of alcohol abuse.

7. **What is hepatorenal syndrome (HRS)? How does it differ from acute kidney injury (AKI) in patients with ESLD?**

   Both types of renal failure occur in cirrhotic patients and are characterized by oliguria and increases in serum creatinine. The etiology in both cases is renal hypoperfusion. Differentiation is important because treatment and prognosis vary.

   HRS occurs in cirrhotic patients with portal hypertension and ascites. HRS is defined as a plasma creatinine of >1.5 mg/dl and a urine sodium <10 mmol/L in the absence of other renal disease. The etiology is thought to be renal hypoperfusion resulting from a decrease in vasodilating prostaglandins and profound splanchnic sequestration of blood. HRS exists in two forms, types I and II. Type I progresses rapidly and requires immediate dialysis and liver transplantation. Type II HRS is less severe and responsive to conservative treatments, including terlipressin and a transhepatic intraportal portosystemic shunt (TIPS) procedure.

   AKI is caused by decreased blood flow to the kidneys. It may be the result of hemorrhage (e.g., ruptured varices), splanchnic sequestration of blood, ascites formation, or dehydration. Restoring blood volume typically corrects AKI, but it can progress to acute tubular necrosis (ATN). In patients with ATN, the ability to retain sodium is lost. Urinalysis will show sodium of 50 to 70 mmol/L and frequent tubular casts.

8. **Describe volume assessment and fluid management in patients with HRS.**

   Optimization of renal blood flow by correction of hypovolemia may prevent further renal injury during surgery in these patients. Volume assessment may be difficult since central venous pressures are often elevated despite relative hypovolemia from increased venocaval backpressure from hepatic enlargement or scarring. A trial of volume expansion, often with albumin, should be undertaken as the initial treatment of oliguria. Although immediate improvement occurs in more than one third of patients treated, HRS leads to progressive renal failure unless hepatic function improves.

9. **What are the gastrointestinal and hematologic derangements that occur with cirrhosis?**

GI complications result from portal hypertension (>10 mm Hg). Portal hypertension leads to the development of portosystemic venous collaterals, including esophagogastric varices. Ruptured varices with hemorrhage account for a third of patient mortality.

Hematologic disorders include anemia, thrombocytopenia, and coagulopathy. Anemia is secondary to GI bleeding, malnutrition, and bone marrow suppression. Thrombocytopenia is caused by splenic sequestration, bone marrow depression, and immune-mediated destruction. Coagulopathy is caused by decreased synthesis of clotting factors, accelerated fibrinolysis, and disseminated intravascular coagulation.

10. **Which liver function tests are used to detect hepatic cell damage?**

The enzymes alanine aminotransferase (ALT) and aspartate aminotransferase (AST) are released into the blood as a result of increased membrane permeability or cell necrosis. They tend to rise and fall in parallel. AST is cleared more rapidly from the circulation by the reticuloendothelial system. Their levels are not affected by changes in renal or biliary function. In contrast to ALT, which is mainly confined to hepatocytes, AST is found in heart and skeletal muscle, pancreas, kidney, and red blood cells. Therefore AST lacks specificity as a single diagnostic test. ALT is more specific but less sensitive for detection of hepatic disease.

11. **Describe the laboratory tests used to assess hepatic synthetic function.**

All clotting factors are synthesized by the liver. Factor VIII, although not produced directly by hepatocytes, is synthesized by hepatic endothelial sinusoidal cells. PT/INR indirectly determines the amount of clotting factors available and therefore is used to assess hepatic synthetic function. Vitamin K deficiency, resulting from intestinal malabsorption, as well as anticoagulant therapy, also result in prolonged PT/INR. Once other disease processes have been excluded, PT/INR becomes a sensitive prognostic indicator for acute hepatocellular injury.

Albumin is synthesized in the liver and also reflects hepatic synthetic ability. However, renal and GI losses can affect plasma levels, as do changes in vascular permeability. A reduction in synthesis caused by liver disease may require 20 days to detect because of the long plasma half-life of albumin. Therefore low serum albumin levels are more useful indicators of *chronic* liver disease.

12. **What laboratory tests are used to diagnosis cholestatic liver disease?**

Alkaline phosphatase (ALP), γ-glutamyltransferase (GGT), and 5′-nucleotidase are commonly used to assess biliary tract function. These enzymes are located in biliary epithelial cell membranes. ALP occurs in a wide variety of tissues and is elevated in a number of conditions, including bone disease and pregnancy. The hepatic origin of an elevated ALP is often suggested by the clinical context and simultaneous elevations of GGT and 5′-nucleotidase.

13. **How can laboratory results be used to stratify perioperative risk in patients with cirrhosis?**

In patients with acute liver disease, plasma transaminase concentrations often increase to 10 to 100 times normal. The higher plasma concentrations are associated with greater hepatocellular death and increased mortality. Relatively normal plasma levels can also be found in patients in the earliest and latest stages of acute liver disease, signifying massive cellular necrosis, and are associated with a very high mortality. PT/INR is usually grossly prolonged, reflecting decreased synthetic ability. Albumin levels are often normal. The mortality for intraabdominal surgery in patients with severe acute hepatic disease approaches 100%.

Liver function tests have also been used to predict outcomes following surgery in patients with chronic hepatic impairment. The Child-Turcotte-Pugh scoring system (Table 39-1) was originally used to stratify risk in patients undergoing portosystemic shunting

Table 39-1. Modified Child-Turcotte-Pugh Score

Presentation	POINTS		
	1	2	3
Albumin (g/dl)	>3.5	2.8–3.5	<2.8
International normalized ratio	<1.7	1.7–2.3	>2.3
Bilirubin (mg/dl)	<2	2–3	>3
Ascites	Absent	Moderate	Tense
Encephalopathy	None	Grade I–II	Grade III–IV

Class A = 5–6 points; Class B = 7–9 points; Class C = 10–15 points.

Box 39-1. Model for End-Stage Liver Disease Equation

MELD score = 3.8 × log (e) (bilirubin mg/dl) + 11.2 × log (e) (INR) + 9.6 log (e) (creatinine mg/dl)
MELD <10 = Low perioperative mortality
MELD 10–14 = Moderate perioperative mortality
MELD >14 = Severe perioperative mortality

INR, International normalized ratio; *MELD*, Model for End-Stage Liver Disease.

Table 39-2. Risk Factors for Liver Disease

RISK FACTOR	EXAMPLE
Viral hepatitis	Intravenous drug abuse, transfusion, tattoos, contact with infected person
Drugs	Alcohol, prescription medications (e.g., acetaminophen, haloperidol, tetracycline, isoniazid, hydralazine, captopril, and amiodarone)
Autoimmune disease	Systemic lupus erythematosus, sarcoidosis, mixed connective tissue disorder
Metabolic disease	Hemochromatosis, Wilson disease, cystic fibrosis, α_1-antitrypsin deficiency, glycogen storage disease
Inflammatory bowel disease	Crohn disease and ulcerative colitis/primary sclerosing cholangitis

procedures. Using this method, 30-day mortality rates of 10%, 14% to 31%, and 51% to 80% were identified in Child class A, B, and C patients, respectively, when undergoing noncardiac surgery. More recently the Model for End-Stage Liver Disease (MELD) scoring system was created as a more objective method for assessing 90-day mortality in cirrhotic patients (Box 39-1). When compared to the Child scoring system, the MELD is a superior predictor of perioperative risk in patients with cirrhosis. MELD is calculated using bilirubin, INR, and creatinine. MELD scores of <10, 10 to 14, and <14 correlate well with the Child A, B, and C classifications.

14. **What risk factors for liver disease can be identified by history and physical examination?**
See Table 39-2. Stigmata of chronic liver disease include ascites, hepatosplenomegaly, spider angiomata, caput medusae, and gynecomastia.

Table 39-3. Causes of Unconjugated Bilirubin

CAUSE	EXAMPLE
Hemolysis	Incompatible blood transfusion, arterial/venous bypass circuit, congenital or acquired defects (e.g., autoimmune and drug-induced hemolytic anemia, glucose-6-phosphatase deficiency)
Hematoma resorption	Retroperitoneal or pelvic hematoma
Enzymatic deficiencies	Congenital deficiency (Gilbert syndrome) to complete absence (Crigler-Najjar syndrome) of hepatic uridine diphosphate glucuronyl transferase

Table 39-4. Causes of Biliary Obstruction/Stasis

EXTRAHEPATIC OBSTRUCTION	INTRAHEPATIC OBSTRUCTION
Tumor (bile duct, pancreas, and duodenum)	Primary biliary cirrhosis
Cholecystitis	Drugs (estrogens, anabolic steroids, tetracycline, and valproic acid)
Biliary stricture	Total parenteral nutrition
Ascending cholangitis	Pregnancy
Sclerosing cholangitis	

15. **What is jaundice?**
    Jaundice is a visible yellow or green discoloration, usually first observed in the sclera, caused by elevation of serum bilirubin. Levels of 2 to 2.5 mg/dl (normal 0.5 to 1 mg/dl) result in jaundice. The oxidation of bilirubin to biliverdin gives the green hue often observed.

16. **Distinguish between unconjugated and conjugated hyperbilirubinemia.**
    The distinction is essential to the differential diagnosis of jaundice. Elevations in the serum unconjugated bilirubin fraction are usually related to changes in the turnover of red blood cells and their precursors. Conjugated hyperbilirubinemia always signifies dysfunction of the liver or biliary tract.

17. **List the common causes of unconjugated and conjugated hyperbilirubinemia.**
    Unconjugated hyperbilirubinemia is defined as an elevation of the total serum bilirubin, of which the conjugated fraction does not exceed 15%. The causes are listed in Table 39-3.
    Elevations of conjugated bilirubin are caused by hepatocyte dysfunction and/or intrahepatic or extrahepatic stasis. See Table 39-4.

18. **What are the main causes of hepatocyte injury?**
    See Table 39-5.

19. **Do volatile anesthetics produce hepatic dysfunction?**
    Rarely inhalational agents can cause inflammation or death of hepatocytes due to their metabolic products. Generally the degree of metabolism of the agents is halothane > sevoflurane > enflurane> isoflurane > desflurane. Halothane, the most extensively metabolized agent, is associated with mild hepatic dysfunction in up to 30% of individuals exposed and manifests as asymptomatic transient elevation of hepatic AST and ALT.
    In rare cases an immunologically mediated idiosyncratic reaction occurs in individuals exposed to volatile anesthetics. The formation of immune complexes is related to the extent of metabolism. As halothane has the greatest degree of metabolism associated with it, hepatitis resulting from halothane exposure is the most common. However, given

Table 39-5. Causes of Hepatocyte Injury

CAUSE	EXAMPLE
Infection	Hepatitis A, B, and C; cytomegalovirus; Epstein-Barr virus
Drugs	Acetaminophen, isoniazid, phenytoin, hydralazine, α-methyldopa, sulfasalazine
Sepsis	Pneumonia
Total parenteral nutrition (TPN)	Abnormal liver function tests in 68%–93% of patients given TPN for longer than 2 weeks
Hypoxemia	Lower arterial oxygen or interference with peripheral use as in cyanide and carbon monoxide poisoning
Ischemia	Increased venous pressure (e.g., congestive heart failure, pulmonary embolus, and positive-pressure ventilation) Decreased arterial pressure (e.g., hypovolemia, vasopressors, and aortic cross-clamp)

that halothane use is now rare in the United States, this problem is not likely to be encountered.

20. **Do inhalational agents alter hepatic blood flow?**
These agents dilate the hepatic artery and preportal blood vessels, decreasing mean hepatic artery pressure and increasing splanchnic pooling. Portal flow decreases. Overall, the result is suboptimal hepatic perfusion. However, at levels below 1 minimum alveolar concentration (MAC), isoflurane, sevoflurane, and desflurane only minimally decrease hepatic blood flow. In addition, autoregulation of the hepatic artery is abolished, and blood flow becomes pressure dependent. This is usually tolerated well in patients with normal hepatic function since these drugs also decrease metabolic demand. Patients with hepatic disease are more susceptible to injury secondary to preexisting impaired perfusion and therefore should be anesthetized at levels below 1 MAC.

21. **What adjustment in IV anesthetics should be made in a patient with liver disease?**
The induction agents propofol, etomidate, and ketamine possess a high hepatic extraction ratio, and their pharmacokinetic profile is relatively unchanged in mild to moderate cirrhosis. With severe hypoalbuminemia, an exaggerated induction response can be seen with thiopental. Although pseudocholinesterase levels are decreased in patients with liver disease, the clinical prolongation of succinylcholine is not significant. Intermediate-acting steroidal nondepolarizing muscle relaxants such as vecuronium and rocuronium display a prolonged effect in patients with cirrhosis. The prolonged duration of these muscle relaxants is accentuated with repeated dosing. Benzyl-isoquinoline relaxants such as atracurium and cisatracurium undergo organ-independent elimination, and their duration is not affected by liver disease.
Benzodiazepines metabolized by phase I oxidative reactions such as midazolam and diazepam have a prolonged duration of action. Lorazepam, cleared by phase II glucuronidation, undergoes normal metabolism. All benzodiazepines should be dosed judiciously in patients with liver disease.
All opioids, with the exception of remifentanil, are metabolized in the liver. Morphine and meperidine have a prolonged half-life in patients with liver disease and can precipitate hepatic encephalopathy. Fentanyl, although completely metabolized by the liver, does not have a prolonged clinical effect in cirrhosis. Therefore fentanyl and remifentanil are the opioids of choice in liver disease.

22. **What are the preoperative management goals in a patient with liver disease?**
The type and severity of liver disease should be determined. Patients with acute hepatitis or Child type C (MELD > 14) cirrhosis should have elective surgeries cancelled. A complete

organ system review should be performed, specifically looking for encephalopathy, ascites, portal hypertension, and renal insufficiency. A complete laboratory evaluation should be performed, including transaminases, bilirubin, albumin, basic metabolic profile, complete blood count with platelets, and a coagulation profile. For major surgery, coagulopathy should be corrected to an INR < 1.5, platelets corrected to >100 × 10^9, and fibrinogen to >100 mg/dl. A thromboelastogram may be useful in guiding component therapy when correcting a preexisting coagulopathy.

23. **What are the intraoperative management goals in a patient with liver disease?**
Preservation of hepatic blood flow and existing hepatic function are key. Hypoxemia, hemorrhage, and hypotension may all reduce hepatic blood flow; thus these should be avoided when possible. Drug selection and dosing should be judicious. The operating room should be warmed and a warming/rapid infusion device available. Consider regional anesthesia if appropriate.

24. **Describe some indications and contraindications for liver transplantation.**
Indications for liver transplantation include ESLD from hepatocellular, cholestatic, or polycystic disease. Some nonresectable hepatic malignancies, metabolic liver diseases, and fulminant hepatic failure are indications (Table 39-6). Over time, relative and absolute contraindications for liver transplantation have evolved (Table 39-7). Because MELD predicts 3-month survival, those with the highest scores have the greatest chance of dying from liver disease and thus have the best risk-benefit ratio for undergoing transplantation.

Table 39-6. Listing Status for Liver Transplantation

Status 1 (MELD score 40 or greater)	Patients with acute liver failure/disease with an estimated survival of less than 7 days (highest priority for liver transplantation).
Status 2a (MELD score >29)	Patients with end-stage liver disease, severely ill, and potentially hospitalized.
Status 2b (MELD score 24–29)	Patients with end-stage liver disease, severely ill, but not requiring hospitalization.
Status 3 (MELD score <24)	Patients with liver disease that is too early for cadaveric transplantation but may be a suitable live donor transplantation candidate.

Table 39-7. Contraindications to Liver Transplantation

ABSOLUTE CONTRAINDICATIONS	RELATIVE CONTRAINDICATIONS
Sepsis outside hepatobiliary tree	Advanced chronic renal failure
Metastatic hepatobiliary malignancy	Age >60 years
Advanced cardiopulmonary disease	Portal vein thrombosis
Moderate to severe pulmonary hypertension refractory to vasodilator therapy	Cholangiocarcinoma
AIDS	Hypoxemia with intrapulmonary right-to-left shunts
	Hepatitis: HBsAg and HBeAg positivity
	Prior portocaval shunting procedure
	Prior complex hepatobiliary surgery
	Active alcohol and/or drug abuse
	HIV positivity without clinical AIDS
	Advanced malnutrition

AIDS, Acquired immunodeficiency syndrome; HIV, human immunodeficiency virus.
Modified from Maddrey WC, Van Thiel DH: Liver transplantation: an overview. Hepatology 8:948, 1988.

25. **What are some preanesthetic considerations in a liver transplant patient?**
Optimal anesthetic management of these complex, critically ill patients requires management of the pathophysiologic changes of liver disease, comorbid conditions, and the physiologic changes associated with the surgery. In some instances (e.g., pulmonary hypertension, HRS), hepatic disease may be overshadowed by the severity of the comorbid conditions. Prior abdominal surgeries and encephalopathy are important features to note, as are coagulation deficits (factor deficiencies and thrombocytopenia). The thromboelastogram (TEG) provides valuable insight into the patient's entire clotting process. The TEG graphs the viscoelastic properties of a clot from the formation of the first fibrin strands to the full hemostatic plug. Thus the TEG is a dynamic test showing the evolution of clot formation. Because the TEG examines multiple phases of clot formation within a single test, it reflects information that is otherwise available only in multiple tests. The TEG is the best laboratory assessment of qualitative platelet function.

Electrolyte abnormalities are common. Hypokalemia is commonly seen in earlier stages of liver disease since hepatic injury leads to hyperaldosteronism. Hyperkalemia may be caused by the use of potassium-sparing diuretics to treat ascites and HRS. Hyponatremia may result from diuretic use, hyperaldosteronism, or volume overload. Renal dysfunction should be assessed since intraoperative dialysis may be necessary. In fulminant hepatic failure, cerebral cytotoxic edema is a common complication, and there must be aggressive preoperative control of intracranial pressure to prevent brainstem herniation, a common cause of death. Patients with cerebral edema should have intracranial pressure monitoring.

Pulmonary hypertension associated with cirrhosis occurs in approximately 8% of patients and is a cause of significant intraoperative morbidity and mortality. Many liver failure patients are hypoxemic secondary to atelectasis and HPS. All potential transplant candidates should undergo a transthoracic echocardiogram to assess pulmonary arterial pressures, left ventricular function, and intrapulmonary shunting. If pulmonary arterial pressures are elevated or right ventricular function is decreased, a right-sided heart catheterization may be indicated.

26. **Describe the three stages of liver transplantation.**
- The **preanhepatic (dissection) stage (stage 1)** includes the surgical incision, dissection, and hepatic mobilization. Surgeons identify the hepatic artery, portal vein, and the inferior vena cava.
- The **anhepatic stage (stage 2)** isolates the liver from the circulation and occludes the hepatic artery and portal vein. Exclusion of the inferior vena cava follows. During the anhepatic stage, the donated liver is reinserted into the circulation by anastomoses to the patient's vena cava, portal vein, and hepatic artery. The anhepatic stage concludes with removal of the vascular clamps, resulting in reperfusion of the donor liver graft.
- The **reperfusion stage (stage 3)** starts during portal vein reperfusion and extends to the conclusion of the operation. Biliary reconstruction takes place during this phase, as does assessment of neohepatic function.

27. **What is the role of venovenous bypass? Are there any alternatives?**
During the anhepatic phase and caval clamping, the preload to the heart declines precipitously. Often a bypass circuit to return venous blood from distal areas is employed. However, use of vasopressors is preferred to venovenous bypass. Another alternative is to place a cross-clamp over part of the vena cava and remove the liver with the part of the vena cava attached to the hepatic veins. Because part of the vena cava remains open to flow, venous return from the lower body is not compromised. Choice of technique depends on the amount of scarring surrounding the liver and surgeon preference.

28. **List some of the anesthetic concerns during the preanhepatic (dissection) phase.**
- Maintaining normothermia is important because the metabolic activity of the liver contributes significantly to maintaining body temperature. Early temperatures are difficult to correct and potentiate coagulation disturbances.
- Hyperkalemia resulting from administration of blood products and impaired excretion caused by HRS may result in cardiac arrest. The donor organ preservative solution contains 150 mEq/dl of potassium. On reperfusion, much of this potassium reaches the

patient's circulation. Therefore it is important to control potassium early in the surgery, maintaining serum levels at approximately 3.5 mEq/dl. This is achieved with loop diuretics (furosemide) and hyperventilation. If these agents fail, intraoperative hemodialysis should be considered.

- Hyponatremia in patients with liver disease should not be corrected rapidly because fluctuations in the serum sodium during transplantation have produced pontine demyelination, resulting in debilitating disease or death.
- Because citrate in banked blood normally undergoes hepatic metabolism, it accumulates during liver transplantation. Citrate binds calcium and can contribute to hypocalcemia.
- Blood loss during this stage can be significant. It should be anticipated in any patient who has had previous intraabdominal surgery, especially in the right upper quadrant.
- Besides preexisting coagulopathies, mechanical reasons for excessive bleeding in liver failure patients include increased portal pressures and splanchnic venous filling. Patients with cirrhosis have splanchnic hypervolemia. Often splanchnic vasoconstrictors such as vasopressin are started in an attempt to return the splanchnic blood to the arterial circulation.
- By the completion of this phase, patients should be warm, have coagulopathies and intravascular deficits corrected, display good urine output, and possess normal electrolytes.

29. **What are some anesthetic concerns that arise during stage 2, the anhepatic phase?**

Once the dissection is finished, blood loss is usually minimal is not the case during the preanhepatic phase. Because the inferior vena cava is typically cross-clamped, half of the patient's blood volume is confined to the lower body. Therefore central filling pressures are a poor representation of total body blood volume. Most therapy in this phase is directed toward achieving hemodynamic stability and preparing for reperfusion by correcting potassium and pH. Steroids are also administered during this stage. Steroids are the initial step for immunosuppression so that rejection is minimized and are administered before reperfusion.

The anhepatic stage has no means of physiologic compensation. Hyperkalemia, hypocalcemia, and metabolic acidosis are common and must be corrected. Hypernatremia caused by administration of sodium bicarbonate for metabolic acidosis is managed by administration of dextrose in water (D_5W). Increases in $PaCO_2$ associated with bicarbonate administration also require adjustments in ventilation. Perhaps a better buffering agent is tromethamine (THAM). THAM is a low-sodium buffer that does not increase sodium or $PaCO_2$. As previously discussed, serum potassium must be aggressively lowered to <3.5 mEq/L to prevent hyperkalemia-induced asystole during reperfusion. Hyperventilation, alkalinizing agents, and insulin are effective interventions.

Although there are no reliable predictors of hemodynamic instability during venous occlusion, an accentuated hyperdynamic circulatory state, severe portal hypertension, and advanced age have been associated with adverse hemodynamic events.

30. **Define reperfusion syndrome and its implications.**

Reperfusion syndrome is characterized by either a decrease of 30% or more in mean arterial pressure (from baseline) for greater than 1 minute and occurring within the first 5 minutes of reperfusion or a mean arterial pressure less than 60 mm Hg under the same circumstances. Following portal vein unclamping, approximately 30% of patients will exhibit profound cardiovascular collapse on reperfusion irrespective of attentive management during stage 2. The bradycardia, myocardial depression, and systemic vasodilation noted during reperfusion are secondary to rapid increases in serum potassium, decreases in temperature, acute acidosis, and release of vasoactive substances by the grafted liver. Increased age, larger donor organs, cold ischemic time, presence of renal disease, and fulminant hepatic failure are risk factors.

Treatment with calcium, atropine, and/or epinephrine improves cardiovascular function. Fluid administration should be judicious because it can aggravate the already increased filling pressures (secondary to myocardial depression), resulting in impaired hepatic perfusion. When pulmonary hypertension, elevated central venous pressure, and hypotension persist, continuous vasopressor infusions such as vasopressin, norepinephrine, and phenylephrine may be necessary to combat the persistent vasodilation.

31. **Describe some of the major anesthetic management issues during the reperfusion stage (stage 3).**
    - Wide swings in blood pressure and arrhythmias can be expected. Hypertension may be caused by a large increase in distal blood flow to the systemic circulation following caval unclamping. Alternatively, release of the portal vein clamp directs blood through the liver graft to the heart, and products of cell death and residual preservation fluid can cause severe hypotension, bradycardia, supraventricular and ventricular arrhythmias, electromechanical dissociation, and occasionally cardiac arrest. Hypotension may also be the result of surgical bleeding since the anastomotic sites are exposed to venous pressure.
    - Mild to severe coagulation defects are commonly observed during stage 3 because the new liver requires time to resume its synthetic functions. The TEG should guide treatment. Clotting variables gradually return to normal by a combination of specific replacement therapy and production by the allograft. Fibrinogen levels should be assessed regularly.
    - Urine output typically improves, even in patients with prior HRS, and inotrope requirements diminish.
    - The procedure is completed by biliary reconstruction, either by direct bile duct-to-duct anastomosis or by a Roux-en-Y choledochojejunostomy.

32. **What are indicators of graft function during stage 3?**
    An important part of the post anhepatic phase is the evaluation of graft function, as demonstrated by the following:

    Maintain normocalcemia without supplementation when the liver is metabolizing citrate; normalize base deficit, implying hepatic acid clearance; achieve normothermia; note bile production; note clot production, implying hepatic synthesis of clotting factors.

    Signs suggestive of poor graft function include unexplained acute deterioration in urinary output, prolonged hypotension requiring pressor support, and recalcitrant coagulopathy. If persistent bleeding is present despite fresh frozen plasma and platelet transfusions, then recombinant factor VIIa or prothrombin complex concentrate (factors II, VII, IX, X, C, and S) should be considered.

KEY POINTS: PERIOPERATIVE HEPATIC DYSFUNCTION AND LIVER TRANSPLANTATION

1. Patients with end-stage liver disease (ESLD) have a hyperdynamic circulation with increased cardiac output and decreased systemic vascular resistance.
2. Although the portal vein supplies up to 75% of total hepatic blood flow, only 45% to 55% of the oxygen requirements are provided by this part of the circulation.
3. Because of the large hepatic reserve, significant impairment of physiologic function must occur before clinical signs and symptoms of hepatic failure become evident.
4. Because of potential perioperative complications of GI hemorrhage, sepsis, renal failure, and volume overload, elective surgery should not be performed in Child class C (MELD > 14) cirrhotic patients.
5. Patients with ESLD have a hyperdynamic circulation characterized by increased cardiac index, decreased systemic vascular resistance, and impaired myocardial function. Coronary artery disease and pulmonary hypertension are common.
6. Patients with liver disease commonly have an increased volume of distribution, necessitating an increase in initial dose requirements. However, because the drug metabolism may be reduced, smaller doses are subsequently administered at longer intervals.
7. Concerns during the preanhepatic stage of liver transplantation include aggressive rewarming; monitoring serum potassium, sodium, and calcium levels; replacing significant blood losses; treating coagulation disturbances; and restoring effective arterial blood volume.
8. Concerns during the anhepatic stage include correction of hyperkalemia, hypocalcemia, and metabolic acidosis and restoration of intravascular volume in anticipation of vascular unclamping and reperfusion syndrome.
9. Wide swings in blood pressure and arrhythmias can be expected during the postanhepatic stage. Surgical bleeding and impaired coagulation are concerns. Urine output typically improves, the biliary tree is reconstructed, and graft function must be assessed.

WEBSITE

United Network for Organ Sharing: http://www.unos.org

SUGGESTED READINGS

Baker J, Yost S, Niemann C: Organ transplantation. In Miller R, editor: Miller's anesthesia, ed 6, Philadelphia, 2005, Churchill Livingstone, pp 2231–2283.
Befeler A, Palmer D, Hoffman M, et al: The safety of intra-abdominal surgery in patients with cirrhosis, Arch Surg 140:650–654, 2005.
Csete M, Glas K: Anesthesia for organ transplantation. In Barash P, editor: Clinical anesthesia, ed 5, Philadelphia, 2006, Lippincott Williams & Wilkins, pp 1364–1367.
Krenn C, De Wolf A: Current approach to intraoperative monitoring in liver transplantation, Curr Opin Organ Transplant 13(3):285–290, 2008.
Millwala F, Nguyen GC, Thuluvath PJ: Outcomes of patients with cirrhosis undergoing non-hepatic surgery: risk assessment and management, World J Gastroenterol 13:4056–4063, 2007.
Mushlin P, Gelman S: Hepatic physiology and pathophysiology. In Miller R, editor: Miller's anesthesia, ed 6, Philadelphia, 2005, Churchill Livingstone, pp 743–775.

CHAPTER 40

RENAL FUNCTION AND ANESTHESIA

James C. Duke, MD, MBA

1. Describe the anatomy of the kidney.

The kidneys are paired organs lying retroperitoneally against the posterior abdominal wall. Although their combined weight is only 300 g (about 0.5% of total body weight), they receive 20% to 25% of the total cardiac output. The renal arteries are branches of the aorta, originating below the superior mesenteric artery. The renal veins drain into the inferior vena cava. Nerve supply is abundant; sympathetic constrictor fibers are distributed via celiac and renal plexuses. There is no sympathetic dilator or parasympathetic innervation. Pain fibers, mainly from the renal pelvis and upper ureter, enter the spinal cord via splanchnic nerves.

On cross section of the kidney, three zones are apparent: cortex, outer medulla, and inner medulla (Figure 40-1). Eighty percent of renal blood flow is distributed to cortical structures. Each kidney contains about 1 million nephrons. Nephrons are classified as superficial (about 85%) or juxtamedullary, depending on location and length of the tubules. The origin of all nephrons is within the cortex.

The glomerulus and capsule are known collectively as the renal corpuscle. Each Bowman capsule is connected to a proximal tubule that is convoluted within its cortical extent but becomes straight limbed within the outer cortex; at this point the tubule is known as the *loop of Henle*. The loop of Henle of superficial nephrons descends only to the intermedullary junction, where it makes a hairpin turn, becomes thick limbed, and ascends back into the cortex, where it approaches and touches the glomerulus with a group of cells known as the *juxtaglomerular apparatus*. The superficial nephrons form distal convoluted tubules that merge to form collecting tubules within the cortex. The renal corpuscles of juxtamedullary nephrons are located at juxtamedullary cortical tissue. They have long loops of Henle that descend deep into the medullary tissue; the loops also reascend into cortical tissue, where they form distal convoluted tubules and collecting tubules. These nephrons (15% of the total) are responsible for conservation of water.

About 5000 tubules join to form collecting ducts. Ducts merge at minor calyces, which in turn merge to form major calyces. The major calyces join and form the renal pelvis, the most cephalic aspect of the ureter.

2. List the major functions of the kidney.

- Regulation of body fluid volume and composition
- Acid-base balance
- Detoxification and excretion of nonessential materials, including drugs
- Elaboration of renin, which is involved in extrarenal regulatory mechanisms
- Endocrine and metabolic functions such as erythropoietin secretion, vitamin D conversion, and calcium and phosphate homeostasis

3. Discuss glomerular and tubular function.

Glomerular filtration results in production of about 180 L of glomerular fluid each day. Filtration does not require the expenditure of metabolic energy; rather it is caused by a balance of hydrostatic and oncotic forces. Glomerular filtration rate (GFR) is the most important index of intrinsic renal function. Normal GFR is 125 ml/min in males, slightly less in females.

Tubular function reduces the 180 L/day of filtered fluid to about 1 L/day of excreted fluid, altering its composition through active and passive transport. Transport is passive when it is the result of physical forces such as electrical or concentration gradients. When

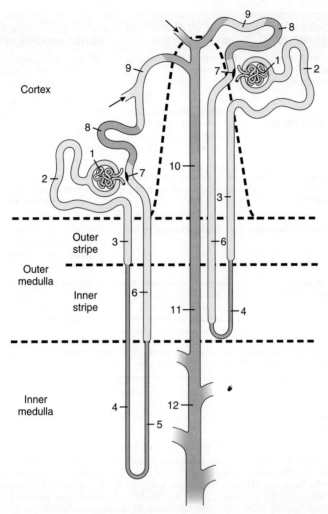

Figure 40-1. This scheme depicts a short-looped and a long-looped nephron together with the collecting system (not drawn to scale). Within the cortex, a medullary ray is delineated by the dashed line. *1*, Renal corpuscle, including Bowman capsule and the glomerulus (glomerular tuft). *2*, Proximal convoluted tube. *3*, Proximal straight tubule. *4*, Descending thin limb. *5*, Ascending thin limb. *6*, Distal straight tubule (thick ascending limb). *7*, Macula densa located within the final portion of the neck of the thick ascending limb. *8*, Distal convoluted tube. *9*, Connecting tubule of the juxtamedullary nephron that forms an arcade. *10*, Cortical collecting tubule. *11*, Outer medullary collecting duct. *12*, Inner medullary collecting duct. *(From Kriz W, Bankir I: A standard nomenclature for structures of the kidney. Am J Physiol 254:F1, 1988, with permission.)*

transport is undertaken against electrochemical or concentration gradients, metabolic energy is required, and the process is termed *active*.

Substances may be either resorbed or secreted from tubules and may move bidirectionally, taking advantage of both active and passive transport. The direction of transit for resorbed substances is from tubule to interstitium to blood, whereas the direction for secreted substances is from blood to interstitium to tubule. Secretion is the major route of elimination for drugs and toxins, especially when they are plasma protein bound.

Table 40-1. Diuretics*

DRUG (EXAMPLE)	SITE OF ACTION	ACTION AND SIDE EFFECTS
Carbonic anhydrase inhibitors (acetazolamide)	Proximal convoluted tubule	Inhibits sodium resorption; interferes with H excretion; hyperchloremic, hypokalemic acidosis
Thiazides (hydrochlorothiazide)	Cortical diluting segment (between ascending limb and aldosterone-responsive DCT)	Inhibits sodium resorption; accelerates sodium-potassium exchange (hypokalemia); decreases GFR in volume-contracted states
Potassium-sparing diuretics (spironolactone, triamterene)	Competitive inhibition of aldosterone in DCT	Inhibiting aldosterone prevents sodium resorption and sodium-potassium exchange
Loop diuretics (furosemide, bumetanide, ethacrynic acid)	Inhibit Cl⁻ resorption at thick ascending loop of Henle	Potent diuretic; acts on critical urine-concentrating process; renal vasodilator; hypokalemia; can produce hypovolemia
Osmotic diuretics (mannitol, urea)	Filtered at glomerulus but not resorbed; creates osmotic gradient in tubules; excretion of water and some sodium	Hyperosmolality reduces cellular water; limited ability to excrete sodium; renal vasodilator

*With the exception of osmotic diuretics, all diuretics interfere with sodium conservation.
DCT, Distal convoluted tubule; GFR, glomerular filtration rate.

4. Review the site of action and significant effects of commonly used diuretics. See Table 40-1.

5. Describe the unique aspects of renal blood flow (RBF) and control.
RBF of about 1200 ml/min is well maintained (autoregulated) at blood pressures of 80 to 180 mm Hg. The cortex requires about 80% of blood flow to achieve its excretory and regulatory functions, and the outer medulla receives 15%. The inner medulla receives a small percentage of blood flow; a higher flow would wash out solutes responsible for the high tonicity (1200 mOsm/kg) of the inner medulla. Without this hypertonicity, urinary concentration would not be possible.

Control of RBF is through extrinsic and intrinsic neural and hormonal influences; a principal goal of blood flow regulation is to maintain GFR. The euvolemic, nonstressed state has little baseline sympathetic tone. Under mild to moderate stress, RBF decreases slightly, but efferent arterioles constrict, maintaining GFR. During periods of severe stress (e.g., hemorrhage, hypoxia, major surgical procedures), both RBF and GFR decrease secondary to sympathetic stimulation.

The renin-angiotensin-aldosterone axis also has an effect on RBF. A proteolytic enzyme formed at the macula densa of the juxtaglomerular apparatus, renin acts on angiotensinogen within the circulation to produce angiotensin I. Enzymes within lung and plasma convert angiotensin I to angiotensin II, which is a potent renal vasoconstricting agent (especially of the efferent arteriole) and a factor in the release of aldosterone. During periods of stress, levels of angiotensin are elevated and contribute (along with sympathetic stimulation and catecholamines) to decreased RBF.

Prostaglandins (PGs) are also found within the kidney. PGE2 and PGE3 are intrinsic mediators of blood flow, producing vasodilation.

6. **Describe the sequence of events associated with decreased renal blood flow.**
   The initial response to decreased RBF is to preserve ultrafiltration through redistribution of blood flow to the kidneys, selective afferent arteriolar vasodilation, and efferent arteriolar vasoconstriction. Renal hypoperfusion results in active absorption of sodium and passive absorption of water in the ascending loop of Henle. Oxygen demand is increased in an area particularly vulnerable to decreased oxygen delivery. Compensatory sympathoadrenal mechanisms redistribute blood flow from the outer cortex to the inner cortex and medulla. If renal hypoperfusion persists or worsens, despite early compensatory mechanisms, and as sodium is resorbed in the ascending loop, increased sodium is delivered to the macula densa, producing afferent arteriolar vasoconstriction and decreasing glomerular filtration. Because GFR is decreased, less solute is delivered to the ascending loop. Because less solute is delivered, less is resorbed (an energy requiring process); thus less oxygen is needed, and the net effect is that afferent arteriolar vasoconstriction decreases oxygen-consuming processes. The result is oliguria. However, the kidney is attempting to maintain intravascular volume and, to that end, the process described has been denoted *renal success*. In reality, oliguria is a poor measure of renal function since more often than not acute renal failure is nonoliguric.

7. **What preoperative risk factors are associated with postoperative kidney injury?**
   Acute kidney injury (AKI) has now increasingly replaced the term *acute renal failure*. Preoperative renal risk factors (increased blood urea nitrogen [BUN] and creatinine and a history of renal dysfunction), left ventricular dysfunction, advanced age, jaundice, and diabetes mellitus are predictive of postoperative renal dysfunction. Patients undergoing cardiac or aortic surgery are particularly at risk for developing postoperative renal insufficiency.

8. **Discuss the major causes of perioperative AKI.**
   AKI is defined as a significant decrease in GFR over a period of 2 weeks or less. Renal failure, or azotemia, can be categorized into prerenal, renal, and postrenal etiologies. Prerenal azotemia is caused by decreased blood flow to the kidney and accounts for about 60% of all cases of AKI. In the perioperative setting, ischemia may be caused by inadequate perfusion from blood and volume losses. Other mechanisms include hypoperfusion secondary to myocardial dysfunction or shunting of blood away from the kidneys, as in sepsis.
   Renal causes account for 30% of all cases of AKI. Acute tubular necrosis (ATN) is the leading cause and may be the result of either ischemia or toxins. In the setting of preexisting renal disease, nephrotoxins include radiocontrast media, aminoglycosides, angiotensin-converting enzyme (ACE) inhibitors, and fluoride associated with volatile anesthetic metabolism. Hemolysis and muscular injury (producing hemoglobinuria and myoglobinuria) are also causes of intrinsic AKI.
   Postrenal causes (10% of cases) are caused by obstructive nephropathy and may be observed in men with conditions such as prostatism and ureteral obstruction from pelvic malignancies.

9. **What laboratory abnormalities are observed in patients with renal failure?**
   Patients have uremia (elevation of BUN and creatinine), hyperkalemia, hyperphosphatemia, hypocalcemia, hypoalbuminemia, and metabolic acidosis. They are also anemic and have platelet and leukocyte dysfunction, rendering them prone to bleeding and infection.

10. **Comment on various laboratory tests and their use in detecting acute renal dysfunction.**
    Indices of renal function can be roughly divided into measures of glomerular or tubular function. Measures of clearance assess glomerular function, whereas the ability to concentrate urine and retain sodium is an index of tubular function. The majority of renal function tests are neither sensitive nor specific in predicting perioperative renal dysfunction and are affected by many variables common to the perioperative environment.
    The ammonia generated from amino acid metabolism in the liver is converted to BUN. Urea is cleared rapidly by glomerular filtration but also resorbed in the tubules. Thus BUN cannot be used as a marker of glomerular filtration, only azotemia. Creatinine is the end product of creatinine phosphate metabolism and is generated from muscle and handled

by the kidney in a relatively uniform fashion. Dietary meat is also a source of creatinine. Serum creatinine (Scr) is a function of muscle mass, and such factors of activity, diet, and hemodilution alter its concentration. Scr can be artifactually increased by barbiturates or cephalosporins. Additional nonrenal variables may also be responsible for elevation of BUN and creatinine, including increased nitrogen absorption, muscle trauma from burns or injury, hypercatabolism, hepatic disease, diabetic ketoacidosis, hematoma resorption, gastrointestinal bleeding, hyperalimentation, and many drugs (e.g., steroids). The usual ration of BUN to creatinine is 10:1, and a ratio greater than 20:1 implies a prerenal syndrome.

Elevation of Scr is a late sign of renal dysfunction. The relationship between Scr and GFR is inverse and exponential. That is to say, a doubling of Scr reflects halving the GRF. This is of greater clinical significance at lower levels of creatinine; an increase of creatinine from 4 to 8 mg/dl does not represent a large absolute decrease in GFR because GFR is already remarkably diminished at 4 mg/dl.

When renal function is stable, using nomograms, creatinine is a reasonable measure of GFR. However, Scr measurements are inaccurate when GFR is rapidly changing. GFR may be reduced by 50% or more before abnormal elevation is observed. Because creatinine production is proportionate to muscle mass, in situations in which substantial wasting has already occurred (e.g., chronic illness, advanced age), creatinine levels may be *normal* despite markedly reduced GFR.

GFR declines with age. A healthy individual of age 20 has a GFR of about 125 ml/min; an otherwise healthy patient at age 60 has a GFR about 60 ml/min. Scr does not begin to increase until GFR falls to about 50 ml/min. GFR can be estimated using population studies based on the patient's age, Scr, sex, and weight. The method of Cockroft and Gault uses the following formula for estimating GFR: GFR = (140 − age) × weight (kg)/(Scr × 72). This is the formula for males, and the result is multiplied by 0.85 to determine the GFR for females. It is obvious that this overestimates GFR in obese patients when total body weight, not ideal body weight, is used. This formula may also overestimate GFR in cachectic patients in whom creatinine production is low.

Creatinine clearance (Ccr) is a sensitive test of renal function. Creatinine is filtered at the glomerulus and not resorbed. There is also some secretion of creatinine with the tubules, and this results in about a 15% overestimation of Ccr. (In actuality, clearance of inulin, a polyfructose sugar, is the gold standard for measurement of GFR because it is filtered at the glomerulus and neither resorbed nor secreted at the tubules.) It has been a long-held belief that measurement of Ccr requires 12- to 24-hour urine collections. In fact, if Scr is rapidly changing, calculations of Ccr based on 24 hours of urine collection and a single creatinine measurement may be inaccurate. In addition, this method requires meticulous urine collection, and failure to accomplish this is a common source of laboratory error. Two-hour spot tests are thought to be reasonably accurate, and serial 2-hour spot tests may be particularly valuable when renal function is acutely deteriorating. Table 40-2 describes various tests of renal function.

11. What are measures of tubular function?

As opposed to the measures of glomerular function previously discussed (creatinine, GFR, Ccr), tests of tubular function describe the ability of the kidney to concentrate urine and handle sodium. Tests of concentrating ability differentiate between prerenal azotemia (dehydration, decreased renal perfusion) and ATN and demonstrate abnormalities 24 to 48 hours before increases in BUN and creatinine. Measures of tubular function give no estimate of renal reserve.

With hypovolemia, renal tubules retain salt and water and result in a relatively hyponatremic, concentrated urine. Concentrating ability is lost during ATN and results in increased volumes of dilute urine high in sodium. As mentioned, in ATN, loss of concentrating ability may be detected 24 to 48 hours before BUN or creatine begins to rise. Other tests of tubular function include urine-to-plasma osmolar ratio, free water clearance, urine-to-plasma creatinine ratio, urine sodium (U_{Na}), and fractional excretion of sodium (FENa). With hypovolemia or dehydration, U_{Na} is less than 20 mEq/L. In ATN, U_{Na} exceeds 60 mEq/L. However, diuretics may increase U_{Na} to this level despite hypovolemia.

Table 40-2. Various Tests of Renal Function

TEST	NORMAL VALUES	ABNORMAL VALUES	COMMENTS
Specific gravity	1.010–1.030	Prerenal azotemia >1.030; loss of concentrating ability <1.010	Nonspecific, affected by glucose, mannitol, diuretics, endocrine disease, radiocontrast
Serum BUN	10–20	>50 definitely associated with renal impairment	Nonspecific, influenced by a wide variety of processes
Serum creatinine (mg/dl)	0.8–1.3 (men) 0.6–1.0 (women)	A doubling of the creatinine value associated with 50% reduction in GFR	A late indicator of renal failure; normal values reflect decreased function as patient ages and muscle mass decreases
Urine-plasma creatinine ratio (U:PCR)— proportion of water filtered by glomerulus that is resorbed	Between 20 and 40:1	ATN <20:1; prerenal azotemia >40:1	Neither sensitive nor specific; of value only at extremes
Urinary sodium (U_{Na}) (mEq/L)	$U_{Na} \approx 20$	ARF >60–80; prerenal azotemia <20	Changes with composition of resuscitation fluid; affected by aldosterone, ADH, diuretics
Fractional of excretion of sodium (FENa)— sodium clearance as a percentage of creatinine clearance	1%–3%	Prerenal azotemia— FENa <1%; ATN—FENa >3%	May not be accurate early in disease process (when most valuable); also nonspecific; affected by diuretics
Creatinine clearance (ml/min)	100–125	Decreased renal reserve 60–100; mild renal impairment 40–60; renal failure <25 ml/min	A good test for measuring GFR; requires 24-hr urine collection but a 2-hr collection may be reasonably accurate

ADH, Antidiuretic hormone; *ARF*, acute renal failure; *ATN*, acute tubular necrosis, *BUN*, blood urea nitrogen; *GFR*, glomerular filtration rate.

12. **At what point is renal reserve lost, and do patients develop laboratory evidence of renal insufficiency?**

   Patients will remain asymptomatic with only 40% of nephrons functioning. Renal insufficiency describes the state in which between 10% and 40% of nephrons remain; and, because there is no renal reserve, these patients are at risk for ARF with any renal insult such as hypovolemia or the administration of nephrotoxins. Patients require dialysis when fewer than 10% of nephrons remain. In terms of Ccr, patients with renal insufficiency have Ccr of less than 40 ml/min, with renal failure they have Ccr less than 25 ml/min, and they require dialysis when Ccr is less than 10 ml/min.

13. **Discuss the usefulness of urine output in assessing renal function.**

Urine output is easily measured through insertion of an indwelling Foley catheter and connection to a urometer. A daily output of 400 to 500 ml of urine is required to excrete obligatory nitrogenous wastes. In adults, an inadequate urine output (oliguria) is often defined as <0.5 ml/kg/hr. GFR is decreased by the effects of anesthesia, sympathetic activity, hormonal influences, and redistribution of blood away from outer cortical nephrons. Invariably urine output decreases as blood pressure falls; thus perioperative oliguria is not uncommon, is usually prerenal in origin, and is not a reflection of ARF. A normal urine output does not rule out renal failure.

14. **What is the best way to protect the kidneys during surgery?**

There are no *magic bullets* to prevent perioperative ARF. The best way to maintain renal function during surgery is to ensure an adequate intravascular volume, maintain cardiac output, and avoid drugs known to decrease renal perfusion.

15. **Does dopamine have a role in renal preservation?**

There is now considerable evidence that dopamine is not renoprotective (i.e., improves renal perfusion); it also does not improve splanchnic perfusion.

16. **Describe the effects of volatile anesthetics on renal function.**

General anesthesia temporarily depresses renal function as measured by urine output, GFR, RBF, and electrolyte excretion. Renal impairment is usually short-lived and completely reversible. Maintenance of systemic blood pressure and preoperative hydration decreases the effect on renal function. Spinal and epidural anesthesia also appears to depress renal function but not to the same extent as general anesthesia.

Fluoride-induced nephrotoxicity has been noted with volatile anesthetics used in the past (e.g., methoxyflurane). Sevoflurane, a volatile anesthetic in current use, has fluoride as a metabolic product (about 3.5% of the total fluoride burden appears in the urine as inorganic fluoride; peak concentrations of about 25 μmol appear within 2 hours of discontinuing the agent). Extensive experience with sevoflurane confirms its safety. Its remarkable insolubility when compared with methoxyflurane may be explanatory; there is simply less sevoflurane deposited in lipid stores to be later metabolized to fluoride, and the overall fluoride burden is less.

An additional breakdown product of sevoflurane is known as compound A and is noted mostly during low-flow anesthetic techniques. Although renal failure has been noted in animal models, no such problems have been observed in humans.

17. **What is the best relaxant for patients with renal insufficiency?**

Muscle relaxants by and large are renally excreted. Atracurium undergoes spontaneous degradation under physiologic conditions (Hofmann degradation and ester hydrolysis) and is preferred. Because atracurium is water soluble, patients with altered body water composition may require larger initial doses to produce rapid paralysis but smaller and less frequent doses to maintain paralysis. Succinylcholine may be used if the serum potassium concentration is <5.5 mEq/L (Box 40-1). Interestingly, patients with chronic renal insufficiency and accustomed to high serum potassium levels may tolerate succinylcholine administration.

18. **How are patients with renal insufficiency managed perioperatively?**

Preoperative preparation is of benefit for patients with end-stage renal disease (ESRD), who have up to a 20% mortality for emergent surgical procedures. Primary causes of death

Box 40-1. Muscle Relaxants and Renal Excretion

Gallamine	90%	Doxacurium	30%
Tubocurarine	45%	Vecuronium	15%
Metocurine	43%	Atracurium	10%
Pancuronium	40%	Rocuronium	10%
Pipecuronium	38%	Mivacurium	10%

include sepsis, dysrhythmias, and cardiac dysfunction. Hemodynamic instability is common. From the standpoint of renal dysfunction, there may be a decreased ability to concentrate urine, decreased ability to regulate extracellular fluid and sodium, impaired handling of acid loads, hyperkalemia, and impaired excretion of medications. Renal impairment is confounded by anemia, uremic platelet dysfunction, arrhythmias, pericardial effusions, myocardial dysfunction, chronic hypertension, neuropathies, malnutrition, and susceptibility to infection. Nephrotoxic agents (e.g., amphotericin, nonsteroidal antiinflammatory drugs, aminoglycosides) should be avoided. If a radiocontrast is contemplated, the real value of the test should be considered. If the contrast study is definitely indicated, the patient should be well hydrated and the contrast dose limited to the minimum needed.

Medications commonly used perioperatively may have increased effects in patients with chronic renal insufficiency. Because these patients are hypoalbuminemic, medications that are usually protein bound, such as barbiturates and benzodiazepines, may have increased serum levels. Both morphine and meperidine have metabolites that are excreted by the kidney. Succinylcholine increases extracellular potassium but can be used if serum potassium is normal. Rapid administration of calcium chloride temporizes the cardiac effects of hyperkalemia until further measures (administration of insulin and glucose, hyperventilation, administration of sodium bicarbonate and potassium-binding resins, and dialysis) can be taken to shift potassium intracellularly and decrease total body potassium.

Before surgery, patients must be euvolemic, normotensive, normonatremic, normokalemic, not acidotic or severely anemic, and without significant platelet dysfunction. Ideally they should have had dialysis the day of or day before surgery. Dialysis usually corrects uremic platelet dysfunction and is best performed within the 24 hours before surgery, although 1-deamino-8-D-arginine vasopressin (DDAVP) may also be administered if bleeding is persistent. However, they may be hypovolemic as fluid redistributes, and they are prone to hypotension. Other indications for acute dialysis include uremic symptoms, pericardial tamponade, bleeding, hypervolemia, congestive heart failure, hyperkalemia, and severe acidosis.

Patients with ESRD who have left ventricular dysfunction or undergo major procedures with significant fluid shifts require invasive monitoring to guide fluid therapy. A sterile technique should be strictly followed when inserting any catheters. In minor procedures, fluids should be limited to replacement of urine and insensible losses. Normal saline is the fluid of choice as it is free of potassium. However, if large fluid requirements are necessary, normal saline administration may result in hyperchloremic metabolic acidosis. It is clear that cases of this magnitude require invasive monitoring and repeated laboratory analysis.

KEY POINTS: RENAL FUNCTION AND ANESTHESIA

1. Preoperative renal risk factors (increased creatinine and a history of renal dysfunction), left ventricular dysfunction, advanced age, jaundice, and diabetes mellitus are predictive of postoperative renal dysfunction.
2. Patients undergoing cardiac or aortic surgery are particularly at risk for developing postoperative renal insufficiency.
3. The majority of renal function tests are neither sensitive nor specific in predicting perioperative renal dysfunction and are affected by many variables common to the perioperative environment.
4. The best way to maintain renal function during surgery is to ensure an adequate intravascular volume, maintain cardiac output, and avoid drugs known to decrease renal perfusion.

---

19. **What is accomplished during hemodialysis?**

   Blood is drawn from the patient and flows toward a semipermeable membrane, the area of which is about 1 to 1.8 m^2. Across the membrane is a dialysate with normal electrolyte concentrations. Electrolytes and waste products move down their concentration gradients. In addition, alkali within the dialysate moves into the patient. Negative pressure within the dialysate results in excess fluid removal. The duration of hemodialysis (HD) depends on flow rates and usually lasts from 4 to 6 hours. High flow rates are associated with rapid changes in electrolytes and volume status that are poorly tolerated by the patient. Usually these patients have dialysis three times weekly. The mortality rate associated with intermittent dialysis is 5% annually.

Critically ill patients in AKI with hypotension and sepsis frequently tolerate HD poorly. In this case, continuous venovenous HD (CVVHD) or filtration (CVVHF) is used. Only fluid is drawn off during CVVHF, whereas during CVVHD waste products, acid metabolites, and potassium are also removed.

SUGGESTED READINGS

Devabeye YA, Van den Berghe GH: Is there still a place for dopamine in the modern intensive care unit? Anesth Analg 98:461–468, 2004.

Moitra V, Diaz G, Sladen RN: Monitoring hepatic and renal function, Anesthesiol Clin 24:857–880, 2006.

Playford HR, Sladen RN: What is the best means of preventing perioperative renal dysfunction? In Fleisher LA, editor: Evidence-based practice of anesthesiology, Philadelphia, 2004, Saunders, pp 181–190.

Wagener G, Brentjens TE: Renal disease: the anesthesiologist's perspective, Anesthesiol Clin 24:523–547, 2006.

INCREASED INTRACRANIAL PRESSURE AND TRAUMATIC BRAIN INJURY

CHAPTER 41

Brian M. Keech, MD, FAAP

1. **Define elevated intracranial pressure (ICP).**
   ICP in humans is normally less than 10 mm Hg. Elevated ICP is usually defined as a sustained pressure of greater than 18 mm Hg within the subarachnoid space.

2. **What are the determinants of ICP?**
   The brain, including neurons and glial cells (75%), cerebrospinal fluid (CSF), extracellular fluid (ECF) (10%), and the blood perfusing the brain (15%), are all contained in the fixed volume of the cranial vault. Once compensatory mechanisms are exhausted (mostly translocation of CSF into the spinal cord), any increase in volume will increase ICP.

3. **How is ICP measured?**
   Techniques used to monitor ICP include intraventricular catheters, subdural or subarachnoid bolts or catheters, various epidural transducers, and brain intraparenchymal fiber-optic devices. All techniques require accessing the intracranial compartment via a small cranial burr hole and thus create the possibility of brain tissue damage, hematoma, and infection. The intraventricular catheter method, in which a plastic catheter is introduced into the anterior aspect of the lateral ventricle, is most commonly used. This catheter is then used to transduce ICP and to drain CSF in an attempt to reduce pressure if needed. Another commonly used method is placement of a subdural or subarachnoid bolt. This technique does not require penetration through brain parenchyma or identification of the lateral ventricle. The pressure transduction device terminates in the subdural or subarachnoid space. Epidural transducers monitor ICP via a pressure-sensitive membrane that sits close to, or in contact with, the dura. A final technique involves the insertion of a fiber-optic bundle directly into the brain parenchyma and monitors ICP by sensing changes in the amount of light reflected off a pressure-sensitive diaphragm at its tip. Newer generations of fiber-optic ICP monitors allow simultaneous measurement of ICP, local cerebral blood flow (CBF) with Doppler, pH, PO_2, and PCO_2 and avoid the potential infectious problems of a fluid-filled transducing system.

4. **Summarize the conditions that commonly cause elevated ICP.**
   See Table 41-1.

5. **Describe the symptoms of elevated ICP.**
   Symptoms associated with increased ICP include headache, nausea and vomiting, papilledema, focal neurologic deficits, behavioral changes, and altered consciousness. Other symptoms such as pathologic (decerebrate) posturing, oculomotor nerve palsy, abnormalities of brainstem reflexes, and abnormal respiratory patterns (including apnea) are likely caused by mechanical brainstem distortion and/or ischemia secondary to impending herniation. The Cushing reflex is the result of brain medullary ischemia and consists of systemic hypertension and reflex bradycardia.

6. **Discuss the possible consequences of elevated ICP.**
   In addition to producing the previously mentioned symptoms, elevated ICP can lead to a decrease in cerebral perfusion pressure, resulting in CBF and possibly ischemia. Further elevations in ICP can cause herniation of brain contents (across the falx cerebri, tentorium, or foramen magnum), resulting in irreversible brain ischemia.

Table 41-1. Common Causes of Elevated Intracranial Pressure

INCREASED CSF VOLUME	INCREASED BLOOD VOLUME	INCREASED BRAIN TISSUE VOLUME
Communicating hydrocephalus	Intracerebral hemorrhage (aneurysm or AVM)	Neoplasm
Obstructing or Noncommunicating hydrocephalus	Epidural or subdural hematoma	Cerebral edema (Cytotoxic vs. vasogenic)
	Malignant hypertension	Cysts

AVM, Arteriovenous malformation; CSF, cerebrospinal fluid; CVA, cerebrovascular accident; ICP, intracranial pressure.

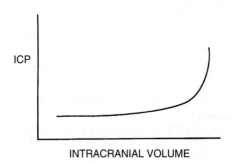

Figure 41-1. Intracranial elastance. *ICP*, Intracranial pressure.

7. **What are the determinants of cerebral perfusion pressure (CPP)?**
   CPP is usually defined as the difference between mean arterial pressure (MAP) and ICP or central venous pressure (CVP), whichever is higher.

8. **What is intracranial elastance? Why is it clinically significant?**
   Intracranial elastance, often incorrectly referred to as intracranial compliance, describes the variation in ICP that occurs with changes in intracranial volume. ICP remains somewhat constant over a limited range of intracranial volumes due to its ability to translocate CSF from the intracranial to the spinal compartments. However, when this compensatory mechanism is exhausted, ICP rises rapidly with further increases in volume (Figure 41-1). Clinically, it is important to appreciate where a patient is along the intracranial elastance curve, as small changes of intracranial volume can lead to catastrophic elevations in ICP when on the steep portion of the curve.

9. **How is CBF regulated?**
   CBF is coupled to cerebral metabolic rate by an incompletely characterized mechanism, probably involving an increase in potassium or hydrogen ions in the ECF surrounding brain arterioles. In general, increases in the cerebral metabolic rate for oxygen ($CMRO_2$) lead to increases in CBF, although the increase is delayed by 1 to 2 minutes. In addition to increases in $CMRO_2$, several other parameters influence CBF. Among them, an increase in the partial pressure of carbon dioxide in arterial blood ($PaCO_2$) is a powerful cerebral vasodilator, with CBF increasing/decreasing 1 to 2 ml/100g/min with a 1-mm Hg change in $PaCO_2$. Similarly, a decrease in the partial pressure of oxygen (PaO_2) in arterial blood below 50 mm Hg greatly increases flow. Variations in MAP also may result in changes in CBF. However, over a broad range (MAP of 50 to 150 mm Hg), flow is nearly constant. This stability of flow over a wide range of pressures is known as autoregulation, and it exists in several organ systems within the body. Chronic hypertension shifts the autoregulation curve to the right, necessitating a higher baseline MAP to adequately perfuse the brain. In

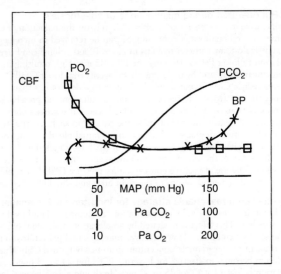

Figure 41-2. Regulation of cerebral blood flow (*CBF*). *BP*, Blood pressure; *MAP*, mean arterial pressure.

addition, following a brain injury such as stroke or trauma, autoregulation may be disrupted, and flow becomes completely pressure dependent (Figure 41-2).

With this being the case, perhaps the next time you are in the operating room or on rounds and are asked a question to which you have forgotten the answer to, instead of saying "I don't know," you should say, "Please just give me a moment, I'll have the answer for you as soon as my CBF increases enough to match the increase in $CMRO_2$ needed to answer your question."

10. **What is the goal of anesthetic care for patients with elevated ICP?**
The goal of anesthetic care is to optimize the cerebral oxygen delivery/demand ratio while preventing secondary insults such as seizure. This is accomplished by reducing $CMRO_2$ and intracranial volume and initiating appropriate seizure prophylaxis medications.

11. **Can this goal be aided by preoperative interventions?**
Several techniques have been utilized to decrease intracranial volume before surgery. Mild fluid restriction (intake of one third to one half of daily maintenance requirements) may decrease ICP over a period of several days. Corticosteroids may be effective in decreasing edema associated with neoplasm. Patients with elevated ICP are frequently placed on seizure prophylaxis prior to coming to the operating room.

12. **How is the goal of reduced intracranial volume achieved at induction of anesthesia?**
Thiopental and propofol are the preferred intravenous induction agents because they reduce both CBF and $CMRO_2$. Ketamine and etomidate are generally avoided. Ketamine has been shown to promote the general disinhibition of inhibitory neurons within the central nervous system and hence will increase $CMRO_2$, CBF, and ICP. Etomidate may induce neurologic deficits in at-risk tissue. Opioids have a variable effect on CBF but are commonly used to blunt the sympathetic response to laryngoscopy and tracheal intubation. However, injudicious administration of opioids in the spontaneously breathing patient may induce hypoventilation and elevated $PaCO_2$ with its consequent increase in CBF and ICP. Commonly used adjuncts at induction include intravenous lidocaine (0.5–1 mg/kg), a cerebral vasoconstrictor that blunts the sympathetic response to intubation. Similarly, short-acting β blockers such as esmolol reduce the systemic hypertension commonly encountered during laryngoscopy.

13. **How is ICP moderated during maintenance of anesthesia?**

   Most intraoperative maneuvers for controlling ICP rely on the reduction of CSF, cerebral blood volume, or total brain water content. CSF can be removed in increments of 10 to 20 ml if a ventriculostomy catheter remains in place. Blood volume can be reduced by hyperventilation to lower $PaCO_2$ (to range of 30 to 35 mm Hg), resulting in transient cerebral vasoconstriction, and by using anesthetic agents that lower $CMRO_2$. Halogenated volatile agents reduce $CMRO_2$ but should be limited to a dose of less than 1 minimum alveolar concentration (MAC) to reduce cerebral vasodilation and preserve systemic hemodynamics. Nitrous oxide is generally avoided because it increases both CBF and $CMRO_2$ and may be neurotoxic. Maintaining the patient in slight reverse Trendelenburg position promotes venous drainage and reduces intracranial blood volume. Brain water can be acutely reduced with diuretics such as mannitol (0.25 to 1.5 g/kg) and/or furosemide (0.5 to 1 mg/kg). In addition, the use of crystalloid intravenous fluid solutions are limited as much as possible. The use of positive end-expiratory pressure (PEEP) may elevate CVP (and ICP) by impeding venous return to the right atria and should be used with caution.

14. **Is hyperventilation a reasonable strategy for long-term ICP management?**

   Hyperventilation induces cerebral vasoconstriction, reducing cerebral blood volume, and hence, it lowers ICP. This effect is mediated by an elevation in cerebral pH and is effective over the course of several hours. However, over time, cerebral pH returns to normal by a gradual decrease in the bicarbonate concentration in newly formed CSF. Thus, hyperventilation becomes ineffective for lowering ICP after 24 to 48 hours. Additionally, hyperventilation below a $PaCO_2$ of 25 to 30 mm Hg should always be avoided out of concern for reducing O_2 delivery (due to profound decreases in CBF) and for restricting the dissociation of O_2 from oxygenated hemoglobin (due to leftward shift of the hemoglobin-oxygen dissociation curve) to at-risk cerebral tissue.

15. **Which intravenous fluids are used during surgery to minimize ICP?**

   In general, hypotonic crystalloid infusions are avoided because they may increase brain water content. Normal saline may be superior to lactated Ringer solution because of its relative isotonicity with ECF. Some centers resuscitate with small volumes of hypertonic saline (4 to 5 ml/kg) to minimize free water administration in the setting of elevated ICP. Glucose-containing solutions are generally avoided due to concerns of worsened neurologic outcome in the setting of ischemia and hyperglycemia. Colloidal solutions (albumin, hetastarch) have not been demonstrated to be superior to isotonic crystalloid solutions.

KEY POINTS: MEASURES TO DECREASE ICP

1. Elevation of head of bed
2. Analgesia and anxiolysis
3. Osmotherapy (mannitol or 3% hypertonic saline)
4. Furosemide
5. CSF drainage
6. Corticosteroids (for tumor-related edema)
7. Avoid hypervolemia
8. Hyperventilation ($PaCO_2$ 30 to 35 mm Hg)
9. Barbiturate coma

---

16. **What are the effects of volatile anesthetics on CBF?**

   All of the commonly used inhaled anesthetics have direct vasodilatory effects that increase CBF. However, the response of CBF to changes in $PaCO_2$ is preserved.

17. **How do neuromuscular blocking agents affect ICP?**

   Succinylcholine has been reported to transiently elevate ICP, but the clinical significance of this is incompletely understood. In general, the routine use of succinylcholine in elective neurosurgical cases is not recommended. However, in patients undergoing emergent surgery who are at high risk for aspiration, rapid-sequence induction with succinylcholine is acceptable. The commonly used nondepolarizing neuromuscular blocking agents (e.g., rocuronium, vecuronium, cisatracurium) have no effect on ICP and can be used safely.

18. **Discuss strategies for controlling ICP at emergence from anesthesia.**
    β Blockers such as esmolol and labetalol can be titrated to attenuate the increased sympathetic tone associated with emergence from anesthesia. They are particularly useful in their ability to effect peripheral dilation without cerebral vasodilation. Intravenous lidocaine may also be of value. Additional measures include elevating the head of the bed and maintaining normo- to slight hypocarbia.

KEY POINTS: FACTORS AFFECTING CBF

1. MAP and CPP
2. PaO_2
3. $PaCO_2$
4. Cerebral metabolic rate ($CMRO_2$)

19. **If the previously mentioned measures fail to control ICP, what else is available?**
    Barbiturate coma has been used in patients who are refractory to other methods of ICP control. Typical doses of pentobarbital are 10 mg/kg given over 30 minutes to load, followed by three hourly doses of 5 mg/kg. This regimen usually provides a therapeutic serum level of 30 to 50 mcg/ml. Maintenance is usually achieved by dosing of 1 to 2 mg/kg/hr.

KEY POINTS: AGENTS TO AVOID IN THE SETTING OF ELEVATED ICP

1. Ketamine
2. Nitrous oxide
3. Hypotonic intravascular fluids
4. Glucose-containing intravascular fluids
5. High concentrations of inhalation agents

20. **What are the mechanisms behind traumatic brain injury (TBI)?**
    Damage to the brain after traumatic head injury can be sustained during the initial injury and as a result of secondary insults such as elevated ICP, hypotension, hypoxemia, and hyperglycemia. The primary mechanism (e.g., blunt or penetrating trauma) can result in focal or global neurologic damage. Focal injuries are primarily caused by penetrating trauma, contusions, or intracranial hemorrhage. Global injuries often occur due to widespread cerebral ischemia or as a result of diffuse axonal injury (DAI), a condition in which rapid deceleration and rotation cause shearing between neocortical gray and white matter. The initial brain injury may not be responsive to therapeutic interventions. However, secondary injuries from hypoperfusion or hypoxemia may be preventable.

21. **What are the anesthetic goals in a patient with TBI?**
    The anesthetic goal of managing a patient with TBI is to prevent the occurrence of secondary injury. The compromised brain is extremely susceptible to hypoperfusion and subsequent hypoxemia. The airway should be rapidly secured and appropriate ventilation and oxygenation commenced. Cerebral perfusion should be closely monitored, but the literature is unequivocal regarding specific goals for CPP or MAP. A systolic blood pressure of <90 mm Hg has been shown to correlate with negative outcome after TBI and should be avoided via adequate resuscitation and the judicious use of vasopressors. Increases in ICP should be addressed by measures previously discussed. Of note, cerebral autoregulation is commonly disrupted in TBI, and uncontrolled hypertension can result in elevated ICP. In addition, after TBI, oxygen demand may be increased secondary to the release of excitatory neurotransmitters, making ischemic damage due to compromised perfusion more likely.

22. **In a patient with TBI, how should intravenous fluid resuscitation be prioritized, and which fluids are beneficial?**

    In general, maintaining hemodynamic stability is a central goal as systemic hypotension has been associated with worse outcomes. If a patient is bleeding and surgical hemostasis has yet to be achieved, packed red blood cells, fresh frozen plasma, platelets, and cryoprecipitate are indicated. As far as differentiating between available balanced salt solutions, this remains an ongoing debate. Traditionally Ringer lactate and normal saline (0.9%) solutions have been used. Ringer lactate has an osmolarity of 273 mOsm/L, hypotonic to ECF. In large volumes, administration of hypotonic solutions can decrease serum osmolarity and result in neuronal edema. Normal saline has an osmolarity of 308 mOsm/L, which is closer to the osmolarity of ECF and is less likely to result in neuronal edema. Occasionally hypertonic saline (3% or 7.5%) is used for fluid resuscitation. Small quantities of hypertonic saline can be used to maintain intravascular volume as they result in the movement of water from the intracellular space to the extracellular space. This may increase intravascular volume and decrease ICP. However, hypertonic saline does not reliably improve cerebral oxygen delivery and can result in electrolyte abnormalities. Colloid solutions (Hextend, albumin) can provide acute intravascular volume expansion. However, albumin has been associated with increased morbidity and mortality in TBI, and hetastarch has been associated with an elevation of prothrombin and partial thromboplastin times when given in volumes >20 ml/kg.

23. **What type of monitoring is generally indicated in patients undergoing intracranial surgery?**

    It is important to have reliable peripheral intravenous access of adequate flow capacity as large blood and evaporative losses can occur quickly during intracranial surgery. In addition to American Society of Anesthesiologists (ASA) standard monitors, an arterial catheter will also be necessary, as beat-to-beat blood pressure monitoring will be useful as well as the need to follow hemoglobin concentration, coagulation status, electrolyte levels, and blood gases. Central venous catheterization may also be helpful. Finally, a precordial Doppler probe may assist with early detection of venous air embolism.

WEBSITE

Brain Trauma Foundation: http://www.braintrauma.org

SUGGESTED READINGS

Bendo AA, Kass IS, Hartung J, et al: Anesthesia for neurosurgery. In Barash PG, Cullen BF, Stoelting RK, editors: Clinical anesthesia, ed 5, Philadelphia, 2006, Lippincott Williams & Wilkins, pp 746–789.

Brain Trauma Foundation, American Association of Neurologic Surgeons, Joint Section on Neurotrauma and Critical Care: Guidelines for the management of severe traumatic brain injury, J Neurotrauma 24(Suppl 1): S1–S106, 2007.

Bulger EM, Nathens AB, Rivara FP, et al: Management of severe head injury: institutional variations in care and effect on outcome, Crit Care Med 30(8):1870–1876, 2002.

Chestnut RM: Care of central nervous system injuries, Surg Clin North Am 87(1):119–156, 2007.

Maloney-Wilensky E, Gracias V, Itkin A, et al: Brain tissue oxygen and outcome after severe traumatic brain injury: a systematic review, Crit Care Med 37(6):2057–2063, 2009.

MALIGNANT HYPERTHERMIA AND OTHER MOTOR DISEASES

James C. Duke, MD, MBA

1. **What is malignant hyperthermia (MH) and its underlying defect?**
   MH is a myopathy characterized by an uncontrolled increase in skeletal muscle metabolism after exposure to a triggering agent. Patients with MH have an uncontrolled release of calcium from the sarcoplasmic reticulum caused by an abnormal ryanodine receptor (RyR1) isoform, a protein crucial for the release of calcium during normal excitation-contraction coupling. RyR1 mutations on chromosome 19 are found in 25% of known MH-susceptible individuals in North America. There are also associations between MH and another protein associated with the calcium channel, the dihydropyridine receptor. The gene for this protein is located on chromosome 7. Other RyR1 mutations have been noted in other countries.

2. **What is the inheritance pattern and what are the triggering agents for MH?**
   MH is inherited as an autosomal-dominant disorder with reduced penetrance and variable expressivity. Succinylcholine and the halogenated inhalational agents may precipitate an episode in a susceptible patient. MH is rare in infants and its incidence decreases after age 50.

3. **Describe the cellular events, presentation, and metabolic abnormalities associated with MH.**
   Hypermetabolism of skeletal muscle leads to hydrolysis of adenosine triphosphate, glycolysis, glycogenolysis, uncoupled oxidative phosphorylation, increase in oxygen consumption, and heat production. The earliest symptom is often unexplained tachycardia. The sine qua non of MH is an unexplained rise in end-tidal CO_2. Patients may demonstrate peculiar rigidity, even after nondepolarizing relaxants have been administered. If untreated, the patient develops numerous metabolic abnormalities, including metabolic acidosis, respiratory acidosis, hypoxemia, hyperthermia, rhabdomyolysis, hyperkalemia, hypercalcemia, hyperphosphatemia, elevations in creatine kinase, myoglobinuria, acute renal failure, cardiac dysrhythmias, and disseminated intravascular coagulation. Death is common if the problem is unrecognized and untreated. Data from the North American Malignant Hyperthermia Registry (NAMHR) show a rate of cardiac arrest of 2.7% and of death 1.4%. Interestingly, although the malady is called MH, temperature increase is a relatively late manifestation.

4. **How is MH treated?**
   - Call for assistance because aggressive therapy requires more than one person.
   - Turn off all triggering agents and hyperventilate the patient with 100% oxygen.
   - Change to a nontriggering anesthetic such as propofol infusion.
   - Notify the surgeon and operating room personnel of the situation at hand and expedite conclusion of the procedure, even if it may require that surgery go unfinished.
   - Administer dantrolene, 2.5 mg/kg; repeat every 5 minutes to a total dosage of 10 mg/kg if needed. Dantrolene sodium inhibits calcium release via RyR1 antagonism.
   - Monitor blood gases. Administer bicarbonate, 1–2 mEq/kg for a pH < 7.1.
   - Cool the patient, using interventions such as iced fluids and cooling blankets, but become less aggressive in reducing body temperature at about 38°C.
   - Promote urine output (2 ml/kg/hr), principally with aggressive fluid therapy, although mannitol and furosemide may also be required.
   - Treat hyperkalemia with calcium chloride, bicarbonate, and insulin.

- Check for hypoglycemia and administer dextrose, particularly if insulin has been administered.
- Treat dysrhythmias with procainamide and calcium chloride, 2 to 5 mg/kg intravenously (calcium chloride is used to treat the hyperkalemia-associated dysrhythmias).

5. **How does dantrolene work? How is dantrolene prepared?**

Dantrolene impairs calcium-dependent muscle contraction. This rapidly halts the increases in metabolism and secondarily results in a return to normal levels of catecholamines and potassium. The solution is prepared by mixing 20 mg of dantrolene with 3 g of mannitol in 60 ml of sterile water. Since dantrolene is relatively insoluble, preparation is tedious and time consuming, and its preparation should not be the responsibility of the primary anesthesiologist involved in the patient's management.

6. **How is MH susceptibility assessed in an individual with a positive family history or prior suggestive event?**

The diagnosis of MH is immensely difficult. There are clinical grading scales that have been used to help determine how likely a suspected episode is a true MH episode. The gold standard for diagnosis is the caffeine-halothane contracture test (CHCT). The patient's muscle is exposed to incremental doses of halothane and caffeine, and the muscle is evaluated for the degree of contracture. The test is offered at only five centers in the United States and two in Canada. The test is 85% to 90% specific and 99% to 100% sensitive. It is important that patients who have experienced MH episodes undergo further evaluation because some of these patients will be found to be MH negative.

Genetic testing for the abnormal RyR1 isoform is now available in the United States and other selected countries. The role for genetic testing is expanding. It is much cheaper than muscle biopsy and CHCT and can be performed on children too young to have CHCT (less than 10 years of age or less than 40 kg). Genetic testing is especially valuable in homogeneous populations in whom the genetic defect is constant. However, if genetic testing is negative in a susceptible individual, a CHCT must be performed.

Exertional heat illness is also a hypermetabolic event characterized by rhabdomyolysis and may suggest a previously undiagnosed patient susceptible to MH.

7. **What are the indications for muscle biopsy and halothane-caffeine contracture testing?**

- Definite indications: suspicious clinical history for MH, family history of MH, prior episode of masseter muscle rigidity
- Possible indications: unexplained rhabdomyolysis during or after surgery, sudden cardiac arrest caused by hyperkalemia, exercise-induced hyperkalemia, moderate to mild masseter muscle rigidity with evidence of rhabdomyolysis
- Probably not indications: diagnosis of neuroleptic malignant syndrome or sudden unexplained cardiac arrest during anesthesia or early postoperative period not associated with rhabdomyolysis

8. **What is masseter muscle rigidity (MMR), and what is its relation to malignant hyperthermia?**

MMR is defined as jaw muscle tightness with limb muscle flaccidity following a dose of succinylcholine. There is a spectrum of masseter response, from a tight jaw to a rigid jaw to severe spasticity, or trismus, otherwise described as "jaws of steel." Of concern, the mouth cannot be opened sufficiently to intubate the patient. If jaws of steel are present, the incidence of MH susceptibility is increased. There is some controversy as to the management of patients experiencing MMR. Most pediatric anesthesiologists agree that, if trismus occurs, the triggering agent should be halted along with the surgical procedure if feasible. The patient should be admitted to the hospital for 24 hours of close observation. Creatine kinase levels should be followed every 6 hours. Creatine kinase levels greater than 20,000 have a 95% predictive value that the patient is MH susceptible.

9. **Describe the preparation of an anesthetic machine and anesthetic for a patient with known malignant hyperthermia susceptibility.**

Clean the anesthetic machine; remove vaporizers; and replace CO_2 absorbent, bellows, and gas hose. Flush the machine for 20 minutes with 10 L/min of oxygen. Have the MH cart in the operating room. Schedule the patient for the first case of the day and notify the postanesthesia care unit to be prepared with an appropriate number of personnel. A cooling blanket should be placed under the patient. Refrigerated saline should be available. A nontriggering anesthetic technique such as continuous intravenous infusion of propofol should be used. The patient should be monitored for 6 to 8 hours after surgery.

10. **Should malignant hyperthermia–susceptible patients be pretreated with dantrolene?**
Dantrolene pretreatment is no longer indicated, providing that a nontriggering agent and appropriate monitoring are used and an adequate supply of dantrolene is available. Dantrolene pretreatment may cause mild weakness in normal patients and significant weakness in patients with muscle disorders. MH-susceptible patients with an uncomplicated intraoperative course should be monitored for at least 4 hours after surgery.

11. **What patients are at risk for redeveloping symptoms of malignant hyperthermia after treatment with dantrolene?**
Review of data from the NAMHR suggests that about 20% of patients redevelop symptoms, known as *recrudescence*. It should be mentioned that the accuracy of these data is limited by their retrospective nature. The mean time until symptoms redeveloped was 13 hours, with a range of 2.5 to 72 hours. Eighty percent manifested symptoms by 16 hours. Patients at risk were more muscular and thus had greater muscle mass, an MH score of 35 or greater (meaning that MH is very likely to be present), and a temperature increase to as high as 38.8°C. There was no strong relationship between use of succinylcholine or a particular volatile anesthetic. Probably the most severely affected patients are likely to develop recrudescence; these findings suggest that all patients who develop MH require at least 24 hours of posttreatment management in a critical care setting.

12. **What drugs commonly administered intraoperatively are safe to use in MH-susceptible patients?**
• Induction agents: barbiturates, propofol, etomidate, ketamine
• Benzodiazepines and opiates
• Amide and ester local anesthetics
• Nitrous oxide
• Nondepolarizing muscle relaxants
• Calcium

13. **Compare neuroleptic malignant syndrome (NMS) with malignant hyperthermia.**
NMS is characterized by akinesis, muscle rigidity, hyperthermia, tachycardia, cyanosis, autonomic dysfunction, sensorium change, tachypnea, and elevated levels of creatine kinase. It is associated with administration of the psychotropic drugs haloperidol, fluphenazine, perphenazine, and thioridazine, to name a few, and is caused by dopamine receptor blockade in the hypothalamus and basal ganglia. NMS is treated with dantrolene or bromocriptine (a dopamine receptor agonist) and has a mortality rate of 10%. Patients with NMS are not prone to MH.

14. **What are the muscular dystrophies (MDs) and their underlying defect?**
MDs are genetically determined degenerative muscle diseases and are divided further into muscular and myotonic dystrophies. Painless muscle degeneration and atrophy are common features. MD is associated with mutations of the gene that codes for the protein dystrophin. Dystrophin attaches muscle fibers to an extracellular matrix. Inadequately tethered muscle fibers are injured by shearing forces, degenerate, and are replaced by adipose and connective tissue. Dystrophin also seems to have other roles, including clustering of acetylcholine receptors on the postsynaptic motor membrane and modulation of ionic channels.

15. **What are the most common MDs and their clinical history?**
Duchenne MD (DMD) is the most common. It is an X chromosome–linked recessive disease with signs and symptoms presenting between 2 and 5 years of age. Death often occurs in late adolescence and is typically caused by heart failure or pneumonia. Degeneration of cardiac muscle, as demonstrated by a progressive decrease in R-wave amplitude on electrocardiogram (ECG), is observed to some degree in 70% of patients with DMD and may lead to a decrease in contractility and mitral regurgitation secondary to

papillary muscle dysfunction. Thus patients with DMD may be sensitive to the myocardial depressant effects of inhaled anesthetics. There is weakness of respiratory muscles, and a restrictive pattern is observed on pulmonary function testing. Smooth muscle may also be affected in patients with DMD, manifesting as gastrointestinal tract hypomotility, delayed gastric emptying, and impaired swallowing, which may lead to increased risk of aspiration. Becker MD has similar, although milder, symptoms and a more protracted course.

16. **Briefly review forms of muscular dystrophy.**
Other forms include the limb-girdle, oropharyngeal, and fascioscapulohumeral MDs. Some of these forms are transmitted as autosomal recessive and/or dominant and thus can be identified in both females and males. Bulbar muscles are usually spared; therefore aspiration is less of a risk, although dysrhythmias, conduction abnormalities, occasional sudden death, and cardiomyopathies are noted. One form, Emery-Dreifuss MD, has posterior nuchal muscle contractures as a feature and may render airway management difficult.

17. **How do patients with MD respond to muscle relaxants and volatile anesthetics?**
Succinylcholine should not be used because of the possibility of severe hyperkalemia and cardiac arrest. Cardiac arrest has been reported in patients with unrecognized MD. Because children with MD may not develop noticeable weakness until they are several years old, many authorities believe succinylcholine should not be used in children except in airway emergencies. Nondepolarizing relaxants are acceptable but may be associated with longer-than-normal recovery times. There is no evidence that MD is a myopathy with an association with MH.
There are reports of massive elevations in creatine kinase, severe myoglobinuria, and cardiac arrest after use of volatile anesthetics. Although not all patients with MD are at risk for MH, some are; thus a nontriggering general anesthetic or regional anesthesia is preferred.

18. **Are patients with MD at risk for MH?**
After succinylcholine administration, children with MH and MD may have similar clinical pictures, including hyperkalemia, elevated creatine kinase, and cardiac arrest, although the mechanism of the diseases is different. There are also reports of children with MD exposed to inhalational agents but not succinylcholine that have demonstrated suggestive signs of MH. However, it is not believed that children with MD are at increased risk for MH, but discussion of a child with a myopathy receiving routine surgery remains a point of debate as far as MH should be a concern.

19. **What is myotonic dystrophy?**
Myotonic dystrophy is an autosomal-dominant disease that usually presents in the second or third decade and is the most common inherited myopathy in adults. It is characterized by persistent contraction of skeletal muscle after stimulation. The contractions are not relieved by regional anesthetics, nondepolarizing muscle relaxants, or deep anesthesia. It is a multisystem disease; deterioration of skeletal, cardiac, and smooth muscle function is progressive.

20. **How does myotonic dystrophy affect the cardiopulmonary system?**
Heart failure is rare, but dysrhythmias and atrioventricular block are common. Mitral valve prolapse occurs in 20% of patients. Restrictive lung disease, with mild hypoxia on room air, a weak cough, and inadequate airway protective reflexes may lead to pneumonia. These patients are also sensitive to medications that depress ventilatory drive.

21. **What are the important muscle relaxant considerations in patients with myotonic dystrophy?**
Succinylcholine produces exaggerated contractions of skeletal muscles. In patients with myotonic dystrophy, these contractions may not subside with skeletal muscle depolarization as is normally seen after the administration of succinylcholine, making mask ventilation and tracheal intubation potentially difficult. The response to nondepolarizing relaxants is normal. Of note, nondepolarizing relaxants will not ablate the contractions noted in patients with myotonic dystrophy.

22. **What is myasthenia gravis?**
Myasthenia gravis is an autoimmune disease of the neuromuscular junction. Antibodies to the acetylcholine receptor may reduce the absolute number of functional receptors by direct destruction of the receptor, blockade of the receptor, or complement-mediated destruction.

23. **Describe the clinical presentation of myasthenia gravis.**

Myasthenic patients present with generalized fatigue and weakness that worsen with repetitive muscular use and improve with rest. Extraocular muscles are very commonly the first affected, and the patient complains of diplopia or ptosis. Of particular concern are myasthenic patients who develop weakness of their respiratory muscles or the muscles controlling swallowing and the ability to protect the airway from aspiration. Depending on whether extraocular, airway, or respiratory muscles are affected, myasthenia gravis may be described as ocular, bulbar, or skeletal, respectively.

24. **How is myasthenia gravis treated? What can lead to an exacerbation of symptoms?**

Cholinesterase inhibitors, corticosteroids, and other immunosuppressants are effective, as is plasmapheresis, although in many patients, thymectomy results in remission. Physiologic stress such as an acute infection, pregnancy, or surgical procedure can lead to exacerbations of myasthenia gravis.

25. **What are some of the principal anesthetic concerns in the management of a myasthenic patient for any operative procedure?**

Principal concerns include the degree of pulmonary impairment, the magnitude of bulbar involvement with attendant difficulty managing oral secretions (risk of pulmonary aspiration), and adrenal suppression from long-term steroid use. Although uncommon, cardiac disease that is related to myasthenia gravis should be considered in the preoperative evaluation. Because symptoms are primarily related to arrhythmias, an ECG should be evaluated. Symptoms of congestive heart failure should be sought as well.

26. **Describe the altered responsiveness of myasthenic patients to muscle relaxants.**

Patients are resistant to succinylcholine. However, the degree of resistance does not appear to be of great clinical significance, and increasing the dose of succinylcholine to 2 mg/kg results in satisfactory intubating conditions.

Myasthenic patients are more sensitive than nonmyasthenic persons to nondepolarizing relaxants. Dosing nondepolarizing relaxants should start at about one tenth the usual recommended doses. Recovery time for these reduced doses varies but may be quite prolonged. Relaxation should be reversed at case conclusion and the patient carefully evaluated for return of strength.

Often at anesthetic induction no muscle relaxant is necessary to achieve endotracheal intubation. These patients are already weak; if volatile anesthetics are administered, suitable muscle relaxation is achieved. The best course of action for myasthenic patients may be to avoid muscle relaxants altogether.

27. **What is Lambert-Eaton myasthenic syndrome? Describe its symptoms, associations, and treatment.**

This is an immune-mediated disease of the neuromuscular junction that frequently arises in the setting of malignancy, often small-cell carcinoma of the lung. Other associated malignancies include lymphoma, leukemia, prostate, and bladder. Antibodies affect the presynaptic junction and result in decreased acetylcholine release. As opposed to myasthenia gravis, weakness improves with motor activity, although frequently the improvement is transient. Proximal muscles are affected more than distal muscles, and legs more than arms. Cranial nerve involvement is also less frequent when compared with myasthenia gravis. Weakness often precedes the cancer diagnosis, although treatment focuses on treatment of the underlying malignancy. Autonomic dysfunction is common and manifests as dry mouth, orthostatic hypotension, and bowel and bladder dysfunction. Corticosteroids, 3,4-diaminopyridine, and other immunosuppressants improve strength.

28. **Review the anesthetic concerns for patients with Lambert-Eaton syndrome.**

These patients are exquisitely sensitive to both depolarizing and nondepolarizing muscle relaxants, and these medications are best avoided. If given, paralysis can last for days and is not reversible with anticholinesterase medications. Volatile anesthetics are safe and often provide the necessary degree of muscle relaxation to facilitate endotracheal intubation. When applicable, regional techniques are encouraged.

KEY POINTS: MALIGNANT HYPERTHERMIA AND OTHER MOTOR DISEASES

1. Malignant hyperthermia (MH) is a hypermetabolic disorder that presents in the perioperative period after exposure to inhalational agents or succinylcholine.
2. Early recognition is critical, and treatment is complex and multifaceted, requiring the assistance of other experienced personnel.
3. The sine qua non of MH is an unexplained rise in end-tidal carbon dioxide in a patient with unexplained tachycardia. A temperature rise is a late feature.
4. Patients with a history of, or susceptibility to, MH must receive anesthesia with a nontriggering agent. The anesthesiologist must have a heightened awareness of MH, have prepared the anesthetic machine, and have the MH cart in the room.
5. Succinylcholine must be avoided in children with muscular dystrophy and should be avoided except in airway emergencies in children.
6. Nondepolarizing muscle relaxants should be used at about one tenth of normal doses (if at all) in patients with myasthenia gravis.
7. Patients with Lambert-Eaton myasthenic syndrome are sensitive to both depolarizing and nondepolarizing muscle relaxants, and these medications are best avoided.
8. Patients with muscular dystrophies are prone to aspiration and respiratory insufficiency and may have dysrhythmias, conduction blockade, and cardiomyopathy.

WEBSITES

Malignant Hyperthermia Association of the United States: http://www.mhaus.org
Myasthenia Gravis Foundation of America: http://www.myasthenia.org

SUGGESTED READINGS

Bhatt JR, Pascuzzi RM: Neuromuscular disorders in clinical practice: case studies, Neurol Clin 24:233–265, 2006.
Brambrink AM, Kirsch JR: Perioperative care of patients with neuromuscular disease and dysfunction, Anesthesiol Clin 25:483–509, 2007.
Brandom BW: The genetics of malignant hyperthermia, Anesthesiol Clin North America 23:615–619, 2005.
Burkman JM, Posner KL, Domino KB: Analysis of the clinical variables associated with recrudescence after malignant hyperthermia reactions, Anesthesiology 106:901–906, 2007.
Hirshey Dirksen SJ, Larach MG, Rosenberg H, et al: Future directions in malignant hyperthermia research and patient care, Anesth Analg 113:1108–1119, 2011.
Larach MG, Brandom BW, Allen GC, et al: Cardiac arrests and deaths associated with malignant hyperthermia in North America from 1987 to 2006, Anesthesiology 108:603–611, 2008.
Litman RS, Flood CD, Kaplan RF, et al: Postoperative malignant hyperthermia. An analysis of cases from the North American malignant hyperthermia registry, Anesthesiology 109:825–829, 2008.
Parness J, Bandschaapp O, Girard T: The myotonias and susceptibility to malignant hyperthermia, Anesth Analg 109:1054–1064, 2009.

CHAPTER 43

DEGENERATIVE NEUROLOGIC DISEASES AND NEUROPATHIES

James C. Duke, MD, MBA

1. **What is amyotrophic lateral sclerosis and its anesthetic considerations?**

   Also known as *Lou Gehrig disease*, amyotrophic lateral sclerosis (ALS) is a disease of both upper and lower motor neurons. It usually affects men in the fourth or fifth decade of life. Patients with ALS develop progressive weakness and eventually die (from pneumonia and pulmonary failure), often in a 3- to 5-year period. Although extremities are involved first, eventually bulbar muscles become affected, increasing the risk of aspiration. The pathogenesis is poorly understood but thought to be caused by mutations in the superoxide dismutase-1 gene. Treatment options are limited.

   Reports of anesthetic difficulties are anecdotal. There is no evidence that either regional or general anesthesia exacerbates the disease. Succinylcholine-induced hyperkalemia and subsequent cardiac arrest have been reported. Nondepolarizing muscle relaxants have a prolonged duration of action. Aspiration is an increased risk, as is the need for postoperative ventilatory support. These patients are not at risk for malignant hyperthermia.

2. **Review the clinical manifestations of Guillain-Barré syndrome.**

   Acute idiopathic polyneuritis (Guillain-Barré syndrome) is currently the most frequent cause of generalized paralysis and usually presents with sudden onset of weakness or paralysis, typically in the legs, that spreads to the trunk, arms, and bulbar muscles over several days. Bulbar involvement may be suggested by facial muscle weakness. Areflexia is also a feature. Respiratory failure requiring mechanical ventilation occurs in 20% to 30% of cases. About half of all cases are preceded by a respiratory or gastrointestinal infection. The pathogenesis is thought to be autoimmune, possibly related to similarities between bacterial liposaccharides and axonal gangliosides. Recovery may occur within weeks, although some residual weakness remains secondary to axonal degeneration. Mortality (3% to 8%) typically results from sepsis, adult respiratory distress syndrome, pulmonary embolism, or cardiac arrest. Plasmapheresis and immunoglobulin therapy result in some improvement, whereas glucocorticoid supplementation does not.

3. **How is the autonomic nervous system affected in Guillain-Barré syndrome?**

   Autonomic dysfunction is a common finding. Patients may experience wide fluctuations in blood pressure, profuse diaphoresis, peripheral vasoconstriction, tachyarrhythmias and bradyarrhythmias, cardiac conduction abnormalities, and orthostatic hypotension. Sudden death has been described.

4. **What are the major anesthetic considerations for patients with Guillain-Barré syndrome?**

   Patients may not handle oral secretions well because of pharyngeal muscle weakness and have respiratory insufficiency secondary to intercostal muscle paralysis. Aspiration is a risk. Secondary to autonomic dysfunction, compensatory cardiovascular responses may be absent, and patients may become hypotensive with mild blood loss or positive-pressure ventilation. Alternatively, laryngoscopy may produce exaggerated increases in blood pressure. The response to indirect-acting vasoactive drugs may also be exaggerated. Because of the unpredictable and wide swings in blood pressure, intraarterial monitoring should be considered. There is no evidence that either general or regional anesthesia worsens the disease.

   Since Guillain-Barré syndrome is a lower motor neuron disease, succinylcholine is contraindicated because of the potential for exaggerated potassium release. Pancuronium should also be avoided because of its autonomic effects. Postoperative ventilation may be necessary because of respiratory muscle weakness.

5. **Review the pathophysiologic features of Parkinson disease.**
Parkinson disease, an adult-onset degenerative disease of the extrapyramidal system, is characterized by the loss of dopaminergic neurons in the basal ganglia. With the loss of dopamine, there is diminished inhibition of the extrapyramidal motor system and unopposed action of acetylcholine.

6. **Describe the clinical manifestations of Parkinson disease.**
Patients with Parkinson disease display increased rigidity of the extremities, facial immobility, shuffling gait, rhythmic resting tremor, dementia, depression, diaphragmatic spasms, and oculogyric crisis (a dystonia in which the eyes are deviated in a fixed position).

7. **What are the effects of levodopa therapy, particularly on intravascular volume status?**
Levodopa, the immediate precursor to dopamine, crosses the blood-brain barrier, where it is converted to dopamine by a decarboxylase enzyme. Treatment with levodopa increases dopamine both in the central nervous system and peripherally. Increased levels of dopamine may increase myocardial contractility and heart rate. Renal blood flow increases, as do glomerular filtration rate and sodium excretion. Intravascular fluid volume decreases, the renin-angiotensin-aldosterone system is depressed, and orthostatic hypotension is a common finding. High concentrations of dopamine may cause negative feedback for norepinephrine production, which also causes orthostatic hypotension.

8. **Review the anesthetic considerations for a patient with Parkinson disease.**
   - Abrupt withdrawal of levodopa may lead to skeletal muscle rigidity, which interferes with adequate ventilation. Levodopa should be administered on the morning of surgery and restarted after surgery.
   - Extremes of blood pressure and cardiac dysrhythmias may occur.
   - Phenothiazines (e.g., chlorpromazine, promethazine, fluphenazine, prochlorperazine) and butyrophenones (e.g., droperidol and haloperidol) may antagonize the effects of dopamine in the basal ganglia. Metoclopramide inhibits dopamine receptors in the brain. These medications should be avoided.
   - Patients may be intravascularly volume depleted; therefore aggressive administration of crystalloid or colloid solutions may be required in the setting of peri-induction hypotension.

9. **What are the clinical signs and symptoms of Alzheimer disease?**
Alzheimer disease accounts for most of the severe cases of dementia in the United States. The disease follows an insidious onset, with progressive worsening of memory and decreased ability to care for oneself and manage the usual activities of daily life.

10. **What is the most significant anesthetic problem associated with Alzheimer disease?**
The inability of some patients to understand their environment or to cooperate with health care providers becomes an important consideration. Sedative drugs may exacerbate confusion and probably should be avoided in the perioperative period. Regional techniques may be used with the understanding that the patient may be frightened or confused by the operating-room environment. Reductions in the level of volatile anesthetic or opioid administered may be of benefit. A lack of cooperation and unanticipated outbursts during the surgical procedure are arguments for general anesthesia.

11. **What are the hallmark features of multiple sclerosis (MS)?**
The corticospinal tract neurons of the brain and spinal cord show random and multifocal demyelination, which slows nerve conduction, resulting in visual and gait disturbances, limb paresthesias and weaknesses, and urinary incontinence. There is increasing evidence that there is demyelination of peripheral nerves as well. The onset of disease is typically between the ages of 15 and 40 years. The cause appears to be multifactorial, including viral and genetic factors. The course of MS is characterized by symptomatic exacerbations and

remissions, although symptoms eventually persist. Female patients often experience remission during pregnancy. Symptoms of MS usually develop over a few weeks, persist for a few months, and resolve to varying degrees over a few months. The etiology is unknown; however, viral infection leading to immunologically mediated destruction of myelin is one hypothesis.

12. **Do steroids have a role in the treatment of MS?**
    Steroids may shorten the duration and severity of an attack but probably do not influence progression of the disease. Other therapies such as immunosuppressive drugs, interferon, and plasmapheresis are also occasionally of benefit.

13. **What factors have been associated with an exacerbation of MS?**
    Emotional stress, fatigue, infections, hyperthermia, trauma, and surgery may exacerbate symptoms. It is thought that elevated temperature causes complete blocking of conduction in demyelinated neurons.

14. **Review some perioperative concerns for patients with MS. Are medications used for most general anesthetics safe?**
    Surgical stress most likely will exacerbate the symptoms of MS. Even modest increases in body temperature (>1°C) must be avoided. There are no known unique interactions between MS and drugs selected for general anesthesia. However, severe disease is often accompanied by varying degrees of dementia. Demented patients will likely have an increased sensitivity to the sedative effects of anesthetic agents, and short-acting agents are recommended. Controlling the known factors associated with MS exacerbation is more important than the choice of medications for general anesthesia.

15. **Are local anesthetics especially toxic for patients with MS?**
    Above threshold concentrations local anesthetics are neurotoxic. This potential may be amplified in the setting of MS because of the loss of the protective effect of the myelin, resulting in the spinal cord and nerves being exposed to higher local anesthetic concentrations.

16. **Are epidural and spinal anesthesias safe for patients with MS?**
    Regional anesthesia may be beneficial in patients with MS because of a decreased stress response to surgery. Epidural anesthesia is considered safe by most authorities. The safety of peripheral nerve blocks cannot be guaranteed as evidenced by a patient with MS sustaining a severe brachial plexopathy after interscalene block (see Koff et al. 2008). Exacerbation of MS symptoms has been reported after spinal anesthesia. This difference in outcomes may be caused by reduced concentrations of local anesthetic at the spinal cord when epidural is compared with spinal techniques and there is less exposure of unmyelinated nerve roots to local anesthetics. When performing an epidural anesthetic or labor analgesic, recommendations are to use the minimum dose necessary and to use shorter-acting agents. Supplementation with epidural opioids will also reduce the local anesthetic requirement. In summary, spinal anesthetic is a technique best avoided in patients with MS.

17. **Are muscle relaxants safe in patients with MS?**
    Since these patients (particularly the patients with severe disease) can have significant motor impairment with associated muscle wasting, succinylcholine might be best avoided because of a potential hyperkalemic response. Lower doses of nondepolarizing relaxants should be used in patients with baseline motor weakness. Shorter-duration nondepolarizing relaxants may be advantageous in this situation.

18. **Describe postpoliomyelitis syndrome.**
    Postpolio syndrome is characterized by progressive weakness of the previously affected muscles that begins years after a severe attack of poliomyelitis. Muscles never affected by polio are less often affected. Common signs and symptoms include fatigue, cold intolerance, joint deterioration, muscle pain, atrophy, respiratory insufficiency, dysphagia, and sleep apnea. Patients with postpolio syndrome who complain of dysphagia may have some degree of vocal cord paralysis. Some patients have decreased lung function, and considerable cardiorespiratory deconditioning may also be present.

19. **What are the anesthetic considerations for patients with postpolio syndrome?**
Patients should be informed about the possibility of postoperative mechanical ventilation. If sleep apnea is present, the patient may have coexisting pulmonary hypertension. Dysphagia and vocal cord paralysis may place patients at increased risk for aspiration. If progressive skeletal muscle weakness is present, succinylcholine should be avoided because of the possibility of exaggerated potassium release.

20. **Review critical illness polyneuropathy and the patient subsets prone to developing it.**
As many as 70% of patients with sepsis, multiple organ dysfunction, or systemic inflammatory response syndrome develop generalized weakness associated with sensory loss and other neurologic findings. This syndrome has been termed *critical illness polyneuropathy* (CIP). The longer the duration of the underlying illness is, the more severe the weakness will be. Patients with mild or moderate underlying critical illness are likely to have improvement in strength once their primary condition improves, although death is not infrequent in those severely affected (and usually related to the primary illness). Although the mechanism is unknown, it is thought to be a disturbance of the microvasculature, resulting in neuronal ischemia and increased capillary permeability. Factors that may be associated with CIP include long-term administration of muscle relaxants, steroids, malnutrition, and hyperglycemia.

21. **Describe the clinical features of CIP.**
Failure to wean is the most common presentation, but coexistent encephalopathy often clouds the clinical picture. Severe cases may present as areflexic quadriparesis. Other clinical characteristics include predominantly distal limb weakness with muscle wasting, decreased or absent deep tendon reflexes, and variable sensory loss, often in a stocking and glove distribution. Cranial nerves are intact. Creatine kinase levels are normal or slightly elevated. Cerebrospinal fluid is normal. Biopsies of nerves show fiber loss with axonal degeneration, whereas muscle biopsies demonstrate denervation atrophy. Electrophysiologic studies reveal an axonal polyneuropathy.

22. **Review the anesthetic concerns in patients with CIP.**
The response to nondepolarizing relaxants cannot be predicted. Succinylcholine should be avoided out of concerns for hyperkalemia. The associated medical problems are probably the greatest risk for patients with CIP.

KEY POINTS: DEGENERATIVE NEUROLOGIC DISEASES

1. Patients with neuropathies often are aspiration risks secondary to bulbar muscle weakness.
2. Similarly, orthostatic hypotension is a common finding.
3. Often these patients require postoperative mechanical ventilation.
4. Because of denervation atrophy, succinylcholine may produce severe hyperkalemia, resulting in cardiac arrest. Thus succinylcholine should be avoided.
5. The response to nondepolarizing muscle relaxants is unpredictable, but most of these patients are probably sensitive to them.
6. Spinal anesthesia should be avoided in patients with multiple sclerosis.
7. With the exception of spinal anesthesia in multiple sclerosis, neither general nor regional anesthesia exacerbates the course of disease in the neuropathies described.

SUGGESTED READINGS

Brambrink AM, Kirsch JR: Perioperative care of patients with neuromuscular disease and dysfunction, Anesthesiol Clin 25:483–509, 2007.

Koff MD, Cohen JA, McIntyre JJ, et al: Severe brachial plexopathy after an ultrasound-guided single-injection nerve block for total shoulder arthroplasty in a patient with multiple sclerosis, Anesthesiology 108:325–328, 2008.

Perlas A, Chan VW: Neuraxial anesthesia and multiple sclerosis, Can J Anaesth 52:454–458, 2005.

ALCOHOL AND SUBSTANCE ABUSE

James C. Duke, MD, MBA

CHAPTER 44

1. **How is alcohol absorbed and metabolized?**

   Alcohol is absorbed across the gastrointestinal mucosa, more so in the small intestine than in the stomach. The volume of distribution (VD) of alcohol is that of body water. Alcohol easily crosses the blood-brain barrier. Arterial blood levels of alcohol correlate well with concentrations in lung alveoli, thus the basis of the breathalyzer test used by law enforcement officers.

   Alcohol is metabolized primarily in the liver. Most consumed alcohol is converted to acetaldehyde by the enzyme alcohol dehydrogenase. Alcohol metabolism follows Michaelis–Menten zero-order kinetics. When alcohol dehydrogenase is saturated with ethanol, the rate of metabolism is constant, although alcohol concentration may increase. A 5% to 10% amount of consumed alcohol is excreted unchanged in the breath and urine.

2. **What are the acute and chronic effects of alcohol on the nervous system?**

   Acutely alcohol depresses the central nervous system by inhibiting polysynaptic function, which is characterized by generalized blunting and loss of higher motor, sensory, and cognitive function. Although the behavioral effects of alcohol consumption may seem excitatory or stimulating to observers and users, this impression is probably caused by a depressive effect on inhibitory pathways (disinhibition).

   Chronic alcohol use is associated with peripheral nerve and neuropsychiatric disorders, many of which (e.g., Wernicke encephalopathy and Korsakoff psychosis) may be linked to nutritional deficiencies. Alcohol-related neuropathy usually involves pain and numbness in the lower extremities, often with concomitant weakness of the intrinsic muscles of the feet. Patients may exhibit hypalgesia in a stocking-foot distribution, and the Achilles tendon reflex may be absent. Generalized weakness in the proximal limb musculature may also be noted.

3. **What are the effects of alcohol on the cardiovascular system?**

   Moderate acute ingestion of alcohol produces no significant changes in blood pressure or myocardial contractility. Cutaneous vasodilation occurs, and heart rate increases. At toxic levels of acute alcohol ingestion, a decrease in central vasomotor activity causes respiratory and cardiac depression.

   The leading cause of death in chronic users of alcohol is cardiac dysfunction. Consumption of 60 oz of ethanol per month (8 pints of whiskey or 55 cans of beer) may lead to alcohol-induced hypertension. An intake >90 oz per month over a 10-year period may result in congestive cardiomyopathy with associated pulmonary hypertension, right-sided heart failure, and dysrhythmias (usually atrial fibrillation and premature ventricular contractions). Ventricular tachydysrhythmias, ventricular fibrillation, and sudden death are also risks.

4. **How does alcohol affect the respiratory system?**

   Acute alcohol intake may cause hyperventilation via disinhibition of central respiratory regulation centers and increases in dead-space ventilation. Despite hyperventilation, alcohol depresses the ventilatory response to carbon dioxide. Aspiration of gastric contents is a risk. Chronic alcohol users are susceptible to pulmonary infections, often by staphylococci or gram-negative organisms. There is also a generalized decrease in all lung capacities (vital, functional residual, and inspiratory capacity).

5. **How does alcohol affect the gastrointestinal and hepatobiliary systems?**

   Acute alcohol use may cause esophagitis, gastritis, and pancreatitis. Chronic alcohol use leads to delayed gastric emptying and relaxation of the lower esophageal sphincter, increasing the risk of aspiration. The liver undergoes transient and reversible fatty infiltration during acute alcohol use. Although such changes resolve with abstinence and the cycle can repeat itself many times, prolonged alcohol exposure leads to chronic infiltration of fat, which, over time, progresses to necrosis and fibrosis of liver tissue. The initial presentation of fatty liver is hepatomegaly. When necrosis, fibrosis, and cirrhosis become apparent, the liver regresses in size. Chronic severe consumption of alcohol leads to irreversible cirrhosis and alcohol-induced hepatitis. Hepatic synthetic function is also impaired. Production of albumin and coagulation factors II, V, VII, X, and XIII is decreased. Reduction of albumin results in lower intravascular oncotic pressure and may lead to tissue edema. A reduction in circulating coagulation factors may predispose to bleeding, which is evidenced by a prolonged prothrombin time.

6. **Which nutritional deficiencies are seen in chronic alcohol users?**
   Deficiency of thiamine leads to Wernicke encephalopathy, polyneuropathy, and cardiac failure characterized by high cardiac output, low systemic vascular resistance, and loss of vasomotor tone. Folic acid deficiency causes bone-marrow depression and thrombocytopenia, leukopenia, and anemia.

7. **What are the effects of alcohol on inhalational anesthetics?**
   In acutely intoxicated, nonhabituated patients, the minimal alveolar concentration (MAC) of inhalational agents is reduced. For chronic users of alcohol, the MAC for inhalational agents is increased.
   Acutely intoxicated patients are more sensitive to the effects of barbiturates, benzodiazepines, and opioids. Cross-tolerance develops to intravenous agents with chronic alcohol exposure.

8. **How does alcohol affect muscle relaxants?**
   Patients with liver disease may have decreased levels of circulating plasma cholinesterase, and the effects of succinylcholine may be prolonged. Cirrhotic patients with poor liver function have a greater V_D for injected drugs and thus require a larger dose of nondepolarizing relaxants. Relaxants that rely on hepatic clearance may have a prolonged duration of action. Muscle relaxants that are metabolized independently of organ function (e.g., cisatracurium) are good choices for patients with liver disease.

9. **Describe special considerations in the perioperative assessment of alcohol-abusing patients.**
   Special consideration must be given to the cardiovascular system of chronic alcohol users. Tachycardia, dysrhythmias, or cardiomegaly may indicate alcohol-related cardiac dysfunction, and a 12-lead electrocardiogram (ECG) should be evaluated. Patients with alcohol-induced cardiac disease are less sensitive to endogenous or parenteral catecholamines. Hypokalemia and hypoglycemia are common, as are anemia, thrombocytopenia, and altered coagulation. These patients are often volume depleted and will require fluid resuscitation. Insert a urinary catheter to follow urine output. Intravascular monitoring should be individualized. Instrumentation of the esophagus should be avoided in patients with known liver disease because of the possibility of rupturing esophageal varices.

10. **How should sober chronic alcohol abusers be anesthetized?**
    Sober chronic alcohol users can tolerate intravenous and inhalational anesthetics. Isoflurane may be the best inhalational agent for maintaining hepatic blood flow. In general, a balanced anesthetic technique using amnestics, opioids, muscle relaxants, and an inhalational agent will suffice.

11. **What are the signs and symptoms of alcohol withdrawal?**
    Alcohol withdrawal presents as anorexia, insomnia, weakness, combativeness, tremors, disorientation, auditory and visual hallucinations, and convulsions. Onset is usually 10 to 30 hours after abstinence, and the symptoms may last for 40 to 50 hours. Prolonged abstinence may lead to delirium tremens or autonomic hyperactivity (tachycardia, diaphoresis, fever, anxiety, and confusion). Alcohol withdrawal syndrome may occur while under anesthesia and manifest as uncontrolled tachycardia, diaphoresis, and hyperthermia. The treatment is administration of benzodiazepines or intravenous infusion of ethanol.

KEY POINTS: CONCERNS IN CHRONIC ALCOHOLICS

1. May have cardiomyopathy and dysrhythmias
2. Predisposed to aspiration and have diminished pulmonary function
3. Portal hypertension and varices (avoid orogastric and nasogastric tubes)
4. Impaired synthetic liver function (important screening tests are albumin and prothrombin time)
5. Alcohol withdrawal may cause seizures.

12. **Review the differences between addiction, dependence, pseudoaddiction, and tolerance according to the American Pain Society.**
    - Dependence implies "a state of adaptation that is manifested by a drug class–specific withdrawal syndrome that can be produced by abrupt cessation, rapid dose reduction, decreasing blood level of the drug, and/or administration of an antagonist."
    - Opioid tolerance is "a state of adaptation in which exposure to a drug induces changes that result in a diminution of one or more of the drug's effects over time."
    - Addiction "is a primary, chronic, neurobiologic disease, with genetic, psychosocial, and environmental factors influencing its development and manifestations. It is characterized by behaviors that include one or more of the following: impaired control over drug use, compulsive use, continued use despite harm, and craving."
    - Pseudoaddiction refers to an iatrogenic state in which the patient displays addiction-type behaviors, but the cause is inadequate treatment of a painful condition. Often the setting is an acute pain condition superimposed on a chronic pain state. Patients on prolonged opioid therapy develop physical dependence and potentially tolerance, but they usually do not develop addictive behaviors.

13. **List complications of chronic opioid abuse.**
    - Cellulitis
    - Pneumonia
    - Adrenal suppression
    - Tetanus
    - Abscess formation
    - Subacute bacterial endocarditis
    - Thrombophlebitis
    - Hepatitis
    - Atelectasis
    - Acute pulmonary edema
    - Anemia
    - Systemic and pulmonary emboli
    - Pulmonary hypertension
    - Acquired immunodeficiency syndrome
    - Sepsis
    - Sclerosing glomerulonephritis
    - Death from overdose

14. **Discuss perioperative problems associated with the chronic opioid abuser.**
    The perioperative period is not an appropriate time to attempt opioid withdrawal. It is necessary to know the patient's usual opioid requirements to avoid undermedication. Associated behavioral and psychologic problems may make general anesthesia a better option than regional or local anesthesia. These patients may be in acute withdrawal and be uncooperative. Intravenous access may be difficult, and central venous catheterization may be necessary. A substantially increased dose of opioids to achieve the desired effect is the norm. Consultation with a pain-management team may help with development of a realistic postoperative pain-management strategy.

15. **Describe the time frame and stages of opioid withdrawal.**
    The onset and duration of withdrawal vary depending on the drug used. For example, meperidine withdrawal symptoms peak in 8 to 12 hours and last for 4 to 5 days. Heroin withdrawal symptoms usually peak within 36 to 72 hours and may last for 7 to 14 days.

Symptoms of withdrawal include restlessness, sweating, nausea, rhinorrhea, nasal congestion, abdominal cramping, lacrimation, and drug craving. Overt withdrawal results in piloerection, emesis, diarrhea, muscle spasms (thus the term *kicking the habit*), fever, chills, tachycardia, and hypertension.

16. **What medications are used to stabilize and detoxify the withdrawing opioid patient?**

    Long-acting medications (e.g., methadone and sustained-release morphine) are used because they have a slower onset of action and the high experienced with rapid-onset medications is less prominent. Autonomic hyperactivity and other symptoms of acute opiate withdrawal are treated with β-adrenergic antagonists and α_2 agonists such as clonidine.

17. **To what arrhythmias are methadone-treated patients prone?**

    There are multiple reports of these patients having prolonged correct QT intervals, torsades de pointes, and sudden death. Other important facts about methadone are that it has no effect on seizure disorders, has no active metabolites, is relatively safe in renal failure, and has not been associated with hepatic toxicity.

18. **What are the various forms of cocaine and routes of administration?**

    A hydrochloride salt of cocaine is a powdery, white crystalline, water-soluble substance that can be sniffed or injected. A lipid-soluble form, called crack or free-base cocaine, is inexpensively manufactured by mixing the hydrochloride salt with an alkali. Crack is more stable on heating, vaporizes readily, and has high bioavailability when smoked.

19. **How is cocaine metabolized and excreted?**

    Peak plasma concentrations occur 15 to 60 minutes after intranasal ingestion; its biologic half-life is about 45 to 90 minutes. Plasma (pseudocholinesterase) and liver esterases hydrolyze cocaine to ecgonine methyl ester (EME) and benzoylecgonine. EME and benzoylecgonine constitute 80% of the metabolites of cocaine and are detected in urine for 14 to 60 hours after cocaine use. Only 1% to 5% is cleared unmetabolized in the urine.

20. **What is the mechanism of action and what are the physiologic effects of cocaine?**

    There is inhibition of the norepinephrine, dopamine, and serotonin transporter mechanisms. However, the physiologic effects are caused principally by increases in norepinephrine levels. At adrenergic nerve endings, cocaine inhibits the reuptake of norepinephrine into the neuron. Increases in serum norepinephrine levels increase systolic, diastolic, and mean arterial pressure; heart rate; and body temperature.

21. **List the common signs and symptoms of acute cocaine intoxication.**
    - Nausea and vomiting
    - Headache
    - Rapid or irregular heartbeat
    - High or low blood pressure
    - Hallucinations
    - Chest pain
    - Convulsions and stroke
    - Mydriasis

22. **What is the most life-threatening toxic side effect and its treatment?**

    Cardiac ischemia and subsequent acute myocardial infarction are present in approximately 6% of all hospital admissions for chest pain secondary to cocaine ingestion. Although acute vasoconstriction with or without thrombus formation has been considered the principal cause, it is now believed to be the result of sympathetic stimulation associated with increased norepinephrine levels. Treatment of cocaine-induced chest pain includes the use of selective β_1-adrenergic blockade, nitrates, calcium channel blockers, and α-adrenergic blockers. Selective β_2 blockade should generally be avoided since it may lead to unopposed α_1-mediated coronary and peripheral vasoconstriction.

23. **List the signs and symptoms of cocaine withdrawal.**
    - Agitation
    - Anxiety and depression
    - Fatigue

- Irritability and disturbed sleep
- Tremors
- Myalgias

24. **What are the anesthetic concerns in the acutely intoxicated cocaine user?**
Preoperative sedation and a deep level of general anesthesia inhibit adrenal release of catecholamines, potentially reducing the dysrhythmic effects of cocaine. The patient should be well anesthetized before airway instrumentation to avoid severe tachycardia and hypertension. Cocaine sensitizes the cardiovascular system to the effects of endogenous catecholamines. Ketamine and pancuronium potentiate the cardiovascular toxicity of cocaine and should be avoided. The MAC of inhalational anesthetic agents is increased in the setting of acute intoxication. Should hypotension require pressor therapy, direct-acting agents such as phenylephrine may be better since these patients may be catecholamine depleted.

25. **Can the nonacutely intoxicated patient who has used cocaine be safely anesthetized?**
A recent study in a large urban public hospital determined that general anesthesia can be safely administered. However, cocaine is known to prolong the QT interval, predisposing the patient to ventricular arrhythmias, including torsades de pointes. Thus an ECG must be obtained before surgery, and, if the QT interval is less than 500 msec, the patient may be anesthetized.

KEY POINTS: CONCERNS IN PATIENTS TAKING COCAINE

1. Myocardial ischemia is not uncommon in cocaine-abusing patients, and selective β_2 blockade should be avoided because it may cause vasoconstriction and worsen the ischemia.
2. Severe hypertension and tachycardia are risks during airway management unless the patient is deeply anesthetized.
3. Cocaine sensitizes the cardiovascular system to the effects of endogenous catecholamines. Ketamine and pancuronium potentiate the cardiovascular toxicity of cocaine and should be avoided.

---

26. **What is crystal methamphetamine, and what are its properties?**
This refers to the synthetic stimulant methamphetamine. Most methamphetamine users are white and young adult. Most users are male, but it is the most common drug of abuse among women. Use of methamphetamine is common among homosexual males, and there is a strong relationship between its use and having the human immunodeficiency virus.

Methamphetamine use produces a rapid pleasurable rush followed by euphoria, heightened attention, and increased energy. These effects are caused by release of norepinephrine, dopamine, and serotonin. It is quite similar to cocaine in its manifestations, and its relatively lower costs may account for its increasing abuse.

Recommendations for anesthetizing a methamphetamine-abusing patient are similar to those for cocaine. Avoid anesthetizing the acutely intoxicated patient for elective procedures. Anesthesia is probably safely started in patients who are chronic users but not acutely intoxicated. There may be an increased incidence of dental trauma because of the common finding of dental decay.

27. **What are the signs of symptoms of methamphetamine intoxication and withdrawal?**
Signs and symptoms of intoxication include anorexia, diaphoresis, hypertension, tachycardia, hyperthermia, agitation, and psychosis. Patients can also have myocardial infarctions, seizures, strokes, rhabdomyolysis, and renal failure. The withdrawing patient will experience fatigue, irritability, insomnia, anxiety, and psychotic reactions. An unusual sign seen in chronic methamphetamine users is dental decay, known as *meth mouth*.

28. **What is ecstasy, and what are its mechanism of action and route of administration?**

    Ecstasy, or 3,4-methylenedioxymethamphetamine, is a synthetic, psychoactive drug similar to the stimulant methamphetamine and the hallucinogen mescaline. It increases the activity of multiple neurotransmitters, including serotonin, dopamine, and norepinephrine. It is taken orally in capsule or tablet form. Its effects last 3 to 6 hours. Additional doses slow its enzymatic degradation, resulting in increased duration of action and increased risk of toxicity.

29. **What are the cognitive, physical, and psychologic effects of ecstasy?**

    Abusers experience a sense of well-being and decreased anxiety. Memory impairment may occur. Physical effects include nausea, chills, involuntary teeth clenching, muscle cramping, and blurred vision. Hypertension, loss of consciousness, and seizures are also frequent. Rarely hyperthermia develops, which may precipitate cardiovascular collapse and multiorgan failure. Withdrawal may involve drug craving, depression, confusion, and severe anxiety. In nonhuman primates, as little as a 4-day exposure has been associated with damage to neurons involved in mood, thinking, and judgment.

30. **What is phencyclidine (PCP), and what is its mechanism of action?**

    PCP is a cyclohexylamine that was developed in the 1950s as an anesthetic but was subsequently taken off the market because of its tendency to produce hallucinations. The precise mechanism of action of PCP is unknown, but it is thought to depress cortical and thalamic function while stimulating the limbic system. PCP may block afferent impulses associated with the affective component of pain perception and suppress spinal cord activity. PCP can also inhibit pseudocholinesterase. Of note, the intravenous anesthetic ketamine is produced by chemical modification of PCP.

31. **Discuss the physical and psychological effects of PCP.**

    PCP produces a dissociative state or out-of-body experience. It crosses the blood-brain barrier to produce amnesia, delirium, disordered thought processes, paranoia, hostility, and delusions. Dissociation may resemble schizophrenia. Nystagmus, ataxia, and difficulty speaking may occur. Autonomic stimulation and cerebral vasodilation are also effects. No significant ventilatory depression is observed, and airway reflexes are maintained. Copious oral secretions may be noted. General anesthesia is preferable in these patients because of their frequent dissociative state and unpredictable violent behavior.

32. **How do you increase clearance of PCP?**

    Clearance is increased by acidification of the urine and nasogastric suction.

KEY POINTS: CONCERNS IN PATIENTS TAKING ECSTASY AND PHENCYCLIDINE

1. Hyperthermia and cardiovascular collapse with ecstasy
2. Dissociative state, severe behavior disturbances, and enhanced sympathomimetic effects with phencyclidine

---

WEBSITES

American Pain Society: http://www.ampainsoc.org
World Health Organization: Management of substance abuse: http://www.who.int/substance_abuse

SUGGESTED READINGS

Hill GE, Ogunnaike BO, Johnson ER: General anesthesia for the cocaine abusing patient. Is it safe? Br J Anaesth 97:654–657, 2006.
Tetrault JM, O'Connor PG: Substance abuse and withdrawal in the critical care setting, Crit Care Clin 24:767–788, 2008.

CHAPTER 45

DIABETES MELLITUS

Robert H. Slover, MD, and Robin Slover, MD

1. **Describe the principal types of diabetes mellitus.**
   - Type 1 diabetes mellitus: An autoimmune disorder in which destruction of the pancreatic islet cells results in the inability to produce insulin. Onset is more common in children and young adults.
   - Type 2 diabetes mellitus: A disorder in the body's ability to use insulin. Early in the course of the disease the patient may be able to make sufficient insulin, but cell-receptor impairment results in hyperglycemia despite normal or high insulin levels. Type 2 diabetes is usually a disease of older adults; onset in the sixth decade and beyond is common. As obesity increases in the population, type 2 diabetes also increases. Type 2 diabetes is now commonly seen in adolescents and young adults with obesity and a sedentary lifestyle.
   - Gestational diabetes: Seen in 2% to 5% of pregnant women, and 40% to 60% of these women will develop type 2 diabetes mellitus later in life.

2. **What is considered ideal (target) glucose control?**
   The American Diabetes Association (ADA) 2008 Clinical Practice Recommendations recommend an A_1C goal for nonpregnant adults in general of <7% (6% or lower is the nondiabetic A_1C range). Less stringent goals apply to children, patients with a history of severe hypoglycemia, and individuals with comorbid conditions.

3. **What comorbidities are frequently observed in patients with diabetes mellitus and to what significance?**
   - Hypertension is seen in 40% of patients with poorly controlled diabetes who undergo surgery. Hypertension is a risk factor for coronary artery disease and cardiac failure. If these patients are treated with potassium-wasting diuretic agents, there is often significant total body loss of potassium.
   - Coronary artery disease is common, occurs in younger patients, and may be silent or present atypically.
   - Autonomic neuropathy may compromise neuroreflexic control of cardiovascular and gastrointestinal function, manifesting as orthostatic hypotension, gastroparesis (increased risk of aspiration), ileus, and urinary retention. Peripheral neuropathies are common.
   - Disturbances in renal function are common, including increased blood urea nitrogen (BUN) and creatinine, protein loss, hypoalbuminemia, acidosis, and electrolyte disturbances.
   - Occult infections are present in 17% of patients with diabetes.
   - Retinal hemorrhages are seen in up to 80% of patients with diabetes over 15 years' duration and may lead to retinal detachment and vision loss.

4. **What oral medications are currently used in type 2 diabetes?**
   There are two categories of drugs used in treating type 2 diabetes: those that enhance the effectiveness of insulin and those that increase the supply of insulin to the cells. These drugs are outlined in Table 45-1.

5. **What insulins are in current use?**
   Modern intensive insulin therapy relies on newly designed insulin analogs. Insulin therapy is given using a basal-bolus construct: long-acting (24-hour) insulin is used to provide a steady basal platform, and rapid-acting insulin is used to provide boluses for carbohydrate intake in meals and snacks. This necessitates giving at least four injections per day or the use of an insulin pump. The specific insulins are outlined in Table 45-1.

Table 45-1. Oral Drugs Used in Type 2 Diabetes

ACTION	GENERIC NAME	BRAND NAME	DOSE	DOSING INTERVAL	SIDE EFFECTS
Enhance Insulin Effect					
Biguanide	Metformin	Glucophage	1000 mg	bid or tid	Transient gastrointestinal symptoms: Lactic acidosis*
Thiazolidinedione "glitazones"	Rosiglitazone Pioglitazone	Avandia Actos	Up to 600 mg daily	Daily or bid	Weight gain, anemia, edema, congestive heart failure,* hepatocellular disease*
α-Glucosidase inhibitors	Acarbose Miglitol	Precose Glyset	Used in combination 50 mg tid (acarbose) 25 mg tid (miglitol)	bid to qid	Flatulence, intestinal disease*
Increase Insulin Supply					
Sulfonylureas	Tolbutamide Chlorpropamide Tolazamide Glipizide Glyburide Glimepiride	Orinase Diabinese Tolinase Glucotrol DiaBeta, Micronase, Glynase Amaryl	2.5–5 mg (Glyburide)	Daily to tid	Hypoglycemia, weight gain, allergy*
Nonsulfonylureas	Repaglinide	Prandin	2 mg tid	bid to qid	Hypoglycemia

*Indicates rare but serious side effects.

6. **Is there an advantage to the use of insulins that are in solution as opposed to insulin that is in a suspension?**

   Insulins in solution provide exact dosing. For example, 10 units of Humalog will always be exactly 10 units. Neutral protamine Hagedorn (NPH), the only remaining insulin that is in suspension, does not provide exact or reproducible dosing but varies by as much as 30% either way. Ten units of NPH could really be 7 to 13 units!

7. **Describe the role of insulin on glucose metabolism and the impact of stress.**

   Insulin enhances glucose uptake, glycogen storage, protein synthesis, amino acid transport, and fat formation. Basal insulin secretion is essential even in the fasting state to maintain glucose homeostasis.

   Surgical procedures lead to increased stress and high counterregulatory hormone activity with a decrease in insulin secretion. Counterregulatory hormones, including epinephrine, cortisol, glucagon, and growth hormone, promote glycogenolysis, gluconeogenesis, proteolysis, and lipolysis. Therefore, in diabetic patients without adequate insulin replacement, the combination of insulin deficiency and excessive counterregulatory hormones can result in severe hyperglycemia and diabetic ketoacidosis, which are associated with hyperosmolarity, increases in protein catabolism, fluid loss, and lipolysis.

8. **Is there evidence that tight glucose control is beneficial in critically ill patients?**

   Recently it was believed that intensive insulin therapy to maintain glucose at or below 110 mg/dl reduces morbidity and mortality in critically ill patients in a surgical intensive care unit (ICU). It has subsequently been determined that extremely tight glucose control in surgical and medical ICUs significantly increases the risk of hypoglycemia and is not associated with significantly reduced hospital mortality. However, tight control does seem to significantly reduce septicemia and improve wound healing.

9. **What are the complications of hyperglycemia in the perioperative setting?**
   - Impaired polymorphonuclear cellular phagocytic function, increased risk of infection, and increased length of hospitalization
   - Osmotic diuresis, dehydration, and hyperosmolarity
   - Ketogenesis and diabetic ketoacidosis
   - Proteolysis and decreased amino acid transport, resulting in retarded wound healing
   - Hyperviscosity, thrombogenesis, and cerebral edema

10. **What considerations are important during the preoperative evaluation?**

    Important considerations include type of diabetes, duration of disease, oral hypoglycemic or insulin therapy, and diabetic complications, including hypertension, renal disease, coronary artery disease (which may be silent or present atypically), and neuropathies (early satiety and reflux suggest gastroparesis). If patients have end-stage renal disease or require dialysis, fluid restrictions may be necessary.

11. **What is the significance of autonomic neuropathy? How can it be assessed?**

    Autonomic neuropathy may affect cardiovascular (silent ischemia), gastrointestinal (gastroparesis with increased risk of aspiration), thermoregulatory (decreased ability to alter blood vessel flow to conserve temperature), and neuroendocrine systems (decreased catecholamine production in response to stimulation). Autonomic neuropathy can be assessed by these tests:
    - An intact sympathetic nervous system can be assessed by the following: A normal response in diastolic pressure (from lying to standing) is a change of at least 16 mm Hg; an affected patient has a response of <10 mm Hg. Autonomic neuropathy is also evidenced by a large change in systolic blood pressure when changing from lying to standing posture. A normal decrease is <10 mm Hg; an affected patient has a decrease of at least 30 mm Hg.
    - An intact parasympathetic nervous system can be assessed by observing heart rate response (i.e., rate variability) to breathing. Normal patients increase heart rate by at least 15 beats/min. Affected patients have an increase of 10 or fewer beats/min. Finally, concurrent with electrocardiogram (ECG) monitoring, the R-R ratio can be measured during a Valsalva maneuver. A normal ratio is >1.2; an abnormal response is <1.1.

Patients with autonomic neuropathy should be considered for preoperative aspiration prophylaxis, which may include an H_2-blocking agent, a gastric stimulant to decrease gastroparesis, and/or a nonparticulate antacid.

12. **What preoperative laboratory tests are appropriate for the patient with diabetes?**
Evaluate electrolytes, phosphate, and magnesium, BUN and creatinine, blood glucose and ketones, urinalysis, and ECG. Proteinuria is an early manifestation of diabetic nephropathy. A cardiac stress test should be considered in sedentary patients with cardiac risk factors. Measuring hemoglobin A_1C will provide valuable information about the level of glucose control. Patients with hemoglobin A_1C >9% are usually noncompliant and have an increased risk of dehydration.

13. **Are there any signs that oral intubation may be difficult?**
Although the remainder of the airway examination may be normal, patients with diabetes may have decreased mobility in the atlanto-occipital joint, which can complicate oral intubation. This can be evaluated radiographically. Patients may also have stiff joint syndrome with anterior fixation of the larynx. Stiff joint syndrome is suggested by the inability to approximate the palmar aspect of the pharyngeal joints of the fingers (also known as the prayer sign, the patient cannot touch the palmar aspects of the fingers together when the palms are together). The palmar print is another way of assessing stiff joints.

14. **How should the patient with diabetes be prepared before surgery? Should all patients with diabetes receive insulin intraoperatively?**
Patients with type 1 diabetes having short or minimally invasive procedures should receive a reduced dose of insulin and have their serum glucose followed. Patients with type 2 diabetes on oral medications should not take these medications the day of surgery. It is ideal to schedule the surgery early in the day.

Patients planned for longer or more stressful surgeries have increased levels of counterregulatory hormones and are likely to benefit from tighter glucose control. Furthermore, insulin requirements are increased by infection, hepatic disease, obesity, steroids, and cardiovascular procedures and pain. An insulin infusion may be considered to establish tighter glucose control. Before surgery, hyperglycemia, fluid and electrolyte imbalances, and ketosis should be corrected. Ideally in patients with renal failure, surgery should occur the day after hemodialysis.

Blood glucose levels under 200 mg/dl in the days preceding surgery are ideal and ensure adequate glycogen stores and insulin sufficiency. On the day before surgery, glucose should be monitored at bedside before each meal, at bedtime, and in the early morning. The goal is to have most glucose between 120 and 180 mg/dl.

15. **How do you make an insulin and glucose infusion?**
Ideally the glucose and insulin infusion should be started at least 1 hour before surgery. Glucose and insulin can be mixed together. They can also be given as separate infusions, but the combination infusion is safer because it is hard to have an accidental bolus of one or the other. Add 8 units regular insulin to 500 ml D_5W. Connect the tubing, shake well, and discard the first 100 ml through the tubing since insulin binds to polyvinyl chloride (PVC) bags and tubing. If a non-PVC bag is used, only 5 units of regular insulin are added to 500 ml of glucose. Again discard the first 100 ml of fluid. The mixture is infused at a rate of 100 ml/hr, and a blood glucose measurement should be obtained 20 minutes after starting the infusion and then hourly. The infusion will usually maintain the blood glucose level, although it may lower the level by 20 to 40 mg/dl.

For longer cases or in more fragile patients, 16 units of regular insulin is added to 1000 ml of D_5W. Consider adding 20 mEq/L of potassium, unless the patient's potassium is >5.5 mEq/L. If the patient's potassium is <4 mEq/L, 40 mEq/L should be added to the infusion. After mixing and discarding the first 100 ml through the tubing, the infusion is run at 100 ml/hr. Again blood glucose measurements are checked 20 minutes after starting the infusion and then hourly. The infusion may be increased or decreased by 4-unit increments.

16. **How fast can the blood glucose be lowered in a markedly hyperglycemic patient?**
    Blood glucose levels should not be lowered more than 100 mg/dl/hr if possible. Since the blood-brain barrier is slower to respond, a rapid drop in blood glucose could lead to cerebral swelling and, in rare cases, to symptomatic cerebral edema.

17. **Describe the postoperative management of the patient with diabetes.**
    In significant procedures with prolonged recovery, it is easier to manage the patient by continuing the insulin and glucose infusion for up to 48 hours, matching increased or decreased insulin needs with changes in rate or concentration of the infusion. Continue bedside monitoring of glucose, electrolytes, and fluids. A blood glucose goal of 120 to 180 mg/dl is reasonable. If total parenteral nutrition is used, the insulin rate may need to increase and should be adjusted based on glucose monitoring.
    With the resumption of oral feeding, insulin is given subcutaneously according to the patient's preoperative schedule. If pain or stress is still significant, it will be necessary to increase the dosage by as much as 20%. Monitor glucose at bedside before meals, at bedtime, and early in the morning, adjusting doses as necessary.

18. **How do you manage patients using subcutaneous insulin pumps?**
    Insulin pumps are now commonly used and can ensure good glucose control. The pumps use one of the newer analog insulins (Humalog, NovoLog, and Apidra) and deliver both basal and bolus insulin doses. Since the basal rate is set to deliver necessary insulin for the fasting state, the pump can be used for insulin delivery during the perioperative and intraoperative periods, continuing the established basal rates. Check blood sugars at regular intervals, every 1 to 2 hours, to ensure that the patient's blood sugar stays between 80 and 180 mg/dl. If the stress of a long surgery raises glucose levels, the basal infusion rate can be safely raised in increments of 0.1 unit per hour. If glucose levels fall, the rate can be safely reduced in increments of 0.1 unit per hour, or the pump can be suspended until glucose levels rise. When the patient is fully recovered, return to normal routines for pump use. The patients may consume a regular diet, as appropriate, when fully alert, awake, and with good bowel sounds.

19. **What insulins are preferred for pump use?**
    The rapid-acting analogs (NovoLog, Humalog, Apidra) are used in the insulin pumps. Interestingly, when insulin is given intravenously, there is no advantage to the analogs compared to regular human insulin. For that reason the less expensive regular insulin is usually used for intravenous therapy.

20. **Describe the management of patients with diabetes requiring urgent surgery.**
    If at all possible, electrolyte and glucose imbalance should be corrected before surgery. Sufficient rehydration, electrolyte replacement, and insulin treatment can be achieved in 4 to 6 hours, improving hyperglycemia, ketosis, and acidosis. Rehydration is initiated with 10 to 20 ml/kg of normal saline (NS). Infuse insulin at 0.1 unit/kg/hr using 0.45 NS (or D_{10} in 0.45 NS if glucose is <150 mg/dl). Patients in ketoacidosis requiring emergency surgery may receive insulin therapy according to the guidelines in Table 45-2.

21. **Are regional anesthetics helpful in patients with insulin-dependent diabetes? Can epinephrine be added to local anesthetic solutions?**
    Regional anesthetic techniques decrease the stress response and may help maintain a more stable blood glucose and decrease stress on the cardiovascular system. Epinephrine should not be used in peripheral nerve blocks (e.g., ankle blocks) because of the risk of decreasing blood flow to an area possibly already affected by impaired microcirculation. In blocks with high systemic absorption, such as brachial plexus or intercostal blocks, low-dose epinephrine may be used.

22. **Is it possible to achieve continuous monitoring of glucose levels in the operating room and in the perioperative period?**
    The technology is commercially available to have continuous glucose monitoring before, during, and after a procedure. Currently there are three continuous glucose-monitoring (CGM) systems that have U.S. Food and Drug Administration approval. Each of these samples interstitial fluid every 30 seconds to report an interstitial fluid glucose level every

Table 45-2. Insulin Therapy Guidelines

	ONSET OF ACTION	PEAK	DURATION OF ACTION
Long-Acting (Basal)			
Lantus (Glargine)	2–3 hr	None	24 hr
Levemir (Detemir)	2–3 hr	None	24 hr
Intermediate-Acting			
Regular	30–60 min	2–4 hr	6–9 hr
NPH (suspension)	4 hr	4–8 hr	8–13 hr
Rapid-Acting			
Humalog (lispro)	10–30 min	30–90 min	3–4 hr
NovoLog (aspart)	10–30 min	30–90 min	3–4 hr
Apidra (glulisine)	10–30 min	30–90 min	3–4 hr

5 minutes. Adjustment to insulin infusions can be made in response to changing glucose levels. Within a few years we expect to use continuous intra- and perioperative glucose monitoring tracings just as we now use continuous glucose tracings.

KEY POINTS: DIABETES MELLITUS

1. Careful attention to glucose control before, during, and after surgery is important to reduce risk of infection, promote more rapid healing, avoid metabolic complications, and shorten hospital stay.
2. The goal for insulin management during surgery is to maintain glucose between 120 and 200 mg/dl.
3. Intraoperative glucose control in all but the shortest cases is best achieved by using a glucose-insulin intravenous infusion or a pump.
4. Patients with diabetes have a high incidence of coronary artery disease with an atypical or silent presentation. Maintaining perfusion pressure, controlling heart rate, continuous ECG observation, and a high index of suspicion during periods of refractory hypotension are key considerations.
5. The inability to touch the palmar aspects of index fingers when palms touch (the prayer sign) can indicate a difficult oral intubation in patients with diabetes.

WEBSITES

American Diabetes Association: http://www.diabetes.org
Children's Diabetes Foundation: http://www.childrensdiabetesfoundation.org
Juvenile Diabetes Research Foundation: http://www.jdrf.org

SELECTED READINGS

Burant CF, Young LA, editors: Medical management of type 2 diabetes, ed 7, Alexandria, 2012, American Diabetes Association, pp 101–103.
Davidson MB: Standards of medical care in diabetes, Diabetes Care 28(Suppl):S4–S36, 2005.
Ferrari LR: New insulin analogues and insulin delivery devices for the perioperative management of diabetic patients, Curr Opin Anaesthesiol 21(3):401–405, 2008.
Fonseca VA: Standards of medical care in diabetes—2008, Diabetes Care 31(Suppl):S12–S54, 2008.
van den Berghe G, Wouters P, Weekers F, et al: Intensive insulin therapy in the critically ill patients, N Engl J Med 345:1359–1367, 2001.
Wiener RS, Wiener DC, Larson RJ: Benefits and risks of tight glucose control in critically ill adults: a meta-analysis, JAMA 300(8):933–944, 2008.

NONDIABETIC ENDOCRINE DISEASE

James C. Duke, MD, MBA

CHAPTER 46

1. **Review thyroid hormones.**
   Thyroid hormone tests include:
   - Total thyroxine (T_4) level
   - Total tri-iodothyronine (T_3) level—formed from the peripheral conversion of T_4
   - Thyroid-stimulating hormone (TSH) level—formed in anterior pituitary
   - Resin T_3 uptake (T_3RU). The T_3RU—useful in conditions that alter levels of thyroid-binding globulin, which would alter total T_4 results (Table 46-1)
   - Thyrotropin-releasing hormone (TRH)—produced by the hypothalamus

2. **What are common signs and symptoms of hypothyroidism?**
   - Symptoms include fatigue, cold intolerance, constipation, dry skin, hair loss, weight gain.
   - Signs include bradycardia, hypothermia, decreased tendon reflexes, hoarseness, periorbital edema.
   - Long-term, untreated hypothyroidism may progress to myxedema coma, which can be fatal. Myxedema is characterized by hypoventilation, hypothermia, hypotension, hyponatremia, and hypoglycemia (the "hypos") as well as obtundation and adrenal insufficiency.

3. **Review causes of hypothyroidism.**
   The most common causes of hypothyroidism include surgical or radioiodine ablation of thyroid tissue in the treatment of hyperthyroidism and, most commonly, Graves disease. Other causes of hypothyroidism include chronic thyroiditis (Hashimoto thyroiditis), drug effects, iodine deficiency, and pituitary or hypothalamic dysfunction.

4. **Which manifestations of hypothyroidism have the greatest anesthetic consideration?**
   Hypothyroidism causes depression of myocardial function. Cardiac output declines as a result of decreased heart rate and stroke volume. Decreased blood volume, baroreceptor reflex dysfunction, and pericardial effusion may also accompany hypothyroidism. Subsequently the hypothyroid patient is sensitive to the hypotensive effects of anesthetics.

   Hypoventilation may be a feature of hypothyroidism. The ventilatory responses to both hypoxia and hypercarbia are impaired, making the hypothyroid patient sensitive to drugs that cause respiratory depression. Hypothyroidism also decreases the hepatic and renal clearance of drugs. In addition, patients are prone to hypothermia because of lowered metabolic rate and consequent lowered heat production.

5. **How does hypothyroidism affect the minimum alveolar concentration (MAC) of anesthetic agents?**
   Animal studies show that MAC is not affected by hypothyroidism. But in clinical cases it has been noted that hypothyroid patients have increased sensitivity to anesthetic agents. This is caused not by a decrease in MAC per se but by the patient's metabolically depressed condition.

6. **Should elective surgery be delayed in a hypothyroid patient?**
   Patients with mild to moderate hypothyroidism are not at increased risk when undergoing elective surgical procedures. Some authorities suggest that elective surgery in patients who are symptomatic should be delayed until the patient is rendered euthyroid. In patients with severe hypothyroidism, elective surgery should be delayed until they have been rendered euthyroid. This may require 2 to 4 months of replacement therapy for complete reversal of

Table 46-1. Usefulness of Thyroid Function Tests in the Diagnosis of Hypothyroid or Hyperthyroid States

DISEASE	T_4	T_3	TSH	T_3RU
Primary hypothyroidism	−	−	+	−
Secondary hypothyroidism	−	−	−	−
Hyperthyroidism	+	+	0	+
Pregnancy	+	0	0	+

T_4, Thyroxine; T_3, tri-iodothyronine; *TSH*, thyroid-stimulating hormone; T_3RU, resin T_3 uptake; +, increased; −, decreased; 0, no change.

cardiopulmonary effects. Normalization of the patient's TSH level reflects reversal of hypothyroid-induced changes.

7. **List common signs and symptoms of hyperthyroidism.**
   - Symptoms include anxiety, tremor, heat tolerance, and fatigue.
   - Signs include goiter, tachycardia, proptosis, atrial fibrillation, weight loss, and weakness.
   - Causes include Graves disease and toxic multinodular goiter.

8. **How is hyperthyroidism treated?**
   - **Antithyroid drugs** such as propylthiouracil (PTU) inhibit iodination and coupling reactions in the thyroid gland, thus reducing production of T_3 and T_4. PTU also inhibits peripheral conversion of T_4 to T_3. Iodine in large doses not only blocks hormone production but also decreases the vascularity and size of the thyroid gland, making iodine useful in preparing hyperthyroid patients for thyroid surgery.
   - **Radioactive iodine,** [131]I, is actively concentrated by the thyroid gland, resulting in destruction of thyroid cells and a decrease in the production of hormone.
   - **Surgical subtotal thyroidectomy**

9. **Review anesthetic effects when patient is in a hyperthyroid state.**
   The metabolic rate is increased, impacting the cardiovascular system, the magnitude of which is proportional to the severity of thyroid dysfunction. Because of the increased oxygen consumption, the cardiovascular system is hyperdynamic. Tachycardia and elevated cardiac output are present, and tachyarrhythmias, atrial fibrillation, left ventricular hypertrophy, and congestive heart failure may develop. Hyperthyroid patients with proptosis are more susceptible to ocular damage during surgery because of difficulty with taping their eyelids closed.

10. **How is MAC affected by hyperthyroidism?**
    As in hypothyroidism, MAC is not affected by hyperthyroidism, although clinically hyperthyroid patients appear to be resistant to the effects of anesthetic agents. Inhalation induction is slowed by the increased cardiac output. The rate of drug metabolism is increased, giving the appearance of resistance.

11. **Review thyrotoxicosis and its treatment.**
    Also known as *thyroid storm*, this is an acute exacerbation of hyperthyroidism usually caused by a stress such as surgery or infection. It is characterized by extreme tachycardia, hyperthermia, and possibly severe hypotension. Perioperatively it usually occurs 6 to 18 hours after surgery but can occur intraoperatively and be mistaken for malignant hyperthermia.
    Treatment consists of judicious β-adrenergic blockade, infusion of intravenous fluids, and temperature control if hyperthermia is present. Corticosteroids should be considered for refractory hypotension because hyperthyroid patients may have a relative cortisol deficiency. Antithyroid drugs should be added after surgery.

12. **What complications may occur after thyroidectomy?**
    Adjacent to the thyroid gland are the trachea and larynx, and cervical hematoma may cause airway obstruction. Chronic pressure on the trachea may lead to tracheomalacia, and

tracheal collapse is a consideration. Inadvertent resection of the parathyroid glands may lead to hypocalcemia and, subsequently, laryngospasm. Damage to recurrent laryngeal nerves (RLNs) may impair vocal cord function and airway obstruction. Bilateral partial RLN injury can result in vocal cord adduction and airway obstruction. Total destruction of the bilateral RLNs results in the vocal cords being in midposition and rarely produces total airway obstruction.

13. **Describe hyperparathyroid function.**
    Parathormone has a significant effect on serum calcium levels, and inadequate parathormone levels are usually associated with hypocalcemia and commonly have observed tetanic effects. Hyperparathyroidism and hypothyroidism are associated with hypercalcemia and hypocalcemia, respectively.

14. **What parathyroid glands are commonly removed?**
    Parathyroid adenomas, a source of hyperparathyroidism, are most commonly removed. Roughly speaking, unplanned total removal of parathyroid glands during thyroidectomy occurs about 0.5% to 5% of the time. On occasion, one parathyroid gland is reinserted in an arm so that parathyroid function persists. One parathyroid gland is thought suitable to maintain serum PTH and calcium levels.

15. **Describe complications post hyperparathyroidectomy.**
    Hypocalcemia may result in laryngospasm. Hematoma may obstruct the airway. Recurrent laryngeal nerves may be transected, affecting vocal cord function, including airway obstruction. Unlike other hormones, there is no replacement analog for parathormone.

16. **Describe the anatomy and physiology of the adrenal gland.**
    The suprarenal adrenal gland is functionally divided into the adrenal cortex and the adrenal medulla. The adrenal cortex principally produces the steroid hormone cortisol (the main glucocorticoid) and aldosterone (the main mineralocorticoid). Aldosterone is secreted by the renal cortex and is regulated by the renin-angiotensin system (discussed in Chapter 40). Mineralocorticoid synthesis may persist during adrenal insufficiency.
    Production of cortisol is regulated by adrenocorticotropic hormone (ACTH) produced by the anterior pituitary. The release of ACTH is promoted by corticotropin-releasing hormone (CRH), derived from the hypothalamus, completing the hypothalamic-pituitary-adrenal (HPA) axis. Cortisol inhibits release of both CRH and ACTH, establishing negative feedback control. Ectopic ACTH can be produced by various neoplasms such as small-cell lung carcinomas.
    The adrenal medulla also secretes epinephrine and norepinephrine. Their release is governed by the sympathetic nervous system, discussed in Chapter 1.

17. **How much cortisol is produced by the adrenal cortex?**
    Normally approximately 20 to 30 mg of cortisol per day is produced. This amount increases dramatically as a response to a stress such as infection or surgery. Under stressful conditions, 75 to 150 mg/day may be produced, with the increase in production being generally proportional to the severity of the stress.

18. **What is the most common cause of HPA axis disruption?**
    Causes of HPA axis disruption include central nervous system mass lesions (tumor or abscess), head injury or subarachnoid hemorrhage, tuberculosis, vascular injury, and adrenal causes (etomidate, ketoconazole, hemorrhage, infection, autoimmune adrenalitis, adrenal hemorrhage, bilateral adrenal metastases), septic shock, and other acute illness.

19. **What is the impact of steroid administration?**
    Exogenous steroids (glucocorticoids) result in HPA axis suppression. Short-term steroid administration—no longer than 7 to 10 days—results in suppression of CRH and ACTH release, which usually returns to normal about 5 days after discontinuation of steroid therapy. Long-term administration of exogenous steroids results in adrenocortical atrophy secondary to a lack of ACTH. This results in prolonged adrenocortical insufficiency, which can last a year or more following steroid discontinuation. Therefore long-term steroid administration should not be terminated abruptly; rather it should be gradually tapered off over a period of 1 to 4 weeks.

Table 46-2. Relative Potency of Cortisol and Exogenous Steroids

STEROID	GLUCOCORTICOID	MINERALOCORTICOID	HALF-LIFE (HOURS)
Cortisol	1	1	8–12
Cortisone	0.8	0.8	8–12
Prednisone	4	0.25	12–36
Methylprednisolone	5	0.25	12–36
Triamcinolone	5	0.25	12–36
Dexamethasone	20–30	—	26–54
Fludrocortisone	5	200	12–36

20. **What is an addisonian crisis?**
Also referred to as *acute adrenocortical insufficiency*, an addisonian crisis is caused by a relative lack of cortisol or other glucocorticoid. It is a shock state characterized by refractory hypotension, hypovolemia, and electrolyte disturbances.

21. **How do exogenous steroids compare with cortisol?**
See Table 46-2.

KEY POINTS: NONDIABETIC ENDOCRINE DISEASE

1. Perioperatively mild to moderate hypothyroidism is of little concern even for elective surgery. Patients with severe, symptomatic hypothyroidism should be treated before surgery.
2. MAC of volatile anesthetics is unchanged in both hypothyroid and hyperthyroid states.
3. Thyrotoxicosis ("thyroid storm") may mimic malignant hyperthermia. It is detected by an increased serum T_4 level and treated initially with β blockade followed by antithyroid therapy.
4. Perioperative glucocorticoid supplementation should be considered for patients receiving exogenous steroids.
5. Chronic exogenous glucocorticoid therapy should not be discontinued abruptly. Doing so may precipitate acute adrenocortical insufficiency.

22. **Is perioperative stress steroid supplementation for patients on chronic steroid therapy necessary?**
Few documented cases of acute perioperative adrenal insufficiency (i.e., addisonian crisis) exist. Studies have shown that patients who have been on long-term steroid therapy undergoing even major surgery rarely become hypotensive because of glucocorticoid deficiency. If observed, hypotension is usually the result of hypovolemia or cardiac dysfunction. Possible side effects of perioperative steroid supplementation include the following:
- Hyperglycemia
- Gastric ulceration
- Fluid retention
- Impaired wound healing
- Aggravation of hypertension
- Immunosuppression

One approach might be that no supplementation is required unless hypotension refractory to standard treatment occurs. Few data indicate any significant problems related to short-term perioperative steroid supplementation. Despite its rarity, acute adrenal insufficiency is associated with significant morbidity and mortality. Therefore, because perioperative steroid supplementation is associated with few risks in itself and because acute adrenal insufficiency can potentially lead to death, supplemental steroids should be given. Currently this seems to be the view of most authorities.

23. **What dosage of corticosteroids should be administered when considered perioperatively?**
Often debated, recent guidelines suggest lower doses and shorter durations than those recommended in the past. Patients ordinarily receiving 5 mg/day or less of prednisone should receive their normal daily replacement but do not require supplementation. For minor surgery, no supplementation or minimal supplementation may suffice. Hydrocortisone, 25 mg, may suffice. For moderate surgery, give 50 to 75 mg of hydrocortisone on the day of procedure and taper the dose quickly over 1 to 2 days. For major surgery, a variety of dosages have been suggested, with none being shown to be superior to the rest. A suggested regimen would be 100 to 150 mg of hydrocortisone on the day of procedure with a quick 1- to 2-day taper. The goal of these regimens is to give the lowest dose that provides sufficient supplementation while avoiding potential side effects.

24. **Review the impact of steroids when patients are critically ill.**
On occasion there is HPA axis suppression and decreased cortisol synthesis though serum cortisol levels may be difficult to interpret. Corticotropin levels are disproportionately elevated relative to plasma cortisol levels. Intravenous hydrocortisone 50 mg every 6 hours should be considered.

25. **Should anabolic steroid use be considered when performing anesthesia on users?**
Anabolic steroids are ingested to enhance physical performance. Increased muscle mass increases oxygen requirements. Cardiomyopathies are common, as is atherosclerosis. Hypertension and diastolic cardiac dysfunction have been noted. Hepatic dysfunction is a risk, as is hypercoagulopathy. Resistance to nondepolarizing muscle relaxants has been reported. Athletes ingesting anabolic steroids may be hyperaggressive and have other behavioral disturbances. Prompt discontinuation of anabolic steroids prior to surgery may result in addisonian effects.

SUGGESTED READINGS

Axelrod L: Perioperative management of patients treated with glucocorticoids, Endocrinol Metab Clin North Am 32:367–383, 2003.

Bouillon R: Acute adrenal insufficiency, Endocrinol Metab Clin North Am 35:767–775, 2006.

Connery LE, Coursin DB: Assessment and therapy of selected endocrine disorders, Anesthesiol Clin North America 22:93–123, 2004.

Cooper MS, Stewart PM: Adrenal insufficiency in critical illness, J Intensive Care Med 22:348–362, 2007.

Kam PC, Yarrow M: Anabolic steroids abuse: physiological and anaesthetic considerations, Anaesthesia 60:685–692, 2005.

Shoback D: Hypoparathyroidism, N Engl J Med 359:391–403, 2008.

Wald DA: ECG manifestations of selected metabolic and endocrine disorders, Emerg Med Clin North Am 24:145–157, 2006.

CHAPTER 47

OBESITY AND SLEEP APNEA

Gillian E. Johnson, MBBChir, BSc, and James C. Duke, MD, MBA

1. **Define obesity.**
   Obesity is defined using the body mass index (BMI) (Table 47-1).

   $$BMI = Weight\ (Kg)/Height\ squared\ (m^2)$$

2. **Discuss the cardiovascular considerations in patients who are obese.**
   Systemic and pulmonary hypertension, as well as left- and right-sided heart failure and coronary artery disease, are all found in obese patients. As body mass increases, so does oxygen consumption. Cardiac output, stroke volume, and circulating blood volume increase to meet increased demand. Systemic hypertension, over time, results in left ventricular hypertrophy. Obese patients with coronary artery disease may have silent myocardial infarctions.

3. **Review some pulmonary and respiratory considerations in obese patients.**
   Considerations include the possibility of a difficult airway, increased asthma, and sleep-disordered breathing or obstructive sleep apnea (OSA), restrictive lung disease, chronic hypoxia with or without polycythemia, and pulmonary hypertension.
   Obesity is typically associated with hypoxemia, the mechanisms of which include:
   - Increased work of breathing. Because of an increased chest wall mass, decreased chest wall compliance, and abdominal cavity adipose tissue decreasing diaphragmatic excursion, work of breathing is 2 to 3 times greater than normal.
   - Restrictive lung disease develops, areas of the lung become underventilated and atelectatic, ventilation/perfusion mismatch occurs, and the lungs compensate by selective vasoconstriction of poorly ventilated regions. Ultimately pulmonary hypertension develops, which leads to right-sided heart failure.
   - Large tissue mass increases the total oxygen consumption and carbon dioxide production.

4. **What are the gastrointestinal and hepatic changes seen in patients who are obese?**
   Obesity increases intraabdominal and intragastric pressures. Hiatal hernias and gastric reflux are common. Despite an 8-hour fast, 85% to 90% of morbidly obese patients have gastric volumes >25 ml, increasing the risk of pulmonary aspiration. These patients typically have fatty infiltration of the liver and may have hepatic inflammation, focal necrosis, or cirrhosis. At present, no causal relationship between fatty infiltration and cirrhotic changes is known. Hepatic enzymes are generally altered, especially after jejunoileal bypass operations. Aminotransferases and γ-glutamyl transpeptidase are increased in this patient population.

5. **Discuss the pharmacokinetic changes found in obese patients.**
   Loading doses of most intravenous (IV) agents are based on volume of distribution. Maintenance dosing is based on clearance. The volume of distribution is usually increased, but clearance approaches normal or is increased compared with that of lean patients (Table 47-2).
   Changes in drug metabolism are unpredictable. Lipophilic intravenous agents (e.g., opioids, benzodiazepines, and barbiturates) have an increased volume of distribution and lower serum drug concentrations. In obese patients, hydrophilic, water-soluble drugs generally have volumes of distribution, elimination half-lives, and rates of clearance similar to those in nonobese patients. Fentanyl shows similar pharmacokinetics in obese and nonobese patients.
   Pseudocholinesterase activity is increased in patients who are obese, and larger doses of succinylcholine are required. Nondepolarizing muscle relaxants are variable in dosing, duration, and recovery, and redosing should be assessed by peripheral nerve stimulation.

Table 47-1. Definition of Obesity

BMI	CLASSIFICATION
18.5–25	Normal range
26–30	Overweight
31–35	Class I obesity
36–40	Class II obesity
41+	Morbid obesity

BMI, Body mass index.

Table 47-2. Loading Dose Strategy for Intravenous Drugs

DRUGS	DOSING STRATEGY
Fentanyl	Loading dose based on TBW; decrease maintenance
Sufentanil	Loading dose based on TBW; decrease maintenance
Remifentanil	Dose based on IBW
Succinylcholine	Dose based on TBW
Atracurium	Dose using TBW
Vecuronium	Dose using IBW
Rocuronium	Dose using IBW
Propofol	Loading dose and maintenance based on TBW
Thiopental	Reduce loading dose
Midazolam	Loading dose based on TBW; adjust maintenance to IBW

IBW, Ideal body weight; TBW, total body weight.

There is no evidence to suggest that any one inhalational anesthetic is superior to another in obese patients.

6. Discuss the appropriate preoperative assessment of the obese population.
   As far as laboratory testing is concerned:
   • An electrocardiogram should be obtained for all obese patients to evaluate for atrial or ventricular enlargement, arrhythmias, and ischemia. Ventricular arrhythmias are common. Stress tests may be required. Echocardiography can quantify cardiac function and pulmonary hypertension.
   • Chest radiographs may not be generally useful without concerning history.
   • A complete blood count and levels of electrolytes, carbon dioxide, blood sugar, blood urea nitrogen, and creatinine suggest associated disease. Elevated bicarbonate suggests carbon dioxide retention. A room air arterial blood gas analysis will identify hypoxemia, hypercarbia, and metabolic compensation.
   • If chronic lung disease is suspected, pulmonary function testing may also be necessary to characterize the extent of disease and amenability to preoperative optimization.

7. What are the advantages or disadvantages of offering regional anesthesia to obese patients?
   Advantages
   • Decreased cardiopulmonary depression
   • Improved postoperative analgesia with decreased need for narcotics
   • Less postoperative nausea and vomiting, shorter post–anesthetic care unit stay (see Chapter 28)

Table 47-3. Respiratory Values Characterized in Morbid Obesity

Respiratory rate	<30 breaths/min
Maximal inspiratory force	−25 to −30 cm H_2O
Vital capacity	10–15 ml/kg
Tidal volume	5 ml/kg (lean body weight)

Disadvantages
- Technical difficulties arise in performing the blocks because of body habitus.
- Failed peripheral nerve or neuraxial blocks may require intubation under suboptimal conditions.
- Positioning is difficult and may not be well tolerated.

8. **Review the challenges in monitoring patients who are obese.**
   American Society of Anesthesiologists standard monitoring devices should be used in all cases. Blood pressure cuffs should span a minimum of 75% of the patient's upper arm circumference. The ankle or wrist may be used as alternate sites for taking blood pressure. Invasive arterial monitoring should be used for severely obese patients and those with significant cardiopulmonary disease or when noninvasive blood pressure cuffs are unreliable. Establishing peripheral intravenous access may be difficult in obese patients, and central venous catheters may prove necessary.

9. **Discuss positioning obese patients.**
   Obese patients have an increased risk of atelectasis, which persists for a greater number of days than in nonobese patients. In addition, they have increased risk of hypoxia for 4 to 7 days after surgery. Postoperative pulmonary physiotherapy is recommended.

10. **What intubation and extubation maneuvers challenge obese patients?**
    Many of these patients do not tolerate a flat, supine position. Placing patients in a head-up position improves airway mechanics by unloading the diaphragm, increasing the functional residual capacity. Obese patients also have an increased risk of atelectasis and are prone to oxygen desaturation. Common respiratory parameters referred to in morbidly obese patients are discussed in Table 47-3.

11. **Describe bariatric surgery as obesity treatment. What are anesthetic concerns?**
    Bariatric surgery broadly encompasses several surgical weight loss procedures used in the treatment of morbid obesity. The most common procedures include gastric banding, adjustable gastric banding, and Roux-en-Y gastric bypass. The surgeries cause weight loss by limiting both the volume of food a person can ingest and the absorption of calories, vitamins, and minerals. Bariatric surgery has become increasingly common, and the surgical candidate population is widening.
    Bariatric surgical procedures are often performed laparoscopically. The increased intraabdominal pressure of morbid obesity combined with a pneumoperitoneum results in venous stasis, reduced intraoperative portal venous blood flow, decreased urinary output, lower respiratory compliance, increased airway pressure, impairment of cardiac function, and hypercapnia. In addition, there is less efficient elimination of carbon dioxide and increased $PaCO_2$ when compared with nonobese patients. As a consequence, pneumoperitoneum is not recommended in morbidly obese patients with severe cardiac, pulmonary, hepatic, or pulmonary dysfunction.
    Preoperative evaluation includes assessment for hypertension, diabetes mellitus, left- or right-sided heart failure, pulmonary hypertension and coronary artery disease. It should also include airway examination and development of a plan for airway management, as these patients often present with difficult airways.
    Intraoperative management to minimize the adverse changes include appropriate ventilatory adjustments to avoid hypercapnia and acidosis, the use of sequential compression devices to minimize venous stasis, and optimized intravascular volume to minimize the effects of increased intraabdominal pressure on renal and cardiac function.

Surgical management results in decreased gastric volumes, with two goals being gastrointestinal restriction and decreased malabsorption. The benefits of bariatric surgical procedures include reduced incidences of OSA, diabetes mellitus and hypertension, as well as an overall reduction in BMI and serum lipid levels. Complications include deep venous thrombosis, anastomotic leaks, wound infection, bleeding, herniation, and small bowel obstruction. Some patients also return to the operating room for panniculectomy and excision of other redundant extremity tissue. These patients are often depleted, and the altered gastric anatomy may predispose the patient to regurgitation of gastric contents at the time of anesthetic induction.

12. What is obesity hypoventilation syndrome (OHS)?

OHS is the triad of obesity, daytime hypoventilation, and sleep-disordered breathing. In addition to the problem of OSA, such patients also have severe upper airway obstruction, restrictive chest physiology, and pulmonary hypertension. Among patients with OHS, 90% have OSA. Morbidity is high but preoperative screening for OHS may be insufficient. Daytime hypercapnia is distinctly common and more prevalent when compared with OSA patients. Arterial blood gases demonstrating chronic carbon dioxide retention may further identify patients considered at risk. Postoperatively, progressive carbon dioxide levels are characteristic if the patient is receiving opioids for analgesia. Cardiac arrest has been noted and is a function of progressive carbon dioxide retention.

13. Is OSA common?

The prevalence of adult sleep apnea is approximately 2% in women and 4% in men. The prevalence of childhood sleep apnea is up to 10%. These children are commonly seen on the otolaryngology surgical schedule for tonsillectomy and adenoidectomy; this is curative in 75% to 100% of cases, even in the obese population. However, it is estimated that nearly 80% of men and 93% of women with moderate to severe sleep apnea are undiagnosed. Undiagnosed OSA may pose a variety of problems for anesthesiologists.

14. Which techniques can be used to identify patients with OSA?

Identifying patients with OSA is the first step in preventing postoperative complications caused by OSA. Questionnaires that have been designed to screen for the presence of OSA include the Berlin questionnaire, the STOP questionnaire, and the American Society of Anesthesiologists checklist. Each of these has been validated in surgical patients as a screening tool for OSA and has demonstrated a moderately high level of sensitivity. All three of the tests evaluate snoring, daytime tiredness, presence of hypertension, and observed apnea. Because of the easy-to-use format and self-administered testing, the STOP questionnaire might be easier for patients to complete and more suitable in busy preoperative clinics. A unique feature is a measured neck circumference of 18 cm or more.

15. What are postoperative risks of OSA patients?

As in patients with OHS, in patients with OSA, carbon dioxide retention is a risk and perhaps made riskier by opioid administration. Respiratory depression has been noted whether the patient has received intravenous, patient-controlled intravenous or epidural analgesia.

16. What are the best treatment modalities for postoperative OSA patients?

Monitoring oxygen saturation, tracking phasic respirations, oxygen therapy, and positive airway pressure to maintain airway patency.

KEY POINTS: OBESITY AND SLEEP APNEA

1. Morbidly obese patients have numerous systemic disorders and physiologic challenges, including restrictive lung disease, obstructive sleep apnea (OSA), coronary artery disease, diabetes, hypertension, cardiomegaly, pulmonary hypertension, and delayed gastric emptying. Safe anesthetic practice requires preparation for diagnosis, monitoring, and emergent treatment of any of these conditions.
2. Obese patients may be difficult to ventilate and intubate, and they may desaturate quickly after anesthetic induction. Backup strategies should always be considered and readily available before airway management begins.

3. In patients who are obese, pharmacokinetic changes secondary to large volumes of adipose tissue require some drugs to be dosed for lean body weight and others based on total body weight.
4. Obese patients often have OSA, requiring appropriate diagnosis and care, especially in the postoperative period.

WEBSITES

Anesthesia Patient Safety Foundation: http://www.apsf.org
Obesity Society: http://www.obesity.org

SUGGESTED READINGS

American Society of Anesthesiologists Task Force on Perioperative Management of patients with obstructive sleep apnea: Practice guidelines for the perioperative management of patients with obstructive sleep apnea: an updated report by the American Society of Anesthesiologists Task Force on Perioperative Management of patients with obstructive sleep apnea, Anesthesiology 120:268–286, 2014.
Brodsky JB, Lemmens HJ: Regional anesthesia and obesity, Obes Surg 17:1146–1149, 2007.
Chau EHL, Lam D, Wong J, et al: Obesity hypoventilation syndrome, Anesthesiology 117:188–205, 2012.
Chung F, Yegneswaran B, Liao P, et al: STOP questionnaire: a tool to screen patients for obstructive sleep apnea, Anesthesiology 108:812–821, 2008.
Chung F, Yegneswaran B, Liao P, et al: Validation of the Berlin questionnaire and American Society of Anesthesiologists checklist as screening tools for obstructive sleep apnea in surgical patients, Anesthesiology 108:822–830, 2008.
DeMaria EJ: Bariatric surgery for morbid obesity, N Engl J Med 356:2176–2183, 2007.
Haque AK, Gadre S, Taylor J, et al: Pulmonary and cardiovascular complications of obesity: an autopsy study of 76 obese subjects, Arch Pathol Lab Med 132:1397–1404, 2008.
Ogunnaike BO, Jones SB, Jones DB, et al: Anesthetic considerations for bariatric surgery, Anesthesiology 2002:1793–1805, 2002.

ALLERGIC REACTIONS
James C. Duke, MD, MBA

CHAPTER 48

1. **Review the four types of immune-mediated allergic reactions and their mechanisms.**
   - **Type I**, or immediate hypersensitivity, is immunoglobulin (Ig) E–mediated hypersensitivity and in its most severe form results in anaphylaxis. Usually there is a previous exposure to the antigen during which IgE is produced and binds to mast cells and basophils. After reexposure, the antigen cross-links two IgE receptors, initiating the cascade that ultimately results in release of potent vasodilating mediators. Type I reactions will be discussed in greater detail subsequently.
   - **Type II** reactions involve IgG, IgM, and the complement cascade to mediate cytotoxicity; an example is Goodpasture syndrome.
   - **Type III** reactions are the result of immune-complex formation, and their deposition in tissue leads to tissue damage; an example is hypersensitivity pneumonitis.
   - **Type IV** reactions, or delayed hypersensitivity, are mediated by T lymphocytes; the best example is contact dermatitis.

2. **What is meant by anaphylaxis?**
   Anaphylaxis is an unanticipated and severe allergic reaction with numerous clinical manifestations, including the following:
   - Hypotension, tachycardia, and cardiovascular collapse
   - Bronchospasm
   - Cutaneous symptoms, including flushing, urticaria, and angioedema
   - Gastrointestinal symptoms, including abdominal pain, nausea and vomiting, and diarrhea
   Because surgical patients are under drapes, the usual presenting features intraoperatively are hypotension, tachycardia, and bronchospasm. Since these are not uncommon problems encountered by anesthesiologists, a degree of clinical acumen is necessary to arrive at the diagnosis of anaphylaxis and quickly institute therapy.

3. **What is an anaphylactoid reaction?**
   Although the symptoms are indistinguishable from anaphylaxis, an anaphylactoid reaction is nonimmune mediated. Release of inflammatory mediators from mast cells and basophils results in activation of the complement cascade.

4. **What are the common causes of anaphylaxis in the operating room?**
   About 80% of all anaphylactic reactions are caused by either muscle relaxants (e.g., succinylcholine, rocuronium, and atracurium) or latex exposure, but there are other causes:
   - **Antibiotics**, usually penicillin and other β-lactam antibiotics (cephalosporins) (see Question 6).
   - **Propofol and thiopental:** The incidence of allergic reaction to the most current preparation of propofol is estimated to be 1 in 60,000 administrations; current evidence also suggests that egg-allergic patients are not at increased risk for allergic reactions. The incidence of anaphylaxis is 1 in 30,000 administrations and may be caused by the presence of sulfur in the compound. Intravenous barbiturates are rarely encountered.
   - **Colloids:** Dextran and gelatin have an allergic reaction incidence of about 0.3%. Hetastarch is the safest colloid.
   - **Morphine and meperidine:** More than likely the reaction seen is to the result of nonimmunologic histamine release.

- **Aprotinin, heparin, and protamine:** Allergic reactions to aprotinin occur in <1% of patients, but reexposure increases the risk. Allergic reactions to unfractionated heparin are rare and to low-molecular-weight heparin are even rarer. The most common reaction to heparin is heparin-induced thrombocytopenia, which is nonimmunologic in origin. Patients with prior exposure to protamine, such as those taking neutral protamine Hagedorn insulin, have the greatest risk of allergic reaction, about 0.4% to 0.76%.
- **Local anesthetics:** Allergies to local anesthetics with amide linkages (e.g., bupivacaine, lidocaine, mepivacaine, ropivacaine) are extremely rare. True allergic reactions to local anesthetics with ester linkages (e.g., procaine, chloroprocaine, tetracaine, benzocaine) are also rare and may be caused by a para-aminobenzoic acid metabolite. Methylparaben, a preservative in local anesthetics, may cause allergic reactions.

5. **Review the issues concerning allergic reactions to muscle relaxants.**
   About 70% of all intraoperative anaphylactic reactions are associated with relaxants. IgE immunoglobulins are sensitive to the tertiary or quaternary ammonium groups found in these compounds. Since such chemical groups are commonly found in foods, cosmetics, and over-the-counter medications, prior exposure to muscle relaxants is often unnecessary. Succinylcholine is more likely to result in anaphylaxis than nondepolarizing relaxants because its smaller, flexible molecular structure can more easily cross-link mast cell IgE receptors. Benzylisoquinolium relaxants are more likely to result in anaphylaxis than are aminosteroid relaxants, and benzylisoquinolium relaxants can also cause nonimmunologic histamine release.

6. **Should a penicillin-allergic patient receive cephalosporins?**
   Authorities disagree on this issue. Although penicillin is the most common cause of anaphylaxis in the general population, only about 10% to 20% of patients reporting a penicillin reaction have a well-documented allergy, and numerous complaints such as gastrointestinal symptoms or rashes of nonimmunologic origin are labeled *allergy*. An oft-quoted statistic is that there is an 8% to 10% risk of cross-sensitivity between penicillin and cephalosporins because they share a β-lactam ring, but this is now disputed.
   In earlier times this may have been true, possibly because earlier generations of cephalosporins contained trace amounts of penicillin. Some authorities believe cephalosporins are safe to be administered to penicillin-allergic patients as long as these patients have not experienced a prior anaphylactic reaction or have a documented positive skin test for penicillin. Clearly there is a lack of consensus on this issue, and the risks of anaphylaxis must be weighed against the benefits of penicillin therapy. A careful and thorough history of what is meant by *penicillin allergy* is important in this decision process.

7. **What is latex?**
   Latex is derived from the sap of the Brazilian rubber tree. There are numerous proteins within this product that may produce allergic reactions. Latex products may differ dramatically in the number of allergens detectable within the product. Unfortunately, with the dramatic increase in need for latex products, quantity has been sacrificed for quality. Chemicals from the manufacturing process of commercial latex products may also result in irritant and allergic contact dermatitis.

8. **What demographic groups are at risk for latex allergy?**
   - Historically patients with meningocele, myelomeningocele, and spina bifida were at increased risk for latex allergy because they required chronic bladder catheterization with latex catheters.
   - Patients with spinal cord injury and developmental abnormalities of the genitourinary system are also at risk.
   - Patients who have had multiple operations may develop a latex allergy.
   - Atopic individuals (i.e., multiple food allergies, eczema, and asthma) are prone as well.
   - Individuals who have problems (rash, itching, edema) with latex products such as condoms, balloons, diaphragms, gloves, or dental dams may be at risk for developing severe latex-associated allergic reactions.

- Sensitivity to certain fruits (e.g., avocado, banana, kiwi, chestnut) and vegetables (e.g., tomato, bell peppers, and carrots) may herald cross-reactivity to Latex.
- Anyone having had a severe allergic reaction during medical care in the past may have latex hypersensitivity.

9. **What is the incidence of anaphylaxis?**
The incidence of anaphylaxis under anesthesia in adults is estimated to be 1 in 6000 to 20,000. The incidence of anaphylaxis in children is 1 in 7700, with latex accounting for 76% of the reactions. True incidence may not be truly defined. In the general population the incidence of latex allergy may be increasing despite improved attempts for recognition of at-risk groups, strategies to avoid latex exposure, and a decrease in latex-containing hospital products. Moreover, in the health care profession, the incidence is increasing. Standard (previously called *universal*) precautions have become an everyday practice for health care workers and there has been vigorous activity to eliminate latex products or carefully protect patients who have a latex-allergic history.

10. **How is a latex allergy developed?**
There are multiple routes by which individuals can be exposed to allergens, including contact with intact or abraded skin and mucous membranes, inhalation, or exposure to an open vascular tree. Latex gloves are the major source of latex proteins and are the primary factor associated with latex-associated allergic reactions. Powderless gloves reduce latex exposure through the inhalational route. Latex gloves can be eliminated from the operating room environment if needed.

11. **How should an operating room be prepared for a latex-allergic patient?**
Surgeries for latex-allergic patients should be scheduled first since the amount of airborne latex particles is least at the beginning of the day. Nonlatex surgical and anesthesia supplies and nonlatex gloves are essential. Increasingly latex-free medical supplies are the standard for all patients, but it is important to be familiar with supplies at hand since a totally latex-free environment for all cases has yet to be achieved. Ordinarily latex-containing supplies are labeled as such.

12. **How should any allergic reaction be treated?**
The typical presentation for a severe reaction is in a patient with prior exposure with symptoms developing soon after repeat exposure, although cross-sensitization with commercial products may permit a severe reaction on initial exposure. Respiratory symptoms include edema, especially of mucous membranes and the larynx; bronchospasm; and pulmonary edema. Cardiovascular symptoms include hypotension and tachycardia. Cutaneous manifestations include flushing and hives. These are the manifestations of the most severe, potentially fatal, IgE-mediated reaction known as *anaphylaxis*. Should a real or likely anaphylactic reaction be recognized, the following recommendations should be followed:
- Call for help and remove the offending stimulus.
- Limit the use of anesthetic agents as much as possible.
- Complete the procedure as quickly as possible or arrive at a suitable stopping point.
- Administer 100% oxygen.
- Aggressive volume expansion may require many liters of crystalloid.
- Epinephrine 5 to 10 mcg initial bolus, increasing up to 500 mcg if ineffective. Consider epinephrine infusions beginning at 1 mcg/min.
- Antihistamines (histamine-1 receptor blocker): diphenhydramine 25 to 50 mg
- Antihistamines (histamine-2 receptor blocker): ranitidine 150 mg or cimetidine 400 mg
- Corticosteroids: hydrocortisone 1 to 5 mg/kg or methylprednisolone 1000 mg
- Nebulized albuterol 0.3% for bronchospasm
- Norepinephrine if epinephrine is insufficient; start about 0.3 mcg/kg/min and increase based on response.
- Vasopressin has also been shown to be effective in doses of 2 to 5 units.

13. **Should patients with a prior history of allergic reaction be pretreated with histamine blockers or corticosteroids?**
Probably not, because pretreatment may delay recognition of early symptoms until a full-blown reaction manifests, but there is disagreement here.

14. **What tests are available to diagnose and characterize a prior allergic reaction? Should patients having a prior anaphylactic reaction be tested?**

    Serum tryptase, a mast cell protease, will be elevated after both immunologic and nonimmunologic mast cell activation, so is probably of little value. In vitro tests such as the radioallergosorbent test (RAST) detect IgE antibodies and can be performed for specific drugs but are insensitive. In vivo testing such as skin prick and intradermal testing is of variable usefulness because many patients in the general population are also cross-sensitized to many drugs. For instance, over 9% of the general population will have a positive skin prick test to muscle relaxants. With regard to latex, there are so many proteins that usual skin testing may not identify the causative allergen. Furthermore, skin testing can induce a systemic reaction severe enough to require therapy! Many authorities believe that the costs, risks, and limited information gained suggest that testing be undertaken only in unusual circumstances. One instance may be the individual suspected of occupation-related allergies.

15. **What are the implications of occupational latex exposure?**

    Currently about 70% of all allergic reactions are reported in health care workers, and it is estimated that 3% to 12% of this group have developed some degree of latex sensitivity. The majority of allergic reactions are probably caused by inhalational exposure from latex particles adhering to the powder of powdered gloves. Since signs and symptoms may be very nonspecific (puffy eyes, nasal congestion, sneezing, wheezing, coughing, hoarseness), the connection may not be made to an occupational exposure. Workers who develop hand dermatitis or have an atopic history may be at increased risk. It is important to note that, although sensitization may occur at work, severe allergic manifestations may occur while these workers are receiving medical care. The key to the protection of health care workers is to reduce work-related exposure (*Stop the Sensitization!*). The use of nonpowdered latex or latex-free gloves is probably the most important intervention. Maintaining good skin care is also important, and workers who develop skin rashes might consider visiting an employee health clinic and undergoing latex sensitivity testing. It is also important not to wear scrub suits home because there are reports of family members developing latex sensitivity by this route.

KEY POINTS: ALLERGIC REACTIONS

1. To prevent severe allergic reactions, it is important to identify patients at risk and to take a good history.
2. The major causes of anaphylactic reactions in the operating room are muscle relaxants, followed by latex allergy.
3. Concerning latex allergy, proper preparation of the operating room environment is critical. Schedule patients at risk as first cases. Latex- and nonlatex-containing supplies should be clearly identified and the former avoided. Powdered gloves should be avoided.
4. The proper medications needed to adequately treat a reaction must be at hand. Treat allergic reactions aggressively. Accelerate epinephrine doses if needed.
5. It is important to recognize that health care workers are at increased risk for latex hypersensitivity. Avoid the use of powdered gloves whenever possible and be alert for the development of symptoms that might signify latex allergy.
6. Health care workers with type I latex allergy should have proper allergy identification and always carry an epinephrine autoinjector device.

SUGGESTED READINGS

Dewachter P, Mouton-Faivre C, Emala CW: Anaphylaxis and anesthesia: controversies and new insights, Anesthesiology 111:1141–1150, 2009.

Hepner DL, Castells MC: Anaphylaxis during the perioperative period, Anesth Analg 97:1381–1395, 2003.

Kelkar PS, Li JTC: Cephalosporin allergy, N Engl J Med 345:804–809, 2001.
Mertes PM, Tajima K, Regnier-Kimmoun MA, et al: Perioperative anaphylaxis, Med Clin North Am 94:761–789, 2010.
Sampathi V, Lerman J: Perioperative latex allergy in children, Anesthesiology 114:673–680, 2011.
Schummer C, Wirsing M, Schummer W: A pivotal role of vasopressin in refractory anaphylactic shock, Anesth Analg 107:620–625, 2008.

CHAPTER 49

HERBAL SUPPLEMENTS

James C. Duke, MD, MBA

1. **How does the U.S. Food and Drug Administration (FDA) regulate herbal medications?**
   The lack of rigorous regulation of herbal medications has resulted in a lack of standardization of doses and purity, contamination with undeclared pharmaceuticals and heavy metals, failure to report adverse events, and no requirement to demonstrate safety or efficacy. However, when presented with a supplement with obvious toxicity issues such as the stimulant effects of ephedra, the FDA does intervene to limit its availability; ephedra is no longer available as an over-the-counter product. The National Center for Complementary and Alternative Medicine, established within the National Institutes of Health in 1998, conducts research and provides information on the usefulness and safety of herbal supplements and complementary health practices.

2. **What is the incidence of herbal medicine use in the surgical patient population? What are commonly used herbal medicines?**
   In 2001 over $4 billion was spent on herbs and other botanical remedies. Reported use varies widely, and the surveys estimate as much as a third of patients who are having surgery ingest herbs and similar medications. Often these are taken without input from a physician. The number of individuals using herbal remedies is rising annually. Use in women is higher than in men, and patients with either neoplastic disease or human immunodeficiency virus have also been noted to use supplements with greater frequency. Supplements most commonly used include vitamins (especially vitamins E and C), garlic (*Allium sativum*), fish oil, ginkgo biloba (ginkgo), ginseng, ginger (*Zingiber officinale*), St. John's wort (*Hypericum perforatum*), *Echinacea angustifolia*, valerian, glucosamine (2-amino-2-deoxyglucose sulfate), chondroitin 4-sulfate, chamomile, kava, and feverfew (*Tanacetum parthenium*). Asian patients who receive preparations from Chinese herbalists often receive more potent compounds with many different herbs contained therein.

3. **How can commonly used herbal medicines adversely affect the surgical patient?**
   Although these supplements are considered natural, they are not free of harmful side effects. They have central nervous system and cardiovascular effects (e.g., ephedra) and interact with prescription drugs. For example, St. John's wort induces the cytochrome P-450 enzymes, accelerating the breakdown of cyclosporine, antiretroviral drugs, digoxin, and warfarin, resulting in a fall in drug levels to subtherapeutic concentrations. Nephrotoxic, hepatotoxic, and carcinogenic effects have been associated with products containing kava or comfrey. Of greatest concern in the perioperative period are effects on coagulation. Vitamin E, garlic, fish oil, ginkgo, ginseng, ginger, and feverfew have anticoagulant potential.

4. **What are the risks involved in consuming ephedra?**
   Ephedra alkaloids have been marketed as a way to boost energy and lose weight. These compounds are powerful cardiovascular and central nervous system stimulants, and severe hypertension, dysrhythmias, myocardial infarction, acute psychosis, seizures, cerebrovascular accidents, and death have been associated with their use. Ephedra may be particularly toxic when combined with caffeine. Many hundreds of people have been hospitalized after using ephedra and, as mentioned previously, the FDA has prevented its over-the-counter availability.

5. **Review the effects of vitamin E.**
   Vitamin E is consumed for the prevention and treatment of cardiovascular disease, diabetes mellitus, and some forms of cancer. Vitamin E is an antioxidant that prevents the formation of free radicals, but high doses may increase bleeding caused by antagonism of vitamin K–dependent clotting factors and platelet aggregation. Concomitant use of vitamin E and

anticoagulant or antiplatelet agents, including aspirin, clopidogrel (Plavix), dalteparin (Fragmin), enoxaparin (Lovenox), heparin, ticlopidine (Ticlid), and warfarin (Coumadin) may potentiate the risk of bleeding.

6. **What are the reported benefits and adverse effects of fish oil?**
Fish oils are used primarily in the treatment of hyperlipidemia, hypertension, and chronic inflammatory states such as rheumatoid arthritis and autoimmune disease. Fish oils contain two long-chain omega-3 fatty acids that compete with arachidonic acid in the cyclooxygenase and lipoxygenase pathways and have antiinflammatory effects, likely caused by the inhibition of leukotriene synthesis. Fish oils decrease blood viscosity and increase red blood cell deformability. The antithrombotic activity of fish oils results from prostacyclin inhibition, vasodilation, reduction in platelet count and adhesiveness, and prolongation of bleeding time. Concomitant use of fish oils and anticoagulant and antiplatelet drugs previously mentioned may increase the risk of bleeding.

7. **What are the beneficial properties and side effects of kava and valerian?**
Kava is antiepileptic, anxiolytic, and sedative in its effects and may potentiate prescribed medications with similar properties. Its action is thought to be through stimulation of γ-aminobutyric (GABA) pathways. Valerian is also a sedative, and discontinuing valerian may result in a benzodiazepine-like withdrawal. Valerian also potentiates the actions of barbiturates and other sedatives, and is probably GABA stimulating. These medications may potentiate the effects of anesthetic medications.

8. **Review the alleged benefits and risks of ginkgo.**
Ginkgo is used for the treatment of dementia, Alzheimer disease, and conditions associated with cerebral vascular insufficiency, including memory loss, headache, tinnitus, vertigo, difficulty concentrating, mood disturbances, and hearing disorders. Active ingredients of ginkgo leaf and its extracts include flavonoids, terpenoids, and organic acids. Although the mechanism of action is only partially understood, there are several theories about how ginkgo works. Ginkgo may protect tissues from oxidative damage by preventing or reducing cell membrane lipid peroxidation and decreasing oxidative damage to erythrocytes, and it may protect neurons and retinal tissue from oxidative stress. Extracts from the ginkgo leaf competitively inhibit platelet-activating factor (decreasing platelet aggregation, phagocyte chemotaxis, smooth muscle contraction, and free radical production) and prevent neutrophil degranulation. A case of bilateral spontaneous subdural hematomas has been linked to chronic ginkgo ingestion. Use of ginkgo may potentiate anticoagulant or antiplatelet agents.

9. **What are the alleged benefits and risks of ginseng?**
Ginseng is a general tonic for improving well-being and stamina and may increase resistance to environmental stress. The active constituents of ginseng are ginsengosides; these compounds may raise blood pressure and act as a central nervous system stimulant. Adrenal function and cortisol release may increase. Ginsengosides are reported to interfere with platelet aggregation and coagulation in vitro, but this effect has not been demonstrated in humans. Ginseng is also associated with hypoglycemia, interferes with warfarin, and may increase partial thromboplastin time.

10. **Review the alleged benefits and risks of garlic.**
Garlic decreases blood pressure and reduces plasma lipids. It may produce smooth muscle relaxation and vasodilation by activation of endothelium-derived relaxation factor. It has been shown to have antithrombotic properties by increasing thrombolytic activity secondary to plasminogen activation and decreasing platelet aggregation through inhibition of thromboxane B_2 formation. Garlic may potentiate the effects of warfarin, heparin, nonsteroidal antiinflammatory drugs (NSAIDs), and aspirin. A spontaneous spinal epidural hematoma associated with excessive garlic ingestion has been reported. However, garlic taken in normal dietary doses does not impair platelet function.

11. **What about ginger?**
Ginger is used for the treatment of arthritis, for a variety of gastrointestinal complaints, for vertigo and motion sickness, and as an antiemetic. It is effective in controlling nausea and vomiting in pregnant women who have hyperemesis gravidarum. Its active component is

gingerol, and its mechanism of action is unclear, although gingerols are thought to inhibit prostaglandin and leukotriene synthesis. Ginger is believed to inhibit thromboxane synthetase, decreasing platelet aggregation. Like garlic, it may potentiate the effect of medications that have anticoagulant properties.

12. **Review the properties and effects of feverfew.**
    Feverfew is used for fever, headache, and prevention of migraine headaches. At least 39 compounds within feverfew have been identified. It is not yet clear how feverfew works in the prevention of migraine. Laboratory evidence suggests that feverfew extracts might inhibit platelet aggregation and serotonin release from platelets and leukocytes. It may inhibit serum proteases and leukotrienes and block prostaglandin synthesis by inhibiting phospholipase, preventing the release of arachidonic acid.

13. **Review the effects of St. John's wort.**
    St. John's wort is used for the treatment of mild to moderate depression through impaired reuptake of serotonin, norepinephrine, and dopamine. As such, when taken in conjunction with selective serotonin reuptake inhibitors (SSRIs) prescribed by a physician, serotonin excess may be an undesired effect. Like SSRIs, St. John's wort should also not be administered to patients who are taking monoamine oxidase inhibitors or β-sympathomimetic amines such as pseudoephedrine. It may alter the metabolism of immunosuppressants (e.g., cyclosporin) and cancer chemotherapy by stimulating cytochrome P-450 3A4. Metabolism of such drugs as warfarin, NSAIDs, local anesthetics, alfentanil, and midazolam may be enhanced.

14. **Since these medications appear to impair coagulation, how can their effect be evaluated clinically?**
    The best means for detecting a coagulation defect secondary to herbal medications is a properly taken clinical history. Especially important are questions related to the hemostatic response during previous surgeries. Also important are questions regarding bleeding tendencies such as easy bruising, gingival bleeding, or excessive bleeding following procedures such as dental extractions. Positive responses to these questions suggest the need for laboratory testing. The most commonly used measures of coagulation include the activated partial thromboplastin time, which evaluates the intrinsic system; the prothrombin time, which evaluates the extrinsic pathway; platelet count; and bleeding time. However, bleeding time, the most commonly used measure of platelet function, is subject to many variables and may not always be reliable. More reliable tests of platelet function are available but are expensive, time-consuming, and not appropriate for routine screening.

KEY POINTS: HERBAL SUPPLEMENTS

1. Herbal does not necessarily mean safe. Few controlled scientific data exist on the risks and benefits of herbal medications.
2. Always ask patients about herbal/alternative medications that they may be taking. Patients may not perceive herbal medications as clinicians might. Do not depend on them to volunteer that information.
3. In situations in which excessive bleeding may prove especially problematic or in patients taking multiple supplements thought to have anticoagulant potential, it may be best to discontinue these medications for 2 to 3 weeks before surgery.
4. Coagulation defects secondary to herbal medicines may not be evident using standard laboratory studies.

15. **What are current recommendations regarding discontinuing use of herbal medications before surgery?**
    Most patients will not admit to the use of herbal medications unless directly questioned, but the use of herbal medications is not necessarily a contraindication to surgery. If regional anesthesia is planned and the patient is on prescribed medications with antiplatelet effects,

it may be wise to discontinue the herbal supplements at least a week before surgery. Some authorities recommend discontinuation of herbal medications for 7 to 14 days. However, it should be noted that the consensus of the American Society of Regional Anesthesia has stated, "Herbal drugs, by themselves, appear to represent no added significant risk for the development of spinal hematoma in patients having epidural or spinal anesthesia."

Finally, it may be of some comfort to clinicians who often do not see patients until just before surgery and do not have an opportunity to make the recommendation to discontinue such supplements before surgery that serious complications associated with use of herbal medications still appear to be distinctly rare events.

SUGGESTED READINGS

Ang-Lee M, Yu CS, Moss J: Complementary and alternative therapies. In Miller RD, editor: Miller's anesthesia, ed 6, Philadelphia, 2006, Churchill Livingstone, pp 605–616.

Horlocker TT, Wedel DJ, Rowlingson JC, et al: Regional anesthesia in the patient receiving antithrombotic or thrombolytic therapy. American Society of Regional Anesthesia and Pain Medicine Evidence-Based Guidelines, Reg Anesth Pain Med 35:64–101, 2010.

Kaye AD, Kucera I, Sabar R: Perioperative anesthesia: clinical considerations of alternative medications, Anesthesiol Clin North Am 22:125–139, 2004.

Lee A, Chui PT, Aun CS, et al: Incidence and risk of adverse perioperative events among surgical patients taking traditional Chinese herbal medicines, Anesthesiology 105:454–461, 2006.

CHAPTER 50

TRAUMA

James C. Duke, MD, MBA

1. **Review conditions that predispose trauma patients to increased anesthetic risk.**
   A depressed level of consciousness may lead to hypoventilation, loss of protective airway reflexes, inappropriate behavior, and decreased ability to examine and interview the patient. Full stomachs increase the risk of pulmonary aspiration of gastric contents. Because of blood loss, hypothermia, alcohol and drug intoxication, and organ injury, these patients are prone to altered responsiveness to anesthetic agents.

2. **Outline the initial management of an unconscious, hypotensive patient.**
   The ABCs (airway, breathing, and circulation) are essential. Unconscious patients require rapid and definitive airway control. The trachea should be intubated in a rapid-sequence fashion. Establish numerous large-gauge sites of intravenous access, using either short 14- or 16-G catheters peripherally or 9-Fr introducers into the central circulation. Establish an arterial catheter for continuous monitoring and blood analysis (arterial blood gases, hematocrit, platelet count, coagulation profiles, and blood chemistries).

3. **What is the significance of a Glasgow Coma Scale (GCS) score of 8?**
   The GCS is an assessment for patients with head injury. The final score is the sum of scores for best eye opening, best motor and best verbal responses; scores range from 3 to 15. Generally, the GCS for severe head injury is 9 or less; for moderate injury, 9–12; and for minor injury, 12 and higher. A patient with a GCS of 8 is sufficiently depressed that endotracheal intubation is indicated (Table 50-1).

4. **Describe the changes in vital signs associated with progressive blood loss.**
   See Table 50-2.

5. **What is the initial therapy for hypovolemic shock?**
   Initially replace estimated blood losses with balanced crystalloid solutions. The crystalloid volume administered is three or four times the estimated blood loss but transfusing red blood cells is essential. Continued hemodynamic instability suggests that there is massive blood loss and intravenous resuscitation with blood products is necessary, although other causes of hypotension such as head injury, hemothorax, tension pneumothorax, or pericardial tamponade should be considered. Contemporary treatment of massively injured patients is described as "massive transfusion protocols" and the usual protocol is a 1:1:1 ratio of red blood cells, plasma, and platelets.

6. **Why is rapid-sequence induction preferred for airway management in trauma patients?**
   Rapid-sequence induction is used because trauma patients are at risk for pulmonary aspiration of gastric contents and it minimizes the time between loss of consciousness and airway protection with a cuffed endotracheal tube (ETT). The usual rapid-sequence induction begins with preoxygenation with 100% oxygen. A cardiostable induction agent in reduced doses is chosen in the unstable patient. The moribund patient may require only paralysis. A rapid-acting relaxant, usually succinylcholine (SCh), is chosen. Before induction, pressure is applied firmly over the cricoid ring (Sellick maneuver) to prevent regurgitation of gastric contents. The patient is intubated as soon as adequate muscle relaxation is achieved (usually around 45 to 60 seconds). The presence of end-tidal CO_2 is confirmed, and breath sounds are assessed before release of cricoid pressure.

7. **How does an uncleared cervical spine modify the approach to the airway?**
   Patients requiring emergent surgical procedures do not have time to have their cervical spines evaluated fully. There is no airway management technique that results in cervical

Table 50-1. Glasgow Coma Scale*

SCORE	MOTOR	VERBAL	EYE OPENING
6	Obeys commands	N/A	N/A
5	Localizes stimulus	Oriented	N/A
4	Withdraws from stimulus	Confused	Spontaneously
3	Flexes arm	Words/phrases	To voice
2	Extends arm	Makes sounds	To pain
1	No response	No response	Remain closed

*Scores from 3 to 15.

Table 50-2. Changes in Vital Signs with Progressive Blood Loss

PARAMETER	<15%	15%–30%	30%–40%	>40%
Heart rate	<100	>120	>120	>140
Systolic blood pressure	Normal	Normal	Decreased	Decreased
Pulse pressure*	Normal to increased	Decreased	Decreased	Decreased
Capillary refill	Normal	Delayed	Delayed or absent	Absent
Respiratory rate	14–20	20–30	30–40	>35
Mental status	Anxious	Anxious	Confused	Lethargic

*Pulse pressure is the difference between systolic and diastolic pressures.
From the American College of Surgeons: Advanced trauma life support manual, *ed 6, Chicago, 1997, American College of Surgeons.*

immobility. These precautions include an appropriately sized Philadelphia collar, sand bags placed on each side of the head and neck, and the patient resting on a hard board with the forehead taped and secured to it. All said, a recent closed claims analysis found that a great majority of cervical spinal cord injuries occurred in the absence of trauma, cervical spine instability, or airway management problems.

Alternative airway management techniques in the traumatized patient include rapid-sequence induction with in-line stabilization, use of the Bullard laryngoscope, blind nasal intubation, and fiber-optic bronchoscopic-assisted ventilation. GlideScope (Verathon, Bothell, WA) is a laryngoscope with a camera lens on its tip and is very useful when a patient's neck must be maintained in a neutral position. Several similar products are available.

When a cervical fracture or cervical spinal cord injury (SCI) is documented, most anesthesiologists choose fiber-optic intubation facilitated by some form of topical anesthesia to the airway and sedation, titrated to effect, keeping in mind the patient's other injuries and hemodynamic status. This allows postintubation assessment of neurologic status before induction of unconsciousness. It would not be advisable to ablate all protective airway reflexes in a patient with a full stomach.

8. **Which induction agents are best for trauma patients?**
Far more important than the particular drug is the dose given because most induction agents produce hypotension through loss of sympathetic tone. Ketamine may be the best agent in the hypovolemic patient because its sympathetic stimulation supports the blood pressure; it should be recognized that, on occasion, its direct myocardial depressant effects may result in hypotension. It is contraindicated in patients with increased intracranial pressure because it increases cerebral blood flow. Etomidate may be used in some trauma

patients because of its minimal effect on hemodynamic variables; however, it will decrease sympathetic tone in patients probably relying on enhanced autonomic tone to maintain cardiac output; thus reductions in usual doses are appropriate. It also depresses adrenal function, although the impact of one dose is unclear.

9. **Why are trauma patients hypothermic?**
Hypothermia results from the same events as in any surgical patient, including loss of hypothalamic regulation, peripheral vasodilation, and exposure within a cold environment. However, trauma patients are often hypothermic on arrival to the hospital because of environmental exposure, are often not well covered during their diagnostic period, and may be receiving unwarmed intravenous fluids and blood. Hypothermia also contributes to coagulopathy. Hypothermia, acidosis, and coagulation disturbances have been described as the "lethal triad." To reduce the potential of hypothermia, the following strategies are recommended:
   - Warm the room before arrival.
   - Warm all fluids and blood products.
   - Use convective air-warming blankets and cover all nonprepped exposed skin surfaces.
   - Warming of gases is not particularly useful because the heat content of gas is negligible.

10. **What is meant by damage control surgery?**
Damage control is the principle of performing the minimum necessary interventions to save life and limb, leaving further reconstructive procedures to a later time, after the patient has obtained hemodynamic stability.
    For a liver laceration the injured surface of the liver is packed with surgical sponges to temporize bleeding while the anesthesia team concentrates on resuscitation. Once stabilized, the patient's abdominal cavity is not fully closed but covered with a sterile dressing, and the resuscitative efforts continue in the intensive care unit. Perhaps only the next day when the patient has stabilized is he or she returned to the operating room and re-explored and further procedures undertaken as indicated. The damage control philosophy has been embraced by other surgical disciplines as well, particularly orthopedics.

11. **How have damage control concepts been applied in orthopedic injuries?**
Many patients with femur or pelvic fractures have multisystem injuries and are hemodynamically unstable. Pulmonary contusions can be problematic in these patients because reaming of the femoral canal for intramedullary nailing can shower the lungs with fat emboli at a vulnerable period, propagating an inflammatory reaction that may lead to increased morbidity (e.g., adult respiratory distress syndrome, prolonged intensive care stays and hospitalizations, and increased ventilator days) and mortality. Rather than perform definitive surgery at the time of injury, damage control is practiced by using temporary external fixation as a bridge until the patients are better able to tolerate internal fixation.

12. **Describe the concept of compartment syndromes.**
Increased pressure within any semi-rigid anatomic structure will increase to the point at which perfusion is diminished by the increasing pressure. This can apply to the cranium (increased intracranial pressure), thorax, pericardium, abdomen, and extremities. Failure to recognize and rapidly treat any compartment syndrome results in increased morbidity and may result in death. Since patients with abdominal trauma are now less likely to be closed completely until much improved over time, abdominal compartment syndromes are now less likely.

13. **What are the manifestations of the abdominal compartment syndrome?**
A victim of polytrauma experiencing hypotension, oliguria, and respiratory failure manifesting as increasing airway pressures and decreasing oxygenation may have abdominal compartment syndrome. Diagnosis is by clinical suspicion and confirmed by measuring bladder pressure (>25 cm H_2O is suspicious).

14. **How does cardiac tamponade present? What is the Beck triad? How should anesthesia be managed in a patient with tamponade?**
Cardiac tamponade may arise from either blunt or penetrating trauma. When bleeding into the pericardial space increases pericardial pressures, cardiac filling is impaired.

Positive-pressure ventilation further decreases venous return and may greatly exacerbate the reduction in cardiac output. Stroke volume decreases, and tachycardia compensates for a time to increase cardiac output. Beck triad consists of hypotension, distant heart sounds, and distended neck veins, the classic signs associated with cardiac tamponade, although neck vein distention may not be observed because of hypovolemia. Electrical alternans, in which the major electrocardiogram (ECG) axis is constantly changing, may be noted. This is because the heart floats freely in the expanded pericardium.

A patient with tamponade is at risk for cardiovascular collapse with anesthetic induction. Because of this, it may be wise to drain the pericardium using local anesthesia at the operative site (a subxiphoid pericardial window) before general anesthetic induction.

15. **What are the significance, clinical presentation, and treatment of a tension pneumothorax?**

Patients may sustain a pneumothorax in association with trauma such as rib fractures, stab wounds, and central line placement. If the pleural cavity does not communicate with the ambient environment, air may accumulate between the chest wall and lung and may expand quickly with positive-pressure ventilation. Eventually a tension pneumothorax decreases venous return to the thorax and causes torsion of mediastinal vessels, leading to cardiovascular collapse.

The chest may rise unevenly with inspiration, breath sounds become unequal, the hemothorax is tympanitic to percussion, and the trachea may shift away from the affected side. Neck veins may become distended if the patient is normovolemic. Airway pressures rise.

The immediate treatment is the placement of a large-bore needle through the chest wall in the second intercostal space in the midclavicular line. A rush of air confirms the diagnosis. The needle should be left in place until a tube thoracostomy is performed. Tension pneumothorax is a clinical diagnosis; do not delay treatment for radiologic confirmation of this life-threatening condition. Nitrous oxide should not be used in trauma patients because it quickly diffuses into any air-filled cavity such as a pneumothorax.

16. **What challenges do spinal cord–injured patients pose?**

Airway management has been discussed briefly. The technique of choice depends on the urgency of the situation but might be direct laryngoscopy or fiber-optic intubation with in-line stabilization. When moved, patients should be *log-rolled*; that is, rolled and moved with care to maintain the neck in a neutral position.

Some degree of neurogenic shock should be expected with injuries above the T6 level. However, hypotension in spinal cord–injured patients is most likely caused by other injuries. Catecholamine surges may produce pulmonary vascular damage, resulting in neurogenic pulmonary edema. There may be some element of myocardial dysfunction. If moderate fluid resuscitation does not result in hemodynamic improvement, central venous catheterization for monitoring may be required. Spinal cord injuries cephalad to midthoracic levels interrupt sympathetic cardioaccelerator fibers, resulting in bradycardia. If accompanied by hypotension, administration of atropine is indicated. Occasionally infusion of vasopressors such as phenylephrine is needed to support blood pressure. Anesthetic agents should be titrated carefully since drug-associated cardiovascular depression cannot be compensated for by increases in sympathetic tone. Doses of 30% to 50% of normal are likely to be sufficient. SCh may be administered in the first 24-hour period after cord injury but not thereafter to avoid the potential for life-threatening hyperkalemia.

Sympathetic tone eventually returns after injury, and sympathetic responses to stimuli distal to the injury may be exaggerated. Despite a loss of sensation, any surgical procedure or distention of a hollow viscus below the injury may produce life-threatening hypertension, termed *autonomic hyperreflexia*. Exaggerated reactions manifest as the patient moves into the period of spastic paralysis (4 to 8 weeks after injury) and beyond. The more distal the stimulus, the more exaggerated the reaction. Urologic procedures or fecal disimpaction, common procedures in chronic spinal cord–injured patients, are examples. All procedures on chronic cord-injured patients require some anesthetic to prevent or attenuate autonomic hyperreflexia. Neuraxial and inhalational anesthetics are usually satisfactory, although occasionally vasodilators such as nitroprusside are necessary to control hypertension.

17. **Should succinylcholine be used in patients with SCI?**

Within 48 to 72 hours after acute SCI, the denervated muscles respond with proliferation of extrajunctional acetylcholine receptors along the muscle cell membrane. When SCh is administered in the presence of extrajunctional receptors, a large release of potassium into the circulation results in dysrhythmias, ventricular fibrillation, and cardiac arrest. Prior administration of a nondepolarizing muscle relaxant does not reliably decrease the potassium release associated with administration of SCh in patients with SCI. SCh should be avoided in patients with SCI.

18. **Describe the presentation of a myocardial contusion.**

Blunt chest trauma may cause cardiac contusion. Associated injuries include sternal fractures, rib fractures, and pulmonary contusion. Dysrhythmias are common, the most common being sinus tachycardia with nonspecific ST segment changes. Conduction blocks and ventricular rhythms may also be observed. Patients may also sustain injury to valves or papillary muscles and sustain thrombosis to coronary arteries, most commonly the right coronary artery (presenting with ischemic changes in inferior ECG leads). The absence of dysrhythmias for 24 hours is reassuring. Pump failure is an ominous finding. Cardiac enzymes add little to the evaluation of a patient suspected of having a contusion. Echocardiography is perhaps the most useful test and, in the presence of contusion, reveals segmental wall motion defects. Urgent surgery need not be delayed in the presence of contusion, although the threshold for invasive monitoring is lower. Myocardial contusion is predominantly a clinical diagnosis.

KEY POINTS: TRAUMA

1. The initial management of a trauma patient requires attention to the ABCs: airway, breathing, and circulation. Ensuring numerous large-gauge intravenous sites for resuscitation is a priority.
2. Precipitous cardiovascular collapse may be caused by unrecognized sources of bleeding, cardiac tamponade, tension pneumothorax, or air embolism.
3. Unstable, hemorrhaging patients should receive O-negative, type-specific, or crossmatched blood if still unstable after resuscitation with 2 L of balanced crystalloid solution.
4. Massive transfusion protocols now mandate aggressive administration of plasma and platelets as well as red blood cells, usually in a 1:1:1 ratio.
5. The triad of hypothermia, acidosis, and coagulopathy is highly lethal; in this scenario damage-control surgical principles should be considered and long operative periods avoided.

19. **Describe the management of a pregnant trauma patient.**

The usual concerns for pregnant women apply. Because of airway edema and large breasts, airway management may be difficult, and these patients are at risk for pulmonary aspiration. The gravid uterus may render the patient hypotensive, especially if there has been blood loss. Patients should be positioned with left uterine displacement. Pregnancy is also a vasodilated state, confounding interpretation of vital signs. Probably because of the effects of progesterone, pregnant women have increased sensitivity to sedatives and local anesthetics. Pregnant women have dilutional anemia, confounding interpretation of the hematocrit. Consult an obstetrician concerning fetal viability. Seat belts may produce uterine rupture. If fetal distress occurs, an emergency cesarean section may be required, depending on fetal age. Aggressive resuscitation of the maternal circulation will improve the fetal circumstances. After surgery the patient may experience premature labor that may be masked by the administration of opioids for surgical pain. Monitoring uterine contractions and fetal heart tones is necessary.

20. **Review concerns for the elderly trauma patient.**

Elderly patients may have significant, life-threatening injuries despite seemingly trivial mechanisms of injury. They have diminished organ reserves and numerous comorbidities. They are on numerous medications that may have led to the injury (e.g., benzodiazepines and other psychotropic medications) or may render them prone to bleeding (e.g., antiplatelet drugs, warfarin). They may easily lose airway protective reflexes, rendering them prone to aspiration, and have blunted cardiovascular reflexes as well. Elderly patients have increased mortality rates when compared with younger cohorts.

21. How might a bronchial or tracheal tear present? What are alternatives for managing ventilation during operative repair?
Large airway injuries usually occur within 2.5 cm of the carina and are usually immediately recognizable; distal bronchial injuries are more difficult to identify. Physical features that may be associated with these injuries include respiratory distress, subcutaneous or mediastinal air, hemoptysis, pneumothorax, and persistent large air leak after tube thoracostomy.
     Any injury near the carina is likely to require lung isolation and single-lung ventilation. A single-lumen ETT might be inserted into the uninvolved mainstem bronchus. Other options include inserting a double-lumen ETT or using a bronchial blocker. A fiber-optic bronchoscope is invaluable for any option chosen.

22. How is air embolism diagnosed and managed?
Penetrating lung injuries may result in systemic air entrainment via bronchovenous or alveolocapillary fistulas. Increased airway pressures associated with loss of pulmonary compliance and reduced venous pressure increase the likelihood of air embolism. Frothy, sanguineous secretions emanating from injured lung surfaces should make one wary of systemic air embolization. Air may be observed within coronary arteries. Systemic air embolism should be suspected whenever unexpected signs of central nervous system or myocardial ischemia and precipitous cardiovascular collapse occur in the appropriate clinical context. When treating patients at risk, minimize inspiratory airway pressure, avoid positive end-expiratory pressure, and administer small tidal volumes.

23. Are regional anesthetic and analgesic techniques valuable for trauma patients?
The sole use of intravenous opioids can lead to hypoventilation. Thoracic epidural analgesia is useful for multiple rib fractures and flail chest injuries. Intercostal nerve blocks are also useful. As long as an extremity should be monitored for development of compartment syndromes (and hypoperfusion of extremity musculature), peripheral nerve blocks with or without indwelling catheters could be beneficial.

SUGGESTED READINGS
David JS, Godier A, Dargaud Y, et al: Case scenario: management of trauma-induced coagulopathy in a severe blunt trauma patient, Anesthesiology 119:191–200, 2013.
Hindman BJ, Palecek JP, Posner KL, et al: Cervical spinal cord, root, and bony spine injuries: a closed claims analysis, Anesthesiology 114:782–795, 2011.
Malbrain ML, De Laet IE: Intra-abdominal hypertension: evolving concepts, Clin Chest Med 30:45–70, 2009.
Stundner O, Memtsoudis SG: Regional anesthesia and analgesia in critically ill patients: a systematic review, Reg Anesth Pain Med 37:537–544, 2012.
Shaz BH, Dente CJ, Harris RS, et al: Transfusion management of trauma patients, Anesth Analg 108:625–648, 2009.

CHAPTER 51

THE BURNED PATIENT, LASER SURGERY AND OPERATING ROOM FIRES

Philip R. Levin, MD, Alma N. Juels, MD, and James C. Duke, MD, MBA

THE BURNED PATIENT

1. **Who gets burned?**
   Approximately 2 million fires are reported each year, which result in 1.2 million people with burn injuries. Approximately 45,000 people are hospitalized in the United States for thermal injury. There are about 5000 fire and burn deaths per year. The majority of burns are thermal injuries. Electrical burns usually cause tissue destruction by thermal and associated injuries. In chemical burns the degree of injury depends on the particular chemical, its concentration, and duration of exposure. Seventy percent of burn patients are men. Mean age for all cases is 35 years old. Scalds are the most common in those below 5 years of age, whereas fire injuries are more common in older patients.

2. **What are the three main factors that correlate with increased mortality with burn injury?**
   Advanced age, burn size, and presence of inhalation injury correlate with increased mortality.

3. **What are the consequences of skin damage?**
   The skin is the largest organ of the human body. It has three principal functions, all of which are disrupted by burn injury:
   - The skin is an important sensory organ.
   - It performs a major role in thermoregulation for the dissipation of metabolic heat.
   - The skin acts as a barrier to protect the body against the entrance of microorganisms in the environment. A burn patient may have extensive evaporative heat and water loss, and loss of thermoregulation may lead to hypothermia. Burn patients have a profound risk of infection and sepsis.

4. **How are burns classified?**
   The severity of the burn is graded by its depth, which depends on the extent of tissue destruction.
   - **Superficial burns** involve the upper layers of the epidermis; the skin is painful and appears red and slightly edematous, much like a sunburn.
   - **Superficial partial-thickness burns** occur when tissue damage extends into the superficial layer of the dermis, which is still lined with intact epithelium that proliferates and regenerates new skin. These burns develop blisters and have red or whitish areas that are very painful.
   - **Deep partial-thickness burns** extend downward into the deeper layer of the dermis. Edema is marked, and sensation is altered.
   - **Full-thickness and subdermal burns** affect every body system and organ. A full-thickness burn extends through the epidermis and dermis and into the subcutaneous tissue layer. A subdermal burn damages muscle, bone, and interstitial tissue. Some centers are now using laser Doppler imaging to better determine burn depth.

5. **What systems are affected by burns?**
   All physiologic functions can be affected by burns, including the cardiovascular and respiratory systems; hepatic, renal, and endocrine function; the gastrointestinal tract; hematopoiesis; coagulation; and immunologic response.

6. **How is the cardiovascular system affected?**
   A transient decrease in cardiac output, as much as 50% from baseline, is followed by a hyperdynamic response. In the acute phase, organ and tissue perfusion decreases because of hypovolemia, depressed myocardial function, increased blood viscosity, and release of vasoactive substances. The acute phase starts immediately after injury; the second phase of burn injury, termed the *metabolic phase*, begins about 48 hours after injury and involves increased blood flow to organs and tissues. Geriatric patients may have a delayed or nonexisting second phase. Hypertension of unknown cause develops and may be quite extensive.

7. **How is the respiratory system affected?**
   Pulmonary complications can be divided into three distinct syndromes based on clinical features and temporal relationship to the injury. Early complications, occurring 0 to 24 hours post burn, include carbon monoxide (CO) poisoning and direct inhalation injury and can lead to airway obstruction and pulmonary edema. Delayed injury, occurring 2 to 5 days after injury, includes adult respiratory distress syndrome. Late complications, occurring days to weeks after the injury, include pneumonia, atelectasis, and pulmonary emboli. The two most common complications of burn injury are pneumonia and respiratory failure.

8. **What is inhalation injury?**
   Inhalation injury occurs when hot gases, toxic substances, and reactive smoke particles reach the tracheobronchial tree. These substances result in wheezing, bronchospasm, corrosion, and airway edema and should be suspected if the burn was sustained in a closed space. The presence of carbonaceous sputum, perioral soot, burns to the face and neck, stridor, dyspnea, or wheezing are indications for complete respiratory tract evaluation. Inhalation injury can cause damage to the upper airway (i.e., airway compromise, nasal obstruction, and acute laryngitis with varying degrees of laryngeal edema), damage to the conducting airway (i.e., tracheitis and bronchitis), and injury to the lower respiratory tract (i.e., pneumonitis, pulmonary edema, and adult respiratory distress syndrome). Chest radiographs during the initial phase usually underestimate the severity of lung damage because the injury is usually confined to the airways. Fiber-optic bronchoscopy has been quite useful in diagnosis of inhalation injury.

9. **What is the best way to treat inhalation injury?**
   Management is generally supportive. Oxygen should be provided as necessary to ensure adequate oxygenation. Bronchospasm usually responds to β agonists. Patients with smoke inhalation can require greater fluid resuscitation than other patients with burns. Respiratory care may be important if there is excessive carbonaceous material in the lungs. Intubation or tracheotomy may be necessary if there is significant upper airway compromise. Patients with heat and smoke injury plus extensive face and neck burns usually all require intubation. Patients with oral burns but no smoke injury should still be intubated early because these patients have significant edema and secretions and it may be nearly impossible to intubate later. If intubation occurs, make sure to secure the endotracheal tube because it may be extremely difficult to replace it if it becomes dislodged. High-frequency percussive ventilation has also been shown to be effective in clearing secretions.

10. **What are the features of CO poisoning?**
    CO toxicity is one of the leading causes of death in fires. CO is produced by incomplete combustion associated with fires, exhaust from internal combustion engines, cooking stoves, and charcoal stoves. Its affinity for hemoglobin is 200 times that of oxygen. When CO combines with hemoglobin, forming carboxyhemoglobin (COHb), the pulse oximeter may overestimate hemoglobin saturation. Symptoms are caused by tissue hypoxia, shift in the oxygen-hemoglobin dissociation curve, direct cardiovascular depression, and cytochrome inhibition. The persistence of a metabolic acidosis in the patient with adequate volume resuscitation and cardiac output suggests the persistent CO impairment of oxygen delivery and use. Treatment is initiated with 100% oxygen, which decreases the serum half-life of COHb. Hyperbaric oxygen (2 to 3 ATM) produces an even more rapid displacement and is most useful in cases of prolonged exposure, when it is more difficult to displace CO from the cytochrome system. The drawback of hyperbaric oxygen use is the inability to *get to the*

burn patient during the crucial period of hemodynamic and pulmonary instability. The vast majority of cases can be managed simply by using 100% oxygen.

11. **How do burns affect the gastrointestinal tract?**
Ileus may occur. Acute ulceration of the stomach or duodenum, referred to as Curling ulcer, may lead to gastrointestinal bleeding. The small and large intestine may develop acute necrotizing enterocolitis with abdominal distention, hypotension, and bloody diarrhea.

12. **How is renal function affected?**
Renal blood flow and glomerular filtration diminish immediately, activating the renin-angiotensin-aldosterone system. Antidiuretic hormone is released, resulting in retention of sodium and water and loss of potassium, calcium, and magnesium. The incidence of acute renal failure in burned patients varies from 0.5% to 38%, depending primarily on the severity of the burn. The associated mortality rate is very high (77% to 100%). Hemoglobinuria secondary to hemolysis and myoglobinuria secondary to muscle necrosis can lead to acute tubular necrosis and acute renal failure.

13. **How is myoglobinuria treated?**
Myoglobinuria is treated by vigorous fluid resuscitation, to the end point of a urine output of 2 ml/kg/hr. Administration of bicarbonate to alkalinize the urine may reduce the incidence of pigment-associated renal failure. Osmotic diuretics (i.e., mannitol) can be used in rare circumstances, except that its use obscures urine output as an indicator of circulating volume.

14. **How is hepatic function affected?**
Acute reduction of cardiac output, increased viscosity blood, and splanchnic vasoconstriction can cause hepatic hypoperfusion, which can result in decreased hepatic function.

15. **Are drug responses altered?**
Drugs administered acutely by any route other than intravenously have delayed absorption. After 48 hours the plasma albumin concentration is decreased, and albumin-bound drugs such as benzodiazepines and anticonvulsants have an increased free fraction and therefore a prolonged effect. The effect of drugs metabolized in the liver by oxidative metabolism (phase I reaction) is prolonged (e.g., diazepam). However, drugs metabolized in the liver by conjugation (phase II) are not affected (e.g., lorazepam). Opioid requirements are increased, most likely because of habituation and hypercatabolism. Ketamine may cause hypotension secondary to hypovolemia and depleted catecholamine stores, exerting its direct cardiodepressant effect. Propofol, thiopental, and etomidate may cause hypotension secondary to hypovolemia in the acute phase. Inhalational agents are likewise poorly tolerated in hypovolemic patients.

16. **What is the endocrine response to a burn?**
The endocrine response to a thermal burn involves massive release of catecholamines, glucagon, adrenocorticotropic hormone, antidiuretic hormone, renin, angiotensin, and aldosterone. Glucose levels are elevated, and patients are susceptible to nonketotic hyperosmolar coma. Patients with larger burns are more highly associated with development of adrenal insufficiency.

17. **What are the hematologic complications that occur with burns?**
Anemia is a common finding in severely burned patients. In the immediate postburn period, erythrocytes are damaged or destroyed by heat and removed by the spleen in the first 72 hours. This decrease in red cell mass is not immediately apparent because of the loss of plasma fluid and hemoconcentration. With fluid resuscitation, the deficit becomes more apparent. In the early postburn period, more red cell loss occurs secondary to decreased erythropoiesis. In addition, ongoing infection can result in subacute activation of the coagulation cascade. Consumption of circulating procoagulants results in various degrees of coagulopathy. Platelet function is both qualitatively and quantitatively depressed. Antithrombin deficiency has been noted in severe burn patients, usually found in the first 5 days after injury. The incidence is higher with increasing burn size and the diagnosis of inhalation injury.

18. **What are the immunologic complications that occur with burns?**

Infection in the burn patient is a leading cause of morbidity and mortality and remains one of the most demanding concerns for the burn team. Initially the burn wound is colonized principally with gram-positive organisms. Within a week they usually are replaced by antibiotic-susceptible gram-negative organisms. If wound closure is delayed and the patient becomes infected, requiring treatment with broad-spectrum antibiotics, these flora may be replaced by yeasts, fungi, and antibiotic-resistant bacteria. As burn wound size increases, bloodstream infection increases dramatically secondary to increased exposure to intravascular catheters and burn wound manipulation-induced bacteremia. Systemic antimicrobials are indicated to treat only documented infections such as pneumonia, bacteremia, wound infection, and urinary tract infection. Prophylactic antimicrobial therapy is recommended only if the burn wound must be excised or grafted in the operating room. It should be used only for coverage of the immediate perioperative period. Fifty percent or more of patients with both a major burn and an inhalation injury develop pneumonia. One of the major concerns is the worldwide emergence of antimicrobial resistance among a wide variety of nosocomial bacterial and fungal burn wound pathogens, which seriously limits the available effective treatment of burn wound infections.

19. **How are patients with burns resuscitated?**

The goal of fluid resuscitation is to correct hypovolemia and optimize organ perfusion. Adequate fluid administration is critical to the prevention of burn shock and other complications of thermal injury. Burns cause a generalized increase in capillary permeability, with loss of fluid and protein into interstitial tissue; this loss is greatest in the first 12 hours. A perfect formula for predicting fluid requirements remains elusive despite decades of research and debate. Two general principles most agree on are to give only what is needed and continuously reassess fluid requirements to prevent under-resuscitation or over-resuscitation. The goal of fluid resuscitation is to maintain a urinary output of 0.5 ml/kg/hr, which is thought to indicate adequate renal perfusion. The most common formula used today is the Parkland formula. The *Parkland formula* involves giving 4 ml of lactated Ringer (LR) solution per kilogram of body weight per percentage of total body surface area (TBSA) burned (4 ml/kg/% TBSA). One half of the calculated amount is given during the first 8 hours, and the remainder is given over the next 16 hours, in addition to daily maintenance fluid. Most burn centers use crystalloid as the primary fluid for burn resuscitation. Another formula that some use is the *modified Brooke formula*: 2 ml/kg/% TBSA LR administered as noted previously. The administration of colloid has been associated with increased risk of lung injury. In the United States most believe that colloid solutions should not be used in the first 24 hours. On the second day after injury capillary integrity is restored, and the amount of required fluid is decreased. Infusion of crystalloid is decreased after the first day, and colloids are administered:

- 0% to 30% TBSA burned: no colloid required
- 30% to 50% TBSA burned: 0.3 ml/kg/%burn/24 hr of colloid required
- 50% to 70% TBSA burned: 0.4 ml/kg/%burn/24 hr of colloid required
- 70% to 100% TBSA burned: 0.5 ml/kg/%burn/24 hr of colloid required

20. **How do you calculate the percent of total body surface burned?**

The severity of a burn injury is based on the amount of surface area covered in deep partial-thickness, full-thickness, and subdermal burns. The *rule of nines* method allows reasonable estimation (Table 51-1). Because of the difference in body habitus (particularly head and neck), the rule of nines must be altered in children (Table 51-2).

21. **Early surgical burn wound intervention has recently been shown to be one of the major reasons for the improved outcome in burn patients. What are the four categories of operations that are common for the burn-injured patient?**

- Decompression procedures (escharotomies and fasciotomies)
- Excision and closure operations
- Reconstruction operations
- Supportive general surgical procedures (tracheostomy, gastrostomy, cholecystectomy, bronchoscopy, vascular access procedures)

Table 51-1. Rule of Nines for Adults

Head and neck	9%
Upper extremities	9% each
Chest (anterior and posterior)	9% each
Abdomen	9%
Lower back	9%
Lower extremities	18% each
Perineum	1%

Table 51-2. Rule of Nines for Children: Percent Body Surface According to Age

BODY PART	NEWBORN	3 YEARS	6 YEARS
Head	18	15	12
Trunk	40	40	40
Arms	16	16	16
Legs	26	29	32

22. **What is important in the preoperative history?**
It is important to know at what time the burn occurred for fluid replacement. The type of burn is also important to assess airway damage, associated injuries, and the possibility of more extensive tissue damage than initially appreciated (electrical burns). A standard preoperative anesthetic history also must be taken, including past coexisting medical conditions, medications, allergies, and anesthetic history.

23. **What should the anesthesiologist look for on the preoperative physical examination?**
In addition to the conventional concerns of any patient about to undergo surgery, the status of the patient's airway should be the number one priority. A complete airway examination is essential. Excessive sputum, wheezing, and diminished breath sounds may suggest inhalation injury to the lungs. The cardiovascular system should also be evaluated, noting pulse rate and rhythm, blood pressure, cardiac filling pressures (if available), and urine output. Special attention should be given to the neurologic examination. It is important to assess the patient's level of consciousness and orientation.

24. **What preoperative tests are required before induction?**
Special emphasis should be placed on correcting the acid-base and electrolyte imbalance during the acute phase. Therefore an arterial blood gas analysis and a chemistry panel are suggested. In the presence of CO poisoning, the pulse oximeter may overestimate the saturation of hemoglobin; therefore a COHb level, determined by co-oximetry, may be helpful to assess the degree of the CO poisoning and to guide treatment. Coagulation tests are also helpful, because such patients often have bleeding diathesis. A urine myoglobin should be done in patients with a history of electrical injury or pigmented urine.

25. **What monitors are needed to give a safe anesthetic?**
Access for monitoring may be difficult. Needle electrodes or electrocardiogram (ECG) pads sewn on the patient may be required for the ECG monitor and nerve stimulator. A blood pressure cuff may be placed on a burned area, but an arterial catheter may be better and allows frequent blood analysis. Temperature measurement is a must because of exaggerated decreases in body temperature. Invasive monitors are placed as deemed necessary, taking into account the patient's previous baseline medical condition. If the procedure involves a large amount of blood loss, central venous pressure (right atrial pressure) should be

monitored through an introducer sheath. If myocardial dysfunction is likely, a pulmonary artery catheter may be necessary, although authorities disagree on this point.

26. **How must the use of muscle relaxants be modified for a burned patient?**
From about 24 hours after injury until the burn has healed, succinylcholine may cause hyperkalemia because of proliferation of extrajunctional neuromuscular receptors. On the other hand, burned patients tend to be resistant to the effects of nondepolarizing muscle relaxants and may need two to five times the normal dose.

27. **What techniques have been used to markedly reduce blood loss in excisional burn surgery?**
Subeschar and subcutaneous epinephrine clysis, extremity exsanguinations, pneumatic tourniquet use, and maintenance of intraoperative euthermia are all simple surgical techniques that have been found to significantly decrease blood loss.

28. **What induction drugs are good for burn patients?**
Various medications have been given successfully to burn patients. In patients who are adequately volume resuscitated and not septic, propofol is an acceptable induction agent. Ketamine offers the advantage of stable hemodynamics and analgesia and has been used extensively for both general anesthesia and analgesia for burn dressing changes. Unfortunately it tends to produce dysphoric reactions. If the patient is hemodynamically unstable, etomidate is a reasonable induction alternative.

KEY POINTS: THE BURNED PATIENT

1. The initial goal of resuscitation in burn patients is to correct hypovolemia. Burns cause a generalized increase in capillary permeability with loss of significant fluid and protein into interstitial tissue.
2. There should be a low threshold for elective intubation in patients suspected of having inhalation injury.
3. From about 24 hours after injury until the burn has healed, succinylcholine may cause hyperkalemia, because of proliferation of extrajunctional neuromuscular receptors.
4. Burned patients tend to be resistant to the effects of nondepolarizing muscle relaxants and may need two to five times the normal dose.

---

29. **Describe specific features of electrical burns.**
Care of electrical burns is similar to care of thermal burns, except that the extent of injury may be misleading. Areas of devitalized tissue may be present under normal-appearing skin. The extent of superficial tissue injury may result in underestimation of initial fluid requirements. Myoglobinuria is common, and urine output must be kept high to avoid renal damage. The development of neurologic complications after electrical burns is common, including peripheral neuropathies or spinal cord deficits. Many believe that regional anesthesia is contraindicated. Cataract formation may be another late sequela of burn injury. Cardiac dysrhythmias and ventricular fibrillation or asystole may occur up to 48 hours after injury. Apnea may result from titanic contraction of respiratory muscles or cerebral medullary injury.

LASER SURGERY AND OPERATING ROOM FIRES

30. **What is a laser?**
Laser stands for light amplification by stimulated emission of radiation. Within a laser, atoms, ions, or molecules are stimulated by an energy source and spontaneously radiate energy in the form of monochromatic light. The radiated light is then amplified and emitted as the laser beam. Laser light has three defining characteristics:
1. **Coherence:** All waves are in phase, both in time and in space.
2. **Collimation:** The waves travel in parallel directions.
3. **Monochromaticity:** All waves have the same wavelength.

Table 51-3. Characteristics of Lasers Commonly Used in the Operating Room

LASER TYPE	WAVELENGTH	ABSORBER	TYPICAL APPLICATIONS
CO_2	10,600 (invisible—far infrared)	All tissues, water	General, precise surgical cutting
Nd:YAG	1064 (invisible—near infrared)	Darkly pigmented tissues	General coagulation, tumor debulking
Nd:YAG-KTP*	532 (visible—emerald green)	Blood	General, pigmented lesions
Argon	488–514 (visible—blue-green)	Melanin, hemoglobin	Vascular, pigmented lesions
Krypton	400–700 (visible—blue-red)	Melanin	General, pigmented lesions

*Neodymium:yttrium-aluminum-garnet:potassium-titanyl-phosphate.

Benefits of using lasers are that they are extremely precise in their excision margins and there is minimal dissipation of damaging heat and energy to surrounding tissues.

31. **What makes lasers behave differently from each other?**
When excited, the source of the laser radiates light of a certain wavelength. The longer the wavelength is, the more strongly it is absorbed by the tissue target and the shallower is the overall lasing effect. Conversely, the shorter the wavelength is, the higher the energy and the deeper the penetration of the laser light. For example, a carbon dioxide (CO_2) laser has a longer wavelength and is absorbed almost entirely at the tissue surface. As a result, precise excision of superficial lesions is possible. Conversely, a neodymium:yttrium-aluminum-garnet (Nd:YAG) laser has a shorter wavelength, deeper penetration, and is useful for heating large tissue masses and tumor debulking (Table 51-3).

32. **What are the hazards of lasers?**
    - The vaporization of tissue and dispersion of diseased particulate matter are hazards for all operating room (OR) personnel. The smoke produced by vaporization of tissues with lasers may be mutagenic, transmit infectious diseases, and cause acute bronchial inflammation.
    - A laser beam in contact with flammable materials such as endotracheal tubes, anesthetic gas tubing, surgical drapes, and sponges may cause fires or explosion. Fires result in minimal or no harm to the patient if the situation is handled swiftly but may be catastrophic if not.
    - Although rare, venous gas embolism may occur, especially during laparoscopic or hysteroscopic procedures. Reported cases have been associated primarily with Nd:YAG lasers, in which coolant gases circulate at the probe tips. It is these coolant gases that embolize.
    - Inappropriate energy transfer: Laser light vaporizes whatever tissue lies in its path. Precise aim by the surgeon and a cooperative (well-anesthetized, paralyzed) patient are mandatory. In addition, laser light is easily reflected by surgical instruments and may be hazardous to all OR personnel. Laser contact with the eyes may impair vision or cause blindness. The nature of ocular damage depends on the wavelength of the laser light. For example, CO_2 lasers cause corneal opacification, whereas Nd:YAG lasers cause damage to the retina. Any plastic lens protects against CO_2 laser injury; contact lenses do not. Other lasers require more specialized eye protection.
    - Perforation: Misdirected laser energy may perforate a viscus or large blood vessel. Laser-induced pneumothorax after laryngeal surgery also has been reported. Sometimes the perforations do not occur until several days after surgery when edema and tissue necrosis are at a maximum.

33. **What are some unique airway considerations for the patient having laser surgery of the airway?**
    - **Upper airway lesions:** In laser resection of upper airway lesions, tracheal intubation is optional. Techniques that do not involve an endotracheal tube allow better visualization of the operative field by the surgeon and also remove potentially flammable materials from the airway. Responsibility for the airway is being shared by surgeon and anesthesiologist, and a discussion of the operative course before the procedure begins is important.
    - **Lower airway lesions:** The CO_2 laser beam is directed at the lesion through a rigid metal bronchoscope, coated with a matte finish to reduce reflected laser light. Ventilation is accomplished through the side arm of the bronchoscope, using saline-soaked gauze to form a seal around the bronchoscope. Jet ventilation is another option. In certain instances (e.g., lower tracheal and bronchial lesions) the laser approach is via fiber optic, and the Nd:YAG laser is required because it can travel through fiber-optic cables, whereas the CO_2 laser cannot.

34. **Describe ventilation techniques commonly encountered during airway laser surgery.**
    - **Jet ventilation:** In this technique the surgeon aims a high-velocity jet of O_2 at the airway opening. The high flow of O_2 entrains room air as a result of the Venturi effect, thus ventilating the lungs with a high volume of O_2–air mixture. Ventilation is accomplished by attaching a suction catheter to wall O_2 and a Sanderson-type jet injector. This apparatus is mounted to the operating laryngoscope. Sometimes the mass of the airway lesion makes this method impossible. If the jet stream is not aimed in the trachea, gastric dilation may occur. Barotrauma to the airway and subsequent pneumothorax are also risks and may in turn lead to mediastinal or subcutaneous air. An intravenous anesthetic is necessary for this procedure.
    - **Spontaneous ventilation:** Allowing the patient to inhale volatile agents via the operating laryngoscope is also an option, although it is not feasible for some procedures. It is difficult to control the depth of anesthesia during spontaneous ventilation, and it is often necessary to paralyze the patient during many airway procedures. Hypoventilation, hypercarbia, and aspiration (surgical debris, secretions, vomitus, and smoke) are additional complications related to both jet and spontaneous ventilation.
    - **Endotracheal intubation:** This method allows excellent ventilation and airway protection of the anesthetized patient but often obscures the operative field and puts flammable materials in the path of the laser beam.

35. **What are the three essential components necessary to create an OR fire?**
    The *fire triad* consists of:
    - Oxidizers. Within the OR environment they are O_2 and nitrous oxide.
    - Ignition sources include electrosurgical or electrocautery devices, lasers, argon beam coagulators, fiber-optic light cables, defibrillator pads, heated probes, and drills and burrs. When not in use, electrocautery devices should remain within appropriate holders, not lying on the surgical drapes. The first three ignition sources listed are the most common ignition sources.
    - Fuel sources include the following: endotracheal tubes, sponges, drapes, gauze, alcohol-containing preparation solutions, the patient's hair, surgical dressings, gastrointestinal tract gases, and packaging materials. When using alcohol-containing preparation solutions, they should be allowed to dry before the patient is draped and ignition sources used. Surgical sponges, gauze, and the like are less likely to be fuel sources when they are wet rather than dry.

36. **What are high-risk procedures for OR fires?**
    They include but are not limited to tonsillectomies, tracheostomies, removal of laryngeal papillomas, cataract or other eye surgery, burr hole surgery, and removal of lesions about the head, neck, or face.

37. **What strategies can reduce the incidence of airway fires?**
    - Laser-resistant endotracheal tubes should be chosen. The cuffs should be filled with saline, not air, and it is also recommended that the saline contain a small quantity of

methylene blue to help identify rupture of the cuff, should this happen (as in an airway laser procedure). Many laser specialty tubes already have dye crystals within the cuffs. Cuffed tubes are also preferable to uncuffed tubes.

- Some authors advocate wrapping the endotracheal tube with metal tape; however, this method limits the pliability of the tube and increases the risk of a reflected laser beam and loss of metal tape fragments in the trachea.
- Nitrous oxide should not be used in high-risk procedures. Use only the lowest possible O_2 concentration necessary to maintain the patient's O_2 saturation.
- Ignition sources such as electrosurgical devices should not be allowed to enter the trachea. If they are required, the anesthesiologist should be warned of this by the surgeon, and a suitable period should allowed to decrease the delivered O_2 concentration to the minimum amount tolerated by the patient.

38. **What are signs that a fire has occurred?**
A flame or flash may be noted; unusual sounds heard (*pop, snap,* or *foomp*); and unusual odors, smoke, discoloration of the drapes or heat detected. Abnormal movements of the surgical drapes have also been noted in some fires.

39. **Should an airway fire occur, what are the recommended practices for its management?**
    - Halt the procedure.
    - Remove the endotracheal tube.
    - Stop the flow of all airway gases.
    - Flood the surgical field with saline and remove all flammable and burning materials.
    - Mask-ventilate the patient with 100% O_2 and reintubate.
    - Perform rigid laryngoscopy and bronchoscopy to assess the damage and remove debris.
    - Monitor the patient for 24 hours.
    - Use short-term steroids.
    - Continue ventilatory support and antibiotics as needed.

KEY POINTS: APPROPRIATE SCHEME TO MANAGE AN AIRWAY FIRE

1. Stop ventilation.
2. Disconnect the O_2 source, remove the endotracheal tube, and flood the surgical field with saline.
3. Mask-ventilate the patient with 100% O_2 and reintubate.
4. Perform rigid laryngoscopy and bronchoscopy (using Venturi jet ventilation) to assess the damage and remove debris.
5. Monitor the patient for 24 hours.
6. Use short-term steroids.
7. Continue ventilatory support and antibiotics as needed.

---

40. **Are there additional recommendations for a fire not involving the airway?**
For an intubated patient it is not necessary to halt the flow of ventilator gases. However, if the patient is receiving O_2 by nasal cannula or mask, stopping the flow of these gases may eliminate the oxidizing source. The burning drapes should be removed. Fire extinguishers of the CO_2 type may be needed. An out-of-control fire may require removal of the patient from the OR. The best way to manage any fire is to have a preestablished, practiced algorithm in which every member of the OR team understands his or her role.

WEBSITES

American Burn Association: www.ameriburn.org
Emergency Care Research Institute, Medical Device Safety Reports: The patient is on fire: http://www.mdsr.ecri.org

SUGGESTED READINGS

American Society of Anesthesiologists: Practice advisory for the prevention and management of operating room fires, Anesthesiology 108:786–801, 2008.

Buckley NA, Isbister GK, Stokes B, et al: Hyperbaric oxygen for carbon monoxide poisoning: a systematic review and critical analysis of the evidence, Toxicol Rev 24:75–92, 2005.
Cone JB: What's new in general surgery: burns and metabolism, J Am Coll Surg 200:607–615, 2005.
Klein MB, Hayden D, Elson C, et al: The association between fluid administration and outcome following major burn: a multicenter study, Ann Surg 245:622–628, 2007.
Pham TN, Cancio LC, Gibran NS: American Burn Association practice guidelines for burn shock resuscitation, J Burn Care Res 29:257–266, 2008.
Rampil IJ: Anesthesia for laser surgery. In Miller RD, editor: Miller's anesthesia, ed 6, Philadelphia, 2005, Churchill Livingstone, pp 2573–2587.

CHAPTER 52

NEONATAL ANESTHESIA

Rita Agarwal, MD, and Laurie M. Steward, MD

1. **Why are neonates and preterm infants at increased anesthetic risk?**
   - **Pulmonary factors.** Differences in the neonatal airway, including large tongue and occiput, floppy epiglottis, small mouth, and short neck predispose infants to upper airway obstruction. The more premature the infant, the higher the incidence of airway obstruction. The carbon dioxide response curve is shifted farther to the right in neonates than in adults (i.e., infants have a comparatively decreased ventilatory response to hypercarbia). Newborn vital capacity is about one half of an adult's vital capacity, respiratory rate is twice that of an adult, and oxygen consumption is two to three times greater. Consequently opioids, barbiturates, and volatile agents have a more profound effect on oxygenation and ventilation in neonates than in adults.
   - **Cardiovascular factors.** Newborn infants have noncompliant ventricles that function at close to maximal contractility. Cardiac output is dependent on heart rate. Neonates are highly sensitive to the myocardial depressant effects of many anesthetic agents, especially those that may produce bradycardia. Inhalational agents and barbiturates should be used cautiously.
   - **Temperature regulation.** Infants have poor central thermoregulation, thin insulating fat, increased body surface area–to-mass ratio, and high minute ventilation. These factors make them susceptible to hypothermia in the operating room. Shivering is an ineffective mechanism for heat production because infants have limited muscle mass. Non-shivering thermogenesis uses brown fat to produce heat, but it is not an efficient method to restore body temperature and increases oxygen consumption significantly. Cold-stressed infants may develop cardiovascular depression and hypoperfusion acidosis.
   - **Pharmacologic factors.** Neonates have a larger volume of distribution and less tissue and protein binding of drugs than do older children and adults. They also have immature livers and kidneys and a larger distribution of their cardiac output to the vessel-rich tissues. Neonates often require a larger initial dose of medication but are less able to eliminate the medication. Uptake of inhalation agents is more rapid, and minimum alveolar concentration is lower.

2. **Do neonates have normal renal function?**
   Glomerular function of the kidneys is immature, and the concentrating ability is impaired. Renal clearance of drugs may be delayed. Extra salt and water are not handled well. Neonates do not compensate for hypovolemia.

3. **Why is it important to provide infants with exogenous glucose?**
   Neonates have low stores of hepatic glucose, and mechanisms for gluconeogenesis are immature. Infants who have fasted may develop hypoglycemia. Symptoms of hypoglycemia include apnea, cyanosis, respiratory difficulties, seizures, high-pitched cry, lethargy, temperature instability, and sweating. Hypoglycemia may be associated with long-term neurologic sequelae.

4. **What are the differences in the gastrointestinal or hepatic function of neonates?**
   Gastric emptying is prolonged, and the lower esophageal sphincter is incompetent; thus the incidence of reflux may be increased. Elevated levels of bilirubin are common in neonates. Kernicterus, a complication of elevated levels of bilirubin, may lead to neurologic dysfunction and even death in extreme cases. Commonly used medications such as furosemide and sulfonamide may displace bilirubin from albumin and increase the risk of kernicterus. Diazepam contains the preservative benzyl alcohol, which also may displace bilirubin. Hepatic metabolism is immature, and hepatic blood flow is less than that in older children or adults. Drug metabolism and effect may be prolonged.

5. **What is retinopathy of prematurity?**
   Retinopathy of prematurity is a disorder that occurs in premature and occasionally full-term infants who have been exposed to high inspired concentrations of oxygen. Proliferation of the retinal vessels, retinal hemorrhage, fibroproliferation, scarring, and retinal detachment may occur, with decreased visual acuity and blindness. Premature and full-term infants should have limited exposure to high concentrations of inspired oxygen. Oxygen saturation should be maintained between 92% and 95%, except during times of greater risk for desaturation. Use of an oxygen blender to control the FiO_2 is useful.

6. **How is volume status assessed in neonates?**
   Blood pressure and heart rate are not reliable measures of volume status in neonates. If the anterior fontanel is sunken, skin turgor is decreased, weight loss is present, the infant cries without visible tears or appears lethargic, then dehydration may be present. Capillary refill after blanching of the big toe should be less than 3 seconds. The extremities should not be significantly cooler than the rest of the body. Finally, the skin should look pink and well perfused—not pale, mottled, or cyanotic.

7. **What problems are common in premature infants?**
   See Table 52-1.

8. **What special preparations are needed before anesthetizing a neonate?**
   The room should be warmed at least 1 hour before the start of the procedure to minimize radiant heat loss. A warming blanket, head cover, and warming lights also help to decrease heat loss. Covering the infant with plastic decreases evaporative losses. Forced-air warming blankets have been shown to be effective at keeping infants warm. They work equally well

Table 52-1. Common Problems in Premature Infants

PROBLEM	SIGNIFICANCE
Respiratory distress syndrome	Surfactant, which is produced by alveolar epithelial cells, coats the inside of the alveolus and reduces surface tension. Surfactant deficiency causes alveolar collapse. BPD occurs in about 20% of cases.
Bronchopulmonary dysplasia (BPD)	Interstitial fibrosis, cysts, and collapsed lung, all impairing ventilatory mechanics and gas exchange, may accompany bronchopulmonary dysplasia.
Apnea and bradycardia (A and B)	This is the most common cause of morbidity in the postoperative period. Sensitivity of chemoreceptors to hypercarbia and hypoxia is decreased. Immaturity and poor coordination of upper airway musculature also contribute. If apnea persists >15 sec, bradycardia may result and worsen hypoxia.
Patent ductus arteriosus (PDA)	Incidence of hemodynamically significant PDA varies with degree of prematurity but is usually high. Left-to-right shunting through the PDA may lead to fluid overload, heart failure, and respiratory distress.
Intraventricular hemorrhage (IVH)	Hydrocephalus may result from IVH. Avoiding fluctuations in blood pressure and intracranial pressure may reduce the risk of IVH.
Retinopathy of prematurity	See Question 5.
Necrotizing enterocolitis	Infants develop distended abdomen, bloody stools, and vomiting. They may present in shock and require surgery to resect ischemic intestines.

if the infant is placed on them or if the blanket is placed on the infant. Temperature should be monitored carefully because it is easy to overheat a small infant.
- Routine monitors in a variety of appropriately small sizes should be available. At least two pulse oximeter probes are helpful in measuring preductal and postductal saturation.
- Listening to heart and breath sounds with a precordial or esophageal stethoscope is invaluable.
- Calculate estimated blood volume, maintenance, and maximal acceptable blood loss.
- Placing 25 to 50 ml of balanced salt solution in a buretrol prevents inadvertent administration of large amounts of fluid.
- Five percent albumin and blood should be readily available.

9. **What intraoperative problems are common in small infants?**
   See Table 52-2.

10. **What are the most common neonatal surgeries?**
   - Tracheoesophageal fistula (TEF)
   - Gastroschisis
   - Congenital diaphragmatic hernia (CDH)
   - Patent ductus arteriosus (PDA)
   - Omphalocele
   - Intestinal obstruction
   - Pyloric stenosis

Table 52-2. Common Intraoperative Problems in Infants

PROBLEM	POSSIBLE CAUSES	SOLUTION
Hypoxia	Short distance from cords to carina may cause hypoxia. Further, ETT is easily dislodged or displaced into bronchus. Pressure on abdomen or chest by surgeons may decrease FRC and vital capacity.	At intubation, place the ETT into right mainstem, carefully listen to breath sounds, pull the tube back so that breath sounds are bilateral. Tape ETT 1-2 cm above level of carina. Inform surgeons when they are interfering with ventilation. Hand ventilation helps to compensate for changes in peak pressure.
Bradycardia	Hypoxia Volatile anesthetics Succinylcholine	Preoxygenate before intubation or extubation. All airway manipulations should be performed expeditiously. Minimize amount of volatile agent administered, especially halothane. Give atropine before administering succinylcholine to blunt vagal effects and ensure oxygenation.
Hypothermia	See Question 1	Facilitate a warm operating room by having a warming blanket, warming lights, warm fluids, and humidifier, and keep the infant covered whenever possible.
Hypotension	Bradycardia Volume depletion	Treat bradycardia with anticholinergics and ensure oxygenation. Many neonatal surgeries are associated with major fluid loss. Volume status should be carefully assessed, with deficits replaced appropriately.

ETT, Endotracheal tube; *FRC*, functional residual capacity.

11. **Discuss the incidence and anesthetic implications of congenital diaphragmatic hernia.**
    • The incidence is 1 to 2 out of 5000 live births.
    • The diaphragm fails to close completely, allowing the peritoneal contents to herniate into the thoracic cavity. Abnormal lung development and hypoplasia usually occur on the side of the hernia but may be bilateral.
    • The majority of hernias occurs through the left-sided foramen of Bochdalek.
    • Associated cardiovascular abnormalities present in 23% of patients.
    • Patients present with symptoms of pulmonary hypoplasia. The severity of symptoms and prognosis depend on the severity of the underlying hypoplasia. Pulmonary hypertension is very common.
    • Mask ventilation may cause visceral distention and worsen oxygenation. The infant should be intubated while awake. Low pressures must be used for ventilation to prevent barotrauma. Pneumothorax of the contralateral (healthier) lung may occur when high pressures are needed. Some patients may require high-frequency ventilation or extracorporeal membrane oxygenation.
    • A nasogastric tube should be used to decompress the stomach.
    • A transabdominal approach is used for the repair.
    • Good intravenous (IV) access is mandatory. An arterial line may be necessary if the infant has significant lung or cardiac abnormalities.
    • Pulmonary hypertension may complicate management by impairing oxygenation and decreasing cardiac output. Most patients need to remain intubated in the postoperative period.
    • Opioids and muscle relaxants should be the primary agents used. Inhalational agents may be used to supplement the anesthetic if tolerated by the infant.

12. **Which congenital anomalies are associated with TEF?**
    TEFs may occur alone or as part of a syndrome. The two most common syndromes are the VATER and the VACTERL syndromes. Patients with VATER have vertebral anomalies, imperforate anus, tracheoesophageal fistula, and renal or radial abnormalities. Patients with VACTERL have all of the above and cardiac and limb abnormalities.

13. **How should patients with TEF be managed?**
    • Patients usually present with excessive secretions, inability to pass a nasogastric tube, and regurgitation of feedings. Respiratory symptoms are uncommon.
    • Positive-pressure ventilation may cause distention of the stomach. In a spontaneously breathing patient, either an awake intubation or inhalational induction may be carried out. Surgeons may perform bronchoscopy prior to intubation to evaluate location of fistula.
    • The endotracheal tube (ETT) should be placed into the right mainstem and gradually withdrawn until bilateral breath sounds are heard. The stomach should be auscultated to ensure that it is not overinflated. If the infant has significant respiratory distress because of overinflation of the stomach, it may be necessary to perform a gastrostomy before anesthetizing the patient.
    • An arterial line is usually not necessary in an otherwise healthy infant with no other congenital anomalies. In selected patients, it may be helpful to monitor blood gas values.
    • Pulse oximetry is invaluable. Probes should be placed at a preductal (right hand or finger) and postductal site (left hand or feet).
    • Once the airway has been secured, the infant is placed in the left lateral decubitus position. Placing a precordial stethoscope on the left chest helps to detect displacement of the ETT.
    • Surgical repair involves either thoracotomy or video-assisted thoracoscopic repair. The fistula is divided. If possible, the esophagus is re-anastomosed; if not, a gastrostomy tube is placed. Maintenance of adequate ventilation and oxygenation can be extremely challenging.
    • It is desirable to extubate the infant as soon as possible to prevent pressure on the suture line.

14. **What are the differences between omphalocele and gastroschisis?**
    An omphalocele is a hernia within the umbilical cord caused by failure of the gut to migrate into the abdomen from the yolk sac. The bowel is completely covered with

chorioamnionic membranes but otherwise usually normal. Patients with omphalocele frequently have associated cardiac, urologic, and metabolic anomalies.

In gastroschisis the bowel is not covered with chorioamnionic membranes; often there is an inflammatory exudate, and the bowel anatomy may be abnormal. The exact cause of gastroschisis is unknown; it may be the result of occlusion of blood supply to the abdominal wall or fetal rupture of an omphalocele.

15. **How are patients with omphalocele or gastroschisis managed in the perioperative period?**
    - It is important to prevent evaporative and heat loss from exposed viscera. The exposed bowel should be covered with warm, moist saline packs and plastic wrap until the time of surgery. The operating room should be warmed before the arrival of the infant. Warming lights and a warming blanket help to decrease conductive and radiation heat loss. Covering the head and extremities with plastic prevents evaporative loss. Placing the baby on a forced air blanket can substantially reduce heat loss.
    - Respiratory distress is uncommon; therefore infants usually arrive in the operating room breathing spontaneously. Rapid-sequence induction quickly establishes airway control.
    - Ventilation is controlled with muscle relaxants to facilitate return of the bowel into the abdomen.
    - After intubation, a nasogastric tube should be placed if not already present.
    - Patients need good IV access to replace third-space and evaporative losses. An arterial line can be helpful.
    - Once the surgeons begin to put the viscera into the abdomen, the ventilatory requirements change. Hand ventilation during this phase allows the anesthesiologist to feel peak airway pressures and changes in airway pressures. If peak airway pressures are greater than 40 cm H_2O, the surgeons must be notified.
    - The abdominal cavity may be too small for the viscera. Venous return from or blood flow to the lower extremity may be compromised. A pulse oximeter on the foot helps to detect such changes. Renal perfusion may decrease and manifest as oliguria.
    - If primary closure is not possible, the surgeons choose either to do a fascial closure or to place a synthetic mesh silo over the defect. Both approaches necessitate return trips to the operating room for the final corrective procedure.
    - Patients usually remain intubated after surgery.
    - Surgeons are increasingly performing placement of a silo device at the bedside in the neonatal intensive care unit and bringing patients to the operating room for the final repair.

16. **How does pyloric stenosis present?**
    Pyloric stenosis is a common surgical problem, occurring in 1 out of 300 live births. First-born males are more commonly affected, and it usually presents between 2 and 6 weeks of age. Patients present with persistent vomiting. Dehydration, hypochloremia, and metabolic alkalosis can develop. Continued severe vomiting and dehydration can lead to metabolic acidosis. An olive-like mass may be felt in the epigastrium. Confirmation of the diagnosis by upper gastrointestinal study has largely been replaced by abdominal ultrasound. Surgeons may choose to repair the pylorus laparoscopically or by an open approach.

17. **Discuss the perioperative management of patients with pyloric stenosis.**
    - Electrolyte and volume imbalances need to be corrected before surgery.
    - A gastric tube should be placed and continuous suction applied. The patient may have a large gastric volume of oral x-ray film contrast.
    - Patients are at risk for aspiration; therefore rapid-sequence intubation or modified rapid-sequence intubation should be performed. Awake intubation in this situation has been associated with greater desaturation and a longer time to intubate.
    - Choice of anesthetic agents and muscle relaxants will be guided by the speed of the surgeon (duration of surgery can be 10 to 60 minutes).
    - Opioids are usually unnecessary and should be avoided intraoperatively.
    - Patients need to be closely monitored for postoperative apnea.

18. **Are there any benefits to specific ventilator strategies in neonates?**
    Evidence has emerged that strongly supports the use of lung protective ventilation (8 ml/ kg) in the management of neonates with respiratory distress syndrome (RDS), meconium aspiration syndrome, or congenital diaphragmatic hernia. Injury that has resulted in heterogeneous lung mechanics may cause a particular susceptibility to overdistention because of small absolute lung volumes and a highly compliant chest wall. Regional overdistention from large tidal volumes and elevated airway pressures may be more significant in neonates because of the difference in chest wall compliance and abdominal compartment pressures. In addition to barotrauma caused by high airway pressure, atelectotrauma, related to repeated alveolar recruitment and derecruitment, has been identified as potentially injurious in patients at risk for RDS.

19. **At what age should the former premature infant be allowed to go home after surgery?**
    Premature infants are at increased risk for the development of postoperative apnea even after relatively minor surgery. Postoperative apnea has been reported in ex-premature infants up to 60 weeks' postconceptual age (PCA). Côté and associates showed that, in ex-premature infants born at a gestational age of 32 weeks undergoing inguinal herniorrhaphy, the risk of postoperative apnea was not less than 1% until 56 weeks' PCA. Anemia appropriate for gestational age or high-for-gestational-age infants and a history of continuing apnea increased the risk of postoperative apnea.

KEY POINTS: NEONATAL ANESTHESIA

1. Neonates are at increased anesthetic risk because:
   - They desaturate quickly.
   - They are prone to airway obstruction.
   - Noncompliant ventricles depend on adequate heart rate to maintain cardiac output.
   - They become hypothermic quickly.
   - Immature kidney and liver function affects the pharmacology of administered medications.
2. Common neonatal surgeries include:
   - Tracheoesophageal fistula
   - Gastroschisis
   - Congenital diaphragmatic hernia
   - Patent ductus arteriosus
   - Omphalocele
   - Intestinal obstruction
   - Pyloric stenosis
3. When anesthetizing neonates, the following procedures are followed:
   - Warm the room and have warming lights, blankets, head covers, and convection air warming blankets available to maintain body heat.
   - Have multiple endotracheal sizes available.
   - Estimate fluid maintenance, deficit, blood volume, and acceptable blood loss before the surgery.
   - Prevent accidental overhydration by limiting the amount of volume in the buretrol.

20. **Does regional anesthesia protect the patient from developing postoperative apnea?**
    Spinal anesthesia without supplemental sedation has been associated with less apnea than general anesthesia. Caudal epidural blockade may also be used. The addition of sedation may increase the incidence of postoperative apnea.

SUGGESTED READINGS

Côté CJ, Zaslavsky A, Downes JJ, et al: Postoperative apnea in former preterm infants after inguinal herniorrhaphy: a combined analysis, Anesthesiology 82:809–822, 1995.

Feldman JM, Davis PJ: Do new anesthesia ventilators deliver small tidal volumes accurately during volume-controlled ventilation? Anesth Analg 106:1392–1400, 2008.

Gregory G, Andropoulos DA: Pediatric anesthesia, ed 5, Oxford, 2011, Wiley-Blackwell.

Schultz MJ, Haitsma JJ, Slutsky AS, et al: What tidal volumes should be used in patients without acute lung injury? Anesthesiology 106:1226–1231, 2007.

Vitali SH, Arnold JH: Bench-to-bedside review: ventilator strategies to reduce lung injury—lessons from pediatric and neonatal intensive care, Crit Care 9:177–183, 2005.

CHAPTER 53

PEDIATRIC ANESTHESIA

Rita Agarwal, MD, and Laurie Steward, MD

1. **What are the differences between the adult and pediatric airways?**
   See Table 53-1.

2. **Are there any differences in the adult and pediatric pulmonary systems?**
   See Table 53-2.

3. **How does the cardiovascular system differ in a child?**
   - Newborns are unable to increase cardiac output (CO) by increasing contractility; they increase CO only by increasing heart rate.
   - Infants have an immature baroreceptor reflex and limited ability to compensate for hypotension by increasing heart rate. Therefore they are more susceptible to the cardiac depressant effects of volatile anesthetics and most intravenous anesthetics.
   - Infants have increased vagal tone and are prone to bradycardia. The three major causes of bradycardia are hypoxia (most commonly), vagal stimulation (e.g., laryngoscopy), and volatile anesthetics. Bradycardia decreases CO.

4. **What are normal vital signs in children?**
   See Table 53-3.

5. **When should a child be premedicated? Which drugs are commonly used?**
   Children may have fear and anxiety when they are separated from their parents and during anesthetic induction. Children who are 2 to 6 years old who have had previous surgery, no preoperative tour or education, or who fail to interact positively with health care providers should be premedicated. Children who are anxious during induction may suffer from negative postoperative behavioral changes. Children who receive premedication with midazolam have fewer negative postoperative changes than children who do not (Table 53-4). Distraction techniques using video games or cartoons are being increasingly utilized to reduce perioperative anxiety.

6. **Should parents be allowed to accompany their children to the operating room (OR)?**
   Young children may become anxious and frightened when they are separated from their parents. Allowing parents to accompany children to the OR may facilitate anesthetic induction in some cases. Parents and children should be educated and prepared for what to expect, and parents should be prepared to leave when the anesthesiologist believes it to be appropriate. Anxious, reluctant, or hysterical parents are a hindrance. An anesthesiologist who is not comfortable with parental presence probably should not allow them to be present. An uncooperative, frightened child may not benefit from parental presence. Although allowing parents to be present during induction of anesthesia is beneficial to the parents, premedication with midazolam is associated with lower levels of anxiety in the child. The benefit of both premedication and parental presence during anesthesia does not appear to be additive.

7. **What medications are available for premedication?**
   See Table 53-4.

8. **Describe the commonly used induction techniques used in children.**
   - Inhalational induction is the most common induction technique in children younger than 10 years of age who do not have intravenous (IV) access. The child is asked to breathe a mixture of 70% nitrous oxide (N_2O) and 30% oxygen for approximately 1 minute; sevoflurane is then added. The sevoflurane concentration can be increased slowly or rapidly.

Table 53-1. Differences Between the Adult and Pediatric Airways

INFANT AIRWAY	SIGNIFICANCE
Obligate nose breathers, narrow nares	Infants can breathe only through their noses, which can become easily obstructed by secretions.
Large tongue	Tongue may obstruct airway and make laryngoscopy and intubation difficult.
Large occiput	Sniffing position may be achieved with roll under shoulder.
Glottis located at C3 in premature babies, C3-C4 in newborns, and C5 in adults	Larynx appears more anterior; cricoid pressure frequently helps with laryngeal visualization.
Larynx and trachea are funnel shaped	Narrowest part of the trachea is at the vocal cords; the patient should have an ETT leak of <30 cm H_2O to prevent excessive pressure on the tracheal mucosa, barotrauma.
Vocal cords slant anteriorly	Insertion of ETT may be more difficult.

ETT, Endotracheal tube.

Table 53-2. Differences in the Pediatric and Adult Pulmonary Systems

PEDIATRIC PULMONARY SYSTEM	SIGNIFICANCE
Decreased, smaller alveoli	Thirteen-fold growth in number of alveoli between birth and 6 years; threefold growth in size of alveoli between 6 years and adulthood
Decreased lung compliance	Increased likelihood of airway collapse
Increased airway resistance, vulnerability to smaller airways	Increased work of breathing and disease affecting small airways
Horizontal ribs, pliable ribs and cartilage	Inefficient chest wall mechanics
Less type 1, high-oxidative muscle	Babies tire more easily
Decreased total lung capacity, faster respiratory and metabolic rate	Quicker desaturation
Higher closing volumes	Increased dead-space ventilation

Table 53-3. Normal Vital Signs in Children

AGE (YEARS)	HR	RR	SBP	DPB
<1	120–160	30–60	60–95	35–69
1–3	90–140	24–40	95–105	50–65
3–5	75–110	18–30	95–110	50–65
8–12	75–100	18–30	90–110	57–71
12–16	60–90	12–16	112–130	60–80

DBP, Diastolic blood pressure; HR, heart rate; RR, respiratory rate; SBP, systolic blood pressure. A good rule of thumb is normal BP = 80 mm Hg + 2 × age.

Table 53-4. Routes of Administration for Premedications in Children

DRUG	ROUTE	COMMENTS	DISADVANTAGES
Midazolam	PO, PR, IN, IV, SL	Quick onset, minimal side effects	Tastes bad when given orally, burns intranasally
Ketamine	PO, PR, IN, IV, SL	Quick onset, good analgesia	May slow emergence, tastes bad, burns intranasally
Fentanyl	OTFC	Tastes good, good analgesic, onset at 45 minutes	Possible hypoxemia, nausea
Diazepam	PO, PR, IM	Cheap, minimal side effects	Long onset time, may prolong emergence
Dexmedetomidine	IN, IV, IM	Does not burn intranasally	Long onset time, may prolong emergence, bradycardia

IM, Intramuscular; IN, intranasal; IV, intravenous; OTFC, oral transmucosal fentanyl citrate; PO, by mouth; PR, per rectum; SL, sublingual.

- Rapid inhalational induction is used in an uncooperative child. The child is held down, and a mask containing 70% N_2O, 30% oxygen, and 8% sevoflurane is placed on the child's face. This unpleasant technique should be avoided if possible. Once anesthesia has been induced, the concentration of sevoflurane is decreased.
- Steal induction may be used if the child is already sleeping. Inhalational induction is accomplished by holding the mask near the child's face while gradually increasing the concentration of sevoflurane. The goal is to induce anesthesia without awakening the child.
- IV induction is used in a child who already has an IV line in place and in children older than 10 years. Typical medications used in children are propofol, 2 to 3 mg/kg, etomidate, 0.2 to 0.3 mg/kg, ketamine, 2 to 5 mg/kg, methohexital, 1 to 2 mg/kg. EMLA cream (eutectic mixture of local anesthesia) applied at least 60 minutes before starting the IV infusion makes this an atraumatic procedure.

9. **How does the presence of a left-to-right shunt affect inhalational induction and intravenous induction?**
A left-to-right intracardiac shunt leads to volume overload of the right heart and pulmonary circulation, resulting in congestive heart failure and decreased lung compliance. Uptake and distribution of inhaled agents are minimally affected; onset time for IV agents is slightly prolonged.

10. **How about a right-to-left shunt?**
Right-to-left shunting causes hypoxemia and left ventricular overload. Patients compensate by increasing blood volume and hematocrit. It is important to maintain a high systemic vascular resistance (SVR) to prevent increased shunting from right to left. Such shunts may slightly delay inhalation induction and shorten the onset time of IV induction agents.

11. **What other special precautions need to be taken in a child with heart disease?**
- The anatomy of the lesion(s) and direction of blood flow should be determined. Pulmonary vascular resistance (PVR) needs to be maintained. If the PVR increases, right-to-left shunting may increase and worsen oxygenation, whereas a patient with a left-to-right shunt may develop a reversal in the direction of blood flow (Eisenmenger syndrome). If a patient has a left-to-right shunt, decreasing the PVR may increase blood flow to the lungs and lead to pulmonary edema. Decreasing the PVR in patients with a right-to-left shunt may improve hemodynamics. Conditions that can increase shunting are listed in Table 53-5.
- Air bubbles must be meticulously avoided. If there is communication between the right and left sides of the heart (ventricular septal defect, atrial septal defect, patent foramen

Table 53-5. Conditions That Can Increase Shunting

LEFT-TO-RIGHT SHUNT	RIGHT-TO-LEFT SHUNT
Low hematocrit	Decreased SVR
Increased SVR	Increased PVR
Decreased PVR	Hypoxia
Hyperventilation	Hypercarbia
Hypothermia	Acidosis
Isoflurane	Nitrous oxide, ketamine

PVR, Pulmonary vascular resistance; SVR, systemic vascular resistance.

Table 53-6. Guidelines for Endotracheal Tube Size

AGE	SIZE—INTERNAL DIAMETER (mm)
Newborns	3.0–3.5
Newborn–12 months	3.5–4.0
12–18 months	4.0
2 years	4.5
>2 years	ETT size = (16 + age)/4

ETT, Endotracheal tube.

ovale), air injected intravenously may travel across the communication and enter the arterial system. This may lead to central nervous system symptoms if the air obstructs the blood supply to the brain or spinal cord (paradoxical air embolus).
- Prophylactic antibiotics should be given to prevent infective endocarditis. Recommendations for medications and doses can be found in the American Heart Association guidelines.
- Avoid bradycardia.
- Recognize and be able to treat a "tet spell." Children with tetralogy of Fallot have right ventricular outflow tract (RVOT) obstruction (pulmonary artery stenosis or atresia), an overriding aorta, ventricular septal defect, and right ventricular hypertrophy. They may or may not have cyanosis at rest. However, many are prone to hypercyanotic spells (tet spells) as they get older. Such episodes are characterized by worsening RVOT obstruction, possibly as a result of hypovolemia, increased contractility, or tachycardia during times of stimulation or stress. Patients are frequently treated with β blockers, which should be continued perioperatively. Hypovolemia, acidosis, excessive crying or anxiety, and increased airway pressures should be avoided. The SVR should be maintained. If a hypercyanotic spell occurs in the perioperative period, treatment includes maintaining the airway, volume infusion, increasing the depth of anesthesia, or decreasing the surgical stimulation. Phenylephrine is valuable in increasing SVR. Additional doses of β blockers may also be useful. Metabolic acidosis should be corrected.

12. **How is an endotracheal tube of appropriate size chosen?**
An endotracheal tube (ETT) a half size above and a half size below the estimated size in Table 53-6 should be available, the leak around the tube should be <30 cm H$_2$O, and the ETT should be placed to a depth of approximately three times its internal diameter.

13. **Can cuffed ETTs be used in children?**
Common teaching was that cuffed ETTs should not be used in children <8 years old. The reasons are twofold:
1. Avoid trauma to the narrowest part of the pediatric airway—the cricoid.
2. Allow a bigger uncuffed ETT to be passed, which would decrease the work of breathing (WOB). Early studies were done in cadavers; in cadaveric models the airway is cone

shaped, with the cricoid at its apex. More recent magnetic resonance imaging studies to measure laryngeal and tracheal parameters in anesthetized, nonparalyzed spontaneously breathing children found that, although the airway was cone shaped, the apex and narrowest diameters were at the vocal cords. In addition, they found that the airway was elliptical and not circular.

Many patients who are intubated (in either the OR or intensive care unit) are mechanically ventilated; thus the WOB is not as much of an issue as it used to be. Newer circuits and anesthesia machines have also helped decrease the problem of WOB.

Tracheal mucosal inflammation and injury are related to a number of factors, including duration of intubation and number of intubation attempts. Several recent studies have found that cuffed ETTs decrease the number of intubation attempts and are associated with decreased air leak (resulting in decreased OR pollution and greater ability to use low fresh gas flows) and provide better protection against aspiration.

Cuffed ETTs can be used in children and neonates. Of course, the cuff takes up space, thus limiting the size of the ETT. Use the cuffed tube one half size smaller than the appropriate uncuffed tube. The advantages of cuffed ETTs are that they avoid repeat laryngoscopy and may allow use of lower fresh gas flows.

New Microcuff ETTs are formulated with microthin polyurethane cuff material that is reputed to seal the airway with half the pressure of conventional cuffed ETTs. Their cuff is short and cylindrical and placed near the tube tip. This positions the cuff lower in the airway.

Laryngeal mask airways (LMAs) are also useful in pediatrics. They can help secure a difficult airway, either as the sole technique or as a conduit to endotracheal intubation. In addition, their use may be instrumental for difficult mask ventilation situations. The LMA is used increasingly for routine airway management in minor procedures and is now included in the Neonatal Resuscitation Program protocol for airway management.

14. **How is an appropriate-size laryngeal mask airway chosen?**
See Table 53-7.

15. **How does the pharmacology of commonly used anesthetic drugs differ in children?**
   - The minimal alveolar concentration (MAC) of the volatile agents is higher in children than in adults. The highest MAC is in infants 1 to 6 months old. Premature babies and neonates have a lower MAC.
   - Children have a higher tolerance to the dysrhythmic effects of epinephrine during general anesthesia with volatile agents.
   - In general, children have higher drug requirements (mg/kg) because they have a greater volume of distribution (more fat, more body water).
   - Opioids should be used carefully in children less than 1 year old who are more sensitive to the respiratory depressant effects.

Table 53-7. Laryngeal Mask Airways for Children

SIZE OF CHILD	LMA SIZE
Neonates up to 5 kg	1
Infants 5–10 kg	$1\frac{1}{2}$
Children 10–20 kg	2
Children 20–30 mg	$2\frac{1}{2}$
Children/small adults >30 kg	3
Children/adults >70 kg	4
Children/adults >80 kg	5

LMA, Laryngeal mask airway.

Table 53-8. Guidelines for Estimated Blood Volume in Children

AGE	EBV (ml/kg)
Neonate	90
Infant up to 1 year old	80
Older than 1 year	70

EBV, Estimated blood volume.

16. How is perioperative fluid managed in children?

- Maintenance is calculated as follows:
  - Infant <10 kg: 4 ml/kg/hr
  - 10 to 20 kg: 40 ml/hr plus 2 ml/kg/hr for every kg over 10
  - Child >20 kg: 60 ml/hr plus 1 ml/kg/hr for every kg over 20
- Estimated fluid deficit (EFD) should be calculated and replaced as follows:
  - EFD = maintenance × hours since last oral intake
  - ½ EFD + maintenance given over the first hour
  - ¼ EFD + maintenance given over the second hour
  - ¼ EFD + maintenance given over the third hour
- All EFDs should be replaced for major cases. For minor cases, 10 to 20 ml/kg of a balanced salt solution (BSS) with or without glucose is usually adequate.
- Estimated blood volume (EBV) and acceptable blood loss (ABL) should be calculated for every case.

17. What is the most common replacement fluid used in children? Why?

A balanced salt solution, such as lactated Ringer with glucose (D_5LR) or without glucose (LR) is recommended. Hypoglycemia is rare in healthy children undergoing minimally invasive procedures, and administration of 5% glucose-containing solutions results in hyperglycemia in the majority of children. Others still use 5% glucose solutions for maintenance but recommend non-glucose–containing BSS for third space or blood loss. In major operations it is prudent to check serial glucose levels and avoid hyperglycemia or hypoglycemia.

18. What is the estimated blood volume in children?

See Table 53-8.

19. How is acceptable blood loss calculated?

$$ABL = [EBV \times (pt\ hct - lowest\ acceptable\ hct)]/average\ hct$$

where ABL = acceptable blood loss, EBV = estimated blood volume, pt = patient, and hct = hematocrit. The lowest acceptable hematocrit varies with circumstances. Blood transfusion is usually considered when the hematocrit is <21% to 25%. If significant blood loss is anticipated, transfusion may need to be started earlier. For example, a 4-month-old infant is scheduled for craniofacial reconstruction. He is otherwise healthy, and his last oral intake was 6 hours before arriving in the OR; weight = 6 kg, preoperative hct = 33%, lowest acceptable hct = 25%.

- Maintenance = weight × 4 ml/hr = 24 ml/hr
- EFD = maintenance × 6 hr = 144 ml
- EBV = weight × 80 ml/kg = 480 ml
- ABL = [EBV × (pt hct − lowest acceptable hct)]/average hct = [480 × (33 − 25)]/29 = 132 ml

20. How do the manifestations of hypovolemia differ in children compared with adults?

Healthy children compensate for acute volume loss of 30% to 40% before blood pressure changes. The most reliable early indicators of compensated hypovolemic shock in a child are persistent tachycardia, cutaneous vasoconstriction, and diminution of pulse pressure.

Table 53-9. Systemic Response to Blood Loss in Children

ORGAN SYSTEM	<25% BLOOD LOSS	25%–40% BLOOD LOSS	>45% BLOOD LOSS
Cardiac	Weak, rapid, pulse; thready pulse	Tachycardia	Hypotension, tachycardia; bradycardia indicates severe blood loss and impending circulatory collapse
Central nervous system	Lethargic and confused	Obtunded, dulled response to pain	Comatose
Skin	Cool, clammy	Cyanotic, decreased capillary refill, cold extremities	Pale, cold
Kidneys	Oliguria	Minimal UOP	Minimal if any UOP

UOP, Urine output.

Table 53-10. Commonly Used Doses of Local Anesthetic for Caudal Block

DOSE (ml/kg)	LEVEL OF BLOCK	SITE OF OPERATION
0.5	Sacral/lumbar	Penile, lower extremity
1	Lumbar/thoracic	Lower abdominal
1.2	Upper thoracic	Upper abdominal

UOP, Urine output.
Data from Gunter JB, Dunn CM, Bennie JB, et al: Optimum concentration of bupivacaine for combined caudal-general anesthesia in pediatric patients. Anesthesiology 75(1): 57–61, 1991.

21. **What are the systemic responses to blood loss?**
   See Table 53-9.

22. **What is the most common type of regional anesthesia performed in children? Which local anesthetic is used, and what dose is appropriate?**
   Caudal epidural block is the most common regional technique. It is usually performed in an anesthetized child and provides intraoperative and postoperative analgesia. It is used most commonly for surgery of the lower extremities, perineum, and lower abdomen.
   Bupivacaine (0.125% to 0.25%) or ropivacaine 0.2% are most commonly used. Bupivacaine 0.25% produces intraoperative analgesia and decreases the required volatile anesthetic, but motor blockade may occur. The toxic dose of bupivacaine in the child is 2.5 mg/kg; in the neonate, 1.5 mg/kg. Commonly used doses are listed in Table 53-10.

23. **Describe the common postoperative complications.**
   - **Postoperative nausea and vomiting** (PONV) is the most common cause of delayed discharge or unplanned admission. Factors associated with PONV in children include age >6 years, length of surgery >20 minutes, previous history of PONV, eye surgery, inner ear procedures, history of motion sickness, tonsillectomy/adenoidectomy, preoperative nausea or anxiety, hypoglycemia, and use of opioids and N_2O. The best treatment for PONV is prevention. Prophylactic administration of an antiemetic should be considered for patients at high risk for PONV. Avoiding opioids decreases the incidence of PONV as long as pain relief is adequate (e.g., patient has a caudal block). Management includes administering IV fluid, limiting oral intake, and administering dexamethasone, metoclopramide, or ondansetron.
   - **Laryngospasm** and **stridor** are more common in children than in adults. Management for laryngospasm includes oxygen, positive pressure ventilation, jaw thrust, succinylcholine,

propofol, and re-intubation if necessary. Stridor is usually treated with humidified oxygen, steroids, and racemic epinephrine.

- **Emergence agitation** has increased in incidence with the use of short-acting volatile agents (sevoflurane and desflurane). Pain can worsen, and analgesics improve agitation. Agitation can occur even in patients undergoing non-painful procedures, although fentanyl, 1 mcg/kg, reduces agitation.

KEY POINTS: PEDIATRIC ANESTHESIA

1. Infants may be difficult to intubate because they have a more anterior larynx, relatively large tongues, and a floppy epiglottis. The narrowest part of the larynx has been found to be below the vocal cords at the cricoid cartilage.
2. Children de-saturate more rapidly than adults because of increased metabolic rate, increased dead space, inefficient chest wall mechanics and, in neonates, immature alveoli.
3. Premedication with midazolam has been shown to be superior in decreasing a child's anxiety when compared with a placebo or parental presence at the time of induction.
4. Children who receive premedication have a lower incidence of postoperative negative behavioral changes than those who do not.

---

24. **What is the significance of masseter muscle rigidity?**

Rigidity of the masseter muscles occurs in 1% of children receiving halothane and succinylcholine. Masseter muscle rigidity (MMR) may be the first symptom of malignant hyperthermia (MH), but it may also occur in patients who are not susceptible to MH. When MMR develops, the major issue is whether or not to continue. Unless other signs of MH develop, or severe masseter muscle spasm impedes intubation, the anesthetic is changed to a non-triggering technique and the surgery proceeds.

After surgery patients should be admitted and followed for signs of MH (tachycardia, hypercarbia, acidosis, blood pressure lability, muscle rigidity, hyperthermia, and myoglobinuria). Hyperthermia is regularly a late sign. If creatine phosphokinase (CPK) is >20,000, the patient should be considered to have MH. If the CPK is <20,000 but still significantly elevated, an MH work-up should be considered, including a muscle biopsy. If CPK is normal or minimally elevated, the patient is probably not at increased risk for MH.

25. **Should children with upper respiratory infections receive general anesthesia?**

The risk of adverse respiratory events is 9 to 11 times greater up to 6 weeks after an upper respiratory infection (URI). Underlying pulmonary derangements include decreased diffusion capacity for oxygen, decreased compliance, increased airway resistance, decreased closing volumes, increased shunting (ventilation-perfusion mismatch), hypoxemia, and increased airway reactivity (desaturation, bronchospasm, laryngospasm). Associated factors predicting an increased likelihood of perioperative complications include airway instrumentation, fever, productive cough, lower respiratory tract involvement, a history of snoring, passive smoking, induction anesthetic agent, copious secretions, nasal congestion, and anticholinesterase use.

General recommendations for a child with a mild URI include the following:
- Discuss increased risk with parents and the surgical team.
- Try to avoid intubation (LMA or mask use has a lower risk).
- Use anticholinergics and/or β agonists to help decrease secretions and airway reactivity.
- Humidification and hydration are thought to decrease airway dryness and maintain ciliary clearance.
- The febrile child with rhonchi that do not clear with coughing, an abnormal chest x-ray film, elevated white count, or decreased activity levels should be rescheduled for an elective procedure.
- The afebrile child with an uncomplicated URI with clear secretions and well appearing may be able to safely undergo anesthesia.

26. **What are the implications of sleep-disordered breathing in children?**

Sleep-disordered breathing (SDB) is a continuum that ranges from normal breathing and oxygenation to chronic intermittent desaturation and obstructive sleep apnea (OSA).

OSA is known to be associated with decreased CO_2 response curve and a higher incidence of perioperative respiratory problems such as desaturation, obstruction, apnea, and opioid sensitivity. It is important to assess the severity and comorbidities present in each patient.

SDB can be caused by upper airway obstruction secondary to adenotonsillar hypertrophy, obesity, neuromuscular problems, or craniofacial abnormalities. Children with SDB can have significant behavioral and school performance issues. Tonsillectomy and adenoidectomy have been shown to eliminate airway obstruction in 85% to 95% of healthy patients with OSA and result in significant improvement in clinical symptoms. Recent studies have challenged the myth of adverse effects from preoperative sedation in these children.

SUGGESTED READINGS

Francis A, Eltaki K, Bash T, et al: The safety of preoperative sedation in children with sleep-disordered breathing, Int J Pediatr Otorhinolaryngol 70:1517–1521, 2006.

Goldstein NA, Pugazhendhi V, Rao SM, et al: Clinical assessment of pediatric obstructive sleep apnea, Pediatrics 114:33–43, 2004.

Gregory GA, Andropoulos DA: Pediatric anesthesia, ed 5, Oxford, 2011, Wiley-Blackwell.

Tait AR, Malviya S: Anesthesia for the child with an upper respiratory tract infection: still a dilemma? Anesth Analg 100:59–65, 2005.

CHAPTER 54

CONGENITAL HEART DISEASE

Lawrence I. Schwartz, MD, and Robert H. Friesen, MD

1. **What is the incidence of congenital heart disease (CHD)?**
   CHD is the most common type of birth defect. Although a variable range can be found in the literature, a reasonable estimate of the incidence in 1 in 250 live births. Ventricular septal defect is the most common type of CHD, comprising 25% of all congenital heart defects.

2. **What are some of the unique features of the neonatal heart?**
   The newborn myocardium is not fully mature at birth. Some features of the neonatal heart can make caring for these patients quite challenging.
   - The newborn myocardium is poorly organized and has fewer myofibrils with fewer contractile elements leading to decreased tension development.
   - Underdeveloped calcium cycling and excitation-contraction coupling lead to cytosolic calcium dependence.
   - Incomplete sympathetic innervation combined with intact parasympathetic system provides the "vagal tone" that can cause bradycardia.
   - Beta-adrenergic receptors are less sensitive and may be downregulated in children with CHD.
   - These cellular differences result in a newborn heart that is less compliant, develops less contractile force, and is less responsive to inotropic support than mature heart. This can contribute to cardiac dysfunction in newborns with CHD presurgical and postsurgical repair. Myocardial maturation is generally complete by 6 to 12 months of age.

3. **How are different types of CHD classified?**
   CHD can be classified in multiple ways, including segmentally, anatomically, and physiologically. Anesthesiologists often use a physiologic classification. Specific CHDs can be classified as acyanotic heart disease or cyanotic heart disease. Acyanotic heart defects can further be divided into acyanotic disease with left-to-right shunt and acyanotic disease without left-to-right shunt. Cyanotic heart disease can be classified as having "ductal-dependent" pulmonary blood flow, "ductal-dependent" systemic blood flow, and mixing lesions without "ductal-dependent" blood flow (Table 54-1).

4. **How are shunts calculated?**
   Using cardiac catheterization data, relative flows in the pulmonary and systemic circulations can be calculated using the Fick principle (flow is inversely related to oxygen extraction):

$$Qp/Qs = (SaO_2 - SvO_2)/(SpvO_2 - SpaO_2)$$

   where Qp = pulmonary blood flow; Qs = systemic blood flow; SaO_2 = systemic arterial oxygen saturation; SvO_2 = systemic mixed venous oxygen saturation; $SpvO_2$ = pulmonary venous oxygen saturation; and $SpaO_2$ = pulmonary arterial oxygen saturation.

5. **What are the anesthetic considerations for patients with left-to-right shunts?**
   A left-to-right shunt will ultimately lead to volume overloading of both ventricles. This may lead to congestive heart failure, which, in the pediatric patient, may present as feeding difficulties, failure to thrive, tachycardia, and poor perfusion. Excess blood flow through the shunt (atrial septal defect or ventricular septal defect) and through the developing pulmonary vascular bed can cause arterialization of blood vessels, leading to increased pulmonary vascular resistance (PVR) and pulmonary hypertension. The anesthetic management of these patients may include:
   - Judicious use of oxygen, so as to not increase the left-to-right shunt and decrease cardiac output in the face of congestive heart failure
   - Treatment of congestive heart failure with inotropic agents such as milrinone, dopamine, or epinephrine

Table 54-1. Classification of Congenital Heart Disease

CLASSIFICATION OF CONGENITAL HEART DISEASE (CHD)	EXAMPLES
Acyanotic CHD with left-to-right shunt	Atrial septal defect, ventricular septal defect, partial anomalous pulmonary venous return
Acyanotic CHD without left-to-right shunt	Coarctation of the aorta, aortic valvar disease, cardiomyopathies
Cyanotic CHD with ductal-dependent pulmonary blood flow	Ebstein anomaly, tetralogy of Fallot + pulmonary atresia, tricuspid atresia
Cyanotic CHD with ductal-dependent systemic blood flow	Hypoplastic left heart syndrome, interrupted aortic arch, critical aortic stenosis
Mixing lesions without ductal-dependent blood flow	Atrioventricular septal defect transposition of the great arteries, double outlet right ventricle

Table 54-2. Treatment of Pulmonary Hypertension

GOAL	METHOD
Increase PO_2	Increase FiO_2 Treat atelectasis Control ventilation
Alkalosis	Hyperventilation Treat metabolic acidosis
Control stress response	Adequate analgesia
Pulmonary vasodilation	Inhaled nitric oxide Intravenous prostacyclin (PGI_2)

FiO_2, Fraction of inspired oxygen; PO_2, partial pressure of oxygen.

- Management of pulmonary hypertension with pulmonary vasodilators such as inhaled nitric oxide
- Management of arrhythmias arising during surgical repair: complete atrioventricular block, junctional ectopic tachycardia

6. **What is a pulmonary hypertensive crisis? How is it treated?**
   In patients with pulmonary hypertension, the pulmonary vasculature is hyperreactive to various stimuli that cause pulmonary vasoconstriction. These stimuli include hypoxia, acidosis, hypercarbia, hypothermia, and the stress associated with pain. When the PVR suddenly increases as a result of such hyperreactivity to a point at which right ventricular pressure equals or exceeds left ventricular pressure, a pulmonary hypertensive crisis is said to occur. This is a dangerous situation in which death can occur as a result of rapidly progressive right ventricular failure, diminishing pulmonary blood flow and cardiac output, and hypoxia. Table 54-2 outlines the treatment of pulmonary hypertension.

7. **What is tetralogy of Fallot?**
   The tetrad of anatomic findings described by Fallot for this congenital heart lesion is ventricular septal defect, overriding aorta, right ventricular outflow tract (RVOT) obstruction, and right ventricular hypertrophy. Depending on the degree of pulmonary obstruction, these patients can present with hypoxemia or normal blood oxygen saturation. When patients present for surgical repair, one of the primary concerns for the anesthesiologist is an acute hypercyanotic episode, or "tet spell."

Table 54-3. Treatment of Hypercyanotic Spells

GOALS	METHODS
Relax the RVOT	Beta blockers Deepening anesthesia (too deep can decrease SVR further)
Increase SVR	Phenylephrine 5-10 mcg/kg (or more)
Decrease PVR	Increase FiO_2 Hyperventilation Sodium bicarbonate
Increase stroke volume	Intravenous fluid balance

FiO_2, Fraction of inspired oxygen; PVR, pulmonary vascular resistance; RVOT, right ventricular outflow tract; SVR, systemic vascular resistance.

8. **What is a "tet spell," and how is it treated?**
   The RVOT obstruction in tetralogy of Fallot can have a dynamic component. The subvalvular RVOT is muscular and contracts in response to inotropic stimuli, such as catecholamine release. When such contraction occurs—or if systemic vascular resistance (SVR) decreases significantly—less blood can flow in the pulmonary artery, and the desaturated blood is shunted right to left across the ventricular septal defect into the left ventricle and out the systemic circulation. The subsequent hypoxemia and acidosis increases PVR and further increases the right-to-left shunt. This acute hypercyanotic episode can create a downward spiral that can lead to cardiopulmonary collapse.
   The treatment of a "tet spell" includes rebalancing SVR and PVR ("reversing the shunt") and overcoming the RVOT obstruction. The goals of therapy are aimed at increasing SVR, lowering PVR, relaxing the hyperdynamic RVOT, and increasing right ventricular stroke volume (Table 54-3).

9. **What are the three shunts of fetal circulation?**
   Fetal circulation is a parallel circulation with three shunts in order to provide the most oxygenated blood to the developing fetus. The ductus venosus shunts well-oxygenated, nutrient-rich blood from the umbilical vein to the right atrium, thereby bypassing the liver. This blood is then shunted from the higher pressure fetal right atrium through the foramen ovale to the left side of the heart where it can provide oxygen to the developing heart and brain. In the presence of atelectatic, amniotic fluid–filled lungs and high PVR, deoxygenated blood returning to the right ventricle is shunted from the main pulmonary artery through the ductus arteriosus to the descending aorta. It can then flow via the low SVR pathway back to the placenta via the umbilical artery for reoxygenation.

10. **What is meant by "ductal-dependent" lesions?**
    In some forms of CHD, there is complete obstruction of either pulmonary or systemic blood flow. The ductus arteriosus is a fetal blood vessel that shunts deoxygenated blood from the right ventricle to the descending aorta in order to return blood to the placenta for reoxygenation. In lesions such as pulmonary atresia or hypoplastic left heart syndrome, a patent ductus arteriosus is the only means of supplying pulmonary or systemic blood flow, respectively. However, the ductus arteriosus is meant to close in the higher oxygen environment following birth. Therefore, an infusion of prostaglandin E_1 is vital to maintaining ductal patency and supporting life until palliative or corrective surgery can be performed.

11. **What is single ventricle physiology?**
    Patients born with single ventricle physiology have only one functional ventricle that provides both pulmonary and systemic cardiac output. Single ventricle physiology is a parallel circulation that, if not repaired, will lead to chronic cyanosis and volume overload congestive heart failure. By definition, single ventricle physiology exists in any CHD that ultimately requires Fontan palliation surgery.

12. **How is a single ventricle congenital heart defect repaired?**
    The ultimate goal of single ventricle repair is to provide a series circulation without intracardiac shunt or obstruction. This is done in a stepwise fashion over the patient's first 2 to 3 years of life. There are classically three surgeries performed to gradually achieve this goal.
    1. Stage I palliation is performed in the newborn period and involves securing pulmonary blood flow. This is often done with a modified Blalock-Taussig shunt. A small Gore-Tex graft is sewn from the subclavian artery to the right pulmonary artery. In the case of hypoplastic left heart syndrome, a neo-aorta is also created in order to stabilize systemic blood flow. This surgery is known as the *Norwood operation*.
    2. Stage II palliation occurs at a few months of life. A cavo-pulmonary anastomosis is created by taking the superior vena cava off the right atrium and connecting it to the branch pulmonary artery. This surgery, commonly called a *modified bidirectional Glenn surgery*, begins the process of reducing the volume overload on the single ventricle. From this point onward, the patient's pulmonary blood flow is dependent on direct venous flow into the lungs.
    3. Stage III palliation in performed at approximately 2 years of life. This is the Fontan completion and involves creating an inferior cavo-pulmonary artery anastomosis. This establishes the series circulation; the single ventricle is now only responsible for providing systemic blood flow. All systemic venous return now flows "passively" and directly to the lungs.
    The anesthetic management of these surgeries is very complex and requires close attention to balancing pulmonary and systemic vascular resistances and blood flows. Additionally, these patients require treatment for myocardial dysfunction and arrhythmia. These patients can provide some of the biggest challenges to pediatric cardiac anesthesiologists.

13. **What are the outcomes of surgery for CHD?**
    Short-term surgical survival is the expected outcome in patients presenting with CHD. As surgical, anesthetic, and postoperative care has improved over the past 50 years, survival following surgical intervention has improved to well over 90% for complex CHD at major CHD centers. However, long-term outcomes are still associated with significant morbidity and mortality. Children with congenital heart disease represent 30–50% of all infant and childhood deaths resulting from birth defects.

14. **Are there adults with CHD?**
    With advances in the care of patients with CHD, many children now survive into adulthood. Currently in the United States, there are more adults than children with CHD. The prevalence of CHD increased greater than 50% between 2000 and 2010. By 2010, adults accounted for two thirds of patients with congenital heart disease in the general population. Although adults with CHD are living longer lives, they are at risk for multiple long-term sequelae and often require lifelong medical surveillance and therapy.

15. **What are the long-term complications related to CHD?**
    Numerous complications can occur in patients with repaired or palliated CHD. Residual shunts, obstructions, heart valve abnormalities, surgical trauma, inflammation, foreign material implants, and myocardial injury can lead to long-term consequences including ventricular failure, cardiac arrhythmia, heart block requiring a pacemaker, pulmonary hypertension, subacute bacterial endocarditis, and chronic cyanosis.

16. **What causes cyanosis in CHD?**
    When at least 5 g/dl of desaturated hemoglobin is present in arterial blood, the lips, nail beds, and mucous membranes appear blue, or cyanotic. Cyanosis occurs in patients with congenital heart lesions involving a right-to-left shunt and decreased pulmonary blood flow (including tetralogy of Fallot, pulmonary stenosis or atresia with septal defect, and tricuspid atresia); in patients with lesions involving mixing of right- and left-sided blood without decreased pulmonary blood flow (including truncus arteriosus, anomalous pulmonary venous return, single ventricle, and double-outlet right ventricle); and in patients with parallel right and left circulations (transposition of the great arteries).

17. Describe the clinical problems associated with cyanotic CHD.
In response to chronic hypoxemia, these patients develop polycythemia. When hematocrit exceeds about 65%, increased blood viscosity is associated with a greater risk of intravascular thrombosis, stroke, coagulopathy, and poor flow in the microcirculation. The combination of hypoxemia and impaired blood flow can lead to tissue ischemia and organ dysfunction. In the heart, ventricular dysfunction occurs as the myocardium is subjected to chronic ischemia and is exacerbated by the hypertrophy associated with ventricular outflow obstruction, as in pulmonary stenosis.

In the presence of right-to-left shunting, air bubbles inadvertently injected into a vein can cross to the left side of the heart and enter the systemic arterial circulation, where they may cause stroke or myocardial ischemia.

KEY POINTS: PATHOPHYSIOLOGIC EFFECTS OF CYANOTIC HEART DISEASE

1. Polycythemia
2. Increased blood viscosity
3. Coagulopathy
4. Decreased tissue perfusion
5. End-organ ischemia

18. What is subacute bacterial endocarditis, and how can it be prevented?
Turbulent or high-velocity blood flow in the heart associated with congenital heart defects can cause damage to the endocardium of the heart or valves. Damaged endocardium can be a nidus for infection in the presence of bacteremia or septicemia. Bacteremia can occur during dental or surgical procedures and can lead to bacterial endocarditis. Prophylactic administration of antibiotics during these procedures can prevent the development of endocarditis. However, the overall risk from surgery is still low, and the latest recommendations from the American Heart Association restrict the use of prophylactic antibiotics to the highest risk population only. Dental and oral surgical procedures carry the greatest risk of infection. Box 54-1 outlines the cardiac population in which it remains currently recommended to treat with antibiotic prophylaxis. Except for the conditions listed, antibiotic prophylaxis is no longer recommended for patients with any other form of CHD.

Patients can be treated with amoxicillin, ampicillin, cefazolin, or clindamycin if they have a penicillin allergy. Patients should continue to receive prophylactic antibiotic treatment as indicated for surgical procedures. In these cases it is reasonable to choose a medication that will also provide prophylaxis for subacute bacterial endocarditis.

19. How much training does a pediatric cardiac anesthesiologist obtain?
Typically a pediatric cardiac anesthesiologist must complete a 1-year internship, a 3-year anesthesiology residency, a 1-year pediatric anesthesiology fellowship, and an advanced

Box 54-1. Cardiac Conditions Associated with the Highest Risk of Adverse Outcome from Endocarditis for Which Prophylaxis with Dental Procedures Is Reasonable[2E]

Prosthetic cardiac valve or prosthetic material used for cardiac valve repair
Previous infective endocarditis
Congenital heart disease (CHD)
  Unrepaired cyanotic CHD, including palliative shunts and conduits
  Completely repaired CHD with prosthetic material or device, whether placed by surgery or catheter intervention, during the first 6 months after procedure
  Repaired CHD with residual defects at the site or adjacent to the site of a prosthetic patch or device
Cardiac transplantation recipients who develop cardiac valvulopathy

fellowship in pediatric cardiac anesthesiology. Many of these anesthesiologists have additional training in pediatric medicine and pediatric critical care medicine. Regardless of the training, pediatric cardiac anesthesiologists must make a lifelong commitment to ongoing education and improvement.

Suggested Readings

Arnon RG, Steinfeld L: Medical management of the cyanotic patient with congenital heart disease, Cardiovasc Rev Rep 6:145–156, 1985.

Fischer LG, Van Aken H, Bürkle H: Management of pulmonary hypertension: physiological and pharmacological considerations for anesthesiologists, Anesth Analg 96:1603–1616, 2003.

Garson A Jr, Bricker JT, Fisher DJ, et al: The science and practice of pediatric cardiology, ed 2, Baltimore, 1998, Lippincott, Williams & Wilkins.

Gilboa SM, Salemi JL, Nembhard WN, et al: Mortality resulting from congenital heart disease among children and adults in the United States, 1999 to 2006, Circulation 122:2254–2263, 2010.

Graham TP Jr: Ventricular performance in congenital heart disease, Circulation 84:2259–2274, 1991.

Hickey PR, Hansen DD, Cramolini GM, et al: Pulmonary and systemic hemodynamic responses to ketamine in infants with normal and elevated pulmonary vascular resistance, Anesthesiology 62:287–293, 1985.

Hickey PR, Hansen DO, Wessel DL, et al: Blunting of stress responses in the pulmonary circulation of infants by fentanyl, Anesth Analg 64:1137–1142, 1985.

Hoffman JI, Kaplan S, Liberthson RR: Prevalence of congenital heart disease, Am Heart J 147(3):425–439, 2004.

Laird TH, Stayer SA, Rivenes SM, et al: Pulmonary-to-systemic blood flow ratio effects of sevoflurane, isoflurane, halothane, and fentanyl/midazolam with 100% oxygen in children with congenital heart disease, Anesth Analg 95:1200–1206, 2002.

Laishley RS, Burrows FA, Lerman J, et al: Effect of anesthetic induction regimens on oxygen saturation in cyanotic congenital heart disease, Anesthesiology 65:673–677, 1986.

Lake CL: Pediatric cardiac anesthesia, ed 3, Stamford, CT, 1997, Appleton & Lange.

Laussen PC, Wessel DL: Anesthesia for congenital heart disease. In Gregory GA, editor: Pediatric anesthesia, ed 4, New York, 2002, Churchill Livingstone, pp 467–539.

Marelli AJ, Ionescu-Ittu R, Mackie AS, et al: Lifetime prevalence of congenital heart disease in the general population from 2000–2010, Circulation 130(9):749–756, 2014.

Marelli AJ, Mackie AS, Ionescu-Ittu R, et al: Congenital heart disease in the general population: changing prevalence and age distribution, Circulation 115:163–172, 2007.

Morray JP, Lynn AM, Mansfield PB: Effect of pH and PCO_2 on pulmonary and systemic hemodynamics after surgery in children with congenital heart disease and pulmonary hypertension, J Pediatr 113:474–479, 1988.

Nudel D, Berman N, Talner N: Effects of acutely increasing systemic vascular resistance on oxygen tension in tetralogy of Fallot, Pediatrics 58:248–251, 1976.

Nussbaum J, Zane EA, Thys DM: Esmolol for the treatment of hypercyanotic spells in infants with tetralogy of Fallot, J Cardiovasc Anesth 3:200–202, 1989.

Rabinovitch M, Haworth SG, Castaneda AR, et al: Lung biopsy in congenital heart disease: a morphometric approach to pulmonary vascular disease, Circulation 58:1107–1122, 1978.

Rivenes SM, Lewin MB, Stayer SA, et al: Cardiovascular effects of sevoflurane, isoflurane, halothane, and fentanyl-midazolam in children with congenital heart disease, Anesth Analg 94:223–229, 2001.

Rudolph AM, Yuan S: Response of the pulmonary vasculature to hypoxia and H+ ion concentration changes, J Clin Invest 45:399–411, 1966.

Tabbutt S, Ramamoorthy C, Montenegro LM, et al: Impact of inspired gas mixtures on preoperative infants with hypoplastic left heart syndrome during controlled ventilation, Circulation 104(12 Suppl 1):159–164, 2001.

Williams W: Surgical outcomes in congenital heart disease: expectations and realities, Eur J Cardiothorac Surg 27:937–944, 2005.

Wilson W: Prevention of infective endocarditis: guidelines from the American Heart Association, Circulation 116(15):1736–1754, 2007.

Wood P: The Eisenmenger syndrome or pulmonary hypertension with reversed central shunt, Br Med J 46:701–709, 1958.

CHAPTER 55

FUNDAMENTALS OF OBSTETRIC ANESTHESIA

Ana M. Lobo, MD, MPH, and Mary DiMiceli, MD

1. **What are the cardiovascular adaptations to pregnancy?**
   Increased progesterone levels associated with pregnancy are presumed to increase the production of nitric oxide and prostacyclin. This, coupled with a decreased response to catecholamine and angiotension, results in an increase in peripheral vasodilation. The subsequent decrease in systemic vascular resistance (SVR) is demonstrated by decreased diastolic blood pressure. Furthermore, levels of relaxin, responsible for increased tissue elasticity, increase, which may lead to aortic dilation, especially in patients with connective tissue disorders. A parturient's plasma volume increases partly as a response to increased water and sodium retention from increased renin levels. Table 55-1 summarizes the major cardiovascular changes.

2. **When is the greatest increase in cardiac output (CO) experienced by parturients?**
   The most notable increase in CO (see Table 55-1) is achieved postpartum as a result of autotransfusion during uterine contractions. This physiologic change is one of the most important changes and can potentially be life threatening in patients with pulmonary hypertension and stenotic valvular lesions. Anatomically, the increase in blood volume results in hypertrophy as demonstrated by an enlarged cardiac silhouette on chest x-ray. Also, a new grade I–II systolic murmur can often be heard on physical exam. By the second half of pregnancy, the third heart sound can commonly be detected on auscultation, with a fourth heart sound heard in up to 16% of patients.

3. **What hematologic changes accompany pregnancy?**
   Table 55-2 summarizes the hematologic changes during pregnancy. Plasma volume increases from 40 to 70 ml/kg near term, and blood volume increases by 1000 to 1500 ml. Red cell mass increases slowly by 23% to 30%, which is offset by the increase in plasma volume resulting in a dilutional anemia. Maternal anemia occurs as a result of iron deficiency, particularly when the hemoglobin and hematocrit levels fall below 10 g and <30%, respectively. Parturients may also experience a noninfectious leukocytosis with a concomitant decrease in cell-mediated immunity, with possible increased risk of developing viral infections.

4. **What hematologic complications are parturients at increased risk for developing?**
   Pregnancy is associated with a hypercoagulable state as a result of increased activity of coagulation factors, particularly I, VII, VIII, IX, X, and XII with a concomitant decrease in activity of anticoagulant factors, such as protein S and acquired activated protein C resistance. Accordingly, parturients are at increased risk for thrombotic events (e.g., deep venous thrombosis and pulmonary embolism). This is counterbalanced by increased fibrinolysis as a consequence of decreased levels of factors XI and XIII, which normally act as antifibrinolytics. Also, there is increased platelet consumption, which is counterbalanced by increased platelet production. As a result, platelet count is usually normal, although thrombocytopenia can occur in 0.9% of normal patients. Thrombocytopenia in pregnancy can also occur in pathologic conditions, specifically with preeclampsia or with hemolysis, elevated liver enzymes, and low platelet count (HELLP) syndrome.

5. **What pulmonary and respiratory changes occur with pregnancy?**
   Parturients experience a cephalad displacement of the diaphragm in addition to an increase in the anteroposterior diameter of the chest wall during pregnancy. These anatomic changes

Table 55-1. Cardiovascular Changes During Pregnancy

Cardiac output	Increase 50% (plateaus by 28 weeks)
During labor	Additional 30%–40% increase
Immediately postpartum	75% increase above prelabor value
48 hours postpartum	At or below prelabor value
2 weeks postpartum	10% above prepregnant value (returns to normal by 12–24 weeks postpartum)
Stroke volume	Increase 25% (between 5 and 8 weeks)
Heart rate	Increase 25% (increases 15% by end of first trimester)
Mean arterial pressure	Decrease 15 mm Hg (normal by second trimester)
Systemic vascular resistance	Decreases 21%
Pulmonary vascular resistance	Decreases 34%
Central venous pressure	No change
Uterine blood flow	10% maternal cardiac output (600–700 ml/min at term)

Table 55-2. Hematologic Changes During Pregnancy

Plasma volume	Increase 45%–50% by term (15% by end of first trimester)
Red blood cell volume	Increase 55% during second trimester
Blood volume	Increase 45%
Hemoglobin	Decrease 15% by midgestation ($\approx$11.6 g/dl)
Platelet count	No change or decrease
PT and PTT	Decreased
Fibrinogen	Increased
Fibrinolysis	Increased
Factors I, VII, VIII, IX, X XII	Increased

PT, Prothrombin time; *PTT*, partial thromboplastin time.

contribute to the decrease in functional residual capacity (FRC) at term as a result of a decrease in expiratory reserve volume and residual volume (RV). This, coupled with increased oxygen consumption, places parturients at increased risk of rapid desaturation with apnea. With an eightfold increase in difficult/failed intubation compared with nonpregnant women, given the precipitous decrease in oxygen saturation with apnea, it is extremely important to ensure adequate and effective preoxygenation and proper ramp positioning prior to induction of general anesthesia (Figure 55-1). Minute ventilation significantly increases in pregnant women as a result of increase in respiratory rate and tidal volume. Oxygen delivery to tissues is enhanced and facilitated by the concomitant increase in CO, 2,3-DPG levels, and P-50 from 27 to 30 mm Hg. Furthermore, there is a decrease in the amount of physiologic shunt and so PaO_2 levels slightly increase (Table 55-3).

Extravascular spaces, including the respiratory tract, become more edematous with significant capillary engorgement secondary to increased intravascular volume. The mucosa becomes very friable and very prone to bleeding with manipulation or trauma. Accordingly, nasal intubations or other manipulation should never be attempted unless in extremely emergent situations.

6. What is a normal arterial blood gas in a pregnant patient?
   Given the rise in minute ventilation, pregnant women develop a respiratory alkalosis (Table 55-4). Hyperventilation during active labor further contributes to the preexisting metabolic

Table 55-3. Respiratory Changes at Term in Pregnancy

Minute ventilation	50% increase (can go up to 140% of prepregnancy values in the first stage of unmedicated labor and up to 200% in the second stage)
Alveolar ventilation	70% increase
Tidal volume	40% increase
Oxygen consumption	20% increase
Respiratory rate	15% increase
Dead space	No change
Lung compliance	No change
Residual volume	29% decrease
Vital capacity	No change
Total lung capacity	5% decrease
Functional residual capacity	15%–20% decrease
FEV_1	No change

FEV_1, Forced expiratory volume in 1 second.

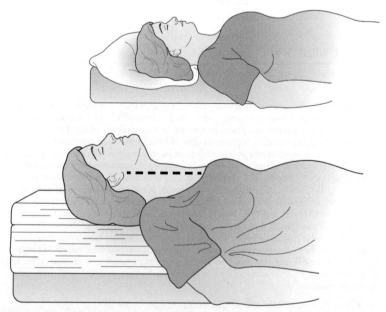

Figure 55-1. Ramp positioning is achieved by alignment of the patients' auditory canal with the sterna notch by placement of multiple folded towels or large foam ramp pillows. *(Illustration by M. DiMiceli, MD.)*

Table 55-4. Normal Arterial Blood Gas Values in Pregnant and Nonpregnant Women

	PH	PAO₂	PACO₂	HCO₃
Pregnant	7.41–7.44	85–109 mm Hg	27–33 mm Hg	21–27 mmol/L
Nonpregnant	7.35–7.45	60–100 mm Hg	35–45 mm Hg	24 mmol/L

disturbance and is the second most important physiologic change during labor as it can result in uterine vasoconstriction and decreased placental perfusion, hypoxemia, and fetal distress.

7. **What gastrointestinal changes occur during pregnancy?**
   The expanding uterus not only displaces the stomach upward, resulting in incompetence of the lower gastroesophageal sphincter (GES) but also increases intragastric pressure. Increased progesterone levels also decrease the tone of the lower GES. These changes place parturients at higher risk for reflux, regurgitation, and possible aspiration, with the risk being almost equal during induction and emergence. Some patients, particularly when in labor or secondary to parenteral opioid use, may experience prolonged gastric emptying time. All pregnant patients are considered to have a full stomach and are managed accordingly.

8. **What renal changes are associated with pregnancy?**
   Renal plasma flow, glomerular filtration rate (GFR), and creatinine clearance increase by the fourth month of gestation. Blood urea nitrogen (BUN) and creatinine are decreased; normal values in pregnancy are 6 to 9 and 0.4 to 0.6 mg/dl, respectively. Glucosuria up to 10 g/dl and proteinuria up to 300 mg/dl are not abnormal. With increased vasodilation seen in pregnancy, in addition to dilation of the renal calyces, pelves, and ureters, renal plasma flow and GFR and creatinine clearance all increase. Autoregulation is, however, preserved. Urinary stasis contributes to the frequency of urinary tract infections seen in pregnancy.

9. **What changes occur in the central nervous system of pregnant patients?**
   Progesterone in both the plasma and cerebrospinal fluid increases tenfold to twentyfold in late pregnancy. Progesterone is sedating and potentiates the effects of volatile anesthetics. Pregnant patients are also more sensitive to local anesthetics and clinically may need dose reductions by as much as 30%. Minimal alveolar concentration has been demonstrated to decrease with pregnancy by 28% in women undergoing termination of pregnancy at 8 to 12 weeks compared with nonpregnant women. An enlarging uterus compresses the inferior vena cava (IVC), with the secondary effect of causing distention of the epidural venous plexus and an increase in epidural blood volume. This must be taken into consideration when providing neuraxial analgesia as there is subsequent smaller potential epidural space with a higher pressure and accordingly increased risk for dural puncture or intravascular catheter placement.

10. **What hepatic alterations occur with pregnancy?**
    Liver size, blood flow, and liver morphology do not change during pregnancy. Lactate dehydrogenase, serum bilirubin, alanine aminotransferase, aspartate aminotransferase, and alkaline phosphatase (of placental origin) increase with pregnancy. Elevated progesterone levels inhibit release of cholecystokinin, thus resulting in incomplete emptying of the gallbladder. When coupled with altered bile acid formation, pregnant women are at increased risk of gallstone formation. Due to elevated plasma volume, total protein, plasma albumin concentration, and oncotic pressure (by about 5 mm Hg) decrease during pregnancy. As a result, free fractions of protein-bound drugs increase with decreasing albumin levels. Plasma cholinesterase concentrations decrease by about 25% before delivery and 33% by day 3 after delivery but are probably not clinically significant.

11. **What is the uterine blood flow at term?**
    Uterine blood flow is approximately 50 to 190 ml/min before pregnancy and reaches approximately 10% of maternal CO (600 to 700 ml/min) at term. Accordingly, the

pregnant patient at risk of or with uterine rupture, uterine atony, placenta previa, or placental abruption has a significantly high risk for peripartum hemorrhage.

12. **How quickly do the physiologic alterations of pregnancy return to normal after delivery?**
    - **Cardiovascular:** CO returns to slightly above prepregnancy values at about 2 to 4 weeks after delivery.
    - **Respiratory:** FRC and RV rapidly return to normal. Alveolar ventilation returns to baseline by 4 weeks after delivery with a gradual rise in maternal PCO_2.
    - **Hematologic:** Dilutional anemia and hematocrit values return to normal within 4 weeks secondary to postpartum diuresis.
    - **Renal:** Serum creatinine, GFR, and BUN return to normal levels in less than 3 weeks.
    - **Gastrointestinal:** The mechanical effects of the gravid uterus on the gastrointestinal system resolve at about 2 to 3 days after delivery.

13. **What are the three stages of labor?**
    - **Stage 1.** Cervical dilation and effacement begin with the onset of regular, painful contractions and end when dilation of the cervix is complete (or 10 cm). The latent phase is characterized by slow cervical dilation and effacement. The active phase is defined as the period of progressive cervical dilation, which usually begins around 4 to 5 cm.
    - **Stage 2.** The second stage ends with delivery of the neonate.
    - **Stage 3.** The third stage ends with delivery of the placenta.

14. **What structures does labor pain derive from? What levels of the spinal cord are involved in transmitting labor pain during stages 1 and 2?**
    Pain during the first stage of labor is caused by uterine contractions and cervical dilation as transmitted by the sympathetic fibers entering the dorsal horn of the spinal cord at T10–L1. As labor progresses and the fetal head descends into the pelvis during stage 2, pain is transmitted from the pelvic floor, lower vagina, and perineum via the pudendal nerve, entering the spinal cord at S2–S4.

15. **What is aortocaval compression syndrome? How is it treated?**
    The IVC and aorta can become compressed by the gravid uterus, resulting in hypotension and tachycardia; this is known as *aortocaval compression syndrome*. Decreases in uterine and placental blood flow may ensue secondary to aortic compression, which may manifest as nonreassuring fetal heart rate (FHR) changes. Accordingly, uterine displacement (lateral position or a wedge under the right hip) is a helpful maneuver used to prevent aortocaval compression and to increase venous return. Symptomatic patients should be placed in left uterine displacement (LUD) position and may be treated with intravenous fluid administration, supplemental oxygen, and sometimes use of a vasopressor.

16. **Describe the anatomy of the placenta and umbilical cord.**
    The maternal side of the placenta is made up of a basal plate. Within the basal plate are spiral arteries, which are divisions from the uterine arteries, and veins. The fetal side is the chorionic plate, made up of villi surrounded by chorion. The space where these two surfaces meet is the intervillous space. The villi contain divisions from two umbilical arteries, which carry blood to the placenta, and divisions from the single umbilical vein, which carries the nutrient-rich blood back to the fetal circulation.

17. **What factors influence uteroplacental perfusion?**
    Aortocaval compression by the gravid uterus can decrease uteroplacental perfusion. Uterine blood flow may also decrease with maternal hypotension, a fall of >25 mm Hg in maternal mean arterial pressure. Additionally, uterine contractions, conditions such as preeclampsia and placental abruption, and administration of some medications, such as ketamine and oxytocin, can all result in significant increases in uterine vascular resistance, which can decrease uterine blood flow. Finally, increased maternal levels of catecholamines (e.g., during labor), maternal hypoxia, hypercarbia, and hypocarbia have all been associated with decreased uteroplacental perfusion.

18. **How should hypotension associated with spinal anesthesia be treated in a cesarean section or laboring patient?**

    Historically treatment of hypotension under spinal anesthesia was guided by the goal to maintain uteroplacental blood flow. Accordingly, ephedrine was the preferred vasopressor of choice because other agents decreased uteroplacental blood flow, but ephedrine did not. However, more recent studies suggest that large doses of ephedrine may be detrimental to the fetus (dose-dependent fetal metabolic acidosis, tachycardia, and abnormal FHR variability), whereas infusions or large doses of phenylephrine did not result in depression of fetal pH. Although α-adrenergic agonism with phenylephrine produces peripheral vasoconstriction, with uterine vascular resistance greater than SVR, it has not clinically been shown to decrease uteroplacental blood flow. Problems observed with ephedrine are likely related to the direct β-agonist activity on fetal metabolism and is less likely secondary to decreased uteroplacental perfusion. However, it is important to note that all of these studies were done in healthy parturients at term undergoing cesarean section. It is reasonable to infer that ephedrine would cause similar metabolic derangements in laboring patients and those with high-risk pregnancies. The routine use of prophylactic ephedrine to prevent any adverse effects of maternal hypotension following spinal anesthesia for cesarean section is also not supported by systematic reviews of the literature.

19. **What is the role of intravenous fluid preloading before regional anesthesia for cesarean delivery?**

    Intravenous fluid preloading before regional anesthesia as a means to prevent hypotension remains controversial. Many studies have been conducted that compare outcomes after crystalloid versus colloid administration as well as comparing outcomes between preload versus co-load timing of administration. Preload or co-load intravenous fluid may prevent hypotension associated with neuraxial analgesia for cesarean delivery; however, to date, no study has definitive conclusive results.

20. **How are drugs and other substances transported across the placenta? What drugs cross the placenta?**

    Placental transfer is accomplished by simple diffusion, active transport, bulk flow, facilitated diffusion, and breaks in the chorionic membrane. Anesthetic compounds cross the placenta mostly by simple diffusion. Compounds that are low in molecular weight, small in spatial configuration, poorly ionized, and lipid soluble have high rates of placental transfer. Most anesthetic drugs are highly lipid soluble and have molecular weights <600, and for this reason their rates of placental transfer are high. Some drugs known to cross the placenta include atropine, scopolamine, β-adrenergic antagonists, nitroglycerin, diazepam, propofol, isoflurane, nitrous oxide, local anesthetics, opioids, neostigmine, and ephedrine. Important to note is that poorly ionized substances cross the placenta more easily than do ionized substances, and a change in pH can change the degree of ionization of the molecule. Accordingly, in the presence of fetal acidosis, poorly ionized local anesthetics delivered via neuraxial technique can cross the placenta and result in ion trapping whereby the molecule becomes highly ionized and remains in the fetal circulation.

21. **What methods are used to evaluate fetal well-being during labor?**

    FHR values and trends are recorded routinely, particularly in conjunction with recordings of uterine activity, either with an external or internal monitor. The baseline (FHR) is measured between contractions and is normally 110 to 160 beats/min. Fetal tachycardia (>160) may indicate fever, hypoxia, use of β-sympathomimetic agents, maternal hyperthyroidism, or fetal hypovolemia. Fetal bradycardia (<110) may be caused by hypoxia, complete heart block, β blockers, local anesthetics, or hypothermia. The beat-to-beat variability is thought to represent an intact neurologic pathway in the fetus. Increased variability is seen with uterine contractions and maternal activity. Decreased variability can be seen with central nervous system depression, hypoxia, acidosis, sleep, narcotic use, vagal blockade, and magnesium therapy for preeclampsia. Absence of beat-to-beat variability, especially in the presence of FHR decelerations or bradycardia, is a particular concern for fetal acidosis (Table 55-5).

Table 55-5. Fetal Heart Rate Pattern Classification

CATEGORY	CHARACTERISTICS
1–Normal	Baseline rate 110–160 bpm Moderate baseline variability Late or variable decelerations: absent Early decelerations: present/absent

2–Indeterminate	All tracings not categorized as 1 or 3, which include examples such as:
	  Baseline variability: minimal or marked
	  Absent variability WITHOUT recurrent decelerations
	  Prolonged deceleration
	  Absence of induced accelerations after fetal stimulation

3–Abnormal	Baseline variability: absent AND recurrent late or variable decelerations Bradycardia

Adapted from Macones GA, Hankins GD, Spong CY, et al: The 2008 National Institute of Child Health and Human Development workshop report on electronic fetal monitoring: update on definitions, interpretation and research guidelines. Obstet Gynecol 112:661–666, 2008.

22. **What is the significance of fetal heart rate decelerations?**
    - Early decelerations: Caused by head compressions (vagal stimulation). Typically, they are uniform in shape, begin near the onset of a uterine contraction with its nadir at the same time as the peak of the contraction, and are benign (Figure 55-2).
    - Variable decelerations: Caused by umbilical cord compression. They are nonuniform in shape and are abrupt in onset and duration (lasting longer than 15 seconds but less than 2 minutes). Although they usually do not reflect fetal acidosis, repetitive variable decelerations can lead to fetal hypoxia and acidosis.
    - Late decelerations: Caused by uteroplacental insufficiency. They are uniform in shape, with a gradual onset (just after onset of contraction) and return to baseline, with their nadir and recovery after the peak and recovery of the contraction. These are associated with maternal hypotension, hypertension, diabetes, preeclampsia, or intrauterine growth retardation, and are an ominous indicator that the fetus is unable to maintain normal oxygenation and pH in the face of decreased blood flow.
      The treatment for nonreassuring neonatal heart rate changes involves administering oxygen to the mother, maintaining maternal blood pressure, and placing the parturient in the left uterine displacement position.

23. **What is the Apgar score?**
    Dr. Virginia Apgar, an anesthesiologist and first female full professor at Columbia University College of Physicians and Surgeons, developed a simple and repeatable method to assess newborn well-being 1 and 5 minutes after birth. It is the most widely accepted and used system to evaluate neonates, determine which neonates need resuscitation, and measure the success of resuscitation (Table 55-6). The score is comprised of separate scores (from 0 to 2) assigned to variables including heart rate, respiratory effort, muscle tone, reflex irritability, and color to provide a total score of 10. The Apgar score can be measured again at 10 and 20 minutes as resuscitative efforts are continued. A score of 0 to 3 indicates a severely depressed neonate, whereas a score of 7 to 10 is considered normal.

24. **Describe the management of the pregnant patient undergoing nonobstetric surgery.**
    Organogenesis occurs as early as the fifth week of gestation; since this is the most crucial time for fetal development, it is best to avoid all nonemergent surgery during this time. The safest period is during the second trimester for this reason and since preterm contractions and spontaneous abortions are least likely. The most common surgical conditions include appendicitis, cholecystitis, pancreatitis, bowel obstruction, ovarian torsion, ovarian cyst rupture, or hemorrhage and trauma. In emergent situations, surgery is obviously unavoidable and the primary goal is maternal safety.

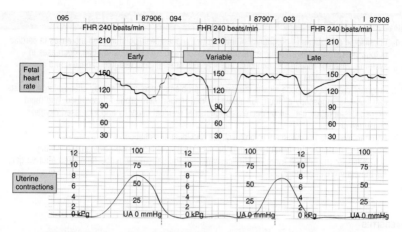

Figure 55-2. Early, variable, and late fetal heart rate (FHR) deceleration during labor.

Table 55-6. Apgar Score

SCORE	HEART RATE	RESPIRATORY EFFORT	MUSCLE TONE	REFLEX IRRITABILITY	COLOR
0	Absent	Apneic	Flaccid	No response	Pale or blue
1	<100	Irregular, shallow, or weak cry	Some flexion of extremities	Grimace or weak cry	Acrocyanosis
2	>100	Good and crying	Active motion	Sneeze, cough, or cry	Pink

There is no evidence that any drug or technique is preferred over another as long as maternal oxygenation and perfusion are maintained. Furthermore, there is no evidence that any anesthetic agent currently in use is associated with teratogenic effects, particularly at standard recommended doses. However, nitrous oxide has been associated with deoxyribonucleic acid synthesis inhibition and probably should be avoided in the first trimester. Although type of anesthesia does not affect outcome, it is recommended to provide regional anesthesia whenever possible. If surgery is performed, particularly when the fetus is deemed viable (24 weeks), fetal monitors are placed to assess fetal well-being intraoperatively to assist in deciding whether delivery is most prudent or necessary, but FHR should be assessed both preoperatively and postoperatively. Obstetric personnel and pediatricians should be involved and informed.

If general anesthesia is chosen, the patient should receive aspiration prophylaxis with ranitidine, sodium citrate, or metoclopramide, before rapid-sequence intubation with cricoid pressure. (Use of cricoid pressure can be controversial and has its limitations.) It is very important to maintain maternal and uteroplacental perfusion and hemodynamics, and as such the patient should be kept in left uterine displacement to avoid aortocaval compression. Hypotension must be treated with an appropriate vasopressor and intravenous fluids; maternal hypoxemia must be avoided in order to prevent fetal hypoxia and metabolic acidosis and ensure fetal well-being.

It is important to keep in mind the parturient's altered responsiveness to local anesthetics if regional anesthesia is provided, as well as the possibility that the onset of labor may be masked by the administration of opioids. Postoperatively, the patient should be monitored for early onset of labor and, if necessary, tocolysis initiated if it occurs.

KEY POINTS: FUNDAMENTALS OF OBSTETRIC ANESTHESIA

1. Physiologic alterations in pregnancy of interest to the anesthesiologist include increases in cardiac output, heart rate, plasma volume, minute ventilation, and oxygen consumption; decreases in systemic vascular resistance; dilutional anemia; loss of functional residual capacity; and a hypercoagulable state.
2. Pregnant patients can pose airway management problems because of airway edema, large breasts that make laryngoscopy difficult, full stomachs that render them prone to aspiration, and rapid oxygen desaturation caused by decreased functional residual capacity and increased oxygen consumption.
3. Pregnant patients are sensitive to both volatile and local anesthetics.
4. Nonemergent surgical procedures should be avoided if possible during pregnancy or ideally scheduled for the second trimester if necessary, and the patient should be monitored after surgery for the early onset of labor.

WEBSITES

American Congress of Obstetricians and Gynecologists: http://www.acog.org
American Society of Anesthesiologists: http://www.asahq.org
Society for Obstetric Anesthesia and Perinatology: http://www.soap.org

SUGGESTED READINGS

American College of Obstetricians and Gynecologists: Obstetric analgesia and anesthesia. ACOG Practice Bulletin No. 36, 2002.
American Society of Anesthesiologists Task Force on Obstetric Anesthesia: Practice guidelines for obstetric anesthesia: an updated report by the American Society of Anesthesiologists Task Force on Obstetric Anesthesia. www.asahq.org (last amended on October 20, 2010).
Cooper DW, Carpenter M, Mowbray P, et al: Fetal and maternal effects of phenylephrine and ephedrine during spinal anesthesia for cesarean delivery, Anesthesiology 97:1582–1590, 2002.
Cyna AM, Andrew M, Emmett RS, et al: Techniques for preventing hypotension during spinal anesthesia for caesarean section, Cochrane Database Syst Rev (4):CD002251, 2006.
Gaiser R: Physiologic changes in pregnancy. In Chestnut DH, editor: Obstetric anesthesia: principles and practice, ed 4, Philadelphia, 2009, Mosby.
Lee A, Ngan Kee WD, Gin T: Prophylactic ephedrine prevents hypotension during spinal anesthesia for cesarean delivery but does not improve neonatal outcome: a quantitative systematic review, Can J Anaesth 49:588–599, 2002.
Macones GA, Hankins GD, Spong CY, et al: The 2008 National Institute of Child Health and Human Development Workshop report on electronic fetal monitoring: update on definitions, interpretation and research guidelines, Obstet Gynecol 112:661–666, 2008.
Ngan Kee WD: Uteroplacental blood flow. In Chestnut DH, editor: Obstetric anesthesia: principles and practice, ed 4, Philadelphia, 2009, Mosby.
Ngan Kee WD, Khaw KS, Ng FF: Comparison of phenylephrine infusion regimens for maintaining maternal blood pressure during spinal anesthesia for caesarean section, Br J Anaesth 92:469–474, 2004.

OBSTETRIC ANALGESIA AND ANESTHESIA

Ana M. Lobo, MD, MPH, and Mary DiMiceli, MD

CHAPTER 56

1. **What modes of analgesia are available to the parturient?**
   Parenteral opioids, inhaled nitrous oxide, epidural, spinal, and combined spinal-epidural are all acceptable modes of analgesia depending on the patient's comorbidities, time of presentation, clinical condition, and personal preference.

2. **What are the most commonly used parenteral opioids for labor analgesia? Which side effects are of special concern to the parturient?**
   While intravenous medications may decrease the intensity of labor pain and make it more tolerable they do not provide complete analgesia and may cause maternal sedation and nausea. Parenteral opioids easily cross the placenta and may cause a decrease in fetal heart rate variability. If opioids are administered in close proximity to newborn delivery, neonatal respiratory depression may occur. Table 56-1 summarizes commonly used parenteral opioids and their side effects. Notably, the newer piperidine derivative, remifentanil, is gaining popularity and has demonstrated significant efficacy.

3. **What advantages does patient-controlled analgesia (PCA) offer over conventional intermittent bolus dosing?**
   PCA has been associated with greater patient satisfaction, less risk of maternal respiratory depression, less need for antiemetic use, and better pain relief despite lower drug doses. PCA is an intravenous form of opioid delivery and is especially useful if epidural anesthesia is contraindicated or not available. The most experience has been gained with meperidine and fentanyl using the regimens noted in Table 56-1. A trial comparing the PCA efficacy of remifentanil and meperidine demonstrated more effective and reliable analgesia as well as improved patient satisfaction scores with remifentanil.

4. **Discuss the benefits of epidural analgesia for labor and delivery.**
   Uterine contractions and labor pain have the effect of increasing catecholamine levels and increasing autonomic activity. High levels of catecholamines such as epinephrine and norepinephrine may prolong labor by decreasing uterine contractility through their β-agonist activity. Increased catecholamine levels may result in decreased placental perfusion and fetal acidosis. Respiratory alkalosis, an effect of hyperventilation, may shift the oxyhemoglobin dissociation curve to the left, decreasing delivery of oxygen to the fetus and creating fetal acidosis. Epidural analgesia provides the most effective pain relief in most laboring women and effectively reduces maternal catecholamine levels, potentially improving uteroplacental perfusion. Finally, epidural analgesia may be converted to epidural anesthesia if cesarean section is indicated, thus avoiding the need for general endotracheal anesthesia.

5. **What are the indications and contraindications for epidural analgesia during labor and delivery?**
   Patient request is an indication and *analgesia* can be readily converted to *anesthesia* by increasing local anesthetic concentration. Labor analgesia is beneficial in patients with hypertension. Some cardiac disease (e.g., mitral stenosis) improves unwanted hemodynamic effects (increased preload, tachycardia, increased systemic vascular resistance, hypertension, and hyperventilation).
   Absolute contraindications to epidural anesthesia include:
   - Patient refusal
   - Coagulopathy
   - Uncontrolled hemorrhage

Table 56-1. Intravenous Analgesics for Labor

DRUG	USUAL DOSE	ONSET	DURATION	PCA DOSING
Meperidine	25–50 mg IV	5–10 minutes	2–3 hours	10–15 mg q5–10min
Comments: Normeperidine is an active metabolite that may last for 3 days; neonatal effects are most likely if delivery occurs 1–4 hours after administration. Half-life of meperidine in the neonate is 18–23 hours and of normeperidine is 60 hours.				
Fentanyl	1–2 mcg/kg IV (1 mcg/kg IM)	3–4 minutes	45 minutes	10–25 mcg q5–12min
Comments: Short acting, no active metabolites, potent respiratory depressant for mother, minimal sedation and nausea. Context-sensitive half-life increases with infusion duration.				
Remifentanil	0.4–0.5 mcg/kg IV	1 minute	5–10 minutes	0.25–0.5 mcg/kg q2–3min
Comments: Short acting, quick onset, and constant short context-sensitive half-life (3–4 min), rapid degradation to inactive metabolites.				
Butorphanol	1–2 mg IV	5 minutes	2–3 hours	N/A
Comments: Sedating for mother, ceiling effect for both analgesia and respiratory depression, dysphoric reactions or withdrawal symptoms in opioid-dependent patients can occur.				
Nalbuphine	10 mg IV	5 minutes	2–3 hours	N/A
Comments: Similar profile as butorphanol.				

IM, Intramuscular; *IV,* intravenous; *N/A,* not applicable; *PCA,* patient-controlled analgesia.

- Elevated intracranial pressure (ICP)
- Severe stenotic valvular disease
- True allergy to local anesthetics
- Infection at the site of needle introduction
    Relative contraindications include:
- Maternal bacteremia
- Prior spinal instrumentation with hardware
- Certain neurologic diseases

6. **Discuss the importance of a test dose and suggest an epidural test dose regimen. When and why is this regimen used?**
The test dose is performed to diagnose subarachnoid or intravenous placement of the epidural catheter, thereby preventing total spinal anesthesia or systemic toxicity from local anesthetics.
    A common test dose is 3 ml of 1.5% lidocaine (45 mg) with 1:200,000 epinephrine (15 mcg). If the test dose of local anesthetic is administered intrathecally, motor and sensory block will appear within 3 to 5 minutes. If the test dose is injected intravenously, tachycardia results within 45 seconds because of the epinephrine additive. If there is any doubt in the practitioner's mind about the exact location of the epidural catheter, the catheter should be removed and replaced.

7. **What are the characteristics of the ideal local anesthetic for use in labor? How does epinephrine affect the action of local anesthetics?**
The ideal local anesthetic for labor would have rapid onset of action, minimal risk of toxicity, minimal motor blockade with effective sensory blockade, and a minor effect on uterine activity and placental perfusion. Bupivacaine and ropivacaine are most commonly used for obstetric epidural analgesia. Lidocaine and chloroprocaine are most commonly used for obstetric surgical anesthesia. Addition of epinephrine (1:200,000) speeds the onset and prolongs the duration of action by decreasing vascular absorption of local anesthetic, but it

Table 56-2. Common Local Anesthetics Used for Obstetric Anesthesia and Analgesia

DRUG	CLASS	ADVANTAGES	DISADVANTAGES
Bupivacaine (0.125–0.5%)	Amide	Limited placental transfer (highly protein bound) Intermediate onset of action (15–20 min to peak effect) Analgesia lasts ≈2 hours	Intermediate motor blockade Cardiovascular toxicity (slower dissociation channels)
Ropivacaine (0.1–0.2%)	Amide	Onset, duration, and sensory block similar to bupivacaine Less motor block Less cardiotoxic	Less potent than bupivacaine More expensive
Lidocaine (0.75–1.5%)	Amide	Quick onset (10 min)	Crosses placenta readily Greater motor blockade Short duration of analgesia (45–90 min)
2-Chloroprocaine (35)	Ester	Rapid onset (6–12 min) Short half-life because rapid metabolism may make it PABA–allergic reaction safer	Rapid onset (6–12 min) Short half-life because rapid

PABA, p-aminobenzoic acid.

also increases the intensity of sensory and motor blockade (not desirable in laboring patients). The addition of epinephrine to a local anesthetic does not appear to affect uterine blood flow adversely, and it decreases the risk of maternal toxicity.

8. **Discuss local anesthetics used for obstetric purposes. Discuss the four most common local anesthetics used in obstetric anesthesia. Describe their advantages and disadvantages.**
   See Table 56-2.

9. **Discuss the complications of epidural anesthesia and their treatments.**
   The most common complication of epidural analgesia/anesthesia is hypotension, defined as a decrease in systolic pressure of 20% to 30% from baseline. This may result in decreased uteroplacental perfusion and fetal hypoxia and acidosis, and so avoidance is paramount to decrease risk of fetal distress. Hypotension results from sympathetic blockade, peripheral venodilation, and decreased venous return to the heart. Also, remember supine hypotension syndrome occurs in ≈10% parturients, but it occurs more frequently after sympathectomy from neuraxial blockade. Therefore, treatment includes volume expansion and placement of the mother in the full lateral position. Phenylephrine (50–100 mcg) or ephedrine (5–10 mg intravenously) should be administered if blood pressure does not promptly return to normal.

   Inadequate analgesia is also very common, occurring in approximately 1 of 8 women. Inadequate analgesia requiring replacement occurs in roughly 5% to 13% of parturients. Other common complications or known side effects include pruritus, nausea/vomiting, and shivering, all of which require supportive care and/or treatment with other medications, such as nalbuphine or butorphanol, ondansetron, and meperidine, respectively.

   The incidence of unintentional dural puncture is quoted anywhere from 0.19% to 3.6%. If cerebrospinal fluid is noted, the needle may be removed and the epidural catheter placed at an alternate interspace or a catheter may be left in the subarachnoid space. Placing an epidural catheter at a different interspace does have the potential risk for local anesthetic that is subsequently injected to pass into the subarachnoid space by the puncture hole previously created, possibly resulting in a block that is unexpectedly high or dense. Leaving the spinal catheter in place for 24 hours may decrease the incidence of headache; however, there are no definitive data to support this.

Intravenous local anesthetic injection may produce dizziness, restlessness, tinnitus, seizures, and loss of consciousness. Cardiovascular collapse may follow central nervous system symptoms. Bupivacaine cardiovascular toxicity secondary to large intravenous doses is especially severe and may be fatal. To treat local anesthetic toxicity:

- Give the patient 100% oxygen and intubate if necessary (to oxygenate, hyperventilate, and protect the airway).
- Stop convulsions with a barbiturate or a benzodiazepine.
- Support blood pressure (intravenous fluids and pressors).
- Use cardiopulmonary resuscitation and advanced cardiac life support protocols as necessary.
- Consider administration of intralipid to act as a lipid "sink" to bind the local anesthetic and remove it from the maternal circulation.
- Treat bradycardia with atropine.
- Treat ventricular tachycardia with amiodarone.
- Treat ventricular fibrillation with vasopressin, epinephrine, and defibrillation.
- Deliver the fetus if an effective rhythm is not restored within 5 minutes so more effective cardiopulmonary resuscitation can be provided to the mother.

The incidence of an unexpected high block or total spinal block is approximately 1 in 4500 lumbar epidurals during labor. Risk is minimized by aspirating the catheter and giving a test dose each time local anesthetic is administered via the catheter. The signs and symptoms of a total spinal block include hypotension, dyspnea, inability to speak, and loss of consciousness. Treatment includes intubation, oxygen administration, ventilation, and support of maternal circulation with vasoactive medications.

10. **Explain the mechanism of action of intrathecal and epidural opioids. What effect do they have on pain perception, sympathetic tone, sensation, and movement?**
Opioids administered intrathecally or epidurally provide excellent analgesia without appreciably affecting sympathetic tone, sensation, or voluntary motor function. Opioids given via these routes bind to presynaptic and postsynaptic receptor sites in the dorsal horn of the spinal cord (Rexed laminae I, II, and V), altering nociceptive transmission. Some of the effects of lipid-soluble opioids may be caused by their systemic absorption.

11. **What opioids are used to provide spinal and epidural analgesia during labor? Name their most common side effects. Do they provide adequate analgesia for labor and delivery when used alone?**
The most commonly used neuraxial (spinal and epidural) opioids are fentanyl (12.5–25 mcg), sufentanil (5 mcg), and morphine (0.1–0.25 mg). Pruritus, nausea, and vomiting are the most common side effects; delayed respiratory depression is the most serious complication, although it is very uncommon in this population. Intrathecal or epidural opioids alone may provide adequate relief for the early stages of labor, but they are unreliable in producing adequate analgesia for the active phase of labor. Very high doses of epidural opioids are required, which leads to excessive side effects. Concurrent administration of local anesthetic is necessary for late cervical dilation and delivery of the infant. Meperidine (10 mg) may also provide effective analgesia and strengthens neuraxial blockade when administered intrathecally secondary to κ-opioid agonism and local anesthetic properties. Finally (although not a narcotic) clonidine, a central α_2 agonist, can be used as an intrathecal and epidural analgesic/anesthetic adjunct. It has also been shown to extend the duration of analgesia and strengthen the degree of sensory and motor blockade.

12. **Does epidural analgesia cause prolongation of labor or result in operative delivery?**
No. This issue *was* highly controversial. It has been reported that epidural analgesia is *associated* with prolonged labor and increased operative delivery, but recent studies do not support this assertion. The association is likely because anesthesiologists and obstetricians

Table 56-3. Drugs Used for Spinal Anesthesia for Cesarean Section

DRUG	DOSE	DURATION (MINUTES)
Lidocaine	75 mg	45–75
Bupivacaine	11 mg	60–120
Tetracaine	7–10 mg	90–120
Adjuvant Drugs Epinephrine	200 mcg	
Morphine	0.1–0.3 mg	
Fentanyl	10–25 mcg	

may be more likely to strongly recommend that the patient receive neuraxial analgesia if she is more at risk for operative delivery (i.e., morbidly obese, significant labor pain in early first stage of labor). Although epidural labor analgesia may prolong the second stage by about 30 minutes, there appears to be no harm to mother or fetus, and the American College of Obstetricians and Gynecologists (ACOG) recommends allowing an extra hour of pushing for mothers with an epidural block in place. ACOG has stated: "Neuraxial analgesia techniques are the most effective and least depressant treatments for labor pain ... more recent studies have shown that epidural analgesia does not increase the risks of cesarean delivery." As a matter of fact, one study compared cesarean section rates before and after institution of regional anesthesia as the primary mode of anesthesia delivery and found no change in the incidence of cesarean deliveries.

13. **Relate the advantages and disadvantages of spinal anesthesia for cesarean section. Which drugs are frequently used in the technique?**
    Spinal anesthesia produces a dense neural blockade, is relatively easy to perform, has a rapid onset, and carries no risk of local anesthetic toxicity. The development of small-gauge, noncutting needles has significantly reduced the incidence of post–dural puncture headache (PDPH) to 1% or less. Hypotension can be very significant and can occur relatively rapidly, requiring rapid intravenous fluid administration, repositioning to avoid aortocaval compression, and use of phenylephrine (50–100 mcg) or ephedrine (5–10 mg IV). Commonly used drugs are summarized in Table 56-3.

14. **What are the advantages and disadvantages of cesarean section with epidural anesthesia versus spinal anesthesia?**
    If epidural analgesia is used for pain relief during labor and delivery, higher concentrations of local anesthetics can provide surgical anesthesia. The local anesthetic should be given in increments, titrating to the desired sensory level. Titration of local anesthetic results in more controlled sympathetic blockade; thus the risk of hypotension and reduced uteroplacental flow may be decreased. Typically epidural anesthesia produces less intense motor and sensory blockade than spinal anesthesia.
    Disadvantages of epidural anesthesia include slower onset, larger local anesthetic dose requirement, occasional patchy block unsuitable for surgery and the risk of total spinal anesthesia or systemic toxicity if the epidural catheter migrates subarachnoid or intravascular. Unintentional dural puncture may occur, and 50% to 85% of such patients experience headache.

15. **How is combined spinal-epidural anesthesia performed? What are its advantages?**
    Combined spinal-epidural anesthesia may be performed either by a needle-through-needle approach or by performing both procedures separately. The needle-through-needle approach involves identification of the epidural space by loss-of-resistance technique with a Tuohy needle, followed by insertion of a long (120-mm), small-gauge (24- to 27-G), noncutting spinal needle until the dura is punctured and clear cerebrospinal fluid is noted.

Subsequently, a spinal dose of local anesthetic (plus narcotic, if desired) is injected into the subarachnoid space, and the spinal needle is removed. Finally, an epidural catheter is threaded into the epidural space. The advantage to a combined spinal-epidural technique is rapid and reliable anesthesia with administration of spinal anesthesia in addition to using the epidural catheter for maintenance of anesthesia, being able to extend duration of anesthesia, and use for postoperative analgesia.

16. List the indications for general anesthesia for cesarean section.
    • Extreme fetal distress (in the absence of a functioning epidural catheter)
    • Significant coagulopathy
    • Inadequate regional anesthesia
    • Acute maternal hypovolemia/hemorrhage
    • Patient refusal of regional anesthesia

17. What concerns the practitioner when administering general anesthesia for cesarean section? How is it performed?
The obstetric population is at greater risk for difficult intubation, rapid oxygen desaturation, and aspiration of gastric contents. The goal is to minimize maternal risk and neonatal depression. This goal is accomplished by following certain guidelines. After monitors are placed, while the patient is being preoxygenated, the abdomen is prepared and draped. When the obstetricians are scrubbed in and ready to make their skin incision, rapid-sequence induction with cricoid pressure is performed, and incision occurs after correct placement of the endotracheal tube is verified. Frequently used induction agents include thiopental, ketamine, propofol, or etomidate. Succinylcholine is the muscle relaxant of choice for most patients (1–1.5 mg/kg). To prevent maternal awareness until the neonate is delivered, a combination of 50% nitrous oxide in oxygen is used with a low end-tidal concentration of a halogenated agent (0.5 minimum alveolar concentration). Larger concentrations of a volatile agent may cause relaxation of the uterus and excessive bleeding.

After delivery of the child, the concentration of nitrous oxide is increased, and opioids are administered. Benzodiazepines and muscle relaxants may also be used at the practitioner's discretion. The concentration of the volatile agent is decreased if uterine atony appears to be a problem. Oxytocin (Pitocin) is also administered to facilitate uterine contraction. At the conclusion of the procedure, the patient is extubated after thorough orogastric and airway suctioning and after the patient has demonstrated return of strength and mentation.

KEY POINTS: OBSTETRIC ANALGESIA AND ANESTHESIA

1. Opioids administered intravenously to the mother easily cross the placenta and may cause a decrease in fetal heart rate variability. In addition, intravenous opioids may cause neonatal respiratory depression and neurobehavioral changes.
2. Intravenous patient-controlled anesthesia has been associated with greater patient satisfaction, less risk of maternal respiratory depression, less need for antiemetic use, and better pain relief with lower drug doses.
3. In most laboring women, epidural analgesia is effective and reduces maternal catecholamine levels, potentially improving uteroplacental perfusion. Pain management is an important component of obstetric care.
4. The contraindications to epidural anesthesia include patient refusal, coagulopathy, uncontrolled hemorrhage, increased intracranial pressure, and infection at the site of needle introduction. Relative contraindications include systemic maternal infection, back surgery with hardware placement, and certain neurologic diseases.
5. Bupivacaine, ropivacaine, lidocaine, and chloroprocaine are the most commonly used local anesthetics in obstetric anesthesia.
6. Spinal anesthesia for cesarean delivery produces dense sensory and motor blockade, is relatively easy to perform, has a rapid onset, and carries no risk of local anesthetic toxicity.

WEBSITES
American Congress of Obstetricians and Gynecologists: http://www.acog.org

SUGGESTED READINGS
American College of Obstetricians and Gynecologists Committee Opinion 339: Analgesia and cesarean
delivery rates, Obstet Gynecol 107:1487–1488, 2006.
American College of Obstetricians and Gynecologists: Obstetric analgesia and anesthesia, 2002. ACOG
Practice Bulletin No. 36.
American Society of Anesthesiologists Task Force on Obstetric Anesthesia: Practice guidelines for obstetric
anesthesia: an updated report, Anesthesiology 106:843–863, 2007.
Cyna AM, Dodd J: Clinical update: obstetric anaesthesia, Lancet 370:640–642, 2007.
Evron S, Glezerman M, Sadan O, et al: Remifentanil: a novel systemic analgesic for labor pain, Anesth Analg
100:233–238, 2005.
Shen MK, Wu ZF, Zhu AB, et al: Remifentanil for labour analgesia: a double-blinded, randomized controlled
trial of maternal and neonatal effects of patient-controlled analgesia versus continuous infusion, Anesthesia
68:236–244, 2013.
Simmons SW, Cyna AM, Dennis AT, et al: Combined spinal-epidural versus epidural analgesia in
labour, Cochrane Database Syst Rev (3):CD003401, 2007.
Weinberg GL: Current concepts in resuscitation of patients with local anesthetic cardiac toxicity, Reg Anesth
Pain Med 27:568–575, 2002.

CHAPTER 57

HIGH-RISK OBSTETRICS

Ana M. Lobo, MD, MPH, and Mary DiMiceli, MD

1. **Define high-risk pregnancy.**
   High-risk pregnancies are those that involve either a maternal or fetal condition that increases the likelihood of maternal or fetal morbidity and/or mortality. They comprise approximately 6% to 8% of total pregnancies (Table 57-1). Substance abuse and withdrawal may also define the parturient as high risk. Providing adequate analgesia and monitoring withdrawal are concerns.

2. **Describe the hypertensive disorders of pregnancy.**
   Hypertensive disorders are associated with 6% to 8% of pregnancies and are the leading cause of maternal morbidity and mortality worldwide. Chronic hypertension (HTN) is often diagnosed prepregnancy but may go undiagnosed until the first prenatal visit. HTN is characterized by an increase in mean arterial pressure before 20 weeks' gestation and does not resolve postpartum. Alternatively, gestational HTN is associated with an increase in mean arterial pressure after 20 weeks' gestation and *does* resolve postpartum. Both are unlikely associated with proteinuria, whereas preeclampsia is characterized by proteinuria in addition to a rise in systemic blood pressure. Preeclampsia is divided into mild and severe forms and, if left untreated, can progress to eclampsia and seizures. Table 57-2 summarizes the types of hypertensive disorders found in pregnant patients.

3. **Describe characteristics of preeclampsia, and review the associated risk factors.**
   Preeclampsia is one of the hypertensive disorders of pregnancy. Associated changes in systemic blood pressure and proteinuria are noted in Table 57-2. Although parturients with preeclampsia demonstrate significant mucosal and peripheral edema (no longer part of the diagnostic criteria), clinically they are hypovolemic. Box 57-1 lists some known risk factors. Interestingly, maternal smoking history has been shown to *reduce* a woman's risk of developing preeclampsia. While preeclampsia is typically associated with vasoconstriction, there is also increased vascular permeability, and these women are at increased risk for pulmonary edema. As a result, careful attention must be paid to volume replacement in these patients since volume overload can easily lead to left ventricular failure. Women whose preeclampsia is diagnosed before 34 weeks' gestation have high systemic vascular resistance (SVR) with low cardiac output, whereas those diagnosed after 34 weeks' gestation have low SVR with high cardiac output. Finally, severe preeclamptic patients are at increased risk for coagulation abnormalities as a result of developing HELLP syndrome (see Question 5). The leading cause of death in these patients is cerebrovascular accidents, most of which are hemorrhagic likely secondary to increased vascular permeability in addition to abolition of cerebral vascular autoregulation and coagulation abnormalities.

4. **What is the etiology of preeclampsia?**
   Although the etiology of preeclampsia is unknown, abnormal placentation likely plays a significant role. Abnormal placentation occurs as a result of failure of trophoblastic invasion of the spiral arteries that causes the spiral arteries to remain vasoconstricted, creating a high resistance placental circulation, in contrast to the normally dilated placenta. Placental perfusion is reduced with subsequent release of vasoactive substances, ultimately resulting in fetal growth restriction, thus increasing risk for preterm delivery and associated complications (e.g., respiratory distress syndrome and intraventricular hemorrhage). This is the asymptomatic first stage, followed by the second stage, which is characterized by systemic endothelial dysfunction and inflammation, resulting in vasoconstriction and possible development of thromboemboli.

5. **What is HELLP syndrome?**
   HELLP (*h*emolysis, *e*levated *l*iver enzymes, and *l*ow *p*latelet count) syndrome occurs as part of severe preeclampsia. Patients develop a microangiopathic hemolytic anemia associated

Table 57-1. High-Risk Conditions in Pregnancy

HIGH-RISK CONDITION	PREVALENCE
Obesity	6%–28%
Preterm birth	5%–10%
Mental disorders	10%
Hypertension (chronic, gestational, preeclampsia, eclampsia)	10%
Diabetes (including gestational DM)	6%–8%
Asthma	3%–8%
Substance abuse	4%–5%
Hypothyroidism	2%–3%
Chorioamnionitis	1%
Cardiac disease	1%
Renal disease	1%
Hyperthyroidism	0.2%–0.4%

DM, Diabetes mellitus.

Table 57-2. Hypertensive Disorders of Pregnancy

TYPE	BLOOD PRESSURE	ONSET	PROTEINURIA
Chronic	≥140/90 mm Hg	Before 20 wk EGA	Absent without resolution PP
Gestational	≥140/90 mm Hg	After 20 wk EGA	Absent
Preeclampsia			
Mild	≥140/90 mm Hg	After 20 wk EGA	>300 mg/24 hr
Severe	≥160/110 mm Hg	After 20 wk EGA	>5 g/24 hr

EGA, Estimated gestational age; PP, postpartum.
From Report of the National High Blood Pressure Education Program Working Group on High Blood Pressure in Pregnancy. Am J Obstet Gynecol 183:S1–S22, 2000.

Box 57-1. Risk Factors of Preeclampsia

Nulliparity
Black race
Extremes of age
Personal history or family history of preeclampsia
Multiple gestation
Maternal obesity

Chronic hypertension
Diabetes mellitus
Thrombotic vascular disease
Assisted reproductive technology
Limited exposure to sperm

with thrombocytopenia and elevated liver enzymes. Symptoms may include headache, nausea/vomiting, and right upper quadrant pain secondary to capsular distention. Interestingly, ≈12% may present normotensive. Parturients who develop HELLP syndrome after 34 weeks, especially when associated with laboratory evidence of disseminated intravascular coagulation, require immediate delivery, regardless of gestational age. However, some women with HELLP may be managed expectantly during which they may receive systemic corticosteroids for fetal lung maturity.

6. **How is preeclampsia managed?**

The mainstay of management is blood pressure control. First-line antihypertensive medications include labetalol and hydralazine. Since cerebral autoregulation is disrupted, antihypertensives are given to maintain blood pressure below severe ranges and should not be given to *normalize* parturients' blood pressure in order to prevent cerebrovascular and cardiovascular complications. Labetalol, a competitive antagonist at both α- and β-adrenergic receptors has an onset of 2 to 5 minutes and has seven times more β- than α-antagonist activity. As a result, there is little if any decrease in SVR. Hydralazine, an arteriolar vasodilator, results in a significant decrease in SVR with very little change in cardiac output.

Oral nifedipine, a calcium channel blocker, has been compared favorably to IV labetalol in reducing SVR while increasing cardiac index in preeclamptic patients. Sodium nitroprusside may also be given in a hypertensive emergency and has the advantage of preserving uteroplacental perfusion. However, nitroprusside can result in cerebral vasodilation and cyanide toxicity.

While there is no proven benefit of invasive hemodynamic monitoring, it should be considered in patients who develop pulmonary edema, refractory HTN, or oliguria unresponsive to fluid challenge, or those with preexisting cardiopulmonary disease.

Magnesium sulfate is given for seizure prophylaxis, although the mechanism by which it prevents seizures is unknown. Magnesium has been shown to dilate vascular beds and attenuate the vascular response to endogenous and exogenous vasopressors. Administration of magnesium sulfate is additionally advantageous for fetal neuroprotection as it has been shown to decrease the incidence of neurologic insult.

7. **What are potential complications of magnesium sulfate administration?**

The therapeutic range of magnesium sulfate is 4 to 8 mEq/L. As plasma concentrations increase, patients develop electrocardiogram (ECG) changes with widening of the QRS complex and prolonged QT interval. Deep tendon reflexes are absent at 10 mEq/L; sinoatrial and atrioventricular block and respiratory paralysis occur when concentrations are 15 mEq/L; cardiac arrest occurs at 25 mEq/L. In therapeutic doses, magnesium sulfate increases sensitivity to muscle relaxants, especially nondepolarizing muscle relaxants. Because magnesium sulfate also crosses the placenta, newborns may demonstrate decreased muscle tone, respiratory depression, and apnea. Magnesium toxicity is treated with intravenous calcium.

8. **What are the anesthetic considerations in patients with preeclampsia?**

A thorough preoperative evaluation, including review of past medical history, airway evaluation, and evaluation of coagulation status, is highly recommended. Given that preeclamptic patients have worsened mucosal, particularly oropharyngeal, edema, the airway evaluation is crucial and should be rechecked because the edema (and Mallampati score) can worsen throughout labor. Accordingly, these patients may have a higher risk for difficulty ventilating and intubating if they become necessary.

Since preeclampsia may be accompanied by signs/symptoms of HELLP syndrome, an evaluation of the patient's coagulation status (prothrombin time and partial thromboplastin time) and platelet count is recommended before initiation of neuraxial anesthesia. The concern is to avoid risk of an epidural hematoma with neuraxial technique. Although an arbitrary platelet count of 100,000 is often suggested, the actual platelet count safe for spinal or epidural placement is unknown, and most anesthesiologists would review the trend in the patient's profile.

With the onset of sympathetic blockade from neuraxial anesthesia, care must be taken to avoid acute hypotension. While spinal anesthesia is more likely to produce sudden hypotension, many recent studies have confirmed its safe administration for cesarean delivery. Certainly, spinal anesthesia may be preferable to general anesthesia as the latter places the parturient at risk for difficult intubation, aspiration, and worsened HTN from heightened sympathetic response to laryngoscopy with potential neurologic complications, such as cerebral hemorrhage, as this is the most common cause of maternal mortality in this patient population. Accordingly, extreme care must be taken to avoid an acute hypertensive response. Furthermore, special attention must be placed on administration of intravenous fluid administration as these patients are prone to developing pulmonary edema secondary to increased vascular permeability.

9. **What is eclampsia?**
Eclampsia, usually preceded by preeclampsia, is the development of peripartum seizures and/or coma not caused by underlying neurologic disease. Patients may often experience headache, visual disturbances, and epigastric pain prior to onset of seizure activity. Parturients may have evidence of cerebral edema and focal hemorrhages, and develop liver necrosis and fulminant hepatic failure. Acute kidney injury, disseminated intravascular coagulation, with coagulation disturbances (both bleeding and thrombosis) are also risks.

10. **How are eclamptic seizures treated?**
Maternal airway management and intrauterine resuscitation are of overriding importance. The patient should be placed laterally and intubated and supplemented with oxygen to minimize fetal hypoxia. Intravenous anticonvulsants include thiopental (50–100 mg), diazepam (2.5–5 mg), midazolam (1–2 mg), and magnesium (2–4 g). A magnesium sulfate infusion should be instituted for seizure prophylaxis. Immediate delivery may be indicated.

11. **Discuss preterm labor. How is it managed?**
Preterm labor is the onset of frequent uterine contractions associated with progressive cervical dilation or effacement occurring before 37 weeks' gestation and often resulting in preterm delivery. Preterm labor is associated with placental abruption, uterine abnormalities, cervical insufficiency, multiple gestations, premature rupture of the membranes, and urinary tract, systemic, or gynecologic infection (Box 57-2). Although preterm delivery occurs in only 5% to 10% of pregnancies, it accounts for the majority of neonatal morbidity secondary to pulmonary immaturity and neonatal deaths. Survival is ≈50% at ≤25 weeks but significantly increases to ≈90% at ≥28 weeks' gestation.
   Although there is no treatment for preterm labor, pregnancy can be prolonged with certain medications, including calcium channel blockers, magnesium sulfate, cyclooxygenase inhibitors, and β-mimetic tocolytics and nifedipine (Table 57-3). Nonsteroidal antiinflammatory drugs (NSAIDs) should be selectively used if patients have NSAID-sensitive asthma, active peptic ulcer disease, or coagulation abnormalities. Magnesium sulfate is a poor tocolytic, but again, it improves fetal neurologic outcome.

12. **Discuss antepartum hemorrhage.**
Placenta previa, placental abruption, uterine rupture, and vasa previa are all causes of antepartum hemorrhage. Placental abruption is a separation of the placenta and is most often accompanied by vaginal bleeding, uterine tenderness, and increased uterine activity. Uterine rupture is a defect in the uterine wall that results in fetal distress and/or maternal hemorrhage. Vasa previa is of no threat to the mother; however, there is a velamentous insertion of the cord where fetal vessels traverse fetal membranes ahead of the presenting fetal part. Rupture of these vessels can cause fetal exsanguination. Patients with antepartum hemorrhage are also at risk for postpartum hemorrhage. In the face of significant blood loss, regional anesthesia is a questionable decision when compared with general anesthesia.

13. **What is placenta previa?**
Placenta previa occurs when placental implants are anterior to the presenting part. Classification depends on the relationship between the cervical os and placenta. Several factors are associated with previa: uterine trauma, multiparity, prior cesarean delivery or uterine surgery, advanced maternal age, and a prior history of placenta previa. Painless vaginal bleeding occurs in the second or third trimester and is not related to any particular

Box 57-2. Risk Factors for Preterm Delivery

Black race	Polyhydramnios (uterine distention)
History of preterm delivery	Trauma
History of tobacco/substance abuse	Abdominal surgery during pregnancy
Acute or chronic systemic disease	Multiple gestation
Low prepregnancy BMI	Low socioeconomic status

BMI, Body mass index.

Table 57-3. List of Common Tocolytics and Side Effects

CLASS	DRUG	MATERNAL SIDE EFFECTS	FETAL SIDE EFFECTS
Cyclo-oxygenase inhibitors (NSAIDs)	Indomethacin	Nausea Heartburn	Closure of PDA Pulmonary HTN Renal dysfunction (reversible) Oligohydramnios IVH
Magnesium sulfate	Magnesium sulfate	Flushing Lethargy Muscle weakness Hypocalcemia/demineralization Hypocalcemia Pulmonary edema Cardiac arrest	Hypotonia Respiratory depression
β-Adrenergic agonists	Terbutaline Ritodrine	Dysrhythmias Pulmonary edema Hypotensive Hyperglycemia Hypokalemia N/V, fever	Tachycardia Hyperglycemia Hypertrophy (Neonatal—hypoglycemia hypocalcemia, hypotension)
Calcium channel blockers	Nifedipine Nicardipine	Transient hypotension Flushing Headache Dizziness	None

HTN, Hypertension; *IVH,* intraventricular hemorrhage; *NSAIDs,* nonsteroidal antiinflammatory drugs; *N/V,* nausea/vomiting; *PDA,* patent ductus arteriosus.

event. A lack of abdominal pain and no change in uterine activity differentiate it from placental abruption. The first episode of bleeding rarely causes shock or fetal compromise.

14. **What is postpartum uterine atony? How is it managed?**
   Uterine atony is a failure of contraction of the uterus and may result in severe hemorrhage. Conditions that cause uterine overdistention, including multiple gestation, fetal macrosomia, and polyhydramnios, may increase the risk of uterine atony. Other conditions of atony include high parity, prolonged labor, chorioamnionitis, precipitous labor, augmented labor, and use of tocolytic agents.
   Obstetric management includes bimanual compression, uterine massage, and uterotonics. Oxytocin, the first-line treatment, is a synthetic hormone structurally similar to vasopressin and is administered IV (20–50 units/1000 ml crystalloid). It is rapid in onset. If atony is severe, 1 or 2 units may be administered as an IV bolus dose of 5 to 10 units. It produces vasodilation resulting in hypotension. Methylergonovine is an ergot alkaloid derivative and is administered (0.2 mg) intramuscularly (IM) but is known to cause HTN. Accordingly, it is contraindicated in hypertensive disorders, peripheral vascular disease, and ischemic heart disease. Methyl prostaglandin $F_{2\alpha}$ (Hemabate) is administered into uterine myometrium or skeletal muscle (250 mcg) for the treatment of refractory uterine atony. Side effects include bronchospasm, disturbed ventilation-perfusion ratios, increased intrapulmonary shunt fraction, and hypoxemia, and it is contraindicated in patients with asthma. Depending on the degree of atony and hemorrhage, management may involve placement of a Bakri balloon that serves as a tamponade to bleeding. Atony refractory to all agents may require uterine arterial ligation or embolization or hysterectomy.

15. **Discuss diabetes and its anesthetic considerations.**
Pregnant patients with diabetes are at risk for spontaneous abortions, stillbirth, preeclampsia, polyhydramnios, fetal macrosomia, fetal malformations, and cesarean delivery. Pregestational diabetes is associated with preterm labor and delivery. Glycemic control and treatment of hypotension with nonglucose-containing crystalloids and ephedrine or phenylephrine are helpful in preserving fetal acid-base status during neuraxial anesthesia for labor and delivery. Placental insufficiency is present in this population, which is further worsened by hyperglycemia. Any additional condition that further worsens placental perfusion may significantly impact fetal oxygenation and acid-base status and may potentially place the fetus at risk for intrauterine growth restriction. Neuraxial technique is preferred, as these patients are at high risk for cesarean or forceps-assisted delivery, but may be challenging, as many of these patients are obese with poor landmarks. Ultrasonic guidance may identify landmarks, improving success of epidural or spinal needle insertion. Finally, these patients are likely more difficult to intubate, and anesthesiologists should be fully prepared to manage a difficult airway.

16. **What causes disseminated intravascular coagulation in obstetric patients?**
Disseminated intravascular coagulation results from abnormal activation of the coagulation cascade with formation of large amounts of thrombin, depletion of coagulation factors, activation of the fibrinolytic system, and hemorrhage. In obstetrics, the most frequent causes are preeclampsia, sepsis, fetal demise, placental abruption, sepsis, and amniotic fluid embolism.

17. **Which cardiac disease most commonly complicates pregnancy?**
Congenital heart disease is the most common cardiac disease in pregnant women in the United States. It accounts for approximately 60% to 80% of cardiac disease during pregnancy.

18. **How is congenital heart disease managed during pregnancy?**
Pulmonary artery catheterization is rarely required for most patients with congenital heart disease. Intrathecal opioid injections are good choices for labor analgesia when patients will not tolerate decreased SVR and decreased venous return. Epidural anesthesia is contraindicated in few, if any cardiac lesions, provided that the induction of anesthesia is slow and hemodynamic changes are treated promptly. Single-injection spinals for cesarean delivery are contraindicated in many patients with congenital heart disease. However, neuraxial anesthesia/analgesia may be very advantageous for these patients as it can blunt the sympathetic response to labor pain and the hemodynamic changes that accompany labor and delivery. As a result, these patients are better able to tolerate the cardiovascular demand postpartum with potential to decrease risk for peripartum cardiomyopathy and subsequent heart failure.

KEY POINTS: HIGH-RISK OBSTETRICS

1. Maternal morbidity and/or mortality from hypertensive disorders most often result from cerebrovascular and cardiovascular complications.
2. Indications for invasive central monitoring in preeclamptic patients include (1) refractory hypertension, (2) pulmonary edema, (3) refractory oliguria unresponsive to fluid challenge, and (4) severe cardiopulmonary disease.
3. Uterine atony is the most common cause of postpartum hemorrhage and often results in substantial blood loss.
4. Obesity and diabetes mellitus increase the parturient's risk for development of preeclampsia, preterm labor and delivery, painful labor, fetal macrosomia, and operative delivery, for which a well-functioning, early placed epidural will increase success for safe delivery and avoid risks for potential general anesthesia.
5. Because there is a growing number of women at child-bearing age with a history of congenital heart disease and repair, the obstetric anesthesiologist must be knowledgeable about the condition and the physiologic changes it incurs on the parturient in order to safely manage and administer anesthesia.

WEBSITE

Society for Obstetric Anesthesia and Perinatology: http://www.soap.org

SUGGESTED READINGS

American Society of Anesthesiologists Task Force on Obstetric Anesthesia: Practice guidelines for obstetric anesthesia: an updated report, Anesthesiology 106:843–863, 2007.

American Society of Anesthesiologists Task Force on Pulmonary Artery Catheterization: Practice guidelines for pulmonary artery catheterization: an updated report, Anesthesiology 99:988–1014, 2003.

Beilin Y, Reid RW: Renal disease. In Chestnut DH, Polley LS, Tsen LC, et al, editors: Obstetric anesthesia: principles and practice, ed 4, Philadelphia, 2009, Mosby, pp 1095–1107.

Harnett M, Tsen LC: Cardiovascular disease. In Chestnut DH, Polley LS, Tsen LC, et al, editors: Obstetric anesthesia principles and practice, ed 4, Philadelphia, 2009, Mosby, pp 881–912.

Mayer DC, Smith KA: Antepartum and postpartum hemorrhage. In Chestnut DH, Polley LS, Tsen LC, et al, editors: Obstetric anesthesia principles and practice, ed 4, Philadelphia, 2009, Mosby, pp 811–836.

Polley LS: Hypertensive disorders. In Chestnut DH, Polley LS, Tsen LC, et al, editors: Obstetric anesthesia principles and practice, ed 4, Philadelphia, 2009, Mosby, pp 975–1007.

Sibai BM: Hypertension. In Gabbe SG, Niebyl JR, Simpson JL, editors: Obstetrics: normal and problem pregnancies, ed 5, Philadelphia, 2007, Churchill Livingstone, pp 864–912.

Visalyaputra S, Rodanant O, Somboonviboon W, et al: Spinal versus epidural anesthesia for cesarean delivery in severe preeclampsia: a prospective randomized, multicenter study, Anesth Analg 101:862–868, 2005.

CHAPTER 58

GERIATRIC ANESTHESIA

Gurdev S. Rai, MD

1. **What is geriatric anesthesia, and why is it important?**
   - Geriatric anesthesia is defined as providing anesthetic care for patients older than 65 years old.
   - The geriatric population of the United States exceeds 35 million people, 12% of the total population. This population accounts for 33% of all surgical procedures performed in the United States.
   - Geriatric patients consume 50% of the U.S. federal health care budget.
   - Their population is expected to double by the year 2050.

2. **What are the overriding characteristics and principles governing age-related physiologic changes as they relate to anesthesia in geriatrics?**
   Basal function of most organ systems is relatively unchanged by the aging process per se, but the functional reserve and ability to compensate for physiologic stresses are reduced. However, because of the diversity of this population, it is difficult to predict the extent of age-related physiologic changes and reduction in functional reserve for any particular individual.

3. **Review age-related changes to the cardiovascular system.**
   - Age-related wall thickening and stiffening of large elastic arteries reduce their compliance and increase afterload on the heart. These vascular changes can occur in the absence of atherosclerosis or hypertension and are independent predictors of mortality.
   - Increased afterload (e.g., from hypertension) produces ventricular hypertrophy, leading to increases in wall stress, myocardial oxygen demand, and risk of ischemia.
   - Diastolic dysfunction secondary to ventricular remodeling minimizes the ability to adjust stroke volume in response to changes in intravascular volume and tone.
   - Stroke volume becomes more dependent on atrial preload for adequate end-diastolic volume.
   - The atrium dilates as a result of impaired outflow secondary to ventricular remodeling, making the elderly more prone to atrial fibrillation. Fatty infiltration and fibrosis of myocardium manifest in conduction abnormalities and decreased heart rate variability.
   - Downregulation of β-adrenergic receptors magnifies the decreased ability of the heart to reach maximal cardiac output acutely in response to stress.

4. **Describe age-related changes to the pulmonary system.**
   - Restrictive pulmonary changes are noted as increased thoracic stiffness increases the work of breathing and decreases maximal minute ventilation.
   - Closing capacity surpasses functional residual capacity by age 65 years, increasing the risk of atelectasis.
   - Decreased cough reflex, ciliary clearance, and compromised swallowing mechanics increase risk of perioperative aspiration and pneumonia.
   - There is a centrally mediated decrease in ventilatory response to hypoxia and hypercapnia.
   - Exposure time to environmental, genetic, and social factors increases the prevalence of lung diseases and further exaggerates the changes noted previously.

5. **Discuss age-related changes to the nervous system.**
   - There is overall cerebral atrophy, decreased complexity of neuronal connections and decreased synthesis of neurotransmitters, increased fibrosis of peripheral sympathetic neurons, and impairment of cardiovascular reflexes.
   - Decreased skeletal muscle innervation (and atrophy) results in decreased strength and fine motor control.
   - There is increased sensitivity to all anesthetic agents.

6. **How is baseline renal function impaired in the elderly?**
   There is a progressive decrease in glomerular filtration rate (GFR) because of a decrease in renal blood flow and renal mass and diminishing tubular dysfunction, impairing sodium homeostasis and the ability to respond to acid loads. Under normal circumstances these have no real clinical implications other than subclinical hyponatremia. However, in the face of surgical stress, the failure to adapt to acute volume changes can lead to hemodynamic instability. Therefore meticulous attention needs to be paid to intraoperative fluid and electrolyte management in the elderly population.

7. **How does serum creatinine change with aging?**
   Despite progressive decreases in GFR, because of an overall decrease in muscle mass in the elderly, serum creatinine should remain normal or decrease.

8. **How do changes in renal function affect anesthetic management?**
   Decreases in GFR and renal blood flow lead to an increased risk for intraoperative fluid and electrolyte disturbances and an increased risk of acute renal failure. Intravascular volume must be replaced to maintain urine output at 0.5 ml/kg/hr or more. Moreover, many medications used intraoperatively and their metabolites that depend on renal clearance have prolonged elimination half-lives and longer durations of action. An example of these would be morphine and its metabolites, which, if not used with renal function in mind, can result in prolonged respiratory depression.

9. **How is liver function affected by aging? What are some anesthetic implications?**
   - Liver mass, hepatic blood flow, and hepatic reserve decrease.
   - Age-related loss of endoplasmic reticulum leads to decreased protein synthesis, including albumin. Thus the serum levels of protein-bound drugs increase.
   - Because of the exceptional reserve of the liver, only in the presence of other comorbidities such as alcohol abuse and hepatitis are clinically relevant decreases in drug metabolism noted.

10. **In what ways does body composition change with aging?**
    - Decreased basal metabolic rate leads to an overall increase in percentage of body fat.
    - Muscle mass decreases with time, especially with inactivity.
    - Total body water decreases by 20% to 30% with age, resulting in decreased total blood volume.

11. **How do these changes in body composition affect anesthetic management?**
    - Increased body fat leads to an increased volume of distribution for lipid-soluble drugs. Thus elderly patients may have an extended elimination time and prolongation of effect.
    - Loss of skeletal muscle leads to a decrease in maximal and resting oxygen consumption, a slightly lowered resting cardiac output, and diminished production of body heat (predisposing to hypothermia). Despite a smaller muscle mass, elderly patients are not more sensitive to muscle relaxants, probably because of fewer receptors at the neuromuscular junction.
    - Decreased total body water leads to a smaller volume of distribution and higher-than-expected plasma concentrations of water-soluble drugs.
    - Elderly patients may have a greater-than-anticipated response to drugs and thus appear to be more sensitive.

12. **Why are these patients prone to hypothermia?**
    Elderly patients have a reduced basal metabolic rate, produce less body heat, and have diminished reflex cutaneous vasoconstriction to prevent heat loss. Aging is also associated with a decrease in β-adrenergic receptors, which are integral to temperature homeostasis.

13. **What is the effect of aging on anesthetic requirements?**
    The minimum alveolar concentration for volatile anesthetics decreases 4% to 5% per decade after age 40. The alveolar concentration of a volatile anesthetic increases more rapidly because of decreased circulation time. The median effective dose (ED_{50}) for intravenous agents decreases as well.

14. **How are the pharmacokinetics and quality of spinal anesthesia affected by age?**
   Elderly patients have decreased blood flow to the subarachnoid space, resulting in slower
   absorption of anesthetic solutions. They also have a smaller volume of cerebrospinal fluid,
   the specific gravity of which tends to be higher than that of younger patients. This leads to
   a higher final concentration for a given dose and may alter the spread of the anesthetic.
   Elderly patients may have accentuated degrees of lumbar lordosis and thoracic kyphosis,
   increasing cephalad spread and pooling in the thoracic segments. Thus one might see
   higher levels of spinal anesthesia accompanied by faster onset of action and prolonged
   duration. Older patients also have a lower incidence of post–dural puncture headaches
   when compared with younger patients.

15. **Review the dynamics of epidural anesthesia change with age.**
   Older patients require a smaller local anesthetic dose to achieve the same level of block
   when compared with younger patients. This may be the result of narrowing of the
   intervertebral spaces.

16. **Do all elderly patients need extensive preoperative testing?**
   Preoperative testing should be tailored to the level of risk of planned surgery, underlying
   illnesses, and functional status. An electrocardiogram is recommended if the patient has
   had a recent episode of chest pain or ischemic equivalent, is at medium to high risk for
   cardiac complications during surgery, or is undergoing intermediate- or high-risk surgery.
   Appropriate laboratory testing should be determined by the patient's prior medical history,
   his or her medications, and the scope of the planned procedure.

17. **Is there a difference in outcome when performing regional versus general
    anesthesia in the elderly?**
   Results of studies are mixed and depend on the outcome measured and the procedure. In
   repair of hip fractures, incidence of deep venous thrombosis, fatal pulmonary embolism, and
   1 month mortality has been shown to be significantly reduced when regional anesthesia was
   used. On the other hand, other large studies of peripheral vascular surgeries have failed to
   consistently detect meaningful differences in outcome between elderly patients receiving
   epidural versus general anesthetics. There is a theoretic benefit of improved graft patency
   with epidural anesthesia, but this has not been demonstrated consistently through clinical
   trials.

18. **What are the most common postoperative complications in elderly patients?**
   Adverse drug reactions are three times more likely in the elderly than in young patients.
   Postoperative cognitive dysfunction (POCD) and delirium are very common among the
   elderly.

KEY POINTS: GERIATRIC ANESTHESIA

1. Implications of age-related changes on anesthetic management are profound, affecting almost
   every aspect of perioperative care.
2. Basal function of most organ systems is relatively unchanged by the aging process, but the
   functional reserve and ability to compensate for physiologic stress are reduced.
3. Not all elderly patients need an extensive preoperative workup; tailor it to their underlying illnesses
   and invasiveness of the surgery.
4. In general, anesthetic requirements are decreased in geriatric patients.
5. There is increased potential for a wide variety of postoperative complications in the elderly; POCD
   is arguably the most common.

19. **What is POCD, and what are its risk factors?**
   POCD is a disorder in thought processes, including memory, language comprehension,
   visuospatial abstraction, and attention. Risk factors include advanced age, lower educational
   level, alcohol use, a prior history of stroke, and Alzheimer disease. Polypharmacy and
   delirium during hospitalization are also predictive of POCD.

The complexity of testing and lack of a standardized diagnostic battery of tests have challenged our understanding of POCD.

20. **What are the implications of POCD on patient mortality?**

The occurrence of POCD is associated with increased mortality during the first year after surgery. A rapid decline in cognitive function with a persistent course (greater than 3 months) further increases mortality in these patients. This is attributed to possible underlying health issues in patients with POCD, decreased compliance after surgery, and a higher rate of depression.

21. **What can anesthesiologists do to limit POCD in *at-risk* patients?**

There are not many well-powered studies laying out a plan for anesthetic management. We do know that POCD is not associated with any particular anesthetic technique and that deeper levels of anesthesia seem to be protective. There is also evidence that patient familiarity with the perioperative experience can be helpful. Other studies have hinted that involving a geriatrician in the preoperative evaluation of elderly patients might decrease the incidence of POCD. The most appropriate management would limit the use of drugs already associated with delirium in the elderly. These include but are not limited to long-acting opiates, benzodiazepines, and anticholinergic medications. It would also be appropriate to continuously reevaluate the elderly patient's list of medications with the purpose of eliminating unnecessary medications and considering undesirable synergistic effects.

22. **Is age itself a predictor of perioperative mortality in the elderly?**

Age itself has proven to be a poor predictor of mortality; more predictive risk factors include the following:

- Emergent abdominal or thoracic surgery
- A low preoperative albumin level (reflective of overall nutritional status)
- The number and severity of coexisting diseases
- POCD
- Lack of exercise tolerance and increased frailty

SUGGESTED READINGS

Bryson GL, Wyand A: Evidence-based clinical update: general anesthesia and the risk of delirium and postoperative cognitive dysfunction, Can J Anaesth 53:669–677, 2006.

Chow WB, Rosenthal RA, Merkow RP, et al: Optimal preoperative assessment of the geriatric surgical patient: a best practices guideline from the American College of Surgeons National Surgical Quality Improvement Program and the American Geriatrics Society, J Am Coll Surg 215:453–466, 2012.

Farag E, Chelune GJ: Is depth of anesthesia, as assessed by the bispectral index, related to postoperative cognitive dysfunction and recovery?, Anesth Analg 103:633–640, 2006.

Monk TG, Weldon BC, Garvan CW, et al: Predictors of cognitive dysfunction after major noncardiac surgery, Anesthesiology 108:18–30, 2008.

Silverstein JH, Rooke GA, Reves JG, et al, editors: Geriatric anesthesiology, ed 2, New York, 2008, Springer.

Wijeysundera DN, Duncan D, Nkonde-Price C, et al: Perioperative beta blockade in noncardiac surgery: A systematic review for the 2014 ACC/AHA guideline on perioperative cardiovascular evaluation and management of patients undergoing noncardiac surgery, J Am Coll Cardiol 2014. doi: 10.1016/j.jacc.2014.07.939.

CHAPTER 59

SEDATION AND ANESTHESIA OUTSIDE THE OPERATING ROOM

Mark H. Chandler, MD, and James C. Duke, MD, MBA

1. **What procedures outside the operating room (OR) require sedation or general anesthesia?**
   - Radiologic procedures, including computed tomography, magnetic resonance imaging (MRI), and interventional radiology. A lack of patient cooperation necessitates the need for anesthesia assistance, especially in children.
   - Cardiac catheterizations, insertion of implantable cardiac defibrillators, coronary arteriography, radiofrequency ablation, and cardioversions
   - Surgical procedures in office settings and other highly stimulating procedures outside the OR
   - Extracorporeal shock-wave lithotripsy and cystoscopy
   - Endoscopy
   - Therapeutic radiation
   - Electroconvulsive therapy
   - Any number of pediatric procedures

2. **What equipment and standards are necessary for safety outside an OR?**
   A simple pneumonic to help one remember all that is required when performing sedation outside of the operating room is MAO IS SAME PEST:
   - A reliable source of oxygen with backup. Air is also preferred.
   - Laryngoscopes, endotracheal tubes, oral airways, and the like. Self-inflating hand resuscitator (Ambu) bags are also needed.
   - Suction, electrical outlets, illumination for system failure.
   - Anesthesia machines are sometimes used. IV infusion pumps are also used.
   - Airway equipment
   - Monitors
   - COR carts with defibrillator and emergency drugs
     M = Machine (with scavenger)
     A = Ambu bag
     O = Oxygen (with backup supply)
     I = Illumination
     S = Suction
     S = Space
     A = Anesthetic drugs and equipment
     M = Monitors
     E = Electricity
     P = Postanesthesia care unit
     E = Emergency cart
     S = Staff
     T = Telephone

3. **What monitoring is necessary for administration of any anesthetic, regardless of whether it is in the OR or elsewhere?**
   The American Society of Anesthesiologists (ASA) has established two basic monitoring standards for all anesthesia care, regardless of where it is administered:

1. Qualified anesthesia personnel must be present during the administration of any general anesthetics, regional anesthetics, and monitored anesthesia care.
2. Oxygenation, ventilation, circulation, and temperature shall be continually evaluated in any patient undergoing an anesthetic. Specifically the ASA requires the following:
   - **Oxygenation:** During all anesthetics, a quantitative method of assessing oxygenation such as pulse oximetry shall be used. When using an anesthesia machine, an oxygen analyzer with a low oxygen concentration limit alarm shall be used.
   - **Ventilation:** At the very least, all patients undergoing an anesthetic will be assessed for qualitative clinical signs of ventilation such as observed chest excursion, movement of the reservoir breathing bag, or auscultation of breath sounds. When an endotracheal tube or laryngeal mask airway is inserted, its correct positioning must be verified by identification of carbon dioxide in the expired gas, and carbon dioxide must be monitored with capnography or capnometry.
   - **Circulation:** Every patient receiving anesthesia shall have an electrocardiogram (ECG) continuously displayed throughout the anesthetic and shall have blood pressure and heart rate evaluated at least every 5 minutes. In addition, every patient receiving general anesthesia will have circulatory function continually evaluated by one of the following methods: palpation of a pulse, auscultation of heart sounds, monitoring of a tracing of intraarterial pressure, or pulse oximetry.
   - **Body temperature:** Whenever clinically significant changes in body temperature are expected, anticipated, or suspected, a patient receiving anesthesia shall have temperature monitored.

4. **Is performing sedation outside the OR a safe practice?**
   Review of sedating events outside the OR has demonstrated adverse events, especially inadequate respiration, oxygen desaturation, and loss of patent airways. Patients scheduled out of the OR who have adverse events tend to be older and sicker (and have higher ASA physical classifications).

5. **Review the role of anesthesiologists for establishing safety standards outside the OR.**
   There are obvious safety concerns and anesthesiologists possess unique knowledge and expertise essential for establishing safe practice. A regulatory body known as The Joint Commission has worked with anesthesiologists to establish standards of safety for nonanesthesiologists.

6. **Explain conscious sedation and the continuum of depth of anesthesia.**
   The ASA Task Force on Sedation and Analgesia by Nonanesthesiologists states that sedation and analgesia comprise a continuum of states ranging from minimal sedation to general anesthesia. Advanced training is essential for ensuring safe, high quality patient sedation (Table 59-1).

7. **Compare moderate and deep sedation.**
   Deep sedation is also known as moderate anesthesia care, or MAC. While the principal discussion concerns treatment outside of the OR, MAC can also be performed in the OR by anesthesiologists or nurse anesthetists. Often medications are administered incrementally, but intravenous infusions are also used to create the desired level of deep sedation.
   There are nonanesthesia physicians who may perform MAC, but they should have airway skills by virtue of training. Emergency physicians, oral and maxillofacial surgeons, and critical care specialists are examples.

8. **What are unique problems associated with MRI?**
   The MRI scanner contains a powerful magnetic field. Nonferrous objects are essential, as iron-containing objects become projectiles in the MRI environment. Besides the challenge of administering MAC or general anesthesia in this remote environment, nonferrous equipment, anesthesia machines, and monitors have been developed to allow safe use in this unusual environment.

Table 59-1. Definition of General Anesthesia and Levels of Sedation/Analgesia*

	MINIMAL SEDATION (ANXIOLYSIS)	MODERATE SEDATION/ ANALGESIA (CONSCIOUS SEDATION)	DEEP SEDATION/ MAC	GENERAL ANESTHESIA
Responsiveness	Normal response to verbal stimulation	Purposeful response[†] to verbal or tactile stimulation	Purposeful response[†] following repeated or painful stimulation	Unarousable even with painful stimulus
Airway	Unaffected	No intervention required	Intervention may be required	Intervention often required
Spontaneous ventilation	Unaffected	Adequate	May be inadequate	Frequently inadequate
Cardiovascular function	Unaffected	Usually maintained	Usually maintained	May be impaired

*Monitored anesthesia care does not describe the continuum of depth of sedation; rather it describes "a specific anesthesia service in which an anesthesiologist has been requested to participate in the care of a patient undergoing a diagnostic or therapeutic procedure." (From the American Society of Anesthesiologists.)
†Reflex withdrawal from a painful stimulus is not considered a purposeful response.
MAC, Monitored anesthetic care.
Adapted from American Society of Anesthesiologists, Task Force on Sedation and Analgesia by Nonanesthesiologists: Practice guidelines for sedation and analgesia by nonanesthesiologists. Anesthesiology 96:1004–1017, 2002.

KEY POINTS: ANESTHESIA OUTSIDE THE OPERATING ROOM

1. Not only anesthesiologists but also nonanesthesiologists increasingly provide sedation in nontraditional settings. Regardless of where an anesthetic is administered, the same standards exist for safety, monitors, equipment, and personnel.
2. Anesthesiologists have been, and continue to be, leaders in developing safety standards for patients sedated for various procedures.
3. Administering anesthesia to a patient undergoing an MRI poses unique challenges. Any ferromagnetic object can become a projectile and all equipment, including gas cylinders, must be nonferrous.

WEBSITES

American Society of Anesthesiologists: Guidelines for nonoperating room anesthetizing locations: http://www.asahq.org
Joint Commission on Accreditation of Healthcare Organizations: Comprehensive accreditation manual for hospitals: www.jointcommission.org

SUGGESTED READINGS

Kotob F, Twersky RS: Anesthesia outside the operating room: general overview and monitoring standards, Int Anesthesiol Clin 41:1–15, 2003.
Metzner J, Posner KL, Domino KB: The risk and safety of anesthesia at remote locations: the US closed claims analysis, Curr Opin Anaesthesiol 22:502–508, 2009.

CHAPTER 60

PACEMAKERS AND INTERNAL CARDIOVERTER DEFIBRILLATORS

Christopher M. Lowery, MD, and James C. Duke, MD, MBA

1. **Explain the letters in the NBG coding system for pacemakers.**
   The first three letters refer to chamber paced, chamber sensed, and response to sensed events. The fourth letter generally refers to programmability and rate responsiveness. The fifth letter is rarely used (Table 60-1).

2. **What do AOO, VOO, and DOO modes mean?**
   AOO means pacing in the atrium alone, VOO means pacing in the ventricle only, and DOO means pacing in the atrium and ventricle without sensing or response. Such a device would simply pace at a set lower rate regardless of underlying rhythm.

   These modes (ending in OO) are known as *asynchronous modes* and are useful in the operating room because they allow pacing to be maintained and prevent interference of electrocautery caused by the absence of sensing.

3. **What is the result of VVI pacing?**
   This mode results in ventricular pacing, with sensing in the ventricle alone, and the response is inhibition. This means that the device will release a pacing stimulus unless a sensed event occurs before the expiration of a timer based on the lower rate. If a sensed event occurs, the only response by the device is to inhibit pacing, allowing for the intrinsic rhythm.

4. **What is the result of DDI pacing?**
   DDI means pacing in the atrium and ventricle, sensing in the atrium and ventricle, and the response is constrained to inhibition. The device will thus pace at a set rate in the atrium unless a sensed event occurs at a faster rate in the atrium, which will result in inhibition. The device will then pace in the ventricle at a set rate unless sensing in that chamber occurs at a faster rate, leading to inhibition. This allows for some atrial and ventricular synchrony to be maintained. However, because the response is only inhibition, the pacemaker will not pace in the ventricle as a result of a sensed event in the atrium, which is known as a tracking or triggered response. Thus competitive atrial pacing and variable atrioventricular (AV) timing can occur. This mode is helpful when atrial arrhythmias would lead to rapid heart rates if tracked and is a frequent default mode.

5. **What does DDD pacing mean?**
   DDD pacing means pacing in atria and ventricles, sensing in atria and ventricles, and a dual response (both triggered and inhibited). This is the most common pacing mode. A sensed atrial event occurring before the lower rate timer has expired will inhibit atrial pacing. If no event is sensed in the atrium above the lower rate, an atrial stimulus is released. Both events will initiate a timer expiring before ventricular pacing. If a ventricular-sensed event occurs before this timer expiring, ventricular pacing is inhibited, and intrinsic conduction is maintained. If the AV timer expires, a ventricular pacing stimulus is delivered and is triggered from the previous atrial paced or sensed event. This is known as tracking. If no underlying sensed events occur, atrial and ventricular sequential pacing occur at the lower programmed rate.

6. **Describe the difference between a unipolar and a bipolar pacemaker.**
   Both pacemakers detect electrical signals between two electrodes. In the case of unipolar pacemakers, one electrode is in the heart at the lead-tissue interface, and the other is

Table 60-1. Coding System Describing Cardiac Pacemakers

I CHAMBER PACED	II CHAMBER SENSED	III MODE OF RESPONSE	IV PROGRAMMABILITY	V ANTITACHYCARDIAC FUNCTIONS
O = none	O = none	O = none	O = none	O = none
A = atrium	A = atrium	T = triggered	P = simple programmable	P = pacing
V = ventricle	V = ventricle	I = inhibited	M = multiprogrammable	S = shock
D = dual (A+V)	D = dual (A + V)	D = dual (T + I)	R = rate responsive	D = dual (P + S)

comprised of the pacemaker generator. Sensing occurs from both electrodes. Thus sensing from the generator may lead to sensing extracardiac signals, muscle myopotentials, external noise, and interference. In the case of bipolar leads, the electrodes are closely spaced at the lead tip within the heart. Sensing between the electrodes is limited mainly to cardiac signals with much less oversensing or external interference.

7. **What is an implantable cardioverter defibrillator (ICD)?**
ICDs are devices much like pacemakers that can pace and support the heart rate in bradycardia. However, these devices have leads with shocking coils, usually one or two, that allow the device to administer internal shocks for tachyarrhythmias (which may be lifesaving). These devices also have complex programming. They allow rapid pacing to terminate regular, fast, more organized arrhythmias in a painless fashion. Algorithms in these devices may even allow differentiation of supraventricular arrhythmias from more serious arrhythmias from the ventricle. These devices are implanted for the treatment of life-threatening arrhythmias and prevention of sudden death.

8. **What are common indications for permanent pacing?**
   - In general, patients with symptoms from slow heart rate of any type that are not reversible require pacing.
   - Patients with AV block located below the AV node require pacing. These patients have wide escape complexes, and their escape mechanisms are unreliable and can lead to asystole or death.
   - Patients with arrhythmias caused by bradycardia such as torsades de pointes responsive to pacing require pacing.
   - Patients with syncope caused by carotid hypersensitivity require pacing.

9. **What are some common indications for implantable cardioverter defibrillator implantation?**
   - Cardiac arrest or ventricular fibrillation not from reversible causes
   - Sustained ventricular tachycardia with associated structural heart disease
   - Patients with left ventricular ejection fraction less than 35%, regardless of etiology
   - Primary electrical disorders such as Brugada syndrome or long QT syndrome

10. **What is the effect of placing a magnet over a device?**
The answer depends on the type of device and its programming. In general, placing a magnet over a device prevents device sensing. In the case of pacemakers, this usually leads to asynchronous pacing at a preprogrammed rate, regardless of underlying rhythm. If the device is an ICD, the default is usually to prevent sensing leading to arrhythmia detection and therapy. This may be used emergently when device malfunction is occurring, leading to inappropriate shocks, or when external noise (i.e., electrocautery) is sensed as a tachyarrhythmia. Be certain that the device is not functioning appropriately at the time of ICD discharge when magnet application may lead to withholding of lifesaving therapy! Application of a magnet over a device may also be useful when emergency surgery is required and the ICD therapies cannot be deactivated in a timely manner.

11. **Do patients with devices need to avoid microwave ovens or other hospital electronics?**

In general, modern devices are shielded against routine electromagnetic interference (EMI). This shielding is inadequate for radiofrequency (intraoperative electrocautery) or transcutaneous electrical nerve stimulation units. This may lead to false detection of extracardiac noise, leading to inappropriate inhibition of pacing or to defibrillation caused by inappropriate arrhythmia detection with ICDs. Other forms of strong magnetic fields, such as arc welding and some short-wave radios, may lead to device reprogramming or other malfunction. Cellular phones generally are not problematic unless in a pocket overlying the device; they should be used in the contralateral hand.

12. **Are there other responses to EMI by devices?**

Some devices are rate responsive. In this mode, the device is programmed to respond to various stimuli by increasing or decreasing heart rate to correct for various metabolic demands of exertion in patients. Some of these sensors function with crystals that deform with impact, increase pacing with changes in chest impedance, or increase pacing in response to changes in momentum. With these sensors, lithotripsy, certain electromagnetic monitoring equipment, or simply chest motion may trigger inappropriate rapid pacing. Rate responsiveness should always be programmed off before surgery.

13. **Can device leads be dislodged?**

Generally, after about 6 weeks, the myocardium has begun to scar around the lead tip, which contributes to lead stability. However, new devices known as biventricular pacemakers and defibrillators have a special lead placed in a vein behind the left atrium and ventricle to improve symptoms of heart failure. These leads are placed in a vein with friction as the only mechanism of retention and may easily be displaced years after placement. The placement and withdrawal of intravascular monitoring catheters should be performed with extreme caution and probably with fluoroscopic guidance.

14. **Can device leads be damaged with intravascular access?**

Device leads are generally wound wires surrounded by silicone that can be torn or damaged with an introducer needle. In general, access should be avoided in the veins where leads are in place.

15. **Do typical anesthetics and intraoperative medications affect the ability of implantable cardioverter defibrillators to defibrillate patients?**

Fentanyl reduces the energy required from the device to convert a ventricular arrhythmia (defibrillation threshold). Most inhalational anesthetics do not appear to change the defibrillation threshold except for enflurane and pentobarbital, which appear to increase it.

16. **Can changes in the patient's clinical status affect pacemaker function?**

In critically ill patients, severe acidosis, hyperkalemia, and/or cardiac ischemia may lead to dramatic increases in pacemaker capture thresholds, resulting in apparent pacemaker malfunction.

17. **Can programming patients to a different mode lead to hemodynamic compromise?**

Certain patients may become hypotensive, diaphoretic and nauseated, or short of breath when programmed to modes that lead to AV dyssynchrony, such as VVI setting in a patient with intact sinus mechanism. This may also occur when prolonged AV timing leads to atrial stimulation immediately following previous ventricular contraction. This is known as pacemaker syndrome and can on occasion be quite dramatic.

18. **Should patients with pacemakers or defibrillators be evaluated before and after surgery?**

Yes—to ensure that the device is functioning properly and that adequate battery life remains. The physician should be aware if the patient is pacemaker dependent. This implies that the patient has no underlying cardiac rhythm when the pacemaker is not functioning. If this is the case or if electrocautery is to be used, the device should be programmed to an asynchronous mode to avoid inadvertent device inhibition by EMI. Patients with ICDs should have the arrhythmia therapy feature turned off. This mandates that an external defibrillator be available for external defibrillation should an arrhythmia occur. After surgery, ICDs and pacemakers should be investigated to ensure that no programming errors were caused by EMI.

19. **Are there any precautions that can decrease the effect of electrocautery on devices?**
Yes. The dispersive electrode should be close to the area of the proposed cautery and as far from the device as possible. Bursts of electrocautery should be as brief as possible to avoid prolonged inhibition. The cautery electrode and dispersive pad should not be parallel to the presumed lead configuration and are best if perpendicular to the lead to avoid current traveling down the device leads. Devices with near end-of-life battery voltage may be permanently inhibited with electrocautery.

20. **If no underlying rhythm is seen when a pacemaker rate is rapidly decreased, does that mean that the patient is pacemaker dependent?**
No. Many patients have their rhythm suppressed by pacing but, when given time, will have a hemodynamically tolerated underlying rhythm. To assess for this, the pacing rate should be slowly reduced to allow for the patient's underlying rhythm to recover. If, after slow reduction in pacing rate, no underlying rate is seen above 30 to 40 beats/min, the patient is likely pacemaker dependent.

21. **No pacer spikes are seen on the monitoring system with your patient with a pacemaker. Does this mean that the pacemaker is not functioning properly?**
Not necessarily. The pacemaker may simply be inhibited because of the patient's underlying rhythm. However, it must be noted that with bipolar pacemakers the pacing spike is extremely small and may not be detected. In fact, with most digital recording systems the pacemaker spike seen is added to the strip by the recording system when electrical frequencies are detected that fall in the range of pacemaker stimuli. This sometimes leads to pacer spikes being seen on monitoring strips for patients without devices!

22. **Does failure of a pacemaker stimulus to capture the heart necessarily imply pacemaker malfunction?**
There are many reasons a pacemaker stimulus may not depolarize the tissue. Assess whether a stimulus is an atrial or ventricular stimulus (Figure 60-1). The tissue may have been refractory from a recent event such as a premature ventricular contraction, which is known as functional loss of capture. Occasionally the paced complex is not seen on a single-lead monitoring system because the axis of the paced rhythm is perpendicular to the monitoring lead. In this case, the paced complex will not be visible on the lead viewed despite normal

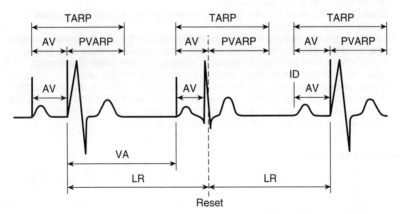

Figure 60-1. Normal atrioventricular pacing (sequential pacing). *AV,* Atrioventricular (paced) interval; *ID,* intrinsic depolarization; *LR,* lower rate (of pacing); *PVARP,* post ventricular atrial refractory period; *TARP,* total atrial refractory period. *(From Zaidan JR: Pacemakers. In Barash PG, editor: Refresher courses in anesthesiology (vol. 21), Philadelphia, 1993, Lippincott, with permission.)*

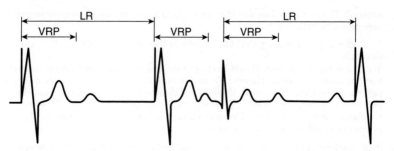

Figure 60-2. Normal VVI pacing. *LR,* Lower rate (of pacing); *VRP,* ventricular refractory period. (*From Zaidan JR: Pacemakers. In Barash PG, editor:* Refresher courses in anesthesiology *(vol. 21), Philadelphia, 1993, Lippincott, with permission.*)

function and normal appearance on other leads if they were monitored. However, if repeated failure to capture is seen or the patient appears compromised, emergent evaluation of pacemaker function should be sought.

23. **If a pacemaker stimulus is superimposed on a native complex, is the pacemaker necessarily malfunctioning?**
No. There are many explanations for the previous finding. Most commonly this is a case in which the pacemaker timer times out before sensing an intrinsic event. In this case the device will release a stimulus. The intrinsic event may have started earlier on a surface lead but was not sensed by the device at the site of the lead until well into the complex. This is a common finding with normal VVI pacing (Figure 60-2). Other programmable behavior may also explain this finding, although inappropriate sensing must also be ruled out.

KEY POINTS: PACEMAKERS AND INTERNAL CARDIOVERTER DEFIBRILLATORS (ICDS)

1. A strong magnet leads to asynchronous pacing at a set rate in pacemakers and prevents inhibition; it also prevents sensing in ICDs and prevents tachycardia therapy.
2. In the pacemaker coding system, the first letter refers to the chamber paced, the second letter to the chamber in which sensing occurs, the third letter to the responses to sensing in chambers, and the fourth letter to rate responsiveness.
3. Bipolar versus unipolar pacing refers to the type of pacemaker and distance between distal sensing electrode and proximal electrode.
4. Unipolar pacemakers pace and sense with the distal electrode at the tip of the lead at the cardiac lead interface, and the proximal electrode generally is the pacemaker generator itself. Sensing occurs between these widely spaced electrodes, predisposing to oversensing of extracardiac noise, and generating large amplitude spikes on recording equipment with pacing.
5. Bipolar pacemakers pace and sense with the distal electrode at the tip of the lead at the cardiac tissue-lead interface and a proximal electrode located usually nearby within 3 cm. Sensing occurs between these closely spaced electrodes and is less susceptible to extracardiac interference. Pacing spikes may not be visible on electrocardiographic recordings.

SUGGESTED READINGS

American Society of Anesthesiologists Committee on Standards and Practice Parameters: Practice advisory for the perioperative management of patients with cardiac implantable electronic devices, Anesthesiology 114(2):247–261, 2011.

Ellenbogen KA, Kay GN, Lau CP, et al: Clinical cardiac pacing, defibrillation, and resynchronization therapy, ed 3, Philadelphia, 2007, Saunders.

Hayes DL, Friedman PA: Cardiac pacing, defibrillation, and resynchronization: a clinical approach, ed 2, New York, 2008, Blackwell.

Kaszala K, Huizar JF, Ellenbogen KA: Contemporary pacemakers: what the primary care physician needs to know, Mayo Clin Proc 83:1170–1186, 2008.

SPINAL ANESTHESIA

James C. Duke, MD, MBA

CHAPTER 61

1. **What are the advantages of spinal anesthesia over general anesthesia?**
   - The metabolic stress response to surgery and anesthesia is reduced by subarachnoid block (SAB).
   - Particularly in elective hip surgery, there may be up to a 20% to 30% reduction in blood loss.
   - SAB decreases the incidence of venous thromboembolic complications by as much as 50%.
   - Pulmonary compromise appears to be less.
   - Endotracheal intubation is avoided.
   - Mental status can be followed.

2. **What are the usual doses of common local anesthetics used in spinal anesthesia and their durations of effect?**
   See Table 61-1.

3. **Where are the principal sites of effect of spinal local anesthetics?**
   The principal sites are the spinal nerve roots and spinal cord. Interestingly nerve roots may have different anatomic configurations (rootlets vs. roots); and there may be variability in fascial compartmentalization of the roots, especially between the dorsal and ventral nerve roots, accounting in part for differences between motor and sensory blockade.

4. **What factors determine the termination of effect?**
   Resorption of the agent from the cerebrospinal fluid (CSF) into the systemic circulation limits duration. Addition of a vasoconstrictor that slows resorption prolongs duration of effect. Vasoconstrictor efficacy decreases with local anesthetics with intrinsic longer durations of effect.

5. **Describe the factors involved in distribution (and extent) of conduction blockade.**
   - Patient characteristics include height, position, intraabdominal pressure, anatomic configuration of the spinal canal, and pregnancy. There is great interindividual variation in lumbosacral CSF volumes; magnetic resonance imaging has shown volumes ranging from 28 to 81 ml. Lumbar CSF volumes correlate well with the height and regression of the block. With the exception of an inverse relation with weight, no external physical measurement reliably estimates lumbar CSF volumes. CSF volumes are also reduced in pregnancy.
   - Needle direction and site when anesthetic is injected are important.
   - The total injected dose of local anesthetic is important, whereas the volume or concentration of injectant is unimportant.
   - The baricity of the local anesthetic solution is important. *Baricity* is defined by the ratio of the density of the local anesthetic solution to the density of CSF. A solution with a ratio >1 is hyperbaric and tends to sink with gravity within the CSF. An isobaric solution has a baricity of 1 and tends to remain in the immediate area of injection. A ratio <1 is a hypobaric solution, which rises in the CSF.

6. **At what lumbar levels should a spinal anesthetic be administered? What structures are crossed when performing a spinal block?**
   The selected level should be below L1 in an adult and L3 in a child to avoid needle trauma to the spinal cord. As an anatomic landmark, the L3-L4 interspace is located at the line intersecting the top of the iliac crests. Either a midline or a paramedian approach can be used. The anatomic layers passed through include skin, subcutaneous structures, supraspinous ligament, interspinous ligament, ligamentum flavum, dura mater, and arachnoid membrane.

Table 61-1. Local Anesthetic Dosing for Spinal Anesthesia

		Suggested Doses (MG) (Minutes)			Duration of Effect	
	USUAL CONCENTRATION	LOWER EXTREMITIES AND PERINEUM	LOWER ABDOMEN	UPPER ABDOMEN	WITHOUT EPINEPHRINE	WITH EPINEPHRINE
Lidocaine	5% in dextrose		30-50	75-100	60-75	75-90
Bupivacaine	0.75% in dextrose		5-10	12-17	90-120	100-150
Ropivacaine	0.25%-1%		8-12	16-18	90-120	90-120
Tetracaine	1% in dextrose		4-8	10-16	90-120	120-240
Ropivacaine	0.5% in dextrose		12-18	18-25	80-110	—
Levobupivacaine		8-10	12-20	90-120	100-150	

7. **What are the most common complications of spinal anesthesia?**

Common complications include hypotension, bradycardia, increased sensitivity to sedative medications, nausea and vomiting (possibly secondary to hypotension), post–dural puncture headache (PDPH), and residual back pain and paresthesias (usually associated with the use of lidocaine. Less frequent but more ominous complications include nerve injury, cauda equina syndrome, meningitis, total spinal anesthesia, and hematoma/abscess formation. Particular issues associated with these complications are discussed subsequently.

8. **What are the physiologic changes and risk factors found with SAB-associated hypotension?**

Hypotension occurs as a result of a loss of sympathetically mediated peripheral vascular resistance. Arterial pressure and central venous pressure decrease with only mild decreases in heart rate, stroke volume, and cardiac output. Hypovolemia, age greater than 40 years, sensory level greater than T5, baseline systolic blood pressure below 120 mm Hg, and performance of the block at or above L3-L4 increase the incidence of hypotension. Hypotension (and possibly decreased cerebral blood flow) may be responsible for nausea and vomiting observed with SAB. Patients should receive a bolus of crystalloid or colloid (250 to 1000 ml) before SAB. Because of the pattern of distribution, colloid is more effective, although more expensive. Volume expansion and intravenous sympathomimetics usually reverse hypotension should it occur. Trendelenburg position may raise the level of blockade and should be used with caution and vigilance. Volume loading should also be used cautiously in patients with limited cardiac reserve. In these patients, as the block recedes, vascular tone increases, raising the central blood volume, which may precipitate heart failure. Strategies to create a unilateral block may also decrease the hypotension associated with SAB. At one time, blocks higher than T4 were thought to be associated with hypoventilation, but now hyperventilation is thought to be common. In fact, hypoventilation is no longer thought to be associated with cardiac arrest.

9. **What are the etiology and risk factors for SAB-associated bradycardia?**

Bradycardia may occur secondary to unopposed vagal tone from a high sympathectomy, blockade of the cardioaccelerator fibers (T1-T4), and the Bezold-Jarisch reflex (slowing of the heart rate secondary to a decrease in venous return). Patients with underlying increased vagal tone (children and adults with resting heart rates <60) are at increased risk. Bradycardia may be treated with anticholinergic agents (atropine) or β-adrenergic agonists such as ephedrine.

10. **Why are patients who have received spinal anesthetics especially sensitive to sedative medications? What is deafferentation?**

Caplan and associates (1988) published a landmark review of healthy patients who, while undergoing elective surgery using spinal anesthesia, experienced a sleeplike state without spontaneous verbalization followed by respiratory and cardiac arrest. Despite the fact that these were witnessed arrests, the patients were difficult to resuscitate and either died or had severe neurologic deficits. Subsequently it has been determined that patients receiving spinal anesthetics are especially sensitive to sedative medications. The cause of this may be loss of peripheral input into the reticular activating system (RAS), that part of the brainstem responsible for maintaining arousal. It appears that motor spinal fibers and afferent sensory input into the RAS contribute to wakefulness and this input is diminished by spinal anesthesia, rendering the patient prone to oversedation. Spinal (and epidural) anesthesia increases the hypnotic potential of midazolam, isoflurane, sevoflurane, and thiopental.

11. **Review the clinical features of total spinal anesthesia.**

Total spinal anesthesia results from local anesthetic depression of the cervical spinal cord and brainstem. Signs and symptoms include dysphonia, dyspnea, upper extremity weakness, loss of consciousness, pupillary dilation, hypotension, bradycardia, and cardiopulmonary arrest. Early recognition is the key to management. Treatment includes securing the airway, mechanical ventilation, volume infusion, and pressor support. The patient should receive sedation once ventilation is instituted and the hemodynamics stabilize. The effects of total spinal anesthesia usually resolve by the conclusion of the surgical procedure, and, unless otherwise contraindicated, the patient can be extubated.

12. **If a patient has a cardiac arrest while having an SAB, how should resuscitative measures differ from standard advanced cardiac life support protocols?**
Overall incidence of cardiac arrest associated with SAB is estimated at 0.07%, a rare incidence. However, standard advanced cardiovascular life support (ACLS) guidelines for cardiac resuscitation are insufficient under this circumstance. Since these patients have loss of sympathetic tone and decreased peripheral vascular resistance, rapidly escalating doses of epinephrine will be necessary to increase peripheral resistance and coronary artery perfusion. Until effective, consider doubling each subsequent dose of epinephrine (e.g., 1 mg, then 2 mg, then 4 mg, and so on).

13. **What are the clinical features of a PDPH, and what is the treatment?**
A potentially severe headache may develop after dural puncture, presumably secondary to the rent in the dura and resultant CSF leak, which may cause traction on the meninges and cranial nerves. The headache typically occurs soon after the puncture. It is characteristically intense, often localized to the occipital region and neck, and worse in the upright position. Diplopia or blurred vision may occur. Newer pencil-point needles have reduced the incidence of PDPH to about 1%. Women, younger patients, parturients, and obese patients tend to have a higher incidence of PDPH, and PDPHs are more closely related to epidural techniques than to spinal techniques. Hydration, analgesics, and caffeine mostly temporize the headache; epidural blood patching (administration of about 20 ml) has >75% success rate. It is important to rule out severe hypertension or central nervous system maladies as a cause of the symptoms before assuming that the patient has a PDPH.

14. **What is the risk of neurologic injury after spinal anesthesia?**
Direct trauma to nerve fibers may occur from the spinal needle and may be heralded by a paresthesia, for which the spinal needle should be redirected. Hematoma formation from epidural venous bleeding (from direct trauma or coagulopathy) or abscess formation is suggested by persistent neurologic deficits or severe back pain. Early recognition and management are imperative to avoid permanent neurologic sequelae. In patients who have received any medication with anticoagulant potential, it is important not to attribute persistent neurologic deficits to residual effects of local anesthesia. Adhesive arachnoiditis has been reported and is presumably caused by injection of an irritant into the subarachnoid space.

15. **What is the effect of spinal anesthesia on temperature regulation?**
Because patients become vasodilated and cannot shiver in response to decreases in body temperature, hypothermia is a risk. Curiously, patients may not perceive cold because the vasodilated extremities are warm. In addition, hypothermia may not be detected by the clinician because temperature monitoring is not widely practiced in patients receiving regional anesthesia and it would be necessary to monitor a site that reflects core body temperature such as the tympanic membrane. Patients receiving regional anesthetics should also be warmed using heated forced air devices.

16. **What are contraindications to spinal anesthesia?**
Absolute contraindications include local infection at the puncture site, bacteremia, severe hypovolemia, coagulopathy, severe stenotic valvular disease, infection at the site of the procedure, and intracranial hypertension. Relative contraindications include progressive degenerative (demyelinating) neurologic disease (e.g., multiple sclerosis), low back pain, and sepsis.

17. **Review the current recommendations for administering regional anesthesia to patients with altered coagulation caused by medications.**
The American Society of Regional Anesthesia and Pain Medicine has defined the risks of regional anesthesia in the anticoagulated patient. Key points include:
- Patients on thrombolytic/fibrinolytic therapy should not receive regional anesthesia except in the most extreme circumstances. Patients who have had regional anesthesia before such therapy has been instituted should receive serial neurologic checks.
- Oral anticoagulants should be stopped 4 to 5 days before the planned procedure, and prothrombin time/international normalized ratio normalized. Bridging doses of low-molecular-weight heparin (LMWH) may be necessary as oral anticoagulants are held.

- Concurrent administration of medications that affect bleeding by different mechanisms (e.g., antiplatelet drugs, aspirin, heparin) complicates the decision to perform regional anesthesia; therefore decisions must be individualized. Patients taking only nonsteroidal antiinflammatory drugs can safely have either single-shot or catheter regional anesthetics.
- Thrombocytopenia and an altered coagulation cascade are likely contraindications to regional anesthesia.

18. **Should spinal (or epidural) anesthesia be performed when unfractionated heparin is administered?**
    - If heparin is to be administered, coexisting thrombocytopenia, antiplatelet medications, oral anticoagulants, and other bleeding dyscrasias suggest that regional techniques should be avoided.
    - The subcutaneous administration of minidoses of unfractionated heparin is not contraindicated, but it is best to time performance of the block when the heparin effect is minimal. Similarly, a heparin dose should be held if it is scheduled soon after performance of the block.
    - In vascular patients who will receive large doses of heparin, avoid regional techniques if other coagulopathies are present, delay heparin administration for at least 1 hour after the procedure, and time removal of the catheter for when heparin effect has diminished (1 hour before subsequent doses or 2 to 4 hours after the last dose). There are no data to guide decision making should a bloody tap occur.
    - Prolonged therapeutic anticoagulation may increase the risk of spinal hematoma, especially if other coagulation abnormalities coexist.

19. **Should spinal (or epidural) anesthesia be performed when LMWH is administered?**
    - Patients who have received LMWH should be believed to have altered coagulation, and a single-shot spinal injection is the safest procedure for these patients. As in the case with unfractionated heparin, other factors that increase the likelihood of bleeding will increase the risk of spinal hematoma when LMWH is administered.
    - Timing of the neuraxial procedure and dosing LMWH is extremely important, as is the dose of LMWH. Needle placement should occur at least 10 to 12 hours after an LMWH dose. Neuraxial procedures should be delayed for 24 hours when the patient is receiving larger LMWH doses: enoxaparin 1 mg/kg q12h, enoxaparin 1.5 mg/kg daily, dalteparin 120 units/kg q12h, dalteparin 200 units/kg daily, or tinzaparin 175 units/kg.
    - A bloody spinal tap should not cause cancellation of the surgery but should delay administration of LMWH by 24 hours.
    - If a patient is to have an epidural catheter for postoperative pain management and is also to receive LMWH after surgery, twice-daily dosing has a greater risk of spinal hematoma formation than single daily dosing, and the benefits of an epidural catheter in a patient receiving twice-daily dosing should be weighed against the risks. Although some authorities are more aggressive, a safe practice is to delay the first dose for at least 24 hours after surgery, and a catheter should be removed a minimum of 10 to 12 hours after the last dose of LMWH.

20. **What are the sites of action, benefits, and side effects of intrathecal opioids?**
    Opioids produce intense visceral analgesia and may prolong sensory blockade without affecting motor or sympathetic function. The major sites of action are the opiate receptors within the second and third laminae of the substantia gelatinosa in the dorsal horn of the spinal cord. Lipophilic agents such as fentanyl and sufentanil have a much more localized effect than do hydrophilic agents such as the hydrophilic opioid morphine. Fentanyl and sufentanil have a rapid onset of action and an effective duration greater than 6 hours. Morphine lasts 6 to 24 hours. Side effects include respiratory depression (which may occur late with hydrophilic agents), nausea, vomiting, pruritus, and urinary retention. Opioid antagonists or agonist/antagonists reverse the complications but, if given in large doses, may also reverse analgesia.

21. **What is transient neurologic syndrome (TNS) and its cause?**
    TNS was first described in 1993. Common findings include pain or dysesthesias in the buttocks radiating to the dorsolateral aspect of the thighs and calves. The pain has been

alternatively described as sharp and lancinating or dull, aching, cramping, or burning. Usually symptoms improve with moving about, are worse at night, and respond to nonsteroidal antiinflammatory drugs. The pain is moderate to severe in at least 70% of the patients with TNS and diminishes over time, resolving spontaneously within approximately a week in about 90% of those affected. It is extremely rare for pain to continue beyond 2 weeks. It is significant to note that no objective neurologic findings are encountered on physical exam.

TNS is associated with the use of spinal lidocaine in the majority of cases, and its incidence, although variable in studies, probably averages about 15%. Much more rarely, TNS has been associated with the use of bupivacaine, prilocaine, procaine, and mepivacaine. The concentration of lidocaine does not appear to be a factor (TNS has been observed with 5% hyperbaric and 2% isobaric lidocaine). There is no association with the presence of dextrose, opioids, epinephrine, or the baricity or osmolarity of the solution. Furthermore, neither gender, weight, age, needle type, difficulty with, nor paresthesias during block placement are factors, although lithotomy positioning may have been a factor. Bupivacaine is not associated with TNS. Interestingly, pregnancy may protect against lidocaine-associated TNS.

KEY POINTS: SPINAL ANESTHESIA

1. Loss of afferent sensory and motor stimulation renders a patient sensitive to sedative medications secondary to deafferentation. For the same reason, neuraxial anesthesia decreases the minimum alveolar concentration of volatile anesthetics.
2. Vagal predominance suggests that a patient may be at risk for cardiovascular collapse during neuraxial anesthesia.
3. Patients with sympathectomies from regional anesthesia require aggressive resuscitation, perhaps with unfamiliarly large doses of pressors, to reestablish myocardial perfusion after cardiac arrest.
4. Suspect transient neurologic syndrome (TNS) in a patient who has received a lidocaine spinal anesthetic and has postanesthetic complaints of pain in buttocks and dorsal lower extremities. Note that there are no objective neurologic findings with this syndrome.

22. **Since lidocaine is associated with TNS, what would be an appropriate local anesthetic selection for an ambulatory procedure?**
Bupivacaine administered in 5- to 7.5-mg doses will achieve peak sensory blocks in the midthoracic region with durations of sensory blockade of about 2 hours, and duration of motor blockade of about an hour and time to discharge may not be appreciably different than if lidocaine is used. Doses of bupivacaine greater than 10 mg will result in delays in voiding. This may not necessarily delay discharge to home if there is not a history of difficulty voiding and the procedure was in a nonpelvic area. Bladder ultrasound has been used to identify patients requiring catheterization. Since TNS was identified, use of spinal lidocaine seems to have disappeared.

23. **Can continuous spinal anesthesia be performed?**
Continuous spinal anesthesia is a technique regaining popularity. In the early 1990s, many cases of cauda equina syndrome were noted after inappropriate dosing of spinal microcatheters. It appeared that the lack of turbulence associated with injecting through microcatheters led to a pooling of local anesthetic caudad to the lumbar lordotic curve, leading to repeated and inappropriate dosing of local anesthetics.

Continuous spinal anesthesia is safe and effective using 18- to 22-G epidural needles and catheters (and improved, specially designed kits). The incidence of hypotension is less, as is the need to rescue with vasopressors. This technique allows for titration of local anesthetics to effect and has been successfully used in elderly patients, patients with aortic stenosis, and trauma patients. This is an attractive technique for the elderly because they tend not to develop PDPH despite dural punctures with large-gauge epidural needles.

WEBSITE

American Society of Regional Anesthesia and Pain Management: http://www.asra.com

SUGGESTED READINGS

Caplan RA, Ward RJ, Posner K, et al: Unexpected cardiac arrest during spinal anesthesia: a closed claims analysis of predisposing factors, Anesthesiology 68:5–11, 1988.

Hocking G, Wildsmith JA: Intrathecal drug spread, Br J Anaesth 93:568–578, 2004.

Kopp SL, Horlocker TT, Warner ME, et al: Cardiac arrest during neuraxial anesthesia, Anesth Analg 100:855–865, 2005.

Moen V, Dahlgren N, Irestedt L: Severe neurological complications after central neuraxial blockades in Sweden 1990–1999, Anesthesiology 101:950–959, 2004.

Pollard JB: Cardiac arrest during spinal anesthesia: common mechanisms and strategies for prevention, Anesth Analg 92:252–256, 2001.

Zaric D, Christiansen C, Pace NL, et al: Transient neurologic symptoms after spinal anesthesia with lidocaine versus other local anesthetics: a systematic review of randomized, controlled trials, Anesth Analg 100:1811–1816, 2005.

CHAPTER 62

EPIDURAL ANALGESIA AND ANESTHESIA

Rachel M. Kacmar, MD, and Andrea J. Fuller, MD

1. **Where is the epidural space? Describe the relevant anatomy.**
   The epidural space lies just outside and encircles the dural sac containing the spinal cord and cerebrospinal fluid (CSF). As the epidural needle enters the midline of the back between the bony spinous processes, it passes through:
   - Skin
   - Subcutaneous fat
   - Supraspinous ligament
   - Interspinous ligament
   - Ligamentum flavum
   - Epidural space
     Beyond the epidural space lie the spinal meninges and CSF. The epidural space has its widest point (5 mm) at L2. In addition to the traversing nerve roots, it contains fat, lymphatics, and an extensive venous plexus (Batson plexus). The epidural space wraps 360 degrees around the dural membrane. Superiorly the space extends to the foramen magnum, where dura is fused to the base of the skull. Caudally it ends at the sacral hiatus. The most anterior boundary of the epidural space is the posterior longitudinal ligament. The epidural space can be entered in the cervical, thoracic, lumbar, or sacral regions to provide anesthesia. In pediatric patients the caudal epidural approach is commonly used (see Question 3).

2. **Differentiate between a spinal and an epidural anesthetic.**
   A spinal anesthetic is performed by puncturing the dura and injecting a small amount of local anesthetic directly into the CSF, producing a rapid, dense, and predictable neural blockade. An epidural anesthetic requires a tenfold increase in dose of local anesthetic to fill the epidural space and penetrate the nerve coverings. The block onset is slower and often less dense, and the anesthesia produced tends to be segmental (i.e., a band of anesthesia is produced, extending upward and downward from the injection site). The degree of segmental spread depends largely on the volume of local anesthetic. For example, a 5-ml volume may produce only a narrow band of anesthesia covering three to five dermatomes, whereas a 20-ml volume may produce anesthesia from the upper thoracic to sacral dermatomes. Placement of an epidural anesthetic requires a larger needle, often includes a continuous catheter technique, and has a subtle end point for locating the space. The epidural space is located by following the feel of the ligaments as they are passed through until there is loss of resistance, whereas the subarachnoid space is definitively identified by CSF flow from the needle following dural puncture.

3. **How is caudal anesthesia related to epidural anesthesia? When is it used?**
   Caudal anesthesia is a form of epidural anesthesia in which the injection is made at the sacral hiatus (S5). Because the dural sac normally ends at S2, accidental spinal injection is rare. Although the caudal approach to the epidural space provides dense sacral and lower lumbar levels of block, its use is limited by major problems:
   - Highly variable sacral anatomy in adults
   - Calcification/ossification of the sacral ligaments in adults
   - Risk of injection into a venous plexus
   - Difficulty in maintaining sterility if a catheter is used
     Caudal anesthesia is used primarily in children (whose anatomy is predictable) to provide postoperative analgesia after herniorrhaphy or perineal procedures. A catheter can be inserted for long-term use if desired.

4. **What are the advantages of epidural anesthesia versus spinal anesthesia?**
   - Epidural anesthesia can produce a segmental block focused only on the area of surgery or pain (e.g., during labor or for thoracic procedures).
   - There is more flexibility in the density of block; if less motor block is desired (for labor analgesia or postoperative pain management), a lower concentration of local anesthetic can be used.
   - The gradual onset of sympathetic block allows time to manage associated hypotension.
   - Duration of anesthesia can be prolonged by continuous infusion or bolus redosing through an indwelling epidural catheter.
   - Theoretically with no hole in the dura there should be no spinal headache; however, an inadvertent dural puncture occurs 0.5% to 4% of the time with the large-bore epidural needle, and about 50% of such patients require treatment for headache. Because newer technology in spinal needles has decreased the incidence of headache requiring treatment to less than 1%, this advantage is probably no longer true.

5. **What are the disadvantages of epidural compared with spinal anesthesia?**
   - The induction of epidural anesthesia is slower because of more complex placement, the necessity of incremental dosing of the local anesthetic, and the slower onset of anesthesia in the epidural space.
   - Because a larger volume of local anesthetic is used, there is risk of local anesthetic toxicity if a vein is entered with the needle or catheter (Figure 62-1).
   - Epidural anesthesia is less reliable; it is not as dense, the block can be patchy or one-sided, and there is no definite confirmatory end point (comparable to seeing CSF in the needle) during placement.

6. **What is a combined spinal-epidural anesthetic? Why use both?**
   To perform a combined spinal-epidural anesthetic, a long spinal needle is passed through an epidural needle that has been placed into the epidural space, and the dura is punctured. When CSF is obtained from the spinal needle, a dose of local anesthetic is deposited in the subarachnoid space, and the spinal needle is removed. The epidural catheter is then threaded into the epidural space, and the epidural needle is removed. This technique combines the advantages of both spinal and epidural anesthesia: rapid onset of an intense spinal block so

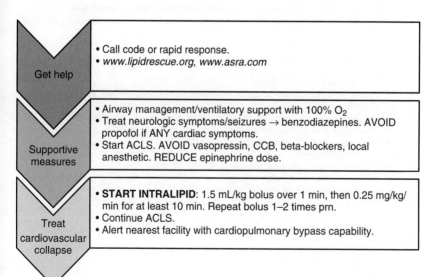

Figure 62-1. Treatment of local anesthetic systemic toxicity (LAST). *ACLS,* Advanced cardiovascular life support; CCB, calcium channel blockers.

that the surgery can proceed quickly and an epidural catheter to extend the duration of the block if necessary for a long surgical procedure or for postoperative pain management.

7. **What are the advantages of using neuraxial (epidural or spinal) anesthesia versus general anesthesia?**
   - Avoidance of initial airway manipulation; useful for asthmatics, known difficult airways, and patients with a full stomach
   - Decreased stress response; less hypertension and tachycardia and cortisol release
   - Less thrombogenesis and subsequent thromboembolism; a proven benefit in orthopedic hip and knee surgery
   - Improved bowel motility with less distention; sympathetic blockade provides relatively more parasympathetic tone
   - The patient can be awake during the procedure; desirable for cesarean deliveries and certain arthroscopic procedures
   - Less postoperative nausea and sedation
   - Better postoperative pain control, especially for thoracic, upper abdominal, and orthopedic procedures
   - Less pulmonary dysfunction, due to better pain control and absence of airway manipulation
   - Faster turnover at the end of the case because there is no emergence time

8. **What are the disadvantages of neuraxial anesthesia compared with general anesthesia?**
   - Initiation of the anesthetic is slower at the beginning of the case.
   - It is less reliable, with a higher failure rate.
   - Emergent management of the airway could result from failed block or patient intolerance to surgery, inadvertent high cervical block, sudden hemorrhage or hemodynamic instability, or other intraoperative complications. In a patient with a difficult airway or a full stomach, this possibility must be considered and planned for.
   - There are occasional contraindications, including coagulopathy, hemodynamic instability, spinal instrumentation, or patient refusal.
   - Prolonged procedures or extremes of position may be uncomfortable or intolerable to patients.

9. **What factors should the anesthesiologist address in the preoperative assessment before performing an epidural anesthetic? Should special laboratory tests be performed?**
   In addition to the general preoperative assessment of every patient before surgery, the following specific items should be assessed before performing epidural anesthesia:
   - **History**
     - Previous back injury or surgery
     - Neurologic symptoms or history of neurologic disease (e.g., diabetic neuropathy, multiple sclerosis)
     - Bleeding tendencies or disease associated with coagulopathy (e.g., preeclampsia)
     - Anticoagulation medication (current or recent, including aspirin)
     - Prior regional anesthesia and any associated problems
   - **Physical examination**
     - Brief neurologic examination for strength and sensation
     - Back examination for landmarks and potential anatomic abnormalities (scoliosis) or pathology (infection at the site of placement)
   - **Surgery**
     - Expected duration and blood loss
     - Positioning required
     - Amount of muscle relaxation necessary
     - Surgeon's preferences (does he/she prefer all, some, or no patients have regional anesthesia as an option?)
   - **General information**
     - The patient should be given a detailed explanation of the procedure, risks, benefits, and options (including general anesthesia if the block fails).
     - Discuss whether the patient desires sedation and how much.

- **Laboratory tests**
  - None is specifically necessary except as based on the history and physical examination.

10. **Describe the technique for performing a lumbar epidural anesthetic.**
    - Resuscitation equipment must be immediately available: oxygen, equipment for positive-pressure ventilation and intubation, and pressors to treat hypotension.
    - Monitor the patient with at least a pulse oximeter and blood pressure cuff.
    - Place a well-running intravenous (IV) line and consider an appropriate co-load of fluid to protect against hypotension after sympathetic blockade.
    - The patient may be sitting or in a lateral position. The spinous processes should be aligned in the same vertical or horizontal plane and maximally flexed. Administer sedation as deemed appropriate.
    - For lumbar epidural placement, visualize a line between the iliac crests to locate the L4 spinous process. Palpate the L2–L3, L3–L4, and L4–L5 interspaces and choose the widest or the closest to the desired anesthetic level. For abdominal or thoracic surgeries, know the appropriate level for catheter placement.
    - Make a skin wheal after sterile preparation and draping of the field. The anesthesiologist must wear a hat, mask, and sterile gloves. The patient should wear a hat. Any additional providers or family members should wear a hat and mask.
    - The epidural needle is inserted in the midline through the skin wheal until increased resistance from ligaments is felt. Remove the needle stylet and attach a syringe with 3 to 4 ml of air or saline. When the barrel of the syringe is tapped, it should feel firm and bounce back while the tip of the needle is in the ligament.
    - Advance several millimeters at a time, tapping the syringe intermittently. The ability to recognize the feel of various layers of ligament comes with experience. Ligamentum flavum is often described as leathery, gritty, or producing a marked increase in resistance. This is the last layer before the epidural space.
    - As the needle passes through ligamentum flavum and enters the epidural space, there is often a *pop* or *give*, and the air or fluid in the syringe injects easily; this marks the loss of resistance.
    - The syringe is removed, and while the nondominant hand grasps the hub of the needle to brace it, the dominant hand threads the catheter about 5 cm into the space (5 cm past the tip of the epidural needle).
    - The epidural needle is withdrawn carefully so as not to dislodge the catheter. After attaching the injector port to the catheter, it is aspirated for blood or CSF; if negative, a test dose may be given. The catheter is then secured in place.

11. **What is the paramedian technique for epidural placement? When is it most useful?**
    - Paramedian epidural placement starts by identifying the spinous process at the desired interspace level and using local anesthetic to create a skin wheal 1 to 2 fingerbreadths lateral to that point.
    - Insert the epidural needle through the wheal perpendicular to the patient's skin until the transverse process of the vertebra is encountered.
    - Walk the epidural needle off the transverse process, moving superiorly and medially (about 15 to 30 degrees, angulation—do not cross midline), until the needle is engaged in the ligamentum flavum.
    - Attach a loss of resistance syringe filled with either air or saline and advance until loss of resistance is achieved.
    - This approach is useful at high thoracic levels (above ≈T9–T10) where the spinous processes are acutely angled making midline approach difficult. It also has advantages in situations where the spaces between spinous processes are small or tight.

12. **Are there any contraindications to epidural anesthesia?**
    Absolute contraindications
    - Patient refusal. Sometimes a more thorough explanation will allay the patient's fears and make the technique acceptable. Some common concerns include:
      - Having to watch surgery or remain wide awake
      - Fear of a needle in the spinal cord and/or fear of paralysis

- Pain (acute or chronic)
- Reassure patients that a curtain will block their view and that the desired degree of sedation can be provided. For lumbar epidural placements, explain that the spinal cord ends at about L1 in adults and that the needle is placed below that level. Compare the procedure to the placement of the IV line, which also uses a 16- or 18-G needle, and explain that a local anesthetic will be used in the skin. Counsel that epidural placement does not cause chronic back pain, and the most common postoperative insertion site discomfort is comparable to the soreness from an intramuscular injection in the arm ("like a flu shot").
- Sepsis with hemodynamic instability. The induction of sympathetic blockade decreases systemic vascular resistance (SVR) even further. There is also a remote risk of epidural abscess if bacteremic blood is introduced into the epidural space without prior antibiotic coverage.
- Uncorrected hypovolemia. With ongoing hemorrhage, the fall in SVR can produce severe refractory hypotension.
- Coagulopathy. If a vessel is injured within the epidural space, an epidural hematoma could form, causing neurologic damage by spinal cord compression.

Relative contraindications
- Elevated intracranial pressure
- Prior back injury with neurologic deficit
- Progressive neurologic disease such as multiple sclerosis
- Chronic back pain
- Localized infection at the injection site

13. **What physiologic changes should be expected after successful initiation of an epidural anesthetic?**
    - **Decrease in blood pressure:** Due to sympathectomy below the level of the block and vasodilation. Afterload reduction can actually be useful for patients with hypertension or congestive heart failure if preload and heart rate are maintained.
    - **Changes in heart rate:** Tachycardia may occur as cardiac output increases to compensate for a drop in SVR. Bradycardia may occur if blockade above T4 disrupts the cardiac sympathetic accelerator fibers.
    - **Ventilatory changes:** In normal patients ventilation is maintained as long as the diaphragm is not impaired (phrenic nerve: C3–C5), but patients may become subjectively dyspneic as they become unable to feel their intercostal muscles. Patients who are dependent on accessory muscles of respiration may be impaired at lower levels of anesthesia. The ability to cough and protect the airway may be lost even if ventilation is adequate. Upper extremity weakness or speech changes are signs of an evolving high block and the possibility of impending ventilatory failure.
    - **Bladder distention:** Sympathetic blockade and loss of sensation may require catheterization for urinary retention.
    - **Intestinal contraction:** Sympathetic blockade with parasympathetic predominance contracts the bowel.
    - **Change in thermoregulation:** Peripheral vasodilation lowers core body temperature if the patient is not covered. Shivering is common during epidural anesthesia, which will increase oxygen consumption.
    - **Neuroendocrine changes:** Neural blockade above T8 blocks sympathetic afferents to the adrenal medulla, inhibiting the neural component of the stress response. Glucose control is better maintained.

14. **What are the potential complications of epidural anesthesia? Can they be anticipated or prevented?**
    - Hypotension caused by sympathetic blockade, which may be prevented by fluid co-load and patient positioning. Have vasopressors such as phenylephrine or ephedrine available.
    - Pruritus secondary to narcotic administration in the neuraxis. This can be treated with a small dose of nalbuphine or naloxone if severe.
    - Subarachnoid injection of a large volume of local anesthetic ("total spinal"). This can be prevented by aspirating the catheter for CSF and giving a small initial dose of local anesthetic to look for rapid onset of sensory block due to the drug entering the

intrathecal space. (Remember: the onset of an epidural anesthetic is slow.) If a total spinal occurs, treat hypotension with pressors and support ventilation with positive pressure by mask or intubation.

- Intravascular injection of local anesthetic. This can be prevented by aspirating the catheter for blood, injecting a marker such as epinephrine that will cause tachycardia if injected into a vessel, and using incremental dosing (no more than 5 ml at a time) (please refer to question 15 below and Figure 62-1).
- Post–dural puncture headache (PDPH). More commonly caused by accidental dural puncture with a large-bore epidural needle, PDPH can also occur after an uncomplicated spinal needle insertion. Although not completely preventable, this can be treated in various ways, depending on the preference of the patient and anesthesiologist. Common therapies include analgesics, caffeine, or an epidural *blood patch*. Factors determining choice of treatment include severity of the headache and how aggressively the patient wishes to be treated. To provide a blood patch, up to 20 ml of the patient's sterile blood is placed in the epidural space to seal the dural hole, prevent further CSF leakage, and elevate low CSF pressure. Prophylactic epidural blood patch is not indicated. PDPH is generally a self-limiting process that should resolve in 7 to 10 days even without intervention.
- Epidural hematomas are extremely rare and usually occur spontaneously in clinical settings outside of the operating room rather than after neuraxial procedures. When they are associated with regional anesthesia, there is almost always a preexisting coagulopathy. Epidural hematomas present as back pain and leg weakness and must be rapidly diagnosed by computed tomography (CT) or magnetic resonance imaging (MRI). If the hematoma is not surgically decompressed in 6 to 8 hours, neurologic recovery is rare.
- Epidural abscess or meningitis. Both are quite rare with proper sterile technique and universal precautions. Several reports link these complications to respiratory bacteria that entered the neuraxis when an anesthesiologist performed an epidural without a mask.
- Nerve root injury. Although rare to have actual injury, paresthesias during epidural placement are not uncommon. If a patient complains of paresthesia, redirect the epidural needle. Never inject medication if the patient feels pain during injection.

15. **What is local anesthetic systemic toxicity (LAST)? How is it treated?**
- LAST occurs after a large dose of local anesthetic is injected intravascularly, or is absorbed from the block site, and overwhelming sodium channel blockade occurs.
- The following blocks are listed from highest to lowest in systemic absorption: intercostal > caudal > epidural > brachial plexus > sciatic nerve.
- Signs, symptoms, and treatment: Depending on the local anesthetic, there may be a stepwise progression of symptoms or sudden, fulminant cardiovascular collapse.
  - Patients may complain of metallic taste, perioral tingling, or lightheadedness.
  - Neurologic symptoms such as tonic-clonic seizures may occur. Stop convulsions with an induction agent or rapid-acting anticonvulsant (benzodiazepine). Intubate the trachea, if necessary, for ventilation and airway protection.
  - Cardiovascular collapse may occur. Initial supportive treatment is with pressors, inotropes, and advanced cardiovascular life support protocols. Start Intralipid (20% lipid emulsion) bolus as soon as possible (1.5 ml/kg over 1 min) followed by infusion at 0.25 ml/kg/min. The bolus may be repeated 1 or 2 times. Avoid propofol (lipid concentration 10%) as it may worsen cardiac instability (see Figure 62-1).
- Intralipid's mechanism of action may be multifaceted. The most commonly accepted thought is that it acts as a lipid sink to remove circulating local anesthetic from the circulation. Other theories include increased mitochondrial uptake of fatty acids, direct lipid interference with local anesthetic binding to sodium channels, cytoprotective action, and calcium channel manipulation with increased inotropy.
- Intralipid should be readily and rapidly available in all locations where neuraxial and regional blocks are performed.

16. **How does one choose which local anesthetic to use?**
The choice of local anesthetic is usually based on the onset, duration, safety profile, and special clinical characteristics of the patient and surgical procedure (Table 62-1).

Table 62-1. Local Anesthetics Used in Epidural Anesthesia for Surgical Procedures

ANESTHETIC	CLASS	CONCENTRATION (%)	ONSET	DURATION	MAXIMAL DOSE WITH EPINEPHRINE	COMMENTS
Chloroprocaine	Ester	3	Rapid	45 min	15 mg/kg	Rapid metabolism, least toxic, intense sensory and motor block
Lidocaine	Amide	2	Immediate	60–90 min	7 mg/kg	Intense sensory and motor block
Bupivacaine	Amide	0.75*, 0.5, 0.25†	Slow	2–3 hr	3 mg/kg	Most cardiotoxic; motor < sensory block
Ropivacaine	Amide	0.75	Slow	2–3 hr	3 mg/kg	Less cardiotoxic than bupivacaine; most expensive

*Not available for obstetric use.
†May not always produce adequate surgical anesthesia.

17. **Why is epinephrine sometimes combined with the local anesthetic? Should it be included in all cases?**
Epinephrine is often added to local anesthetic solutions in a concentration of 5 mcg/ml (1:200,000) or less. There are several benefits to this practice:
- Local α_1 receptor–mediated vasoconstriction reduces uptake into the bloodstream and delays local anesthetic metabolism.
- Improves quality and reliability of blockade, either by increasing the available local anesthetic through decreased uptake or by an intrinsic anesthetic mechanism on central α_2-adrenergic receptors
- Reduces peak blood levels and risk of toxicity by slowing vascular absorption
- Helps to identify an intravascular injection when used as the marker in a test dose. If the epinephrine-containing solution is unintentionally injected into a blood vessel, tachycardia usually results.

Epinephrine may be added to the local anesthetic solution for all blocks except those involving end arteries (digits, penis) or for patients in whom the tachycardia and hypertension may be detrimental (coronary artery disease, preeclampsia).

18. **When should opioids be included in the epidural anesthetic?**
Opioids may be combined with local anesthetic to improve the quality of the surgical block or to manage postoperative pain, either alone or with a dilute local anesthetic solution. Examples of epidural bolus doses are fentanyl 50 to 100 mcg, sufentanil 20 to 30 mcg, and morphine 2 to 5 mg. The opioids act at the μ receptors in the substantia gelatinosa of the spinal cord. The more lipophilic opioids, such as fentanyl and sufentanil, have a fast onset (5 minutes), short duration (2 to 4 hours), and lower incidence of side effects. Morphine is hydrophilic and does not attach to the receptor as easily. It has a long onset (1 hour), long duration (up to 24 hours), and a high incidence of side effects such as itching and nausea. Respiratory depression, although rare, is the most serious concern and requires special monitoring for the duration of the drug.

KEY POINTS: EPIDURAL ANALGESIA AND ANESTHESIA

1. Epidural anesthesia is segmental (i.e., it has an upper and a lower level). The block is most intense near the site of catheter or needle insertion and diminishes with distance.
2. Advantages include avoidance of airway manipulation, decreased stress response, less thrombogenesis, improved bowel motility, awake patient, less postoperative nausea and sedation, better postoperative pain control, and faster turnover.
3. Disadvantages include slower initiation and higher failure rate than general anesthesia.
4. Contraindications include coagulopathy, hemodynamic instability, some types of spinal instrumentation, and patient refusal.
5. Complications include hypotension caused by sympathetic blockade, intravascular injection of local anesthetic, subarachnoid injection of a large volume of local anesthetic (*total spinal*), post–dural puncture headache, and neurologic injury.

19. **Why can some patients with epidural blocks move around and even walk, whereas others have a dense motor block?**
Preserving motor function is especially important in postoperative patients and laboring women. The degree of motor block can be decreased by lowering the concentration of local anesthetic and by choosing a local anesthetic with favorable sensory-motor dissociation. As local anesthetic concentration decreases, the intensity of the block decreases, and fewer motor nerves are affected. Sensory block can be augmented by the addition of epidural opioids if desired. Depending on the surgical site, the rate of infusion can also be adjusted to avoid motor blockade of the lower extremities while still providing analgesia. Bupivacaine and ropivacaine provide relatively less motor block for a given amount of sensory block (so-called sensory-motor dissociation). This property accounts for much of their popularity in obstetric anesthesia. For example, a common epidural infusion for postoperative pain or labor analgesia is 0.1% bupivacaine with 2 to 5 mcg/ml fentanyl.

20. **When is analgesia preferable to anesthesia?**

Anesthesia implies an intense sensory and motor blockade, which is necessary to perform a surgical procedure. It is usually obtained by using the highest available concentration of local anesthetic (e.g., 2% lidocaine or 3% chloroprocaine). Analgesia implies sensory blockade only, usually for postoperative pain management or labor analgesia, and may be achieved with dilute local anesthetic or epidural opioids or a combination of the two.

21. **How do you determine the level of anesthesia needed for different types of surgeries? What is a segmental block? When is it used?**

To provide adequate surgical blockade with an epidural anesthetic, it is necessary to know the innervation of the structures stimulated during the procedure. For example, a transurethral resection of the prostate requires a T8 level because the bladder is innervated by T8 through its embryologic origins. A laparotomy such as a cesarean delivery requires a T4 level to cover the innervation of the peritoneum.

Epidural anesthesia is segmental (i.e., it has an upper and lower level). The block is most intense near the site of catheter insertion and diminishes with distance. The needle and catheter should be placed as close to the site of surgery as possible (e.g., a thoracic injection is used for chest surgery, whereas a midlumbar injection is used for hip surgery). In labor, the lower limit of block can be kept above the sacral nerve roots until the second stage of labor to preserve pelvic floor tone and the perineal reflex.

22. **How do you determine the amount of local anesthetic solution used for different procedures? What factors affect spread in the epidural space?**

The extent of epidural blockade is determined primarily by the volume of local anesthetic; more dermatomes are blocked by more milliliters of local anesthetic. To achieve a T4 level from a lumbar epidural catheter, 20 to 30 ml of solution is required. Other factors that may affect spread in the epidural space include:

- Age: older patients require less local anesthetic
- Pregnancy: requires approximately 30% less
- Obesity: may or may not require less; unpredictable dosing
- Height: taller patients may require more
- Altered spinal anatomy (scoliosis/kyphosis): may have patchy block; may require more or less

23. **What is a combined epidural-general anesthetic? Why give the patient two anesthetics?**

In some surgical procedures, controlled ventilation may be safer or more comfortable for the patient or may be necessary for the surgical procedure. Examples would be intrathoracic or upper abdominal operations. Because these procedures often result in moderate to severe postoperative pain, an epidural anesthetic can be an ideal way to provide pain relief and aid in postoperative mobilization to prevent pulmonary and thromboembolic complications. The epidural anesthetic is placed before induction of general anesthesia. By using the epidural catheter intraoperatively, smaller amounts of general anesthetic agents are required, which may result in fewer hemodynamic effects and faster awakening. At the same time, the patient's airway can be protected, ventilation controlled, and hypnosis and amnesia provided. A specific example of improved outcomes with this combined technique is for patients with chronic obstructive pulmonary disease in whom epidural analgesia contributes to lower postoperative pulmonary complications through faster ventilator weaning and decreased splinting. New evidence also supports that use of epidural anesthesia during breast, ovarian, and colon cancer surgery may improve patient survival.

24. **What should the anesthesiologist ask the patient postoperatively after an epidural anesthetic?**

- **Satisfaction with the anesthetic:** Was there anything that the patient thought should have been done differently? Assess patient satisfaction and try to correct any misunderstandings.
- **Regression of sensory and motor block:** Is there any residual blockade? Can the patient ambulate? Does the patient have any problem with bowel or bladder function? Any of these complaints requires a thorough neurologic examination to localize the deficit. Although the complaint is usually caused by residual local anesthetic or nerve

compression during the surgical procedure (which often resolves with time), in rare instances further evaluation may be needed. Depending on the pattern and severity of the neurologic dysfunction, a formal neurology consultation, electromyogram, or CT may be needed to rule out pathology in the epidural space (such as hematoma).

- **Complaints of back pain:** Examine the site for bruising, redness, or swelling.
- **Complaints of headache:** If an accidental dural puncture occurred, the patient should be followed for several days; such headaches can appear up to 1 week later.
- **Adequacy of postoperative pain relief:** Did any side effects of epidural narcotics (itching, nausea) require treatment? Was pain control acceptable at rest and with movement?

WEBSITES

American Society of Regional Anesthesia and Pain Medicine: http://www.asra.com
LipidRescue™ Resuscitation: www.lipidrescue.org
New York Society of Regional Anesthesia: http://www.nysora.com

SUGGESTED READINGS

Apfel CC, Saxena A, Cakmakkaya OS, et al: Prevention of postdural puncture headache after accidental dural puncture: a quantitative systematic review, Br J Anaesth 105:255–263, 2010.
Berde CB, Strichartz GR: Local anesthetics. In Miller RD, editor: Miller's anesthesia, ed 7, Philadelphia, 2009, Churchill Livingstone, pp 932–934.
Bernards CM, Hostetter LS: Epidural and spinal anesthesia. In Barash PG, Cullen BF, Stoelting RK, et al. editor: Clinical anesthesia, ed 7, Philadelphia, 2013, Lippincott Williams & Wilkins, pp 905–933.
Brown DL: Spinal, epidural and caudal anesthesia. In Miller RD, editor: Miller's anesthesia, ed 7, Philadelphia, 2009, Churchill Livingstone, pp 1611–1638.
Horlocker TT, Wedel DJ, Rowlingson JC, et al: Regional anesthesia in the patient receiving antithrombotic or thrombolytic therapy: American Society of Regional Anesthesia and Pain Medicine evidence-based guidelines, Reg Anesth Pain Med 35:64–101, 2010.
Weinberg G: Lipid infusion resuscitation for local anesthetic toxicity, Anesthesiology 105:7–8, 2006.
Weinberg G: Lipid emulsion infusion: resuscitation for local anesthetic and drug overdose, Anesthesiology 117:180–187, 2012.

1. **What are the advantages of peripheral nerve blocks (PNBs)?**
   PNBs share many of their advantages with neuraxial (spinal and epidural) anesthetic and analgesic techniques, first of which is the lack of need for airway instrumentation. This feature makes PNBs useful in cases in which airway management will be difficult or in which the patient has borderline respiratory function. PNB allows for shorter discharge times in ambulatory settings because of the decreased incidence of nausea, vomiting, and severe pain. PNB may diminish or prevent the development of chronic pain syndromes because of the lack of central nervous system sensitization that occurs after acute injury. Finally, patients with PNB have minimal if any opioid requirements in the immediate postoperative phase.

2. **What basic principles should be followed to ensure a safe and successful PNB?**
   Patients should be informed about the potential risks and benefits of PNB and allowed to decide on the anesthetic they prefer. Not all patients are good candidates for regional anesthetics. For example, performing PNB after high-velocity trauma to a lower extremity might obscure the diagnosis of a compartment syndrome. Sedation should be carefully titrated while performing a PNB because the patient should be able to communicate and give feedback to the clinician. This helps in confirming correct needle placement and giving an early warning of local anesthetic toxicity.
   The clinician must have knowledge of the anatomy, technique, and equipment necessary to perform the most appropriate block for a given situation. The use of aseptic technique, correct equipment (B-bevel needles, nerve stimulators, ultrasound), and basic physiologic monitoring is mandatory. The area in which the PNB is performed should have immediate access to resuscitative equipment and medications.

3. **What are the risks of performing a PNB?**
   - There may be inadvertent damage to anatomic structures by the advancing needle. Examples include direct trauma to the nerve or spinal cord by intraneural injection of local anesthetic, nerve laceration, vascular injury with resulting hematoma formation, or pneumothorax.
   - The drugs that are injected may have undesirable local and systemic effects. Allergic reactions to local anesthetics are rare. Ester local anesthetics are derivatives of *p*-aminobenzoic acid, a known allergen, and therefore are more likely to cause allergic reactions than the amide local anesthetics. Any local anesthetic injected intravascularly has the potential for systemic reactions, including seizures and cardiovascular collapse.

4. **How can the risks from a PNB be minimized?**
   It is essential to ensure correct needle placement. Knowledge of the anatomy of the target region and the surrounding structures is necessary. Knowledge of the equipment and of the pharmacology of local anesthetics is also required. Do not perform a PNB with which you are unfamiliar or not trained to do.

5. **Describe a good technique for advancing the needle and injecting the local anesthetic solution.**
   Continuous aspiration is mandatory while advancing the needle; flow of blood or cerebrospinal fluid is an obvious sign that the needle needs to be redirected and the landmarks reevaluated. Be attentive to reports of symptoms experienced by the patient. A paresthesia indicates close proximity to a nerve; and, depending on the technique being used, it might constitute the end point.
   Once it is determined that the needle is correctly positioned, a 1-ml test dose is administered. Severe pain during injection might be a sign of intraneural needle placement.

Evidence suggests that monitoring the injection pressure is useful in preventing intraneural injection. After the test dose is administered, slow incremental injection of the local anesthetic solution is started. This is a very important safety feature since it allows recognition of signs of local anesthetic toxicity before cardiac collapse occurs.

6. **How are peripheral nerves localized?**
The use of ultrasound has rapidly become the preferred mode to localize nerves. The identification of structures such as blood vessels and fascial planes and their relationship to peripheral nerves facilitates the correct identification of the target nerves. The use of anatomic landmarks to allow precise identification of correct skin insertion sites has been relegated by the use of ultrasound guidance. After the needle is inserted, the nerves can be identified by ultrasonic imaging, nerve stimulation, the presence of paresthesia, or a combination of these modalities. In the nerve stimulation technique, the clinician looks for a known motor response during electrical stimulation of 0.5 mA or less to signal correct needle position.

7. **Is one technique to localize nerves better or safer than any other?**
Improvements in ultrasound equipment have made ultrasonic guidance more popular over the past few years. The safety of PNB may also have been improved by the introduction of ultrasound, although no study has demonstrated this. In experienced hands there seems to be no significant difference between nerve stimulator, landmark techniques, and ultrasound-guided PNB in terms of success rate or complications. If nothing else, ultrasound guidance is responsible for a resurgence of interest in regional anesthesia in many anesthesia practices.

8. **When using ultrasound guidance, what is the difference between an in-plane and an out-of-plane approach?**
The in-plane approach means that the shaft of the needle is visualized while the needle is advanced (Figure 63-1). This technique allows the operator to observe the tip of the needle as it advances through the different anatomic structures. The out-of-plane approach relies

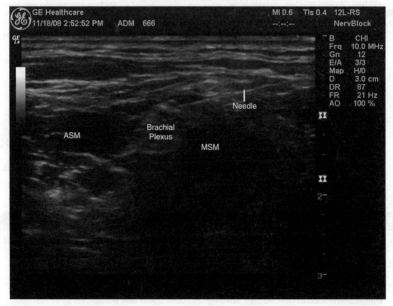

Figure 63-1. A good example of an in-plane approach. Note the needle shaft and tip as it comes in contact with the brachial plexus between the anterior scalene muscle (ASM) and the middle scalene muscle (MSM).

on known anatomic relationships and careful injection (which can be observed in real time) to evaluate the adequacy of needle placement. In the out-of-plane approach, the short axis (transverse cut) of the needle is visualized.

9. **Is there a way to extend the duration of nerve blocks?**
It is possible to extend the duration of a block by adding epinephrine or clonidine to the injected local anesthetic. The results vary and, in many cases, are short lived. If prolonged duration of a nerve block is needed, then placement of a peripheral nerve catheter should be considered. The peripheral nerve catheter can be left in place for days and is even used in outpatients. With the introduction of liposomal preparations of local anesthetics, it is conceivable that single-shot blocks could last several days.

10. **Review upper-extremity nerve blocks, including their indications, limitations, and complications.**
See Table 63-1. The volumes of local anesthetic solutions for an adult are between 20 and 30 ml.

11. **What is the Bier block, and how is it performed?**
The Bier block is also known as intravenous regional anesthesia. It is used mostly for anesthesia of the wrist and hand and usually for nonosseous procedures such as carpal tunnel release, trigger finger release, and ganglion resection. The Bier block works by local anesthetic diffusion from the intravenous space to the nerve fibers traversing the vicinity of the vessels in the upper extremity. The duration of the Bier block is up to 90 minutes, has a high patient satisfaction, and allows for rapid discharge of the patient.
    The first step in performing a Bier block is securing intravenous (IV) access to the limb that is to be anesthetized. (The patient should also have an IV line in the opposite extremity for administration of fluids and medications.) A small-gauge needle is enough, but care should be taken to place the IV line as distally as possible, usually in the back of the hand. A double tourniquet is placed around the upper arm. The arm is exsanguinated by elevating and wrapping it tightly with a wide elastic (Esmarch) band. The distal, then proximal, tourniquet is then inflated to 250 mm Hg. The Esmarch is removed, the distal tourniquet cuff is then deflated, and 40 to 50 ml of 0.5% lidocaine is injected through the IV line. Anesthesia sets in within minutes, and the surgical procedure can begin.

12. **How is local anesthetic toxicity avoided when performing a Bier block?**
Local anesthetic toxicity will happen if the injected local anesthetic solution rapidly enters the central circulation. Local anesthetics can gain access to the circulation only if the tourniquet cuffs are purposefully or accidentally deflated. The anesthesiologists should have immediate access to the tourniquet, tubing, and pressuring device being used while performing a Bier block. Tubing should be secured and situated to avoid any accidental disconnection.
    If the procedure lasts less than 30 minutes, the tourniquet is slowly and repeatedly deflated and reinflated. The brief deflations allow some of the local anesthetic into the circulation. The patient is quizzed for signs of local anesthetic toxicity. Perioral numbness, a metallic taste, and ringing in the ears are common early symptoms of mild toxicity. Should they occur, they should be allowed to resolve before further local anesthetic is released centrally. This should prevent more severe manifestations of local anesthetic toxicity such as seizures and cardiovascular collapse. Other mild symptoms include disinhibition as manifested by agitation and/or tearfulness.

KEY POINTS: PERIPHERAL NERVE BLOCKS

1. There are multiple ways to localize peripheral nerves, including use of nerve stimulator, ultrasound guidance, paresthesia, and relationship to other structures such as arteries or fascial planes.
2. To date no particular technique to localize peripheral nerves has been demonstrated to produce fewer complications or a higher success rate when performed by appropriately trained personnel.
3. The correct use of peripheral nerve block can decrease the incidence of perioperative complications such as pain, nausea, vomiting, and other opioid side effects caused by the decreased use of such drugs.

Table 63-1. Upper-Extremity Nerve Blocks

	INTERSCALENE	SUPRACLAVICULAR	INFRACLAVICULAR	AXILLARY
Indications	Shoulder procedures (i.e., rotator cuff, total shoulder arthroplasty)	Complete anesthesia of the upper extremity; midhumerus to fingers	Anesthesia from the elbow down; peripheral nerve catheter placement	Anesthesia from the elbow down
Limitations	Ulnar nerve commonly missed; therefore should only be used for shoulder procedures	Difficult to perform without ultrasound guidance	Deep block that requires deeper sedation; could potentially miss the musculocutaneous nerve	Need to block the musculocutaneous nerve separately; might be difficult to perform in patients unable to move the upper extremity
Complications	Risk for intraspinal injection, injection into vertebral artery, 100% paralysis of ipsilateral phrenic nerve	Pneumothorax risk is somewhere between 3% and 6% when performed without ultrasound guidance	Puncture of the subclavian vessels	Puncture of the axillary vessels

13. **What PNB can be performed for surgery of the lower extremity?**
The first step in deciding what block is indicated for anesthesia or analgesia is appreciating the innervation of the lower extremity and the requirements of the proposed procedure. The lumbar plexus (L1–L4) gives origin to the ilioinguinal, genitofemoral, obturator, femoral, and lateral femorocutaneous nerves and mainly innervates the inguinal region and the anterior aspect of the thigh. The remainder of the lower extremity is innervated by the sacral plexus. This includes the posterior aspect of the thigh and all the area distal to the knee except for the medial aspect, which is the territory of the saphenous nerve, a branch of the femoral nerve. The main nerve arising from the sacral plexus is the sciatic nerve. The sciatic nerve is actually formed by union of the tibial and peroneal nerves. These two nerves separate in or slightly above the cephalad region of the popliteal fossa. Table 63-2 describes the most common indications, limitations, and complications of the most commonly performed PNB to the lower extremity.

14. **What PNB can be used to provide anesthesia or analgesia to the chest wall?**
A thoracic paravertebral block can be performed to provide anesthesia for breast procedures such as lumpectomy or total mastectomy. Thoracic paravertebral analgesia is also used in patients undergoing thoracic surgical procedures and in patients with multiple unilateral rib fractures as an alternative to thoracic epidural catheter placement.

Table 63-2. Lower-Extremity Nerve Blocks

	LUMBAR PLEXUS	FEMORAL	SCIATIC	ANKLE
Indications	Hip procedures such as THA, hip fractures; in conjunction with a proximal sciatic block provides total anesthesia to the lower limb	Procedures in the anterior thigh, including TKA, and ACL reconstruction and analgesia for femur fractures	Below-the-knee procedures such as foot and ankle procedures, proximal and mid-tibia fractures, BKA	Foot procedures such as toe amputations, hammer toe corrections
Limitations	Difficult to perform, deep block that requires the patient to be placed in the lateral decubitus position	When trying to perform a three-in-one block (lateral femorocutaneous, femoral, and obturator), the obturator is frequently missed	Misses the internal aspect of the leg (saphenous nerve, branch of the femoral nerve)	Requires at least three different injections
Complications	Reports of retroperitoneal hematomas in patients on LMWH; epidural or spinal spread; injury to kidney or ureter	Injury to femoral vessels	Hematoma formation because of its deep position	Minimal

ACL, Anterior cruciate ligament; BKA, below-knee amputation; LMWH, low-molecular-weight heparin; THA, total hip arthroplasty; TKA, total knee arthroplasty.

15. **What PNB can be used to provide anesthesia or analgesia to the anterior abdominal wall?**

    Anesthesia or analgesia to the lower quadrants or the inguinal region can be accomplished by performing intercostal blocks. This procedure is effective at the last three levels or blocking the genitofemoral and the ilioinguinal nerves. A more recently described approach, the transverse abdominis plane (TAP) block, is reported to cover the entire anterior abdominal wall, making it very useful in patients in whom epidural analgesia is impractical. TAP block requires ultrasound guidance to ensure correct needle placement.

WEBSITE

New York Society of Regional Anesthesia: http://www.nysora.com

SUGGESTED READINGS

Brull R, McCartney CJ, Chan VW, et al: Neurological complications after regional anesthesia: contemporary estimates of risk, Anesth Analg 104:965–974, 2007.

De Tran QH, Clemente A, Doan J, et al: Brachial plexus blocks: a review of approaches and techniques, Can J Anaesth 54:662–674, 2007.

Ilfeld BM, Malhotra N, Furnish TJ, et al: Liposomal bupivacaine as a single-injection peripheral nerve block: a dose-response study, Anesth Analg 117:1248–1256, 2013.

Koscielniak-Nielsen ZJ: Ultrasound-guided peripheral nerve blocks: what are the benefits? Acta Anaesthesiol Scand 52:727–737, 2008.

McDonnell JG, O'Donnell B, Curley G, et al: The analgesic efficacy of transversus abdominis plane block after abdominal surgery: a prospective randomized controlled trial, Anesth Analg 104:193–197, 2007.

Tran D, Clemente A, Finlayson RJ: A review of approaches and techniques for lower extremity nerve blocks, Can J Anaesth 54:992–1034, 2007.

Tsai TP, Vuckovic I, Dilberovic F, et al: Intensity of the stimulating current may not be a reliable indicator of intraneural needle placement, Reg Anesth Pain Med 33:207–210, 2008.

CHAPTER 64

PRINCIPLES OF ANESTHESIA IN HEART TRANSPLANTATION

Tamas Seres, MD

1. **What are the common diagnoses indicating heart transplantation in adults?**
   Based on the latest database (January 2005 to June 2010) there is a shift from an equal split between ischemic and nonischemic cardiomyopathy as a cause of heart failure to a significantly greater proportion of patients with nonischemic cardiomyopathy (53% vs. 38%). Valvular heart diseases (3%), re-transplantation (3%), adult congenital heart diseases (3%), and miscellaneous conditions (0.8%) are the remaining indications for heart transplantation.

2. **What is the bridge-to-transplant management of patients with heart failure?**
   In the time period of 2002 to 2010 at the time of transplant, 45% of adult recipients were receiving intravenous inotropic support and 31% were on some type of mechanical support device. This represents a significant change compared to the time period between 1992 and 2001 (55% and 9%, respectively). Between 2002 and 2010, substantially fewer recipients were hospitalized immediately prior to transplant, signifying the current practice of outpatient management with inotropic support and left ventricular assist device use in bridge-to-transplant patients.

3. **What are the indications and contraindications for cardiac transplantation?**
   Absolute indications in appropriate patients
   - For hemodynamic compromise due to heart failure:
     - Refractory cardiogenic shock
     - Documented dependence on IV inotropic support to maintain adequate organ perfusion
     - Peak oxygen uptake (VO_2) <10 ml/kg/min
   - Severe symptoms of ischemia that consistently limit routine activity and are not amenable to coronary artery surgery or percutaneous intervention
   - Recurrent symptomatic ventricular arrhythmias refractory to all therapeutic modalities

   Relative indications
   - Peak VO_2 11 to 14 ml/kg/min or 55% of predicted and major limitation in daily activities
   - Recurrent unstable ischemia not amenable to other intervention
   - Recurrent instability of fluid balance/renal function not due to patient noncompliance with medical regimen

   Insufficient indications
   - Low ventricular ejection fraction
   - History of NYHA III-IV heart failure
   - Peak VO_2 >15 ml/kg/min or greater than 55% of predicted without other indications

   Absolute contraindications
   - Increased nonreversible pulmonary vascular resistance
   - Active malignancy of any kind
   - Active infection (hepatitis and HIV are still under debate)

   Relative contraindications
   - Age
   - Diabetes
   - Obstructive or restrictive lung disease
   - Recent pulmonary embolism

- Cirrhosis
- Impaired renal function

4. What are the priority criteria for the selection of the recipients?

To ensure equitable distribution of donor hearts, the United Network for Organ Sharing (UNOS) has created an organ allocation system. Although many patients qualify for cardiac transplantation, actual donor heart allocation is based on UNOS priority status, ABO blood group compatibility, body-size match, and distance from the donor center. UNOS priority status represents the urgency of the transplantation based on the severity and treatment modalities of the heart failure:

Status 1A: Inpatient with at least one of the following:
- Assisted mechanical support for acute decompensation
- Assisted mechanical circulatory support for >30 days with significant device-related complications
- Mechanical ventilation
- Continuous infusion of a single high-dose IV inotrope or multiple inotropes
- Life expectancy without transplantation of <7 days

Status 1B: Patients with at least one of the following:
- Assisted mechanical circulatory support for >30 days
- Continuous infusion of IV inotropes

Status 2: A candidate who does not meet the criteria for status 1A or 1B

Status 3: A candidate who is considered temporarily unsuitable to receive a thoracic organ transplant

Geographic sequence of thoracic organ allocation: Thoracic organs are to be allocated locally first, then within one of the five zones in the sequence described by the UNOS allocation policy.

This UNOS policy resulted in a major decrease in the mortality rate of patients on the waiting list.

5. What is the significance of maximum oxygen uptake (peak VO₂) measurement?

In general, the peak VO_2 (maximum oxygen uptake in ml/kg/min) appears to provide the most objective assessment of functional capacity in patients with heart failure. Peak exercise capacity is defined as the maximum ability of the cardiovascular system to deliver oxygen to exercising skeletal muscle and of the exercising muscle to extract oxygen from the blood. As a result, exercise tolerance is determined by three factors: pulmonary gas exchange, cardiac performance, and skeletal muscle metabolism. Exercise capacity can be quantitated clinically by measurement of VO_2, carbon dioxide production (VCO_2), and minute ventilation. The VO_2 eventually reaches a plateau despite increasing workload. At this point, peak VO_2 has a strong linear correlation with both cardiac output and skeletal muscle blood flow. The relationship between cardiac output and O_2 consumption also forms the basis for the Fick theorem to measure cardiac output:

$$\text{Cardiac output} = O_2 \text{ uptake} \div \text{Arteriovenous } O_2 \text{ difference}$$

6. What is the role of peak VO₂ in the decision-making process of heart transplantation?

Patients with a profoundly reduced exercise capacity of ≤10 ml/kg/min are likely to experience the most pronounced improvement in survival with transplantation; thus these patients can step forward on the priority list. With optimal pharmacologic and device therapy, the 1-year survival is increasing in low exercise capacity groups; however, the observations suggest that patients with persistent peak VO_2 <10 ml/kg/min may be warranted as an indication for heart transplantation.

7. What are the absolute contraindications for the selection of the recipients?

Malignant tumor; active infection; HIV-positive serology; irreversible, severe hepatic, renal, or pulmonary disease; and alcohol or intravenous drug abuse are absolute contraindications for heart transplantation. High, irreversible pulmonary vascular resistance (PVR) (>6 Wood units/m²) and high transpulmonary gradient (mean pulmonary artery [PA] pressure − pulmonary capillary wedge pressure [PCWP]) (>15 mm Hg) also exclude patients from heart transplantation.

8. **What are the criteria for donor selection?**

   Acceptance of a potential organ donor requires confirmation of brain death and organ viability. Echocardiographic evaluation of cardiac function and coronary angiography for male donors older than 45 years and female donors older than 50 years are recommended. Although cardiac transplant recipients are screened preoperatively for the percentage of reactive antibodies against human leucocyte atigens (HLA), donors and recipients are matched only on ABO blood group and weight ratio unless the percentage of reactive antibodies is greater than 20%.

9. **How is anesthesia managed for organ harvesting?**

   Anesthetic management of the donor during organ harvesting is an extension of preoperative management, with continued monitoring of volume status and systemic arterial and central venous pressures. An inspired oxygen concentration (FiO_2) of 1.0 is optimal for organ viability, unless the lungs are to be retrieved. To decrease the possibility of oxygen toxicity in the case of donor lung retrieval, the lowest possible FiO_2 that will maintain the arterial oxygen partial pressure (PaO_2) greater than 100 mm Hg should be used. Although intact spinal reflexes still may result in hypertension, tachycardia, and muscle movement, these signs do not indicate cerebral function or pain perception. Nondepolarizing muscle relaxants are commonly used to prevent spinal reflex–mediated muscle movement in response to noxious stimuli.

10. **How is the heart retrieved and preserved for transplantation?**

    After initial dissection, the patient is fully heparinized. The perfusion-sensitive organs (kidneys and liver) are removed before the heart. The donor heart is perfused with cardioplegia solution and excised via median sternotomy. After excision, the donor heart is placed in a plastic bag containing ice-cold saline and transported in an ice-filled cooler. Optimal myocardial function after transplantation is achieved when the donor heart ischemic time is less than 4 hours.

11. **Describe the medical management of heart failure patients awaiting heart transplantation.**

    Patients who are waiting for heart transplantation have heart failure managed by different ways as follows:

    - Patients with heart failure who are on oral medications including angiotensin-converting enzyme (ACE) inhibitors, β-receptor blockers, diuretics, vasodilators, digoxin and warfarin. These patients usually have low priority on the heart transplantation list.
    - Patients on IV inotropes with or without vasodilators. The most frequently used inotropes are dobutamine and/or milrinone with or without nitroprusside. None of these medications can be used chronically because they decrease the long-term survival. Decision should be made to use mechanical assist devices or wait for a new heart for a limited time.
    - Patients on mechanical assist device. Intraaortic balloon pump or ventricular assist devices can support left or right ventricular function or both. These patients have high priority for heart transplantation.
    - Patients who have failing transplanted heart and are waiting for re-transplantation.

12. **What are the hemodynamic characteristics of the heart of the recipients?**

    Cardiac transplant recipients typically have hypokinetic, dilated, noncompliant ventricles sensitive to alterations in myocardial preload, afterload, and contractility.

13. **How is anesthesia induced for patients with heart failure?**

    Hemodynamic goals for anesthetic induction are to maintain heart rate and contractility and avoid acute changes in preload and afterload. Inotropic support is often required during anesthetic induction and throughout the pre-CPB (cardiopulmonary bypass) period. As a general rule, induction agents have negative inotropic effects on the heart. In clinical situations where the sympathetic nervous system is activated to maintain the hemodynamic stability of the patient, even etomidate or ketamine can promote cardiovascular collapse.

    Rapid-sequence anesthetic induction is advisable in these cases. Full stomach should be considered because of short notice before the surgery. Furthermore, mask ventilation can be relatively ineffective and the increasing CO_2 level elevates PA pressure, which decreases the cardiac output in certain cases.

Etomidate in combination with fentanyl or sufentanil can be used in these patients with small doses of versed, ketamine, or scopolamine to ensure amnesia. Succinylcholine is appropriate for induction because of the concern of full stomach. Timely administration of vasoactive agents is necessary in these patients because of prolonged onset of the effect of medications. Epinephrine, phenylephrine, atropine, or glycopyrrolate vials should be available to keep the blood pressure and heart rate at the level that is appropriate for organ perfusion.

14. **How is anesthesia maintained for heart transplantation?**
    Patients with relatively stable hemodynamic status or on mechanical assist devices tolerate high-dose narcotics or a combination of anesthetic gases and narcotics. Patients with low cardiac output syndrome do not tolerate anesthetic gases well. Careful titration of narcotics can be the choice in this situation. Muscle relaxants, including vecuronium, rocuronium, or cisatracurium, which do not influence the hemodynamic status, can be used safely. Due to its vagolytic and mild sympathomimetic properties, the muscle relaxant pancuronium is commonly used to counteract high-dose narcotic-induced bradycardia.

15. **What monitors should be used for heart transplantation?**
    Noninvasive monitoring should include a standard five-lead ECG, noninvasive blood pressure measurement, pulse oximetry, capnography, and nasopharyngeal and bladder temperature. Invasive monitoring should include systemic arterial, central venous, and PA pressure measurements. A PA catheter is helpful in the post-CPB period, permitting monitoring of CO and ventricular filling pressures and calculation of systemic and pulmonary vascular resistance. These indices are particularly useful for assessment and treatment of post-CPB pulmonary hypertension and right ventricular dysfunction. Intraoperative transesophageal echocardiography (TEE) is an important tool in evaluation of air in the transplanted heart as well as in monitoring left and right ventricular function.

16. **Are there specific preparations for CPB?**
    Many cardiac transplant recipients have undergone previous cardiac surgery and are at increased risk for inadvertent trauma to the great vessels or preexisting coronary artery bypass grafts during repeat sternotomy.
    • Patients undergoing repeat sternotomy should have external defibrillator pads placed, and cross-matched, irradiated, packed red blood cells should be available in the operating room before anesthetic induction.
    • The potential for a prolonged surgical dissection time in patients undergoing repeat sternotomy often necessitates that anesthesia be induced at an earlier than usual time to coordinate with donor heart arrival.
    • Femoral or axillary CPB cannulation can be necessary because of the potential for increased perioperative bleeding.
    • Moderate hypothermia (28°C to 30°C) is commonly used during CPB to improve myocardial protection.
    • Hemofiltration is common during CPB, because patients with congestive heart failure often have a large intravascular blood volume and coexistent renal impairment.
    • High-dose intravenous glucocorticoids such as methylprednisolone are administered before reperfusion of the new heart to reduce the likelihood of hyperacute rejection.

17. **What is the reason for coagulation abnormalities?**
    Potential etiologies include hepatic dysfunction secondary to chronic hepatic venous congestion, preoperative anticoagulation, CPB-induced platelet dysfunction, hypothermia, and hemodilution of clotting factors. Evaluation of prothrombin time, partial thromboplastin time, platelet number, and/or the parameters of the thromboelastography can help in assessing the coagulation status and planning the administration of appropriate blood products if there is clinical need.

18. **What antifibrinolytic agents can be used for decreasing bleeding?**
    Antifibrinolytics such as tranexamic acid and ε-aminocaproic acid are commonly administered after anesthetic induction or heparin administration to prevent postoperative bleeding. Aprotinin, a polypeptide protease inhibitor with platelet-preserving properties, has been shown to decrease perioperative blood loss in patients undergoing repeat sternotomy. However, this agent was removed from the market because of adverse effects on long-term survival and renal function.

19. **What preparation should be made before termination of CPB?**

    Before termination of CPB, the patient should be normothermic, and all electrolyte and acid-base abnormalities corrected. Complete de-airing of the heart before aortic cross-clamp removal is essential because intracavitary air may pass into the coronary arteries, resulting in significant ventricular dysfunction, or into the cerebral arteries, causing cognitive impairment or stroke. TEE is particularly useful for assessing the efficacy of cardiac de-airing maneuvers. Inotropic agents should be commenced before CPB termination. A heart rate of 100 to 120 beats/min, a mean systemic arterial blood pressure greater than 65 mm Hg, and ventricular filling pressures of approximately 12 to 16 mm Hg (central venous pressure [CVP]) and 14 to 18 mm Hg (pulmonary capillary wedge pressure [PCWP]) are required in the immediate post-CPB period.

20. **What is the implication of autonomic denervation of the transplanted heart?**

    During orthotopic cardiac transplantation, the cardiac autonomic plexus is transected, leaving the transplanted heart without autonomic innervation. The newly denervated heart does not respond to direct autonomic nervous system stimulation or to drugs that act indirectly through the autonomic nervous system (e.g., atropine). Instead, the denervated transplanted heart only responds to direct-acting agents such as catecholamines. Because transient, slow nodal rhythms are common after aortic cross-clamp release, a direct-acting β-adrenergic receptor agonist and/or epicardial pacing is commonly commenced before CPB termination to achieve a heart rate of 100 to 120 beats/min. Infusions of dopamine, dobutamine, milrinone, or epinephrine are effective for inotropic support.

21. **What is the cause of the immediate left ventricular (LV) dysfunction after CPB?**

    Post-CPB LV dysfunction may be a result of a prolonged donor heart ischemic time, inadequate myocardial perfusion, intracoronary embolization of intracavitary air, or surgical manipulation. The incidence of post-CPB LV dysfunction is greater in donors requiring prolonged, high-dose inotropic support before organ harvest.

22. **What is the cause of right ventricular (RV) failure after CPB?**

    RV failure is a significant cause of early morbidity and mortality, accounting for nearly 20% of early deaths. Therefore, prevention, diagnosis, and aggressive treatment of RV dysfunction after CPB are essential. Acute RV failure after cardiac transplantation may be due to preexistent pulmonary hypertension in the recipient, transient pulmonary vasospasm, tricuspid or pulmonic valve insufficiency secondary to early postoperative RV dilation, and donor–recipient size mismatch. Additional factors that may contribute to postoperative RV dysfunction include a prolonged donor heart ischemic time, inadequate myocardial protection, and surgical manipulation of the heart.

23. **How can RV function be evaluated during the surgery?**

    RV distention and hypokinesis may be diagnosed by TEE or direct observation of the surgical field. Another finding suggesting RV failure is elevation in CVP with decreasing PA pressure. The pressure difference between CVP and mean PA pressure is a valuable parameter in evaluation of RV function. Decreasing difference or a difference <5 mm Hg may indicate failing RV.

24. **What are the treatment options for RV failure?**

    Increased FiO_2, correction of acid-base abnormalities, and hyperventilation ($PaCO_2$ of 25 to 30 mm Hg) may reduce PVR. RV function may be improved by inotropic support and pulmonary vasodilation (dobutamine, milrinone). Pharmacologic agents commonly used for pulmonary vasodilation include nitrates, prostacyclin (prostaglandin I2 [PGI2]), prostaglandin E1 (PGE1), phosphodiesterase-III inhibitors, and inhaled nitrous oxide (NO).

25. **What is the advantage of NO in transplantation?**

    In contrast to nonselective vasodilators such as nitroglycerin and sodium nitroprusside that typically produce systemic hypotension, inhaled NO (20 to 40 ppm) selectively reduces PVR in the ventilated area of the lung, thus improving ventilation-perfusion (VQ) mismatch. NO has little systemic effect because it is inactivated by hemoglobin and has a 5- to 10-second half-life.

26. **What are the side effects of NO?**

NO administration results in the formation of nitrogen dioxide and methemoglobin, and the levels of these toxic metabolites should be monitored. In the presence of severe LV dysfunction, selective dilation of the pulmonary vasculature by NO may lead to an increase in PCWP and pulmonary edema. Thus, agents producing both pulmonary and systemic vasodilation, like intravenous or inhaled PGI2, may be a better choice in this setting.

27. **What are the concerns in anesthesia management of patients after heart transplantation for noncardiac surgery?**

Cardiac denervation is an unavoidable consequence of heart transplantation, and reinnervation is absent or incomplete. Baseline cardiac function is normal, but the response to demands for increased cardiac output is altered. Heart rate increases only gradually with exercise, and this effect is mediated by circulating catecholamines. Increases in cardiac output in response to exercise are mostly mediated via an increase in stroke volume. Therefore, maintenance of adequate preload in these patients is crucial. Lack of parasympathetic innervation is responsible for the gradual decrease in heart rate after exercise. Drugs that act indirectly on the heart via either the sympathetic (ephedrine) or parasympathetic (atropine, pancuronium) nervous system will generally be ineffective.

KEY POINTS: PRINCIPLES OF ANESTHESIA IN HEART TRANSPLANTATION

1. Treatment modalities of heart failure include medical therapy, ventricular assist devices, and heart transplantation.
2. More and more patients with heart failure will be on a ventricular assist device before heart transplantation.
3. Anesthesia for patients with heart failure requires assessment of hemodynamic status, invasive monitoring, and careful selection and titration of anesthetic agents.
4. There is a high risk for cardiovascular collapse during induction and maintenance of anesthesia because of the negative inotropic effect of anesthetic agents.
5. Before emergence from cardiopulmonary bypass, left and right ventricular function, cardiac rhythm, and bleeding diathesis should be assessed and treated if necessary.
6. Right ventricular function plays a central role in successful emergence from cardiopulmonary bypass after heart transplantation.

WEBSITES

Heart transplantation: www.uptodate.com
United Network for Organ Sharing: Organ Procurement and Transplantation Network: www.unos.org

SUGGESTED READINGS

DiNardo JA: Anesthesia for heart, heart-lung, and lung transplantation. In DiNardo JA, editor: Anesthesia for cardiac surgery, ed 2, Stamford, CT, 1998, Appleton & Lange, pp 201–239.

Hunt SA, Abraham WT, Chin MH, et al: ACC/AHA 2005 Guideline Update for the Diagnosis and Management of Chronic Heart Failure in the Adult: a report of the American College of Cardiology/ American Heart Association Task Force on Practice Guidelines, Circulation 112:e154–e235, 2005.

Jerome LF, Ileana LP, Gary JB, et al: Assessment of functional capacity in clinical and research applications, Circulation 102:1591–1597, 2000.

Quinlan JJ, Murray AW, Casta A: Anesthesia for heart, lung and heart-lung transplantation. In Kaplan JA, Reich DL, Lake CL, et al, editors: Kaplan's cardiac anesthesia, ed 5, Philadelphia, 2006, Saunders, pp 845–851.

Stehlik J, Edwards LB, Kucheryavaya AY, et al: The Registry of the International Society for Heart and Lung Transplantation: Twenty-eighth Adult Heart Transplant Report—2011, J Heart Lung Transplant 30:1078–1094, 2011.

Taylor DO, Edwards LB, Aurora P, et al: The Registry of the International Society for Heart and Lung Transplantation: Twenty-fifth Official Adult Heart Transplant Report—2008, J Heart Lung Transplant 27:943–956, 2008.

Zacharian T, Rother AL, Collard CD: Anesthetic management for cardiac transplantation. In Hensley FA, Martin DE, Gravlee GP, editors: A practical approach to cardiac anesthesia, ed 4, Philadelphia, 2008, Lippincott Williams & Wilkins, pp 439–463.

CHAPTER 65

CARDIOPULMONARY BYPASS

Barbara Wilkey, MD, and Nathaen Weitzel, MD

1. **What are the main functions of a cardiopulmonary bypass (CPB) circuit?**
   A CPB circuit functions as the temporary equivalent of the native cardiopulmonary system. The CPB circuit allows for perfusion of the patient's vital organs, while oxygenating the blood and removing carbon dioxide (CO_2). Isolation of the cardiopulmonary system allows for surgical exposure of the heart and great vessels along with cardiac electrical silence and a bloodless field.

2. **What are the basic components of the CPB circuit?**
   A CPB circuit has a venous line that siphons central venous blood from the patient into a reservoir. Blood generally reaches the venous reservoir via gravity or vacuum assist. This blood is then passed through an oxygenator and CO_2 is removed before being returned to the patient's arterial circulation. Pressure to perfuse the arterial circulation is supplied by either a roller head or a centrifugal pump, usually resulting in nonpulsatile arterial flow, though some roller pumps can deliver pulsatile flow. The machine also has roller head pumps for cardioplegia administration, a ventricular vent to drain the heart during surgery, and a pump sucker to remove blood from the surgical field. Additionally, the circuit contains filters for air and blood microemboli, because both can cause devastating central nervous system injury if delivered to the arterial circulation. A heat exchanger is present to produce hypothermia on bypass and warm the patient before separating from CPB. The venous reservoir must never be allowed to empty while on CPB because a life-threatening air embolism could result.

3. **Define the levels of hypothermia. What are adverse effects of hypothermia?**
   - Mild: 32°C to 35°C
   - Moderate: 26°C to 3°C
   - Deep: 20°C to 25°C
   - Profound: 14°C to 19°C. This level of hypothermia is achieved if total circulatory arrest is planned.
   - Typical CPB temperatures range from 28°C to 34°C. Adverse effects of hypothermia include platelet dysfunction, reduction in serum ionized calcium concentration due to enhanced citrate activity, impaired coagulation, arrhythmias, increased risk of infection, decreased oxygen unloading, potentiation of neuromuscular blockade, and impaired cardiac contractility.

4. **Why is hypothermia used on CPB?**
   Systemic oxygen demand decreases 9% for every degree of temperature drop. Hypothermia therefore allows for lower CPB pump flows while providing adequate oxygen supply to vital organs. The main concern of CPB is the prevention of myocardial and central nervous system injury, along with renal and hepatic protection.

5. **What are the risk factors for renal insufficiency in the peri-bypass period?**
   These risk factors include advanced age, female gender, preoperative renal insufficiency, ejection fraction less than 40%, diabetes mellitus, hemodilution on CPB, use of intraaortic balloon pump, a long CPB run, and combined valve/coronary artery bypass graft surgery.

6. **What can be done to reduce renal insufficiency?**
   There is no tried and true method for preservation of renal function. Appropriate strategies include maintaining cardiac output and renal perfusion pressure and avoiding nephrotoxins.

7. **Discuss the traditional cannulation sites for bypass.**
   Venous blood is typically obtained through cannulation of the right atrium, using a dual-stage cannula that drains both the superior and the inferior vena cava. Alternatively, for open-heart procedures, bicaval cannulation is used with direct, separate cannulation of the superior and inferior vena cavae. Arterial blood is returned to the ascending aorta

proximal to the innominate artery. The femoral artery and vein can be used as alternative cannulation sites. Drawbacks to femoral bypass include ischemia of the leg distal to the arterial cannula, inadequate venous drainage, possible inadequate systemic perfusion secondary to a small inflow cannula, and difficulty in cannula placement owing to atherosclerotic plaques. Axillary artery cannulation can be used for repeat sternotomies and is often carried out before the sternotomy to allow for arterial fluid or blood administration from the CPB machine during the sternal dissection if necessary. Cannulation of the brachiocephalic artery may be used if circulatory arrest is planned.

8. **How does cannulation for minimally invasive valve operations differ from traditional cannulation for bypass?**
   Venous drainage is generally achieved by placing a single-stage catheter in the right atrium or superior vena cava via the femoral vein (See Figure 65-1). The drainage holes in the catheter should always sit in the right atrium. Venous drainage can be augmented using a vacuum assist system on the bypass machine. If needed, additional drainage may be achieved by placing a venous cannula via the internal jugular vein. In lieu of an internal jugular cannula, an endopulmonary vent catheter may be placed for additional drainage if the surgical approach is through the left atrium. Arterial cannulation can be peripheral (generally femoral) or direct (through thoracotomy). There are three general systems for antegrade cardioplegia administration: (1) either placement of a balloon in the aortic root that occludes and delivers cardioplegia, (2) cross-clamping through the sternotomy with direct placement of an aortic root vent, or (3) if the surgery is an aortic valve replacement (AVR), the surgeon can directly apply cardioplegia to the coronaries after the root is opened. Retrograde cardioplegia can be delivered by direct cannulation of the coronary sinus through the thoracotomy incision or via a percutaneous technique (See Figure 65-2).

9. **What are the basic anesthetic techniques used in CPB cases?**
   Anesthetic choice takes into consideration the degree of systolic dysfunction, extent of coronary disease, magnitude of valvular disease, and overall exercise tolerance. Patients undergoing CPB have been identified as a high-risk group for intraoperative awareness, likely a result of previously popular high-dose opioid techniques. Currently, amnestic agents

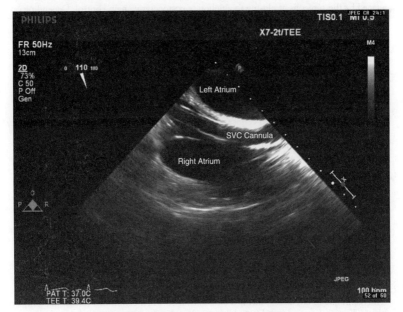

Figure 65-1. Venous drainage cannula in the SVC.

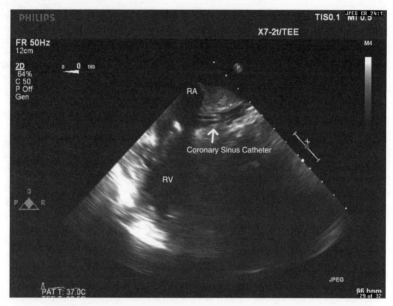

Figure 65-2. Coronary sinus catheter for deliver of retrograde cardioplegia.

such as midazolam are routinely used along with inhalational agents, which are administered by the perfusionist during CPB. Neuromuscular blocking agents prevent patient movement and shivering, increasing systemic oxygen demand during bypass, as well as contraction of the diaphragm during the surgical procedure. Parasternal blocks can be placed by the surgeons at closing to ameliorate postoperative pain control. Depending on the surgery and patient comorbidities (e.g., renal disease), intravenous ketorolac and/or Tylenol can be considered.

10. **What steps does an anesthesiologist need to take during conventional cannulation?**
For a primary sternotomy, ventilation should be held. During aortic cannulation, hypertension should be avoided to minimize the risk of aortic dissection, with a target systolic blood pressure of 110 mm Hg or less. During venous cannulation, use of low tidal volume ventilation may improve surgical access, as the lungs will not encroach on the surgical field. Transesophageal echocardiography (TEE) is routinely used to guide coronary sinus catheter placement. In general, the anesthesiologist should be visually following progress on the field from sternotomy through cannulation, as this can be a time of significant blood loss and hemodynamic shifts.

11. **Are there additional anesthetic considerations with minimally invasive and robotic techniques?**
Minimally invasive and robotic techniques require one-lung ventilation. Additionally, external defibrillation pads must be employed since access for internal defibrillation is challenging. If the patient fibrillates during one-lung ventilation, the lung should be reexpanded before defibrillation so the electrical current has tissue to travel through. Intercostal blocks can be placed by the surgeon for postoperative pain control if a thoracotomy is used for the surgical approach. Additionally, preoperative paravertebral blocks or even a thoracic epidural catheter can be considered.

12. **When and how is circulatory arrest utilized?**
The technique of circulatory arrest is *most often* used when conditions (either anatomy or planned surgical procedure) do not allow for flow through bypass circuits. A common

example is surgery on the aortic arch. Generally, in aortic arch surgery, the patient is placed on CPB until (1) he or she is cooled to the desired temperature and (2) the surgeon is ready to place the aortic graft. At that point, flow is stopped through the bypass circuit. Hypothermia is used to decrease metabolic demand, but the degree of hypothermia used varies by each surgeon's clinical practice. Circulatory arrest can be accompanied by isolated cerebral perfusion. This perfusion may be antegrade or retrograde: antegrade is delivered via a catheter that directs blood up the carotid artery, whereas retrograde is delivered via a catheter in the superior vena cava.

13. **What are the additional anesthetic considerations associated with circulatory arrest?**
    Patients who undergo hypothermic circulatory arrest are at increased risk for coagulopathy, neurologic sequelae, renal failure, and pulmonary dysfunction. In addition to standard case-based monitoring during CPB, one should have some sort of neurologic monitoring such as an electroencephalogram (EEG) or bispectral index (BIS). In theory, obtaining an isoelectric EEG before circulatory arrest will even further decrease cerebral oxygen demand during this low to no-flow state. Packing the head in ice and administering lidocaine and steroids may also be neuroprotective. α-Stat pH management is often used during the time of circulatory arrest. Magnesium may be administered for cardiac protection.

14. **List the two basic types of oxygenators.**
    1. Bubble oxygenators work by bubbling oxygen (O_2) through the patient's blood and then de-foaming the blood to minimize air microemboli.
    2. Membrane oxygenators utilize a semipermeable membrane that allows for diffusion of O_2 and CO_2. They have a significantly lower risk of gas microemboli, reduce damage to blood elements, and are the standard type of oxygenator used in clinical practice today.

15. **What is meant by "pump prime"? What is the usual hemodynamic response to initiating bypass?**
    Priming solutions (crystalloid, colloid, or blood) are used to fill the CPB circuit. When bypass is initiated, the circuit must contain fluid to perfuse the arterial circulation until the patient's blood can circulate through the pump. Priming volumes historically were 1.5 to 2 liters, but newer CPB circuits can achieve priming volumes as low as 650 to 800 ml for an open circuit, and even less with a so-called closed or mini-bypass circuit. Reductions in priming volume have resulted in decreased inflammatory response and a reduction in transfusion requirements. The acute hemodilution from the patient's circulating blood volume mixing with the prime volume can cause an acute reduction in mean arterial pressure and the hemoglobin concentration. If the patient's hemodynamics and starting hemoglobin permit, the perfusion may ask to "RAP." RAP (retrograde autologous prime) is a technique of allowing the patient's blood to prime the circuit in the reverse direction, effectively reducing the pump prime even further to limit hemodilution. Hemodynamic support is occasionally required to facilitate RAP. Bolus doses of phenylephrine are generally sufficient to maintain perfusion pressure.

16. **Why is systemic anticoagulation necessary?**
    Contact activation of the coagulation system occurs when nonheparinized blood contacts the synthetic surfaces of the CPB circuit, resulting in widespread thrombosis, oxygenator failure, and death. In a dire emergency, a minimum standard dose of 300 units/kg of heparin must be given through a central line before the initiation of bypass. Following separation from the CBP machine, protamine is used to bind heparin and reverse the anticoagulant effect.

17. **What are the options for a patient with heparin-induced thrombocytopenia (HIT) antibodies who needs emergent cardiac surgery requiring CPB?**
    Anticoagulant options other than heparin exist for patients with HIT antibodies, but most of these options are not safe during CPB. Danaparoid and fondaparinux have long half-lives and are not reversible. Argatroban and hirudin have been used; however, they have been associated with thrombotic complications and are not reversible. Argatroban has also been associated with thrombotic complications. Bivalirudin may be the safest, as it has a half-life of 25 minutes and is removable by hemofiltration. Monitoring drug levels during bivalirudin therapy can be an issue, however, as the ecarin clotting time (ECT) is unavailable in the

United States and the ACT may not be accurate at high doses. A key issue with bivalirudin is that when blood is stagnant, it will clot; thus venous reservoir blood must be circulated. Use of cardiotomy-suctioned blood has been associated with postoperative hypotension and coagulopathy; therefore, one should stick to a cell saver. There are case reports and series outlining the use of plasmapheresis before or during CPB in those HIT antibody positive. These patients were successfully given unfractionated heparin for CPB.

18. **How is the adequacy of anticoagulation measured before and during bypass?**
An ACT is measured about 3 to 4 minutes after heparin administration and every 30 minutes on CPB. An ACT of 400 seconds or longer is considered acceptable. Heparin levels are frequently measured, but only the ACT is a measure of anticoagulant activity. This is particularly important in patients with heparin resistance (seen with preoperative heparin infusions) and antithrombin III deficiency.

19. **What must be ascertained before placing the patient on CPB?**
   • Adequate arterial inflow of oxygenated blood with acceptable line pressures
   • Sufficient venous return to the bypass pump
   • ACT of at least 400 seconds
   • Appropriate placement of retrograde cardioplegia cannula if being used.
   • Arterial line monitor of mean blood pressure
   • Core temperature monitoring
   • Adequate depth of anesthesia

20. **Why is a left ventricular vent used?**
Left ventricular distention during bypass can be caused by aortic regurgitation or blood flow through the bronchial and thebesian veins. The resultant increase in myocardial wall tension can lead to serious myocardial ischemia by precluding adequate subendocardial cardioplegia distribution and elevating myocardial oxygen demands. A left ventricular vent, placed through the right superior pulmonary vein, decompresses the left side of the heart and returns this blood to the CPB pump.

21. **What are the characteristics of cardioplegia?**
There are several types of cardioplegia, a complete discussion of which is out of the scope of this text. The most common type of cardioplegia used in the United States is a hyperkalemic solution containing various metabolic energy substrates. Perfused through the coronary vasculature, cardioplegia induces diastolic electromechanical dissociation. Myocardial oxygen and energy requirements are reduced to those of cellular maintenance. Cardioplegia is perfused either anterograde via the aortic root coronary ostia or retrograde through the right atrial coronary sinus.

22. **Discuss myocardial protection during CPB. What elements should be in place to optimize myocardial protection?**
Cellular integrity must be maintained during CPB to ensure cardiac performance after CPB. A critical factor to prevent cellular damage is intraoperative myocardial protection. Preservation of the balance between myocardial oxygen consumption and delivery is essential, and the following are key elements in achieving this:
   • Adequate cardioplegia
   • Hypothermia, specifically myocardial hypothermia with myocardial temperature goals below 12° C to 15° C
   • Topical cooling of the heart with icy saline slush
   • Left ventricular venting to prevent distention
   • Insulating pad on the posterior cardiac surface to prevent warming from mediastinal blood flow
   • Minimizing bronchial vessel collateral flow (which also rewarms the arrested heart)
   • Inadequate preservation manifests after CPB as impaired cardiac output, ischemic electrocardiogram (ECG) changes, wall motion abnormalities on TEE, dysrhythmias, and the requirement for inotropic support.

23. **What is the function of an aortic cross-clamp?**
Clamping across the proximal aorta isolates the heart and coronary circulation. The arterial bypass inflow enters the aorta distal to the clamp. Cardioplegia is infused between the

clamp and aortic valve, thus entering the coronary circulation. This isolation of the heart from the systemic circulation allows for prolonged cardioplegia activity, diastolic arrest of the heart, and profound myocardial cooling.

24. **Review the physiologic responses to CPB.**
    - Stress hormones, including catecholamines, cortisol, angiotensin, and vasopressin increase due in part to decreased metabolism of these substances.
    - Exposure of blood to the CPB circuit results in complement activation, initiation of the coagulation cascade, and platelet activation. A systemic inflammatory response is also initiated.
    - Platelet dysfunction associated with CPB may contribute to post-CPB bleeding.
    - Hemodilution associated with onset of CPB decreases the serum concentrations of most drugs, but decreased hepatic and renal perfusion during CPB will eventually increase the serum concentration of drugs administered by continuous infusion.

25. **What are the pH-stat and α-stat methods of blood gas measurement?**
    There are differing opinions as to whether blood gases should be corrected for the temperature during CPB because the solubility of gases decreases with hypothermia. All blood gases are analyzed at 37°C. In pH-stat measurements, the obtained value is corrected on a nomogram, and the reported values refer to the partial pressure at the hypothermic temperatures. CO_2 is then added to the system to correct the acid-base status. More commonly, blood gases are reported uncorrected for temperature, a method referred to as α-stat blood gas management. Studies comparing the two methods show conflicting results, with the main concern being the alteration in cerebral vascular tone due to the CO_2 management. In adults, α-stat management trends toward improved neurologic outcomes and is commonly employed. Neonatal data seem to trend toward neurologic improvement using pH-stat management; thus that method is used in this population.

26. **Develop an appropriate checklist for discontinuing bypass.**
    - Check acid-base balance, ensuring neutral pH, base deficit, PCO_2, hemoglobin or hematocrit, and electrolytes.
    - Ascertain adequate systemic rewarming, typically 37°C.
    - Recalibrate ("zero") all pressure transducers.
    - Ensure adequate cardiac rate and rhythm (may require pacing)—ideally, atrioventricular synchrony.
    - Reexamine the ECG for rhythm and ischemia.
    - Evaluate TEE looking for signs of ischemia (regional wall motion abnormalities) along with evaluation of valves, specifically in cases of valve replacement or repair.
    - Remove intracardiac or intraaortic air if the aorta or cardiac chambers were opened (TEE evaluation is invaluable for this).
    - Initiate ventilation of lungs.

27. **How is the heparin effect reversed? What are potential complications?**
    Protamine, a positively charged protein molecule, binds the negatively charged heparin and this complex is removed from the circulation by the reticuloendothelial system. Although there are different regimens to determine how much protamine should be administered, the simplest and most common method is to dose protamine based on the heparin administered (roughly 1 mg protamine per 100 units heparin). The efficacy of heparin reversal should be assessed by ACT but can also be determined using thromboelastography. Protamine has been associated with systemic hypotension due to histamine release or true anaphylaxis, along with catastrophic pulmonary hypertension due to anaphylactoid thromboxane release. Risk factors include preexisting pulmonary hypertension, diabetics treated with NPH insulin preparations, bolus protamine administration, and central administration of protamine.

28. **Why is cardiac pacing frequently useful after bypass?**
    Between the ischemic insult of bypass, the residual effect of cardioplegia, and effects from hypothermia, cardiac conduction may be impaired and myocardial wall motion suboptimal. Sequential cardiac pacing at a rate of 80 to 100 beats per minute can significantly improve cardiac output.

29. **What are some of the things to consider if a patient has difficulty weaning from CPB?**

From a surgical standpoint, the adequacy of the surgical procedure (whether it be coronary artery bypass, valve replacement, or otherwise) should be reconsidered. TEE can evaluate regional wall motion abnormalities and valvular competency. Filling pressures should be assessed by both TEE and invasive monitors. Hemodynamic variables (cardiac index, mixed venous oxygen concentration, pulmonary artery pressure, pulmonary artery occlusion pressure, systemic vascular resistance) must be interpreted.

30. **What are some therapies for the patient with impaired cardiac performance or difficulty weaning from CPB?**

Typical scenarios encountered during the weaning process include reduced vascular resistance (so-called vasoplegia), which often requires vasopressor support. Contractility problems with the heart itself necessitate inotropic agents or possibly an aortic balloon pump to assist in the weaning from bypass. Right heart dysfunction and/or pulmonary hypertension may also complicate weaning from bypass. Agents such as nitric oxide or vasodilator therapy targeted toward the pulmonary system can be useful in this situation. TEE is invaluable in guiding these decisions along with interpretation of the pulmonary artery catheter. Inotropic and vasodilator therapies are discussed elsewhere.

31. **Review the central nervous system complications of CPB.**

There is about a 1% to 3% incidence of new neurologic events, defined as stroke (including vision loss), transient ischemic attack, or coma. There is also about a 3% incidence of deterioration in intellectual function, memory defects, or seizures, though close neurocognitive testing reveals a much higher incidence (20%–60%) of cognitive dysfunction at 1-month and 6-month intervals. Much of the cognitive dysfunction will resolve over a number of months. Cerebral microemboli, in particular platelet microemboli, are believed to be a contributing factor.

32. **What might be done to decrease the incidence of such complications?**

- Reversible factors may be identified before surgery involving CPB. For instance, patients with significant carotid stenosis may require correction of this problem before undergoing CPB (perhaps at the same surgery). Significant aortic atherosclerosis is an independent risk factor for stroke. Avoiding aortic cross-clamping is therefore important, so an off-pump surgical strategy may benefit these patients. Alternatively, an epi-aortic probe may be used to find an atheroma-free area for cross-clamping.
- Initially, it was thought that off-pump coronary artery bypass graft (CABG) would result in improved neurologic outcomes compared with patients undergoing CABG with CPB. Although study results vary, the majority of the data do not support improved neurocognitive outcomes in patients who have undergone off-pump CABG.
- Decrease cerebral oxygen consumption through hypothermia. Maintenance of perfusion pressure and mixed venous oxygen levels may optimize cerebral supply and demand.
- TEE may identify patent foramen ovale, significant atheromatous disease at the site of aortic cannulation, left atrial thrombi, and intracardiac air, all of which may contribute to a change in subsequent management.
- Avoiding hypoglycemia and hyperglycemia is likely beneficial.
- In the future some pharmacologic interventions may decrease the incidence of neurologic complications.

KEY POINTS: CARDIOPULMONARY BYPASS

1. There are multiple approaches to the anesthetic technique during cardiopulmonary bypass (CPB). The overall cardiac reserve based on the exercise tolerance and severity of disease (valvular or ischemic) should guide the choice of anesthetic, and cardiac depressant agents should be used cautiously.
2. Patients must be completely anticoagulated before CPB is initiated; otherwise, patients face the risk of massive intravascular clot formation.
3. Patients with positive HIT antibodies can undergo emergent CPB procedures.

4. The CPB reservoir should never be allowed to empty during CPB, as massive air embolism is a consequence.
5. Factors involved in myocardial preservation include cardioplegia, myocardial hypothermia, and ventricular venting. Consequences of inadequate myocardial preservation include decreased cardiac output, ischemia, dysrhythmias, and failure to wean from CPB.
6. Always consider inadequate surgical technique (kinking of graft, valve failure, etc.) for the patient failing to wean from CPB.
7. Neurologic complications, in particular neurocognitive deficits, are surprisingly common after CPB.
8. ALWAYS run through your mental checklist before initiating or finishing CPB.

SUGGESTED READINGS

Dorrotta I, Kimball-Jones P, Applegate R II: Deep hypothermia and circulatory arrest in adults, Semin Cardiothorac Vasc Anesth 11:66–76, 2007.

Gravlee G: Cardiopulmonary bypass; principles and practice, ed 3, Philadelphia, 2008, Lippincott Williams & Wilkins.

Hindman BJ, Lillehaug SL, Tinker JH: Cardiopulmonary bypass and the anesthesiologist. In Kaplan JA, editor: Cardiac anesthesia, ed 4, Philadelphia, 1999, Saunders.

Hogue CW Jr, Palin CA, Arrowsmith JE: Cardiopulmonary bypass management and neurologic outcomes: an evidence-based appraisal of current practices, Anesth Analg 103:2–37, 2006.

Kumar A, Suneja M: Cardiopulmonary bypass-associated acute kidney injury, Anesthesiology 114:964–970, 2011.

McMeniman WJ, Chard RB, Norrie J, et al: Cardiac surgery and heparin induced thrombocytopenia (HIT): a case report and short review, Heart Lung Circ 21:295–299, 2012.

Murphy GJ, Angelini GD: Side effects of cardiopulmonary bypass: what is the reality? J Card Surg 19:481–488, 2004.

Uyasl S, Reich D: Neurocognitive outcomes of cardiac surgery, J Cardiothorac Vasc Anesth 27:958–971, 2013.

Vernick W, Woo J: Anesthetic considerations during noninvasive mitral valve surgery, Semin Cardiothorac Vasc Anesth 16(1):11–24, 2012.

Welsby IJ, Um J, Milano CA, et al: Plasmapheresis and heparin reexposure as a management strategy in cardiac surgical patients with heparin-induced thrombocytopenia, Anesth Analg 110:30–35, 2010.

CHAPTER 66

LUNG ISOLATION TECHNIQUES

Mark D. Twite, MB, BChir, FRCP, and Lawrence I. Schwartz, MD

1. What are the indications for lung isolation?

There are five areas for which lung isolation may be required:

1. Thoracic surgery
   Lung surgery: Thoracoscopy, lobectomy, pneumonectomy, lung transplantation, lung volume reduction
   Bronchial surgery: Intraluminal tumors, bronchopleural fistula
   Pleural surgery: Pleurectomy, pleurodesis, decortication
2. Surgery on the great vessels, heart, and pericardium
   Heart: Via thoracotomy (as opposed to sternotomy) approach
   Thoracic aorta: Descending aortic aneurysm, patent ductus arteriosus, coarctation of the aorta, vascular ring
   Pulmonary artery: Rupture, embolectomy
   Pericardium: Pericardiectomy, pericardial window
3. Esophageal surgery
4. Nonthoracic surgical procedures: Anterior thoracic spinal fusion
5. Nonsurgical procedures: Pulmonary lavage, split lung ventilation, isolation of hemoptysis, or pulmonary infections

2. What are the techniques for lung isolation?

There are three basic techniques for lung isolation:

1. Left or right double-lumen endotracheal tube (DLT)
2. Single-lumen endotracheal tube with a bronchial blocker
3. Single-lumen endotracheal tube placed in a mainstem bronchus

3. Describe DLTs.

A DLT has two tubes of unequal length molded together with high-volume, low-pressure cuffs. The DLT is bifurcated with endotracheal and endobronchial lumens, each of which can be used to isolate, selectively ventilate, or deflate the right or left lung independently as indicated by surgical and pathologic requirements. The two lumens are color-coded: white for tracheal and blue for bronchial, at the connection sites, cuffs, and pilot balloons. The tracheal cuff is proximal to the tip of the endotracheal lumen and is placed above the carina; the smaller blue bronchial cuff is proximal to the endobronchial lumen and is placed in the mainstem bronchus. Left and right DLTs are designed to have the bronchial side placed in the corresponding mainstem bronchus, with the length and shape appropriate for the anatomy of that side.

4. Describe bronchial blockers.

A bronchial blocker can be placed in either bronchus to achieve complete isolation and atelectasis of the ipsilateral lung. A bronchial blocker may also be used for selective lobar blockade on the surgical side. Bronchial blockers can be placed through or alongside the endotracheal tube. Examples of available bronchial blockers include:

- Arndt wire-guided endobronchial blocker (Cook Medical)
- Cohen tip-deflecting endobronchial blocker (Cook Medical)
- Fuji Univent™ (endotracheal tube with built-in side channel housing the blocker) and Fuji Uniblocker™ (bronchial blocker alone) (Fuji Systems Corporation)
- Rüsch EZ-Blocker™ (Teleflex)

   Each of these bronchial blockers has a high-volume, low-pressure balloon at the tip and a hollow center channel that can be used to apply continuous positive airway pressure (CPAP) or suction to assist lung collapse. A fiber-optic bronchoscope (FOB) should be used to position the bronchial blocker.

5. **How can a single-lumen endotracheal tube be used to achieve lung isolation?**
   A standard single-lumen endotracheal tube can be selectively placed in the nonoperative bronchus. The operative lung will become atelectatic. This is a simple and fast procedure that can be useful in infants and small children. Remember that pediatric micro-cuffed endotracheal tubes may be less useful for elective right mainstem intubation as they lack a "Murphy eye" and, as a result, right upper lobe ventilation may be compromised. An uncuffed endotracheal tube with a Murphy eye avoids this problem.

6. **What are the advantages and disadvantages of each technique for lung isolation and one-lung ventilation?**
   See Table 66-1.

7. **How do you choose the appropriate size double-lumen endotracheal tube?**
   There are right- and left-sided DLTs to account for the anatomic differences between the right and left mainstem bronchi. Left-sided tubes are more commonly used. The optimal tube size for a particular patient is the largest tube that will pass atraumatically through the glottis, advance down the trachea, and fit in the bronchus with a small air leak detectable when the cuff is deflated. Using the largest possible tube is associated with the least airway resistance and ensures that a bronchial seal is obtained with small cuff volumes. A DLT that is too small requires a large endobronchial cuff volume, which may result in cuff herniation across the carina. Many anesthesiologists select 41-Fr and 39-Fr DLTs for tall and

Table 66-1. Advantages and Disadvantages of Three Techniques Used for Lung Isolation

TECHNIQUE	ADVANTAGES	DISADVANTAGES
Single-lumen tube in nonoperative bronchus	Simple Fast No special equipment needed Useful for small children	Cannot suction operative lung Cannot apply CPAP to operative lung Right upper lobar collapse with right mainstem placement Left-sided OLV can be difficult
Balloon-tipped bronchial blockers (Arndt, Cohen, Fuji, Rüsch)	Varied sizes Easily added to regular ETT Continue ventilation during placement Postoperative two-lung ventilation easy CPAP to operative lung Selective lobar isolation Best device for patients with difficult airways	Time needed for placement Repositioning often required Bronchoscopy necessary for placement Small channel for suctioning High-maintenance device with frequent dislodgment and loss of seal during surgery
Double-lumen endotracheal tube	Quick to place Can place without bronchoscopy (but recommended to use it) Can access both lungs for bronchoscopy and suctioning CPAP to operative lung Less repositioning Best device for absolute lung separation Conversion from two-lung to one-lung ventilation easy and reliable	Difficult to select appropriate size Difficult to place during laryngoscopy Damage to tracheal cuff during placement Major tracheobronchial injuries Not suitable for postoperative ventilation

CPAP, Continuous positive airway pressure; *ETT*, endotracheal tube; *OLV*, one-lung ventilation.

short men, respectively, and 39-Fr and 35- to 37-Fr DLTs for tall and short women, respectively. There is considerable variation in left mainstem bronchi diameters and a relatively weak predictive value of gender and height.

8. **How is the right mainstem bronchus different from the left, and how does this affect right-sided double-lumen endotracheal tube design?**
   The adult trachea is 11 to 13 cm long and begins at the level of the cricoid cartilage and bifurcates behind the sternomanubrial joint. The main differences between the right and left mainstem bronchi include the following:
   - The wider right bronchus diverges away from the trachea at a 25-degree angle, whereas the left bronchus diverges at a 45-degree angle.
   - The right bronchus has upper, middle, and lower lobe branches, whereas the left bronchus divides into only upper and lower lobe branches.
   - The orifice of the right upper lobe bronchus from the carina is 15 mm in women and 20 mm in men, whereas that of the left upper lobe bronchus is 50 mm from the carina.
   - Therefore right-sided DLTs must have a slit in the bronchial cuff for ventilating the right upper lobe. It is more difficult to correctly position a right-sided DLT because of anatomic variations between individuals in the distance between the right upper lobe orifice and the carina, often resulting in difficulties ventilating the right upper lobe (Figure 66-1).

9. **Describe the placement and positioning of DLTs.**
   Using laryngoscopy, the DLT is passed with the distal curvature concave anteriorly and is rotated 90 degrees toward the side of the bronchus to be intubated after the tip passes the larynx. There are then two options to position the tube: auscultation or flexible FOB. With the auscultation method, the DLT is blindly advanced until resistance is felt as the endobronchial lumen enters the bronchus. The endobronchial and tracheal cuffs may then be inflated and the lumens clamped in turn while the chest is auscultated. However, auscultation alone is often unreliable for proper DLT placement. Using the FOB technique, the DLT is placed in the mid-trachea, and the FOB is then placed through the endobronchial lumen and advanced until the carina and mainstem bronchi are identified. The FOB is then advanced into the appropriate bronchus and, using the FOB as a stylet, the DLT is slid over the FOB until its bronchial lumen comes into view just beyond the tip of the FOB. When positioning a right-sided DLT, it must be ensured that the endobronchial cuff does not block the right upper lobe orifice. Finally the FOB is passed through the tracheal lumen of the DLT to check for a carinal or subcarinal position of the bronchial cuff and ensure patency of the opposite mainstem bronchus.

10. **What complications may be caused by DLTs?**
   - **Malposition:** Most often occurs when a patient is turned from the supine to the lateral position. Usually there is cephalad movement of the DLT by 1 cm. Malposition can be avoided by maintaining the head in a neutral position with folded blankets to avoid

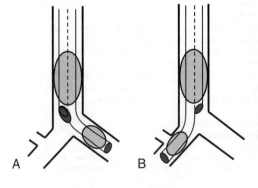

Figure 66-1. A, Double-lumen endotracheal tube correctly positioned in the left mainstem bronchus. **B,** Double-lumen endotracheal tube correctly positioned in the right mainstem bronchus, but notice the position of the bronchial cuff on the endotracheal tube and the right upper lobe bronchus take off.

flexion and extension. After repositioning the DLT, the FOB should be used to confirm that the DLT is still in good position.

- **Airway trauma**: Inflation of the bronchial cuff beyond its resting cuff volume may result in high cuff pressures and bronchial rupture. The cuff volume depends on the size of the DLT. Postoperative hoarseness and vocal cord lesions are significantly more frequent in patients intubated with a DLT compared to when a bronchial blocker is used to achieve lung isolation. There is, however, no difference in the incidence of bronchial injuries between the two groups.
- **Other complications**: Include stapling the endobronchial lumen in the bronchus during pneumonectomy (an argument for placing right-sided DLT for left pneumonectomy) and right upper lobe collapse when using right-sided DLTs.

11. How would you place a bronchial blocker?

Bronchial blockers are placed through or alongside standard endotracheal tubes, or they may be used with nasotracheal or tracheostomy tubes. Each type of bronchial blocker has a unique mechanism to assist in placement, but all require FOB guidance:

1. Arndt blocker™: The tip consists of a nylon wire loop through which the FOB is threaded and then used to directly guide the blocker into position.
2. Univent tube™: This is a single-lumen tube with an external channel that houses a built-in bronchial blocker. This blocker is composed of malleable material that allows the preshaped tip to be positioned with FOB guidance. The blocker of the Univent tube is also available separately as the Uniblocker.
3. Cohen blocker™: The tip can be deflected by turning a wheel at the proximal end of the blocker, which is guided into position using the FOB.
4. Rüsch EZ-Blocker™: This bronchial blocker is unique, as the tip has a "Y" shape that sits at the carina with a balloon in each mainstem bronchus. It may be used for bilateral thoracic surgery without repositioning.

All four bronchial blockers provide equivalent surgical exposure, but they require longer to position at the start of surgery and more intraoperative repositioning compared with DLTs.

12. Describe lung isolation techniques for patients with a difficult airway.

In patients who present with a difficult airway and require one-lung ventilation (OLV), the safest approach is to establish an airway with a single-lumen endotracheal tube while the patient is awake with the aid of an FOB. Lung isolation may then be achieved by using a bronchial blocker. An alternative technique is to use a DLT with an airway catheter exchange technique. For patients with a tracheostomy in place, a bronchial blocker or a short DLT intended for tracheostomies may be used.

13. Describe the physiology of OLV.

During normal ventilation, ventilation and perfusion are well matched anatomically because dependent portions of the lungs receive both greater blood flow (a result of gravity) and greater ventilation (from gravitational effects on lung compliance). The initiation of OLV stops all ventilation to one lung, which would create a 50% right-to-left shunt and relative hypoxemia if perfusion were unchanged. However, the actual shunt fraction is usually around 25% for the following reasons:

- Surgical manipulation of the atelectatic lung obstructs vascular flow to the nonventilated lung.
- Lateral positioning of the patient leads to a gravitational increase in perfusion to the dependent, ventilated lung.
- Hypoxic pulmonary vasoconstriction (HPV) modulates blood flow to hypoxic regions of the lungs.

14. How is the lateral decubitus position different for children?

Children possess a soft, compliant, compressible rib cage, which cannot fully support the dependent lung. This pushes functional residual capacity (FRC) closer to tidal volume, resulting in airway and alveolar closure at tidal volume breathing. There is a lower hydrostatic pressure gradient between nondependent and dependent lungs, leading to relatively less perfusion of the dependent lung compared with adults. Children have a smaller FRC and higher rate of oxygen consumption. All of these factors contribute to more pronounced hypoxemia in children placed in the lateral decubitus position.

Table 66-2. Factors Affecting HPV

HPV IS POTENTIATED (CAUSING LESS SHUNT, IMPROVING OXYGENATION)	HPV IS DECREASED (CAUSING INCREASED SHUNT, WORSENING OXYGENATION)
Metabolic acidosis	Metabolic alkalosis
Respiratory acidosis	Respiratory alkalosis
Hypercapnia	Hypocapnia
Decreased mixed venous oxygenation (lower CO)	Increased left atrial pressure
Hyperthermia	Hypothermia
	Inhalational anesthetic >1 MAC
	Hemodilution

CO, Cardiac output; HPV, hypoxic pulmonary vasoconstriction; MAC, minimal alveolar concentration.

15. **Explain HPV.**

    HPV reduces blood flow through the nonventilated lung by 50% during OLV, moderating the degree of hypoxemia. Alveolar hypoxia triggers the pulmonary vessels to constrict, directing blood away from nonventilated areas to better-ventilated segments, thereby improving ventilation-perfusion (V/Q) matching. The onset of HPV is two-phased, with an initial rapid onset (minutes) and a delayed phase (hours). HPV offset may take several hours and is an important consideration in the case of bilateral sequential thoracic procedures, such as bilateral wedge resections for lung metastases, in which patients will become more hypoxemic during OLV of the second lung.

16. **What factors affect HPV?**

    See Table 66-2.

17. **How do anesthetic agents affect HPV?**

    All volatile anesthetic agents inhibit HPV in a dose-dependent fashion. Older agents tend to be more potent inhibitors. Modern inhaled anesthetics used at doses less than 1 minimal alveolar concentration (MAC) have little clinical effect on HPV and oxygenation. Total intravenous anesthesia has not been shown to have any clinical advantage over inhaled anesthesia.

18. **Describe ventilation strategies for OLV.**

    Smaller tidal volumes of 6 ml/kg are useful for avoiding overdistention, high airway pressures, and lung trauma. Application of 4 to 6 cm H_2O of positive end-expiratory pressure (PEEP) will help maintain FRC in the dependent, ventilated lung, as well as keep pulmonary vascular resistance to a minimum, thus maximizing V/Q matching. It is prudent to avoid long inspiratory-to-expiratory time ratios so as to avoid auto-PEEP and lung overdistention. Increasing minute ventilation (respiratory rate) is also useful for maintaining appropriate gas exchange during OLV. Pressure control ventilation may be safer in avoiding lung injury caused by sudden changes in compliance during OLV. Permissive hypercapnia may be advantageous in OLV as hypercapnia potentiates HPV and causes a rightward shift of the oxyhemoglobin dissociation curve, enhancing oxygen delivery to the tissues.

19. **How should you manage hypoxemia during OLV?**

    During OLV the change in PaO_2 is usually greater than that in $PaCO_2$ because of the greater diffusibility of CO_2. When the patient is hypoxemic on OLV, a sequence of actions should happen:
    - Increase the FiO_2 to 1.0.
    - Optimize tidal volumes and peak inspiratory pressures.
    - Check DLT or bronchial blocker placement with an FOB.
    - Suction airway as needed.
    - Optimize cardiac output.
    - Recruit ventilated lung and apply 5 cm H_2O of PEEP.
    - Apply 5 to 10 cm H_2O of CPAP to the nondependent, nonventilated lung. This supplies oxygen to some of the alveoli that are perfused in the nondependent lung, decreasing shunt.

- If severe hypoxemia continues, alert the surgeon. The surgeon may be able to help by ligating or clamping the pulmonary artery to the nondependent lung, thus eliminating the shunt.
- Consider a return to two-lung ventilation.

20. **How should you prepare a patient for postoperative two-lung ventilation following surgery using OLV?**
    In patients who require postoperative mechanical ventilation, a disadvantage of DLTs is they generally need to be exchanged with a standard single-lumen endotracheal tube after surgery. This may be difficult after prolonged thoracic surgery that has caused bleeding, increased secretions, and airway edema. If DLTs are left in place, it is essential that staff be familiar with the design and function of the different lumens and cuffs to avoid difficulties such as complete airway occlusion.

KEY POINTS

1. One-lung ventilation (OLV) can be achieved with double-lumen endotracheal tubes (DLTs), bronchial blockers, and standard single-lumen endotracheal tubes.
2. After repositioning the patient, one should reassess optimal positioning of lung isolation using a fiber-optic bronchoscope (FOB).
3. A malpositioned tube or bronchial blocker is suggested by an acute increase in ventilator pressures and hypoxemia.
4. DLTs should be exchanged at the end of surgery for conventional single-lumen endotracheal tubes if postoperative ventilation is expected to be prolonged.
5. For patients with a difficult airway, consider awake FOB intubation and then use a bronchial blocker to achieve OLV.
6. Choice of anesthetic (inhalational vs. Total Intravenous Anesthesia, with or without epidural placement) does NOT have a significant clinical effect on oxygenation during OLV.
7. During OLV, protective ventilation strategies include low tidal volume ventilation (6 ml/kg), PEEP 5 cm H_2O, limited peak airway pressures, and permissive hypercapnia.
8. Methods to improve oxygenation during OLV include increasing FiO_2, checking DLT and bronchial blocker placement, applying PEEP to the ventilated lung and CPAP to the nonventilated lung, asking the surgeon to restrict pulmonary blood flow to the nonventilated lung and returning to two-lung ventilation.

WEBSITES

Cook Medical: www.cookmedical.com. Information on Arndt and Cohen bronchial blockers.
Fuji Systems Corporation: www.fujisys.co.jp. Information on Fuji Univent and Uniblocker.
Teleflex: www.teleflex.com. Information on Rüsch EZ-Blocker.
Thoracic Anesthesia: www.thoracic-anesthesia.com. Excellent site with many articles and an online bronchoscopy simulator.

SUGGESTED READINGS

Brodsky JB: Lung separation and the difficult airway, Br J Anaesth 103:i66–i75, 2009.
Campos JH: Lung isolation techniques for patients with difficult airway, Curr Opin Anaesthesiol 23:12–17, 2010.
Campos JH: Which device should be considered the best for lung isolation: double-lumen endotracheal tube versus bronchial blockers, Curr Opin Anaesthesiol 20:27–31, 2007.
Hammer GB: Single-lung ventilation in infants and children, Pediatr Anesth 14:98–102, 2004.
Ishikawa S, Lohser J: One-lung ventilation and arterial oxygenation, Curr Opin Anesthesiol 24:24–31, 2011.
Karzai W, Schwarzkopf K: Hypoxemia during one-lung ventilation: prediction, prevention, and treatment, Anesthesiol 110:1402–1411, 2009.
Knoll H, Ziegeler S, Schreiber J, et al: Airway injuries after one-lung ventilation: a comparison between double-lumen tube and endobronchial blocker, Anesthesiol 105:471–477, 2006.
Módolo N, Módolo M, Marton M, et al: Intravenous versus inhalational anaesthesia for one-lung ventilation, Cochrane Database Syst Rev (7):CD006313, 2013.
Narayanaswamy M, McRae K, Slinger P, et al: Choosing a lung isolation device for thoracic surgery: a randomized trial of three bronchial blockers versus double-lumen tubes, Anesth Analg 108:1097–1101, 2009.
Pedoto A: How to choose the double-lumen tube size and side: the eternal debate, Anesthesiol Clin 30:671–681, 2012.

CHAPTER 67

SOMATOSENSORY-EVOKED POTENTIALS AND SPINAL SURGERY

Daniel J. Janik, MD Colonel (Retired), USAF, MC

1. **What are somatosensory-evoked potentials (SSEPs)?**
   SSEPs are the electrophysiologic responses of the nervous system to the application of a discrete stimulus at a peripheral nerve anywhere in the body. They reflect the ability of a specific neural pathway to conduct an electrical signal from the periphery to the cerebral cortex.

2. **How are SSEPs generated?**
   Using a skin surface disc electrode or subcutaneous fine-needle electrode placed near a major peripheral mixed (motor and sensory) function nerve (such as the median nerve), a square-wave electrical stimulus of 0.2 to 2 ms is applied to the nerve at a rate of 1 to 2 Hz. The stimulus intensity is adjusted to produce minimal muscle contraction (usually 10 to 60 mA). The resulting electrical potential is recorded at various points along the neural pathway from the peripheral nerve to the cerebral cortex.

3. **What major peripheral nerves are most commonly stimulated?**
   In the upper extremity, the common sites of stimulation are the median and ulnar nerves at the wrist. In the lower extremity, the common peroneal nerve at the popliteal fossa and the posterior tibial nerve at the ankle are used. Less commonly the tongue, trigeminal nerve, and pudendal nerve have been studied.

4. **Trace the neurosensory pathway from the peripheral nerves to the cerebral cortex.**
   The axons of the peripheral sensory nerves enter the spinal cord via the dorsal spinal roots. These first-order neurons continue rostrally in the ipsilateral posterior column of the spinal cord until they synapse with nuclei at the cervicomedullary junction. Second-order neurons from these nuclei immediately decussate to the contralateral side of the brainstem, where they continue their ascent via the medial lemniscus through the midbrain, synapsing in the thalamus. Third-order neurons then travel via the internal capsule to synapse in the postcentral gyrus, the primary somatosensory cortex.

5. **At what points along the neurosensory pathway are SSEPs most commonly recorded?**
   After upper limb stimulation, potentials are recorded at the brachial plexus (Erb point, 2 cm superior to the clavicular head of the sternocleidomastoid muscle), the cervicomedullary junction (posterior midline of the neck at the second cervical vertebra), and the scalp overlying the somatosensory cortex on the contralateral side.
   After stimulation of the lower extremity, potentials are recorded at the popliteal fossa, lumbar and cervical spinal cord, and somatosensory cortex. It is important to record nerve and subcortical potentials to verify adequate stimulation and delineate anesthetic effects.

6. **Describe the characteristics of the SSEP waveform.**
   The SSEP is plotted as a waveform of voltage versus time. It is characterized by:
   • Amplitude (A), which is measured in microvolts from baseline to peak or peak to peak
   • Latency (L), which is the time, measured in milliseconds, from onset of stimulus to occurrence of a peak or the time from one peak to another

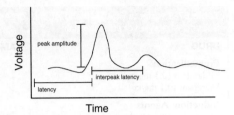

Figure 67-1. Characteristics of the somatosensory-evoked potential waveform.

Table 67-1. Characteristic Peaks for Evaluation of Median Nerve Stimulation

PEAK	GENERATOR
N9	Brachial plexus (Erb point)
N11	Dorsal root entry zone (cervical spine)
N13, 14	Posterior column (nucleus cuneatus)
P14	Medial lemniscus
N20	Somatosensory cortex

Table 67-2. Characteristic Peaks for Evaluation of Posterior Tibial Nerve Stimulation

PEAK	GENERATOR
N20	Dorsal root entry zone (lumbar spine)
N40	Somatosensory cortex

- Morphology, which is the overall shape of the waveform, described as positive (P, below the baseline) or negative (N, above the baseline)
  A waveform is identified by the letter describing its deflection above or below the baseline followed by a number indicating its latency (e.g., N20) (Figure 67-1).

7. **Name several characteristic peaks important for the evaluation of SSEPs.**
   See Table 67-1 and Table 67-2.

8. **What is the central somatosensory conduction time?**
   The central somatosensory conduction time is the latency between the dorsal column nuclei (N14) and the primary sensory cortex (N20) peaks and reflects nerve conduction time through the brainstem and cortex.

9. **What are the indications for intraoperative use of SSEP monitoring?**
   SSEP monitoring is indicated in any setting with the potential for mechanical or vascular compromise of the sensory pathways along the peripheral nerve, within the spinal canal, or within the brainstem or cerebral cortex. SSEP monitoring has been used in the following:
   - Orthopedic procedures
     - Correction of scoliosis with Harrington rod instrumentation
     - Spinal cord decompression and stabilization after acute spinal cord injury
     - Spinal fusion
   - Brachial plexus exploration
   - Neurosurgical procedures
     - Resection of a spinal cord tumor or vascular lesion
     - Tethered cord release

Table 67-3. Effects of Anesthetic Agents on Amplitude and Latency of Somatosensory-Evoked Potentials

DRUG	AMPLITUDE	LATENCY
Premedication		
Midazolam (0.3 mg/kg)	↓	0
Diazepam (0.1 mg/kg)	↓	↑
Induction Agents		
Thiopental (5 mg/kg)	↑/0	↑
Etomidate (0.4 mg/kg)	↑↑↑	↑
Propofol (0.5 mg/kg)	0	↑
Ketamine (1 mg/kg)	↑	*
Opioids		
Fentanyl	↓	↑
Sufentanil	↓	↑
Morphine	↓	↑
Meperidine	↑/↓	↑
Inhaled Anesthetics		
Nitrous oxide	↓	↑
Isoflurane	↓	↑
Halothane	↓	↑
Enflurane	↓	↑
Desflurane	↓	↑
Sevoflurane	↓	↑
Others		
Droperidol	↓	↑
Muscle relaxants	0	0

↑, Increase; ↓, decrease; 0, no change; *, not known.

- Resection of a sensory cortex lesion (e.g., aneurysm or thalamic tumor)
- Carotid endarterectomy
- Vascular surgery
- Repair of a thoracic or abdominal aortic aneurysm

10. **What constitutes a significant change in the SSEP?**
    Any decrease in amplitude greater than 50% or increase in latency greater than 10% may indicate a disruption of the sensory nerve pathways. The spinal cord can tolerate ischemia for about 20 minutes before SSEPs are lost.

11. **Summarize the effects of anesthetic agents on the amplitude and latency of SSEPs.**
    See Table 67-3. Generally, the effects of opioids on the amplitude and latency of the SSEP are not clinically significant.

12. **What is the take-home message of the effects of anesthetic agents on SSEPs?**
    - All of the halogenated inhaled anesthetics probably cause roughly equivalent dose-dependent decreases in amplitude and increases in latency that are further worsened by the addition of 60% nitrous oxide. It is best to restrict the use of volatile anesthetics and nitrous oxide to levels below 1 minimum alveolar concentration (MAC) and not to combine the two.
    - If possible, bolus injections of drugs should be avoided, especially during critical stages of the surgery. Continuous infusions are preferable.

13. **What other physiologic variables can alter SSEPs?**
    - **Temperature:** Hypothermia increases latency, whereas amplitude is either decreased or unchanged. For each decrease of 1° C, latency is increased by 1 ms. Hyperthermia (4° C) decreases amplitude to 15% of the normothermic value.

- **Hypotension:** With a decrease of the mean arterial blood pressure (MAP <40 mm Hg), progressive decreases in amplitude are seen. The same change is also seen with a rapid decline in MAP to levels within the limits of cerebral autoregulation.
- **Hypoxia:** Decreased amplitude caused by hypoxia has been reported.
- **Hypocarbia:** Increased latency has been described at an end-tidal CO_2 <25 mm Hg.
- **Isovolemic hemodilution:** Latency is not increased until the hematocrit is <15%, and amplitude is not decreased until the hematocrit is <7%. This effect is likely caused by tissue hypoxia.

KEY POINTS: SOMATOSENSORY-EVOKED POTENTIALS AND SPINAL SURGERY

1. Somatosensory-evoked potentials (SSEPs) are used when spinal cord or brain parenchyma is at risk for ischemia during surgery.
2. Volatile anesthetics have the most profound effects on SSEP waveforms.
3. An anesthetic technique that minimizes volatile anesthetic exposure is best—an opiate-based technique with low-dose (<1 MAC) volatile or a total intravenous anesthetic.
4. During distraction of the spinal column in scoliosis surgery (or other critical parts of surgery), minimize interventions that will lower mean arterial blood pressure or deepen anesthetic levels acutely to allow differentiation of changes in SSEP waveforms from anesthetic effect.

14. **If SSEPs change significantly, what can the anesthesiologist and surgeon do to decrease the insult to the monitored nerves?**
    - The anesthesiologist can:
      - Increase mean arterial blood pressure, especially if induced hypotension is used.
      - Correct anemia, if present.
      - Correct hypovolemia, if present.
      - Improve oxygen tension.
      - Correct hypothermia, if present.
    - The surgeon can:
      - Reduce excessive retractor pressure.
      - Reduce surgical dissection in the affected area.
      - Decrease Harrington rod distraction, if indicated.
      - Check positioning of associated instrumentation (e.g., screws, hooks).
    If changes in the SSEPs persist despite corrective measures, a wake-up test may be performed to confirm or refute the SSEP findings. The patient's anesthetic level is lightened, and a clinical assessment of neurologic function is performed.

15. **Despite *normal* SSEPs, can patients awaken with neurologic deficits?**
    Although SSEP monitoring is a useful tool in preventing neurologic damage during spinal surgery, it is by no means foolproof. Because motor tracts are not monitored, the patient may awaken with preserved sensation but lost motor function. However, the reported incidence of false-negative monitoring in a large (>50,000) series of cases is 0.06% (1 in 1500). The monitoring of motor-evoked potentials along with SSEPs provides a more complete assessment of neural pathway integrity.

16. **Is blindness a possible complication of spine surgery?**
    Loss of visual acuity (postoperative visual loss [POVL]) can occur following spine surgery and may appear with or without obvious signs of ocular trauma. Visual deficits range from blurring to complete blindness. The four types of visual losses encountered are central retinal artery occlusion, central retinal vein occlusion, cortical blindness, and ischemic optic neuropathy (ION). Occlusions of the central retinal artery or vein are most commonly associated with direct trauma to the globe of the eye (direct pressure on the globe) and less commonly with embolic events. Proper positioning of the patient with careful attention to protection of the eyes is important to prevent this injury. Although ION has occurred following other surgical procedures, most commonly it follows prone spine surgery. Estimated incidence of ION after spine surgery ranges from 0.01% to 0.2%.

17. **What is the cause of this loss of vision?**
Occlusion of the ophthalmic vasculature mostly follows trauma to the eye. Cortical blindness is caused by ischemia of the visual cortex of the brain or the optic tracts within the cranium. The causes of ION are unknown, but the optic nerve and its blood supply are at risk within the orbit and at the lamina cribrosa where it penetrates the thick sclera. The blood supply is variable among individuals, and a watershed area exists along the midsection of the nerve between the zones of perfusion from the more posterior hypophyseal branches of the carotid artery and the short posterior ciliary artery anteriorly. The nerve is damaged when there is a decrease in perfusion pressure to the optic nerve below the threshold of autoregulation, and severity and duration of the ischemia will influence the resulting injury.

18. **What can be done to avoid this devastating complication?**
In a recent analysis of 80 patients from the American Society of Anesthesiologists (ASA) Postoperative Visual Loss (ASA POVL) registry, patients undergoing prone spine surgery were studied with the goal to identify independent risk factors for the development of ION. Those factors are increasing duration of surgery, male sex, use of the Wilson frame for patient positioning, obesity, and lower percentage of colloid to crystalloid fluid replacement. That males are at higher risk suggests a protective effect of estrogen. Anemia, intraoperative blood pressure, and the presence of chronic hypertension, atherosclerosis, smoking, or diabetes were not found to affect risk. This suggests that intraoperative physiologic changes have a greater influence on the development of ION and that venous congestion plays a significant role in precipitating these physiologic perturbations. There is no known treatment for ION. The ASA practice advisory for POVL associated with spine surgery states the following:
   1. There are no identifiable preoperative patient characteristics that predispose to ION, but the risk may be increased in patients undergoing prolonged procedures, those with large blood loss, or both.
   2. Consider informing these patients that there is a small, unpredictable risk of POVL.
   3. Colloids should be used along with crystalloids to maintain intravascular volume in the face of substantial blood loss.
   4. There is no documented lower limit of hemoglobin concentration associated with the development of ION; therefore no transfusion threshold that eliminates the risk of POVL can be established.
   5. Direct pressure on the eye should be avoided to prevent central retinal artery occlusion.
   6. High-risk patients should be positioned so that the head is above or level with the heart, and the head should be in a neutral forward position.
   7. Consideration should be given to the use of staged procedures in high-risk patients.

KEY POINTS: POSTOPERATIVE VISUAL LOSS

1. Ischemic optic neuropathy (ION) can follow spine surgery and is caused by decreased blood flow to the optic nerve at select vulnerable locations.
2. Independent risk factors for ION include male sex, prolonged surgery, use of the Wilson frame, obesity, and low percentage of colloid compared to crystalloid for fluid replacement.
3. Anemia, intraoperative blood pressure, and preexisting disease do not influence the incidence of ION.
4. When positioning the patient prone, avoid direct pressure on the eye and place the head above the level of the heart.

SUGGESTED READINGS

American Society of Anesthesiologists: Practice advisory for perioperative visual loss associated with spine surgery, Anesthesiology 116:274–285, 2012.
Holy SE, Tsai JH, McAllister RK, et al: Perioperative ischemic optic neuropathy: a case control analysis of 126,666 surgical procedures at a single institution, Anesthesiology 110:246–253, 2009.
Jameson LC, Janik DJ, Sloan TB: Electrophysiologic monitoring in neurosurgery, Anesthesiol Clin 25:605–630, 2007.

Postoperative Visual Loss Study Group: Risk factors associated with ischemic optic neuropathy after spinal fusion surgery, Anesthesiology 116:15–24, 2012.

Seubert CN, Mahla ME: Neurologic monitoring. In Miller RD, Eriksson LI, Fleischer LA, et al, editors: Miller's anesthesia, ed 7, Philadelphia, 2013, Churchill Livingstone, pp 1477–1514.

Shen Y, Drum M, Roth S: The prevalence of perioperative visual loss in the United States: a 10-year study from 1996 to 2005 of spinal, orthopedic, cardiac, and general surgery, Anesth Analg 109:1534–1545, 2009.

Sloan TB, Jameson LC, Janik DJ: Evoked potentials. In Cottrell JE, Young WL, editors: Cottrell and Young's neuroanesthesia, ed 5, Philadelphia, 2010, Mosby, pp 115–130.

Williams EL: Postoperative blindness, Anesthesiol Clin North America 20(3):367–384, 2002.

CHAPTER 68

ANESTHESIA FOR CRANIOTOMY

Daniel J. Janik, MD Colonel (Retired), USAF, MC

1. **Are there particular anesthetic problems associated with intracranial surgery?**
Space-occupying intracranial lesions are associated with disturbed autoregulation in adjacent tissue, vascular malformations and aneurysms are accompanied by altered vasoreactivity (particularly if preceded by subarachnoid hemorrhage [SAH]), and traumatic injuries sometimes require contradictory efforts to minimize brain swelling while maximizing systemic resuscitation. Intraoperative concerns include control of cerebral blood flow and volume, anticipation of the effects of surgery and anesthetic management on intracranial pressure (ICP) dynamics, and maintenance of cerebral perfusion. In addition, the patient should be unconscious and unaware of intraoperative stimuli, adrenergic responses of the patient to intraoperative events must be attenuated, and the surgeon's approach to the operative site must be facilitated.

2. **How is the anesthetic requirement different in the brain and related structures?**
During anesthesia for craniotomy, the level of nociceptive stimulus varies greatly. Laryngoscopy and intubation require deep anesthesia to block harmful increases in heart rate, blood pressure, and brain metabolic activity, which may increase cerebral blood flow and brain swelling. Except for placement of pins in the skull for head positioning, considerable time may pass during positioning and operative preparation with no noxious stimulus. Incision of scalp, opening of the skull, and reflection of the dura provide increased surgical stimulus, only to be followed by dissection of the brain or pathologic tissue, which is almost completely free of nociceptive nerve fibers. Occasionally, vascular structures of the brain may respond with an adrenergic surge during surgery, particularly if an SAH has occurred in the region of the procedure.

3. **What types of patient monitoring are used during a craniotomy?**
The usual noninvasive monitors are used for every patient, including pulse oximetry, stethoscope, noninvasive blood pressure cuff, temperature, electrocardiogram, end-tidal and inspired gas monitors, and peripheral nerve stimulator. Continuous arterial pressure monitoring is used routinely to assess hemodynamic changes and intravascular volume status. A central venous catheter is used when there is a high risk of venous air embolism or a likelihood of using vasoactive infusions perioperatively. Other monitors potentially used by the surgeon include continuous electroencephalogram (EEG); somatosensory, motor, and brainstem auditory evoked potentials; and subdural, intraventricular, or cerebrospinal fluid pressure monitors. Jugular bulb venous oxygen saturation and transcranial oximetry have been described as monitors of oxygen delivery and metabolic integrity of the brain globally but are not used regularly in intraoperative settings.

4. **Discuss the considerations for fluid administration during craniotomy.**
Volume depletion from overnight fasting and volume redistribution from anesthetic agents result in relative hypovolemia. Before opening of the dura, sudden increases in intravascular volume may cause deleterious increases in ICP, especially in situations involving intracranial masses, contusions, or intraparenchymal, subdural, or epidural hematomas. Therefore, fluids must be given to avoid hypovolemia and hypotension, but exuberant bolus administration is to be avoided.

An iso-osmolar intravenous fluid should be used. Unless hypoglycemia is documented, glucose-containing solutions should be avoided. In both clinical and experimental settings in which glucose is used in the resuscitation fluids after head injury, outcome is worse. Saline and balanced salt solutions are appropriate for use during craniotomy if their osmolarity approximates or exceeds that of the serum. Colloid solutions such as 5% albumin or 3% NaCl are equivalent solutions for acute volume replacement before packed red cell administration. Often 25% albumin is used for pressure support when blood replacement is not needed. Hetastarch solutions should be used with caution since larger quantities are associated with impaired coagulation in vitro.

5. **When are measures for brain protection required?**
Brain protection refers to the maneuvers by the anesthesiologist to maintain a balance between brain metabolism and substrate delivery and to prevent secondary injury to regions of the brain after an episode of ischemia. The need for brain protection should be anticipated after head trauma and brain contusion and during procedures for the correction of intracranial aneurysms or arteriovenous malformations. Of primary importance is adequate delivery of oxygen and energy substrates to brain tissue by ensuring optimal blood oxygen content and cerebral blood flow.

6. **How can the brain be protected?**
Historically, long-acting barbiturates have been used for metabolic suppression for refractory intracranial hypertension. The goal is suppression of brain activity with resultant reduction of metabolism, which is reflected by a flat EEG.

   In the intraoperative setting, metabolic suppression is needed when a major artery is temporarily clipped to facilitate access to an aneurysm. The EEG correlate is "burst suppression," and this can be achieved by rapid infusion of thiopental, propofol, or etomidate. Profound hypothermia reduces brain metabolism. Mild to moderate hypothermia (32.5° to 34° C) is not useful for intraoperative brain protection. The global metabolic suppression secondary to hypothermia decreases neuronal electrical activity and the energy needed for cellular homeostasis and membrane integrity. Production of excitatory neurotransmitters during reperfusion of ischemic tissue is also suppressed by hypothermia.

   Attention has been directed to suppressing the neuroexcitation that occurs with reperfusion after brain ischemia. Calcium influx into glial cells and vascular smooth muscle may be suppressed by calcium channel blockade, free radicals that are generated may be *scavenged* by mannitol, and avoiding systemic hyperglycemia prevents increased intracellular hyperglycemia.

7. **How is the choice of anesthetic agent made?**
It is based on an understanding of the pharmacologic properties of hypnotic agents, inhalation agents, opioids, and muscle relaxants and on a balancing of beneficial and potentially adverse effects. Whichever agents are chosen, the goals are postoperative hemodynamic stability associated with an awake, neurologically assessable patient.
   - **Hypnotic agents:** Thiopental effectively blocks conscious awareness and reduces the functional activity of the brain, ICP, cerebral blood flow, and brain metabolism. Propofol has similar effects and is eliminated more rapidly. Etomidate and midazolam are only slightly less effective in metabolic suppression and are also useful.
   - **Inhalation agents:** The differences between isoflurane, desflurane, and sevoflurane concerning metabolic suppression and cerebral blood flow are slight. All cause suppression of brain activity while preserving or enhancing cerebral blood flow. Cost and speed of elimination are concerns in selection. Nitrous oxide has been shown to increase ICP and cerebral blood flow, although this effect is modified by the co-administration of other hypnotic, analgesic, and anesthetic agents.
   - **Opioids:** All opioids have negligible effects on cerebral blood flow and small effects on cerebral metabolism. They block the adrenergic stimulation that increases brain activity. Morphine and hydromorphone are eliminated slowly and cause respiratory depression after the procedure is completed. Hypercarbia results in increases in cerebral blood flow and potentially also ICP, which must be avoided after a craniotomy. Shorter-acting synthetic opioids may also cause residual respiratory depression after prolonged infusion.
   - **Muscle relaxants:** Depolarizing muscle relaxants are generally not used in the setting of intracranial pathology unless emergent control of the airway is necessary. The main criteria for choosing a nondepolarizing muscle relaxant are the duration of neuromuscular blockade desired, route of elimination, and cost.

8. **What are the concerns for patient positioning during a craniotomy?**
Because these are lengthy procedures, protecting vulnerable peripheral nerves and pressure-prone areas from injury is essential. Provisions must be made to prevent preparation solutions from entering the eyes. Generally the head is fixed in position with

pins clamped against the outer table of the skull. Because the head is held in a fixed position, any patient movement will stress the cervical spine. Muscle paralysis must be maintained during the time the head is secured in the holding device.

In every craniotomy, the risk of air entrainment into the venous system must be estimated. Whenever the head is positioned 10 cm above the midthorax (>20 degrees elevation), a potential negative pressure exists between the venous sinuses of the head and the central venous system. Air entrained in the central venous system may collect in the right side of the heart and interfere with preload and pulmonary flow. Air can potentially cross the intraatrial septum and, if a patent foramen ovale is present (20% of patients), become a paradoxical air embolus to the systemic circulation. This risk is very significant in sitting-position craniotomies. End-tidal CO_2, end-tidal nitrogen, transesophageal echocardiography, and precordial Doppler are sensitive indicators of venous air. In high-risk situations, a multiorificed right atrial catheter should be placed for removal of air bubbles.

9. **Why do some patients awaken slowly after a craniotomy?**
   Continuous infusion of opioid as part of balanced anesthesia leads to prolonged redistribution and persistent sedation. Residual volatile anesthetic or barbiturate may contribute to slow awakening. However, all residual anesthetic effects are overcome simply by waiting and providing respiratory support. Use of agents of short duration is beneficial. Slow awakening that persists for more than 2 hours is rarely an effect of residual anesthesia. The patient who is unresponsive for several hours after a craniotomy should be evaluated for increased ICP, embolic phenomenon, brainstem ischemia, or intracranial masses. Evaluation should be a joint effort of the neurosurgeon and anesthesiologist. The anesthetic technique should be tailored to facilitate a rapid emergence for early testing of neurologic function.

10. **What anesthesia problems are unique to surgery on the intracranial blood vessels?**
    - **SAH:** Aneurysms of the intracerebral arteries may be diagnosed after SAH. Neurologic impairment after SAH ranges from headache and stiff neck (Hunt-Hess grade I) to deep coma (Hunt-Hess grade V). Initial resuscitation includes observation, tight control of blood pressure, and support of intravascular volume (hypervolemic, hyperosmolar, normotensive). The optimal time for surgical clipping of the aneurysm is within the first few days of hemorrhage. After 5 to 7 days following SAH, the risk of rebleeding remains high, but the risk of vasospasm of the vessel feeding the aneurysm markedly increases because of irritation from the breakdown of old blood. Invasive monitoring of arterial pressure and central venous pressure is required to facilitate maintenance of hemodynamic stability and guide volume replacement. The minimal approach to brain protection is to maintain normal oxygen delivery to the brain tissue. Metabolic suppression by electroencephalographic burst suppression may be done at the time of temporary vessel clipping but may result in poor outcome when accompanied by hypotension.
    - **Rebleeding:** Approximately 30% of intracranial aneurysms that have bled will rebleed at some time if untreated. In the initial few days the hydrodynamic forces on the aneurysm wall are caused by the systolic blood pressure resisted by the tension of the aneurysmal wall. Larger aneurysms have less wall tension for any part of the aneurysmal surface. Rebleeding of the aneurysm before the opening of the dura is catastrophic, requiring the surgeon to approach the bleeding vessel blindly, perhaps temporarily clipping major feeding vessels. Although it might seem reasonable to induce hypotension during the opening of the dura, if a rebleed occurs, hypotension will adversely affect regional perfusion and may promote vasospasm.
    - **Vasospasm:** Vasospasm can occur after any SAH, regardless of clinical stage. The end result of persistent vasospasm is ischemic stroke in the region of distribution of the aneurysmal artery, resulting in permanent neurologic damage. Diagnosis is by angiography or Doppler ultrasonography. Maintaining hypervolemic normotensive hemodynamic status is the first line of prevention of vasospasm and should be continued intraoperatively. Vasospasm is a response to hemoglobin in the interstitium, with calcium influx into the vascular smooth muscle cells. Calcium channel blockade has been

advocated but has shown mixed results. Thromboplastin activators have been used experimentally by irrigation in the region of the aneurysmal bleed with some success. The main lines of prevention are intraoperative irrigation of the hematoma early in the SAH course and maintenance of favorable hemodynamics after surgery.

11. **Are there special anesthetic problems associated with brain tumors?**
Mass lesions of the brain cause problems for the anesthesiologist because of their size and location. Frontal tumors grow to large size without producing neurologic symptoms or increased ICP. Patients with supratentorial tumors of the motor and sensory cortical regions may have seizures, localizing neurologic signs, and increased ICP. Posterior fossa masses in adults cause disturbances in gait, balance, proprioception, or cranial nerve impingement. There is a *penumbra* around all intracranial tumors where the adjacent brain loses autoregulatory function. Thus on induction, regional blood flow in these areas may increase in response to aggressive fluid replacement or increased systolic blood pressure. After the resection is completed, this penumbra may respond to reperfusion with swelling. The end result may be either preincisional or postoperative increases in ICP. Posterior fossa tumors cause particular problems. The tumors are generally small but may surround complex vascular channels of the basilar, posterior communicating, and cerebellar arteries. Simple dissection of a brainstem tumor can cause disturbance of heart rate and rhythm or blood pressure when nerve roots are retracted. The surgical approach to the posterior fossa involves awkward positioning, from sitting to lateral to prone to park bench. These positions require careful attention to the position of the endotracheal tube to avoid migration to an endobronchial position or out of the glottis. The plan for anesthesia must also allow for intraoperative monitoring of auditory-evoked potentials, somatosensory-evoked potentials, or motor-evoked potentials if indicated.

12. **Are there other anesthetic concerns during craniotomies?**
Transsphenoidal surgery, although not strictly a craniotomy, involves manipulation of ventilation to raise the $PaCO_2$ and ICP, which forces the pituitary into a more easily visualized position.
    Rapidly deteriorating neurologic status after closed head injury often leads to emergency intubation, neuroradiologic studies, and emergent craniotomy. The increase in ICP that causes the clinical deterioration may progress to involve brainstem compression. The physiologic response to increased ICP is systemic hypertension and, later, bradycardia (Cushing reflex). This should be treated by reducing ICP as opposed to the hypertension per se. Typically, when the cranium is opened and brainstem pressure is reduced, the blood pressure decreases, but if aggressive treatment of elevated blood pressure has been undertaken, the drop in blood pressure may be precipitous.
    Craniotomies in pediatric patients are rarer. The pathology that is most common in the pediatric group is the posterior fossa tumor, particularly cerebellar astrocytoma. Positioning, cranial nerve root stimulation, and venous air embolus are concerns during posterior fossa resections in children.

KEY POINTS: ANESTHESIA FOR CRANIOTOMY

1. Maintain a cerebral perfusion pressure of at least 50 mm Hg but preferably 70 mm Hg or higher.
2. If intracranial pressure (ICP) is high, avoid volatile anesthetics and opt instead for a total intravenous anesthetic technique.
3. Remember that patients with profound mental status changes require little or no sedation before induction of general anesthesia.
4. Ensure deep anesthesia before intubation to avoid abrupt increases in cerebral blood flow.
5. Patients with large mass lesions may exhibit cardiovascular instability on induction of anesthesia because of intravascular volume reduction as a consequence of aggressive treatment of intracranial hypertension.
6. Rapid emergence from anesthesia facilitates early testing of neurologic function.

Special Considerations in Craniotomy
- Judicious fluid administration with iso-osmotic solutions or colloid will minimize cerebral edema and ICP increases.
- Avoid abrupt increases in systemic blood pressure prior to aneurysm clip placement.
- Preexisting cerebral vasospasm may be worsened by systemic hypotension during surgery.
- If the patient is in a head-up position of >30 degrees, venous air embolism risk justifies the use of a right atrial air-retrieval catheter.

SUGGESTED READINGS

Avitsian R, Schubert A: Anesthetic considerations for intraoperative management of cerebrovascular disease in neurovascular surgical procedures, Anesthesiol Clin 25:441–463, 2007.

Drumond JC, Patel PM: Neurosurgical anesthesia. In Miller RD, Eriksson LI, Fleischer LA, et al, editors: Miller's anesthesia, ed 7, Philadelphia, 2013, Churchill Livingstone, pp 2045–2087.

Pasternack JJ, Lanier WL: Diseases affecting the brain. In Hines RL, Marschall KE, editors: Stoelting's anesthesia and coexisting diseases, ed 5, Philadelphia, 2008, Churchill Livingstone, pp 218–254.

Rozet I, Vavilala MS: Risks and benefits of patient positioning during neurosurgical care, Anesthesiol Clin 25:631–653, 2007.

CHAPTER 69

MINIMALLY INVASIVE SURGERY

Prairie N. Robinson, MD, and James C. Duke, MD, MBA

1. **What are the benefits of minimally invasive procedures?**
   Improvements in scope technology have allowed many procedures to be performed without large surgical incisions, affording the patient rapid recovery of function, less postoperative pain and fewer analgesic requirements, improved pulmonary function, smaller incisions, fewer wound infections, decreased postoperative ileus, decreased length of hospitalization, and a rapid resumption of normal daily activities.

2. **What are some currently practiced minimally invasive procedures?**
   - **General surgery:** Laparoscopic procedures on the gastrointestinal tract, liver, gallbladder and bile ducts, and the spleen, pancreas, and adrenals. In addition, hernia repairs, diagnostic laparoscopy, gastric bypass, gastric banding, Nissen fundoplication, and feeding-tube placement can be performed laparoscopically.
   - **Gynecologic procedures:** Diagnostic procedures for chronic pelvic pain, hysterectomy, tubal ligation, pelvic lymph node dissection, hysteroscopy, myomectomy, oophorectomy, and laser ablation of endometriosis
   - **Thoracoscopic procedure/video-assisted thoracic surgery:** Lobectomy, pneumonectomy, wedge resection, drainage of pleural effusions and pleurodesis, evaluation of pulmonary trauma, resection of solitary pulmonary nodules, tumor staging, repair of esophageal perforations, pleural biopsy, excision of mediastinal masses, transthoracic sympathectomy, pericardiocentesis, and pericardiectomy
   - **Cardiac surgery:** Coronary artery bypass and valve repair
   - **Orthopedics:** Various joint procedures
   - **Urologic procedures:** Laparoscopic nephrectomy, pyeloplasty, orchiopexy, cystoscopy/ureteroscopy, and prostatectomy
   - **Neurosurgery:** Ventriculoscopy, microendoscopic diskectomy, spinal fusion, and image-guided techniques to approach masses/tumors easily
     However, the focus of this chapter will be the physiologic concerns associated with abdominal laparoscopy since they are of utmost importance to the anesthesiologist.

3. **Are there any contraindications for laparoscopic procedures?**
   Relative contraindications for laparoscopy include increased intracranial pressure, patients with ventriculoperitoneal or peritoneojugular shunts, hypovolemia, congestive heart failure, or severe cardiopulmonary disease and coagulopathy.

4. **Why has carbon dioxide (CO_2) become the insufflation gas of choice during laparoscopy?**
   The ideal gas would be physiologically inert, colorless, inflammable, and capable of undergoing pulmonary excretion (Table 69-1). The choice of an insufflating gas for the creation of pneumoperitoneum, pneumothorax, and so on, is influenced by the blood solubility of the gas and its tissue permeability, combustibility, expense, and potential to cause side effects. CO_2 has become the gas of choice because it offers the best compromise between advantages and disadvantages.

5. **How does CO_2 insufflation affect the partial pressure of carbon dioxide ($PaCO_2$)?**
   CO_2 insufflation increases $PaCO_2$. The degree of increase in $PaCO_2$ depends on the intraabdominal pressure (IAP), the patient's age, underlying medical conditions, patient positioning, and mode of ventilation. In healthy patients the primary mechanism of increased $PaCO_2$ is absorption via the peritoneum. Increases in intraabdominal pressure also result in diaphragmatic dysfunction and increased alveolar dead space, leading to ventilatory impairment and subsequent increases in $PaCO_2$. $PaCO_2$ rises approximately 5 to 10 minutes after CO_2 insufflation and usually reaches a plateau after 20 to 25 minutes. The

Table 69-1. Comparison of Gases for Insufflation

	ADVANTAGES	DISADVANTAGES
CO_2	Colorless Odorless Inexpensive Decreased risk of air emboli compared with other gases because of its high blood solubility	Hypercarbia Respiratory acidosis Cardiac dysrhythmias, in rare cases resulting in sudden death More postoperative neck and shoulder pain resulting from diaphragmatic irritation (compared with other gases)
N_2O	Decreased peritoneal irritation Decreased cardiac dysrhythmias (compared with CO_2)	Supports combustion and may lead to intraabdominal explosions when hydrogen or methane is present Greater decline in blood pressure and cardiac index (compared with CO_2)
Air		Supports combustion Higher risk of gas emboli (compared with CO_2)
O_2		Highly combustible
Helium	Inert Not absorbed from abdomen	Greatest risk of embolization

gradient between $PaCO_2$ and end-tidal CO_2 does not change significantly during insufflation, but it may do so in patients with advanced cardiopulmonary disease.

6. **What is considered a safe increase in IAP?**
The current recommendation for IAP is less than 15 mm Hg, and most laparoscopic procedures are performed with IAPs in the 12- to 15-mm Hg range. In general IAPs less than 10 mm Hg have minimal physiologic effects. Insufflation pressures above 16 mm Hg result in undesirable physiologic changes (e.g., increased systemic vascular resistance [SVR] and decreased compliance of the lung and chest wall). At pressures greater than 20 mm Hg, renal blood flow (RBF), glomerular filtration rate, and urine output also decline. Insufflation pressures of 30 to 40 mm Hg have significant adverse hemodynamic effects and should be avoided. Many insufflation machines are set to alarm at 15 mm Hg. If the machine alarms when the surgeon is not insufflating with high pressure, the anesthesiologist should consider insufficient abdominal wall relaxation as one possible cause of the high-pressure alarm. Low-pressure pneumoperitoneum (7 mm Hg) and gasless laparoscopy have been advocated as means of decreasing the magnitude of hemodynamic derangement.

7. **Describe pulmonary and cardiac changes associated with pneumoperitoneum. What is the influence on visceral organs?**
CO_2 insufflation and the resultant increase in IAP result in cephalad displacement of the diaphragm, reducing functional residual capacity (FRC) and compliance. Trendelenburg position further aggravates these changes. When the FRC is reduced relative to the patient's closing capacity, hypoxemia may result from atelectasis and intrapulmonary shunting. Positive end-expiratory pressure of 10 during pneumoperitoneum decreases cardiac output and preload. Hypoxemia is uncommon in healthy patients but becomes a concern in obese patients or those with underlying cardiopulmonary disease since it can be difficult to ventilate against the pressure of the pneumoperitoneum adequately in compromised patients (Table 69-2 and Table 69-3).
An IAP of 12 to 14 mm Hg decreases RBF, glomerular filtration rate, and urine output. The reduction in RBF is related to the decreased cardiac output and compression of the renal vein. Hepatoportal arterial and venous blood flow is gradually decreased with increasing IAP, and elevated liver enzymes have been noted after prolonged laparoscopic cases. Splanchnic microcirculation is decreased.

Table 69-2. Hemodynamic Changes During Laparoscopy

INCREASED	DECREASED	NO CHANGE
SVR	Cardiac output (initially, then increases)	Heart rate (may increase because of hypercapnia or catecholamine release)
MAP	Venous return (at IAP >10)	
CVP		
PAOP		
Left ventricular wall stress		
Venous return (at IAP <10)		

CVP, Central venous pressure; IAP, intraabdominal pressure; MAP, mean arterial pressure; PAOP, pulmonary artery occlusion pressure; SVR, systemic vascular resistance.

Table 69-3. Pulmonary Changes Associated with Laparoscopy

INCREASED	DECREASED	NO SIGNIFICANT CHANGE
Peak inspiratory pressure	Vital capacity	PaO$_2$ (in healthy patients)
Intrathoracic pressure	Functional residual capacity	
Respiratory resistance	Respiratory compliance pH	
PaCO$_2$		

PaCO$_2$, Partial pressure of carbon dioxide; PaO$_2$, partial pressure of oxygen.

KEY POINTS: ANESTHESIA FOR MINIMALLY INVASIVE SURGERY

1. Judicious fluid administration with iso-osmotic solutions or colloid will minimize cerebral edema and ICP elevation.
2. Avoid abrupt increases in systemic blood pressure prior to aneurysm clip placement.
3. Preexisting cerebral vasospasm may be worsened by systemic hypotension during surgery.
4. If the patient is in a head-up position of >30 degrees, venous air embolism risk justifies the use of a right atrial air-retrieval catheter.

8. **Should inhaled nitrous oxide (N$_2$O) be used as an anesthetic adjuvant during laparoscopy?**
There are no clinically significant differences in bowel distention and postoperative nausea and vomiting when N$_2$O/O$_2$ combinations were compared to air/O$_2$ combinations, and no conclusive evidence suggests that N$_2$O cannot be used during laparoscopy.

9. **Describe anesthetic techniques used for minimally invasive surgery.**
Local anesthesia with intravenous (IV) sedation, regional techniques, and general anesthesia have all been used with favorable results. The unexpected conversion from a laparoscopic to an open procedure must be considered when choosing an anesthetic technique. General endotracheal anesthesia is the most frequently used technique. Advantages include optimal muscle relaxation, amnesia, ability to position the patient as needed, ability to control ventilation, protection from gastric aspiration, and a quiet surgical field. Urinary bladder and gastric decompression should be performed to decrease the risk of visceral puncture and improve the surgical field.

10. **Can laparoscopy be performed on children or pregnant women?**
Laparoscopic surgery is now commonly performed in pediatric populations. Children undergo similar physiologic changes and experience similar benefits of laparoscopic procedures as adults. CO_2 absorption in infants may be faster and more profound than in adults because of a greater peritoneal surface area–to–body weight ratio.

Pregnancy was initially considered to be a contraindication to laparoscopic surgery because of concerns regarding decreased uterine blood flow, increased intrauterine pressure, and resultant fetal hypoxia and acidosis. Multiple reports have since determined that laparoscopic surgery is safe in pregnancy and does not result in increased rates of fetal morbidity or mortality. Procedures should be performed in the second trimester if possible. Body positioning should avoid inferior vena cava compression. Abdominal insufflation pressure should be kept as low as possible in pregnant patients.

11. **What complications are associated with laparoscopic surgery and CO_2 pneumoperitoneum?**
Complications are most likely to occur during placement of the trocar through the abdominal wall and CO_2 insufflation.
- **Intraoperative complications:** Major vessel injury, hemorrhage, organ perforation, bladder and ureter injury, burns, cardiac arrhythmias (atrioventricular dissociation, nodal rhythms, bradycardia, and asystole), hypercapnia, hypoxemia, CO_2 subcutaneous emphysema, pneumothorax, gas embolism, endobronchial intubation, increased intracranial pressure, and aspiration are all risks. Other complications are possible, depending on the specific procedure performed.
- **Postoperative complications:** Postoperative nausea and vomiting, pain, shoulder and neck pain secondary to diaphragmatic irritation, deep venous thrombosis, delayed hemorrhage, peritonitis, wound infection, pulmonary dysfunction, and incisional hernia have all been noted.
- As laparoscopy has matured as a technique, procedures have become more complex, and patients are more likely to be older and more debilitated than in the past. Despite the increasing complexity of patients and procedures, complications and mortality rates have decreased for most procedures.

WEBSITES
Society of Gastrointestinal and Endoscopic Surgeons: http://www.sages.org
Society of Laparoendoscopic Surgeons: http://www.sls.org

SUGGESTED READINGS
Ahmad S, Nagle A, McCarthy RJ, et al: Postoperative hypoxemia in morbidly obese patients with and without obstructive sleep apnea undergoing laparoscopic bariatric surgery, Anesth Analg 107:138–143, 2008.
Antonetti M, Kirton O, Bui P, et al: The effects of preoperative rofecoxib, metoclopramide, dexamethasone and ondansetron on postoperative pain and nausea in patients undergoing elective laparoscopic cholecystectomy, Surg Endosc 21:1855–1861, 2007.
O'Rourke N, Kodali BS: Laparoscopic surgery during pregnancy, Curr Opin Anaesthesiol 19:254–259, 2006.
Salihoglu Z, Demiroluk S, Demirkiran O, et al: The effects of pneumothorax on the respiratory mechanics during laparoscopic surgery, J Laparoendosc Adv Surg Tech A 18(3):423–427, 2008.
Sammour T, Kahokehr A, Hill AG: Meta-analysis of the effect of warm humidified insufflation on pain after laparoscopy, Br J Surg 95:950–956, 2008.
Tzovaras G, Fafoulakis F, Pratsas K, et al: Spinal vs general anesthesia for laparoscopic cholecystectomy: interim analysis of a controlled randomized trial, Arch Surg 143:497–501, 2008.

ELECTROCONVULSIVE THERAPY

Philip R. Levin, MD, and Alma N. Juels, MD

1. **What are the major indications for electroconvulsive therapy (ECT) treatment?**
   In the United States, ECT is used mainly to help treat patients with severe major depressive disorder, largely as a secondary treatment, after one or more trials of psychotropic medications have failed. ECT treatment can also be the primary treatment when the clinical situation demands urgent symptomatic improvement. In many countries, ECT is used much more commonly for the treatment of schizophrenia than it is in the United States. Some studies have shown ECT to be more effective than antidepressant medications alone in treating the psychotic subtype of depression.

2. **What are the downsides of antidepressant psychotropic medication?**
   Although antidepressant medications are effective for many patients, the rate of response to the first agent administered can be as low as 50%. The elderly may not be able to tolerate depressant medications because of the inability to tolerate the many side effects associated with antidepressant medications. In addition, certain neuronal changes in the elderly can decrease the response to medications.

3. **What are the proposed mechanisms by which ECT is effective?**
   Although its mechanism of action remains unclear, the four main theories of ECT's mechanism of action are the monoamine neurotransmitter theory, the neuroendocrine theory, the anticonvulsant theory, and the neurotrophic theory. The monoamine neurotransmitter theory suggests that ECT works by increasing dopamine, serotonin, and adrenergic, and possibly GABA and glutamate, neurotransmission. The neuroendocrine theory suggests that ECT induces a release of hypothalamic or pituitary hormones, including prolactin, thyroid-stimulating hormone, adrenocorticotropic hormone, and endorphins. It is hypothesized that the release of these hormones results in the treatment's antidepressant effect. The anticonvulsant theory proposes that ECT's beneficial effects are a result of the anticonvulsant nature of the treatment. Evidence for this theory includes the observations that seizure threshold rises, and seizure duration decreases, over a course of ECT. The neurotrophic theory proposes that ECT's mechanism of action is by inducing neurogenesis and increasing neurotrophic signaling in the brain.

4. **Has ECT always been considered a good treatment for depression?**
   ECT was first used as a treatment for psychiatric disorders in the 1930s. However, complications such as fractures and cognitive impairment raised serious concerns. If not dangerous (use of insulin to cause a hypoglycemic seizure), it was barbaric (no anesthetic agents or muscle relaxants were used). Its use declined when antidepressant medications were introduced. In recent decades further research and technical advances have led to a renewed interest in the role of ECT.

5. **How safe is ECT?**
   ECT treatment is given to approximately 100,000 people each year. Interestingly, ECT appears to have less morbidity and mortality compared with many antidepressant medications. Because of this strong safety record, patients with significant comorbidities are often candidates for ECT.

6. **What is the physiologic response to ECT?**
   ECT has a dramatic effect on blood pressure and heart rate. Between the stimulus and the onset of the seizure, bradycardia, premature atrial or ventricular contractions, or asystole may last for more than 5 seconds due to increased vagal tone. After the seizure, tachycardia and hypertension usually occur secondary to a catecholamine surge. The duration of the tachycardia tends to correlate with the seizure duration as measured by electroencephalography (EEG), although hypertension often persists and requires therapy.

During the seizure, an acute increase in cerebral blood flow and an associated increase in intracranial pressure (ICP) can occur. In addition, increases in adrenocorticotropic hormone, cortisol, epinephrine, vasopressin, prolactin, and growth hormone can be noted. Intraocular pressure and intragastric pressure also transiently increase.

7. **What patients are at increased risk for complications after ECT?**
   There are no absolute contraindications for ECT. However, ECT should be used cautiously, if at all, when the effects on cerebral blood flow, ICP, heart rate, and blood pressure may prove problematic to the patient because of coexisting disease. Thus patients with cerebral space-occupying lesions or cerebrovascular disease are at increased risk. However, in a recent case series, patients with known intracranial lesion who have normal neurologic examinations and minimal or no edema or mass effect on neuroimaging have safely undergone ECT. Consultation with neurology, neurosurgery, or both, is highly recommended for any patients with intracranial masses or vascular lesions. Similarly patients with unstable cardiac disease, including patients with uncompensated congestive heart failure, severe valvular disease, unstable angina, recent myocardial infarction, and uncontrolled hypertension are all at increased risk of complications. Patients with pheochromocytoma should not receive ECT because massive amounts of epinephrine or norepinephrine may be released into the circulation. Patients with recent stroke should delay ECT treatment until at least 1 month after acute stroke. ECT has been used safely in persons with cardiac pacemaker or implantable cardio defibrillators and during pregnancy.

8. **What type of preoperative evaluation is necessary before ECT treatment?**
   A standard preoperative anesthetic history must be taken, including identifying medications, allergies, and prior adverse anesthetic events. Presumably the patient has failed a course of antidepressant medications. The significant comorbidities discussed in Question 7 should be identified and the stability of these conditions assessed. A prior history of response to ECT (both symptomatically and physiologically) is valuable. A physical examination is also considered extremely important. Remember to include an assessment of the patient's teeth and mouth, since the ECT stimulus will result in brief yet intense masseter contraction. There are no absolute requirements for laboratory testing. A decision to order laboratory tests should be based on the stability of the patient's comorbidities and medications. A pregnancy test in women of childbearing age is also reasonable. ECT is equivalent to a low-risk procedure (the short duration of anesthesia, the absence of significant fluid shifts, and the relatively low rate of major cardiac complications) as defined in 2007 in the clinical guidelines issued by the American College of Cardiology and the American Heart Association (ACC–AHA) for the perioperative care of patients undergoing noncardiac surgery. In patients with no active cardiac conditions (e.g., decompensated congestive heart failure, unstable angina, significant arrhythmias, and valvular disease), noninvasive cardiac testing is not indicated, and practitioners can proceed with risk-factor adjustment as appropriate. Patients with active cardiac conditions, once cardiovascular conditions are stable, can safely complete full courses of ECT. Optimal medical therapy in preparation for ECT is advised to minimize risk during and after treatment, although the patient's psychiatric condition may not allow this. In general, the patient's medications should be continued.

9. **Describe the technique of ECT, including appropriate monitors and medications.**
   Commonly a psychiatrist, anesthesiologist, and nurse attend the patient. An intravenous line is established, and routine monitors, including electrocardiogram, intermittent blood pressure, and pulse oximetry are placed. On rare occasions, predicated on the patient's comorbidities, arterial cannulation and continuous monitoring may be required. The psychiatrist places EEG leads to measure the cortical seizure. An additional blood pressure cuff is placed on a leg. This cuff will be inflated before administering muscle relaxants so that the muscles are isolated from the circulation and after the ECT stimulus the duration of the motor seizure can be measured. Before inducing anesthesia, the patient is preoxygenated for a number of minutes with 100% oxygen.
   Anticholinergic medications may be administered to lessen the effects of the initial parasympathetic discharge. In addition, they have antisialagogue properties. The medication most commonly used is glycopyrrolate, 0.2 to 0.4 mg intravenously.

Methohexital is the most common anesthetic induction agent used because it has a rapid, short duration of action, low cardiac toxicity, and, most important, minimal anticonvulsant properties. Side effects include hypotension, myoclonus, and pain on injection. A typical dose of methohexital is 0.75 to 1 mg/kg. In patients with left ventricular dysfunction, etomidate is an effective induction agent since it has minimal effects on myocardial contractility and cardiac output. Etomidate may also enhance seizure duration in patients who had prior ECT but whose seizure durations were thought inadequate to achieve a therapeutic effect. Side effects include pain on injection, nausea and vomiting, and delays in return of cognitive function. A typical dose of etomidate is 0.15 to 0.3 mg/kg.

Propofol has a rapid onset and a short duration of action and allows cognitive function to return soon. Although propofol use is associated with shorter seizure durations, recent investigations suggest that there is no difference in outcome when compared with methohexital. A typical dose of propofol is 0.75 to 1 mg/kg.

Although ketamine has also been used in ECT, compared with methohexital the EEG seizure duration is decreased; ketamine has the additional effects of increasing ICP and myocardial oxygen consumption. It does not seem to be an agent of choice.

The short-acting opioid remifentanil has been used for its anesthetic-sparing effects, providing a stable anesthetic when swings in heart rate and blood pressure are undesirable while having no effect on seizure duration. Potent volatile anesthetic agents offer no advantage over intravenous agents, with the possible exception of late in pregnancy, during which time ECT has been noted on occasion to produce titanic uterine contractions.

After anesthetic induction, the blood pressure cuff on the leg is inflated and acts as a tourniquet. The patient is hyperventilated by Ambu bag to lower seizure threshold. Typically the short-acting muscle relaxant succinylcholine (0.5 to 1.5 mg/kg) is administered. Before administering the electroconvulsive stimulus, a compressible mouth oral guard protector is inserted to protect the patient's teeth, lips, and tongue from injury during the associated severe masseter contraction. Only rarely, based on patient circumstances, is the patient intubated. During the seizure, the patient receives positive-pressure ventilation with 100% oxygen until spontaneous ventilation returns and the patient awakens. When stable, monitoring continues in the postanesthetic care unit until the patient is oriented and meets discharge criteria. Often the patient is confused or complains of a headache; benzodiazepines or opioids are appropriate treatments for these problems. However, benzodiazepines should be avoided before ECT because they increase seizure threshold.

Finally, it is common over a course of therapy that anesthetic medications require modification in their dosing; usually more medication is required. These adjustments must be made based on review of prior records and whether the patient experienced a seizure of therapeutic duration.

10. What additional medications are used to address hypertension and tachycardia?

The cardioselective β-adrenergic blocker esmolol is sometimes given by either bolus or infusion to blunt the sympathetic response of ECT. One must be careful since β blockers may reduce seizure duration. Better choices to attenuate the increase in blood pressure and provide coronary vasodilation are nitroglycerin (3 mcg/kg) IV given 2 minutes before ECT, or 2% nitroglycerin ointment applied 45 minutes before ECT.

For persistent hypertension, the mixed α- and β-adrenergic blocker labetalol or hydralazine is frequently administered.

11. What is an optimal seizure duration?

ECT-induced seizure activity lasting from 25 to 50 seconds is alleged to produce the best response. Patients experiencing an initial seizure lasting less than 15 seconds or greater than 180 seconds have been found to achieve a less favorable response to ECT.

12. What can be done to prolong a seizure of inadequate duration or terminate a prolonged seizure?

Etomidate is the induction drug of choice in patients experiencing inadequate seizure activity. The proconvulsant caffeine (500 mg) is often administered in situations in which the seizure duration during prior electroconvulsive treatments has been suboptimal.

Aminophylline has also been used for this purpose. Prolonged ECT-induced seizures can be terminated with a benzodiazepine or bolus of propofol, 40 to 80 mg.

13. **How many ECT treatments are usually necessary?**
ECT is given as a course of treatments. The total number needed to successfully treat psychiatric disturbance varies from patient to patient. For depression the typical range is from six to twelve treatments. In successful cases initial clinical improvement is usually evident after three to five treatments. In the United States, ECT is typically administered three times a week. In other countries, a twice-a-week schedule is more common. Recent evidence suggests that outcomes are comparable between the two schedules, and that a three-times-per-week schedule may produce results slightly more swiftly but cause more cognitive deficits.

14. **What are some of the adverse effects of ECT?**
Some common adverse side effects include headache (including precipitation of migraine headaches), musculoskeletal pain, jaw pain and worsening of temporomandibular joint issues, nausea, fatigue, and possible injury to the teeth and tongue if a bite block is not properly placed. Infrequent but serious complications include emergence delirium, which is characterized by restless agitation, aimless repetitive movements, grasping objects in view, or restless attempts to remove the monitors and intravenous line. Emergence delirium usually lasts from 10 to 45 minutes or more after the seizure and responds to benzodiazepines. An induced seizure lasting longer than 2 or 3 minutes is considered prolonged and can result in increased cognitive deficits. Prolonged apnea is said to occur if it takes longer than 5 minutes to regain spontaneous ventilations after ECT treatment and may be caused by a pseudocholinesterase deficiency, resulting in prolonged succinylcholine activity.

Anterograde amnesia may occur immediately after an ECT treatment but tends to resolve usually within an hour. Retrograde amnesia is the most common persistent adverse effect of ECT. It is more commonly seen in elderly patients and those with preexisting cognitive impairment. Memory loss of events several months or years in the past can occur. Usually retrograde amnesia improves during the first few months after ECT, although many patients have incomplete recovery.

15. **Is ECT curative?**
ECT is an extremely effective acute treatment for major depressive episodes. However, a permanent cure is extremely rare. Maintenance therapy with occasional (weekly or monthly) ECT treatments in combination with antidepressant pharmacotherapy decreases the relapse rate, but more effective strategies for relapse prevention in mood disorders are urgently needed.

KEY POINTS: ELECTROCONVULSIVE THERAPY

1. Electroconvulsive therapy (ECT) treatment is recommended for patients with severe major depressive disorder, psychotic subtypes of depression, possibly schizophrenia, and patients who cannot tolerate the side effects of, or are treatment-refractory to, antidepressant medications.
2. Typical physiologic responses to ECT include transient parasympathetic discharge resulting in bradyarrhythmias, followed by a sympathetic stimulus resulting in hypertension and tachycardia. Increases in cerebral blood flow and intracranial pressure are also noted.
3. Methohexital is the most common induction agent used during ECT because it has minimal anticonvulsant properties, a rapid onset, short duration of action, and low cardiac toxicity.
4. Succinylcholine is the most common muscle relaxant used during ECT because of its short duration of action.

SUGGESTED READINGS

American Psychiatric Association Work Group on Major Depressive Disorder: Practice guideline for the treatment of patients with major depressive disorder, third edition. http://psychiatryonline.org/guidelines.aspx. 2010.

Dawkins K: Refinement in ECT techniques. Psychiatric Times. http://www.psychiatrictimes.com/electroconvulsive-therapy/refinements-ect-techniques. Apr 29, 2013.

Goodman WK: Electroconvulsive therapy in the spotlight, N Engl J Med 364(19):1785–1787, 2011.

Keller CH, Greenberg RM, Murrough JW, et al: ECT in treatment-resistant depression, Am J Psychiatry 169:1238–1244, 2012.

Narayan VB, Kumar JM: Review of anaesthetic management for electroconvulsive therapy, Anaesth Clin Pharmacol 24:259–276, 2008.

Tess AV, Smetana GW: Medical evaluation of patients undergoing electroconvulsive therapy, N Engl J Med 360(14):1437–1444, 2009.

CHAPTER 71

ACUTE PAIN MANAGEMENT

Robin Slover, MD, Jennifer A. Zieg, MD, and Rachel G. Clopton, MD

1. **Define acute pain.**
   Pain is defined as "an unpleasant sensory and emotional experience associated with actual or potential tissue damage, or described in terms of such damage." Pain is now considered the fifth vital sign. Acute pain refers to pain of short duration (<3 months), usually associated with surgery, trauma, or an acute illness. Acute pain differs from chronic pain because its cause is usually known, it is usually temporary, and it usually resolves with healing.

2. **Why has acute pain been undertreated?**
   Physicians get very little education regarding pain management during the course of medical school and residency training. Many providers overestimate the risks associated with the use of opiates, such as respiratory depression and addiction. The recognition that poorly treated postsurgical pain leads to chronic pain is recent, and this knowledge is not routine in education and training.

3. **How is pain assessed?**
   Pain is subjective and cannot be measured even with the most sophisticated medical equipment. Changes in vital signs such as blood pressure or heart rate may be one indication of pain, but they often correlate poorly with the degree of pain without other measurements for pain.
   The magnitude of pain and the response to treatment can be monitored in several ways. Numbers from 0 (no pain) through 10 (maximal pain) are commonly used as a verbal report. A scale of 10 faces, ranging from very happy to very sad, can be used with young children (Figure 71-1). The child points to the face matching the way he or she feels. Functional ability is also a useful measure of pain. Pain scores with activity may be a more sensitive measure of analgesia because it is easier to control pain at rest than with activity.

4. **What medications are useful in treating acute pain?**
   The medications useful in treating acute pain are similar to those used in treating other types of pain. The World Health Organization analgesic ladder for treating cancer pain also provides a useful approach to treating acute pain (Figure 71-2). For mild pain, non-opioid analgesics such as nonsteroidal antiinflammatory drugs (NSAIDs) (e.g., ibuprofen or acetaminophen) are useful. Such drugs have an analgesic ceiling; above a certain dose, no further analgesia is expected. For moderate pain, compounds combining acetaminophen or aspirin with an opioid are useful. The inclusion of acetaminophen limits the amount of such agents that should be used within a 24-hour period because toxic accumulations can occur. Tramadol should also be considered at this level. With severe levels of pain, an opioid such as morphine or hydromorphone is a better choice; such opioids have no analgesic ceiling. Most postoperative or trauma patients initially respond better to opiates than to milder agents. Intravenous agents are usually faster than oral. Table 71-1 lists the intravenous and oral equivalent doses of common opiates. By the time the patient is eating and ready for discharge, opioid-acetaminophen agents or NSAIDs are often adequate.

5. **Do all types of pain respond equally to medication containing opioids?**
   Not all types of pain respond equally to the same medication. Opioid analgesics are helpful in controlling somatic (well localized) or visceral (poorly localized) pain. Bone pain may be helped partially by opioids. NSAIDs, bisphosphnates, and steroids are highly effective in treating bone pain. Neuropathic pain, often described as pain with a burning, hyperesthetic quality, responds to a diverse group of drugs, including antidepressants, anticonvulsants, muscle relaxants (baclofen), intravenous infusions such as lidocaine and ketamine, and

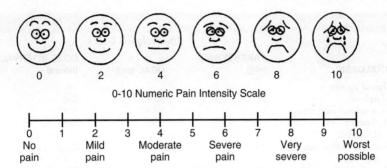

0-10 Numeric Pain Intensity Scale

Figure 71-1. Pain scales for children and adults. (*From Wong D, Whaley L:* Clinical manual of pediatric nursing, *St. Louis, 1990, Mosby.*)

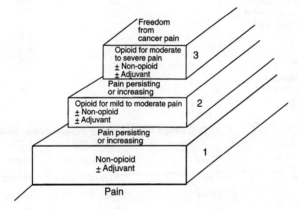

Figure 71-2. World Health Organization analgesic ladder.

α-adrenergic agonists (clonidine). Opiates may also be useful. Adjuvant medications (listed above) may also help to control somatic or visceral pain. Drugs that control pain by different mechanisms may be synergistic when used together (such as NSAIDs and opioids). Another option for mild to moderate pain is use of topical agents such as patches impregnated with lidocaine (Lidoderm) or diclofenac (Flector). In addition, topical gels or ointments can be considered, including 2% to 5% lidocaine, 1.3% diclofenac gel, or various compounded ointments often including ketamine.

6. **What is the risk of addiction with opiates?**
   Addiction (or psychologic dependence) needs to be differentiated from physical dependence. Physical dependence, a physiologic adaptation of the body to the presence of an opioid, develops in all patients maintained on opioids for a period of several weeks. If the opioid is stopped abruptly without tapering, the patient may show signs of withdrawal. Symptoms include sweating, nausea, vomiting, diarrhea, rhinorrhea, pruritus, and tachycardia. Tolerance is the need for higher doses of opiates to produce the same pharmacologic effect. Neither physical dependence nor tolerance indicates addiction. The psychological dependence seen with addiction is characterized by a compulsive behavior pattern involved in acquiring opiates for nonmedical purposes (psychic effects) as opposed to pain relief. The risk of iatrogenic addiction is very low; several studies have shown it to be less than 0.1%. Patients who are inadequately treated may seem to be drug seeking, because they repeatedly request opiates and are concerned with the timing of their next dose. Such *pseudo addiction* may mimic addictive behavior but is caused by inadequate pain

Table 71-1. Equianalgesic Doses

	Equianalgesic Doses		
ANALGESIC	**PARENTERAL (mg)**	**ORAL (mg)**	**DOSE INTERVAL (hours)**
Opioid agonist			
Morphine	10	30–60	3–6
Slow-release morphine	—	30–60	8–12
Hydromorphone (Dilaudid)	1.5	7.5	3–5
Fentanyl (Sublimaze, Innovar)	0.1	—	0.5–1
Transdermal fentanyl (Duragesic)	12 µg transdermal patch	—	72
Methadone (Dolophine)	10	20	4–6
Oxymorphone (Opana)	1	10	3–6
Oxymorphone extended release (Opana ER)		10	12
Oxycodone		30	3–6
Codeine	130	200	3–6
Hydrocodone		30	3–4
Agonist–antagonist			
Nalbuphine (Nubain)	10	—	3–6
Buprenorphine (Butrans)	5-10 µg transdermal patch		
Oral Drugs Approximately Equianalgesic to Aspirin (650 mg)			
Codeine	50 mg	Propoxyphene	65 mg
Hydrocodone	5 mg	Acetaminophen	650 mg
Meperidine	50 mg	Ibuprofen	200 mg
Oxycodone	5 mg	Naproxen	275 mg

treatment. Current studies report that patients with a past history of other substance abuse are at higher risk for opioid addiction. About 4% of patients treated for trauma had problems with opiates but showed other indications of addictive behavior that correlated with their increased use.

7. **How should opiates be given? Are some opiates better than others?**
   Oral administration is usually the easiest and least expensive. Tablets should be provided on a schedule (e.g., oxycodone-acetaminophen tablets every 4 hours) rather than on an *as needed* (PRN) or *as requested* basis initially. Many studies have shown that PRN schedules usually provide only 25% of the maximal possible daily dose of opiates, despite the patient's repeated requests. If a patient cannot take medication orally, opioids can be administered intramuscularly, intravenously (including patient-controlled analgesia [PCA] pumps), subcutaneously, rectally, transdermally, epidurally, intrathecally, through iontophoresis, and through buccal mucosa. Because PCA pumps are safe and effective, they are often used when the patient cannot take oral medication. The daily PCA dose is helpful in converting to an appropriate daily oral opiate dose (see Table 71-1).
   Morphine has an active metabolite (morphine-6-glucuronide) that is analgesic and has a longer half-life than its parent compound. In patients with decreased renal function, the accumulation of an active metabolite may lead to increased side effects, including an increased risk of respiratory depression. Morphine is dysphoric. Fentanyl acts more rapidly than morphine or hydromorphone, is one hundred times more potent, is euphoric, and has no active metabolites. It is a safer choice for patients with impaired renal or liver function.

Hydromorphone is also euphoric, is five times as potent as morphine, and has no active metabolites. Methadone can be given intravenously, and the intravenous dose is equivalent to the oral dose, unlike other opioids (which are more potent intravenously). Methadone is more potent that morphine, but potency varies—between two and ten times as potent— depending on opiate history. While the blood level of methadone is stable for 24 hours, the analgesic dose needs to be given every 6 to 12 hours. Oxymorphone is a newer opioid that is three to ten times more potent than morphine, is euphoric, and has no active metabolites. Tapentadol is a new oral opioid drug approved for moderate to severe acute pain that is half as potent as morphine. Tapentadol is a combination of an opioid binding drug with a norepinephrine reuptake inhibitor. Codeine is not a good analgesic since studies show that metabolism varies greatly due to genetic factors. In up to 10% of patients, it is not analgesic at all.

In a hospital setting, the general guideline should be to schedule pain medications for the first 1 to 2 days after surgery or injury. After that period of time the medication can be transitioned to an *as needed* status. Assessment should continue by pain score and function to determine appropriate dosing. In an outpatient setting, one day of scheduled pain medications is reasonable before transitioning to a PRN dosing schedule.

8. **When treating acute pain in a chronic pain patient, how should the approach differ?**
After an acute injury or surgical procedure, a chronic pain patient's baseline opiate dose should be tripled for the first 1 to 2 days postoperatively (post injury). In the preoperative preparation for a chronic pain patient, a one-time dose of gabapentin (900 to 1200 mg) or pregabalin (75 to 100 mg) coupled with a one-time dose of an NSAID or acetaminophen has been shown to improve pain control. Duloxetine has also been shown to be helpful. After surgery, gabanoids, duloxetine, and NSAIDs (if okay) can be continued as a regular oral dose, and additional adjuvant drugs such as ketamine, clonidine, and steroids may be added. Regional blocks should be used whenever possible and continued at least 24 hours after surgery. Pumps are available for at-home use delivering a fixed dose of local anesthetic that lasts 2 to 3 days.

9. **How should a PCA pump be set?**
Morphine, hydromorphone, and fentanyl are the commonly used opiates. If connected to an epidural as a PCEA, a combination of local anesthetic and opiate is used. Next, decide if the pump will deliver a continuous (basal) dose or only an incremental patient-controlled dose. Finally, decide how often the pump will be able to deliver medications (the lockout period). Chronic pain patients having acute pain could receive their baseline opiate dose as a basal dose if they need PCA.

10. **What are common side effects of opiates? How are they treated?**
The common side effects of opiates are sedation, pruritus, constipation, nausea and vomiting, urinary retention, and respiratory depression. In patients who have taken opiates previously, the risk of respiratory depression and sedation is less. Pruritus is treated by applying lotion to the affected area, by intravenous or oral delivery of diphenhydramine (25 to 50 mg), and in severe cases by using an opioid antagonist (naloxone) or agonist– antagonist (e.g., nalbuphine, 5 mg every 6 hours). Constipation can be treated by methylnaltrexone. Urinary retention is treated by urinary catheter drainage or nalbuphine. Nausea and vomiting respond to a decrease in opioid dose, nalbuphine, clonidine, and antiemetics such as ondansetron, 4 mg intravenously. Respiratory depression is treated by stopping the opiate temporarily and using naloxone or an agonist–antagonist.

11. **How do neuraxial opiates work?**
Opioid receptors are present in levels I and II of the substantia gelatinosa of the dorsal horn. Opiates given either intrathecally or epidurally bind to these receptors. A 300-mg oral dose of morphine is equal to 100 mg of intravenous morphine, which is equal to 10 mg of epidural morphine, which is equal to 1 mg of intrathecal morphine.

Neuraxial morphine is hydrophilic, spreads throughout the spinal fluid, lasts 12 to 24 hours, and can be associated with delayed respiratory depression. Hydromorphone is somewhat lipophilic, spreads over 8 to 10 dermatomes, and lasts 8 to 10 hours. Fentanyl is very lipophilic, spreads over 5 dermatomes, and lasts 2 to 3 hours.

12. How do agonist–antagonists differ from opiates such as morphine?

μ-, δ-, and κ-opioid receptors have been identified in the central nervous system. Most opiates are primarily μ-agonists, with some δ and κ effect. Agonist–antagonists are μ antagonists and κ agonists. Because κ receptors provide weaker analgesia, agonist–antagonists are adequate for mild to moderate pain, whereas μ agonists are adequate for moderate to severe pain. Suboxone is a newer oral combination of buprenorphine and naloxone. Patients using this agent can be given μ-acting opioids but will need much higher doses.

KEY POINTS: ACUTE PAIN MANAGEMENT

1. Acute pain can progress to chronic pain, especially chronic postsurgical pain (CPSP).
2. Multimodal (preventative) analgesia can decrease postoperative complications and CPSP.
3. Multimodal analgesia may include gabanoids, NSAIDs, ketamine, clonidine, opioids, other membrane stabilizers, steroids, antidepressants, and regional blocks.
4. Psychological interventions (pain coping skills) are helpful.
5. Chronic patients with acute pain need at least three times their baseline dose of opiates postoperatively.

13. Is there a role for IV infusions in acute pain management?

Ketamine is an N-methyl-D-aspartate (NMDA) receptor antagonist that alters pain transmission without respiratory depression. Postoperatively it is used as an infusion, typically 100 to 300 mcg/kg/hr. Some patients may need a small dose of a benzodiazepine daily (0.25 to 0.5 mg clonazepam) to prevent hallucinations. Hemodynamic changes are small at these doses. Antidepressant effects are seen at doses between 300 and 500 mcg/kg/hr. Ketamine can decrease opiate requirements and decrease acute pain, especially in patients with preoperative pain. It can also be used intraoperatively.

Lidocaine can also be used as an infusion: 1 to 1.5 mg/kg given as a bolus, followed by 2 mg/min. Lidocaine infusions decrease opiate requirements and associated side effects. This may be particularly important in abdominal postsurgical patients. Lidocaine infusions have decreased efficacy compared with that of neuraxial blocks. Although there is a potential for neurotoxicity, the doses are low and no serious complications have been reported in studies.

14. How is pediatric acute pain management different from adult acute pain management?

Pain assessment can be more challenging in infants and small children than in adults. In addition to visual and photographic scales, caregivers may be helpful in interpreting behavioral clues. Functional scales are used in very young patients. Vital signs, activity level, and feeding can help determine adequacy of pain control. Most medications used in the adult population are used in pediatrics but are dosed by weight. Multimodal strategies are employed early to reduce side effects; regional blocks are utilized whenever possible. Nurse-controlled analgesia (NCA) or caregiver-controlled analgesia (CCA) can be used when the child is unable to use a PCA button to request medication. Most PCA pumps are set with 75% of the daily dose scheduled and 25% available as needed for breakthrough pain. Nonpharmacologic interventions such as distraction, play therapy, pain psychology, coping skills, and meditation are emphasized.

15. What is chronic postoperative pain syndrome?

Chronic postoperative pain syndrome refers to patients who continue to have significant pain for at least 2 months after surgery. Studies show that 10% to 50% of patients following thoracotomies, inguinal hernia repairs, breast surgeries, cholecystectomies, and amputations are at highest risk. Recent studies using multimodal or preventative analgesia have shown a decrease in the incidence of CPSP following high-risk surgeries. The most important predictive factor shown in studies for developing CPSP is persistent moderate to severe postoperative pain on postoperative day 4. Other predictive factors are the presence of pain preoperatively, repeat surgery, intraoperative nerve injury, and psychological factors.

Table 71-2. Multimodal Dosing

DRUG	STARTING DOSE	DAILY DOSE	IDEAL DURATION POSTOPERATIVELY
Gabapentin	900, 1200 mg	900, 1200 mg	8–10 days
Pregabalin	75, 50 mg bid	75, 50 mg bid	5 days
Duloxetine	60 mg	60 mg	1 day
Ketorolac	30 mg	15, 30 mg	3 days
Celebrex	200 mg	100 mg	2–4 days
Ketamine	0.2–0.5 mg/kg	100–300 mcg/kg/hr	1–5 days
Clonidine	0.1 mg	0.1 mg	
Dexamethasone	0.11–0.21 mg/kg		

16. **What is preventive or multimodal analgesia?**
   Preventive analgesia refers to the practice of anticipating pain from surgery and using regional or neuraxial techniques with a combination of synergistic medications started preoperatively and continuing as long as possible postoperatively to control pain and decrease the risk of CPSP. Gabanoids, steroids, opiates, NMDA antagonists (ketamine), clonidine, antidepressants, NSAIDs, and other anticonvulsants have all been used for this purpose. Typical dose ranges are given in Table 71-2. The usual combination would be a gabanoid or other anticonvulsant, NSAID (if possible), opiate, ketamine, and a regional block (if possible). Just using a gabanoid and an NSAID has been helpful with an observed decrease in CPSP.

17. **What other techniques can be used for acute pain management?**
   In addition to multimodal analgesia and regional blocks, psychological approaches have been shown to have an effect on acute pain. Studies on pain coping skills such as breathing techniques, visualization, hypnosis, biofeedback, and cognitive-behavioral therapy have shown benefits. Acupuncture can help headaches and decrease anxiety. Treating the anxiety and depression that frequently accompany pain may be also helpful.

18. **How does good acute pain management affect outcomes?**
   Pain is a form of stress and produces an elevation in stress hormones and catecholamines. Good pain management has been shown to result in shorter hospital stays, improved mortality rates (especially in patients with less physiologic reserve), better immune function, fewer catabolism and endocrine derangements, and fewer thromboembolic complications. In addition, specific benefits have been shown for patients undergoing specific procedures. Patients who undergo amputation under a regional block with local anesthetic have a decreased incidence of phantom pain. Patients in whom a vascular graft is placed have a lower rate of thrombosis. A decreased mortality rate has been shown in patients with flail chests who have epidural analgesia.
   Recent studies have shown the value of preemptive analgesia in some surgical situations. The blockade of the pathways involved in pain transmission before surgical stimulation may decrease the patient's postoperative pain. Local infiltration along the site of skin incision in patients having inguinal hernia repairs with general anesthesia is beneficial if the infiltration is done before the skin incision. Similar results have been found for preoperative local infiltration along the laparoscopic port sites. Several studies using intravenous or epidural opiates in patients having thoracotomies and hysterectomies have also shown a preemptive effect. The use of local anesthetic in spinals and epidurals has not been shown to be preemptive. NSAIDs have not shown a preemptive effect. Further studies with larger patient groups are needed to provide definitive answers regarding preemptive analgesia. Studies looking at preventive (multimodal) analgesia and CPSP have shown benefit from decreasing pain transmission pathways, as discussed above.

Proper pain management not only keeps patients more comfortable but also may decrease the risk of morbidity and mortality, thus improving use of health resources.

SUGGESTED READINGS

American Society of Anesthesiologists Task Force on Acute Pain Management: Practice guidelines for acute pain management in the peri-operative setting: an updated report by the American Society of Anesthesiologists Task Force on Acute Pain Management, Anesthesiology 100:1573–1581, 2004.

Benzon HT, Raja SN, Lui SS, et al, editors: Essentials of pain medicine, ed 3, Philadelphia, 2011, Saunders.

Clarke H, Bonin RP, Orser BA, et al: The prevention of chronic postsurgical pain using gabapentin and pregabalin: a combined systematic review and meta-analysis, Anesth Analg 115:428–442, 2012.

Vollmer TL, Robinson MJ, Risser RC, et al: A randomized, double-blind, placebo-controlled trial of duloxetine for the treatment of pain in patients with multiple sclerosis, Pain Pract 2013. [E-pub ahead of print].

CHAPTER 72

CHRONIC PAIN MANAGEMENT

Ronald Valdivieso, MD, and Jason P. Krutsch, MD

1. **What is the definition of pain?**

   The International Association for the Study of Pain defines *pain* as "an unpleasant sensory and emotional experience associated with actual or potential tissue damage, or described in terms of such damage." Acute pain is associated with an identifiable cause (e.g., surgery, trauma, acute illness) and usually resolves with healing. Chronic pain is more difficult to define. It is believed that pain becomes chronic if it persists beyond 1 month of the usual course of an acute problem. However, other authors do not believe that duration should be identified as one of the distinguishing features of chronic pain and point to cognitive-behavioral aspects as essential criteria in any chronic pain syndrome.

2. **How does normal pain perception occur?**

   Nociceptors are structures located at the ends of axons that are depolarized by noxious thermal, mechanical, or chemical stimuli. The distal ends of most A-δ and C fibers are nociceptors. These axons are the ones that carry nociceptive information to the dorsal root and trigeminal ganglion and enter the spinal cord via the posterior root. The A-δ fibers are myelinated, rapidly conducting sharp, stabbing, and well-localized pain. C fibers are unmyelinated and conduct dull, aching, and poorly localized pain. Once in the spinal cord, these afferent fibers synapse with cells in Rexed laminae I and V preferentially but also in laminae II and X. Axons from the previously mentioned neurons that travel to the contralateral side of the spinal cord will eventually form the spinothalamic tract, spinoreticular tract, and spinomesencephalic tract. Axons that enter the dorsal column will form the postsynaptic dorsal column tract. These ascending nociceptive tracts will eventually synapse with superior structures such as the periaqueductal gray, hypothalamus, and thalamus. The ventroposterolateral, ventroposteromedial, and ventroposteroinferior nuclei of the thalamus then send projections to the somatosensory cortex and cingulated cortices.

3. **What is the classification of pain based on neurophysiologic mechanisms?**

   Pain can be classified according to its neurophysiologic mechanism:

   - **Nociceptive pain:** Occurs when nociceptors are stimulated by noxious stimuli. This category is divided into somatic and visceral pain. Somatic pain sensation originates from trauma, burns, and ischemia, to name the most common ones. It is transmitted via somatic nerves. Visceral pain, as its name implies, originates from visceral structures. It is transmitted preferentially via the sympathetic fibers and is usually produced by distention, ischemia, or spasm of hollow viscera.
   - **Neuropathic pain:** Is pain produced by an alteration in structure or function of the nervous system. Neuropathic pain can be divided into peripheral and central. Examples of peripheral neuropathic pain include complex regional pain syndrome (CRPS) II (causalgia), postherpetic neuralgia, diabetic neuropathy, and radicular pain from mechanical compression. Central neuropathic pain syndromes include poststroke pain, postparaplegic pain, and pain syndromes from multiple sclerosis.
   - **Psychogenic pain:** Is quite controversial in the sense that it is very difficult to define. One popular definition is that this pain is better described and understood in psychological rather than physical language and is pain for which an adequate physical explanation cannot be found.

Table 72-1. Commonly Used Groups of Medications for Treatment of Chronic Pain

GROUP	DRUG EXAMPLES	MODE OF ACTION	POTENTIAL SIDE EFFECTS
TCAs	Amitriptyline Nortriptyline	Norepinephrine and 5-hydroxytryptamine uptake inhibition Descending inhibition pathway activation	Anticholinergic actions Decreased seizure threshold Cardiac dysrhythmias Weight gain
NSAIDs	Ibuprofen Rofecoxib	Inhibit production of prostaglandin	Gastrointestinal bleeding Platelet dysfunction Bronchospasm Coronary thrombosis
SSRIs	Fluoxetine Paroxetine Sertraline	Inhibit serotonin reuptake	Anxiety Nausea Weight loss Increase in levels of TCAs
Anticonvulsants	Carbamazepine Valproic acid Gabapentin Pregabalin	Reduce Na, K conductance Increase GABA activity	Blood dyscrasias Liver dysfunction Gastrointestinal symptoms Sedation Ataxia
Neuroleptics	Fluphenazine Haloperidol	May alter perception of pain	Extrapyramidal symptoms Orthostatic hypotension
Benzodiazepines	Diazepam Lorazepam	Reduce anxiety	Sedation Great addiction potential
Opioids	Morphine Meperidine Oxycodone Methadone	μ-Receptor agonists	Sedation Constipation Addiction
Muscle relaxants	Baclofen Cyclobenzaprine	Interaction with GABA receptor	Sedation Anticholinergic action Orthostatic hypotension Conduction block
Others	Mexiletine β Blockers	Na-channel blocker β-Receptor blocker	Bronchospasm Congestive heart failure

GABA, γ-Aminobutyric acid; NSAIDs, nonsteroidal antiinflammatory drugs; SSRIs, selective serotonin reuptake inhibitors; TCAs, tricyclic antidepressants.

4. Name the most commonly used groups of medications for the treatment of chronic pain.
   See Table 72-1.

5. How are nerve blocks helpful in the treatment of chronic pain?
   • **Diagnosis:** Nerve blocks can help identify the nerve site responsible for the symptoms.
   • **Therapy:** Nerve blocks temporarily reduce pain and therefore facilitate physical therapy. Based on the response to a diagnostic block, it might be possible to determine if a neuroablation procedure is appropriate to treat a given condition.

6. Are psychosocial factors important in the diagnosis and treatment of pain?
   Painful disorders can present with associated psychological or psychiatric symptoms. These can vary from mild depression to obvious substance abuse problems to suicidal thoughts. It is necessary to address such issues to improve the patient's chance for recovery.

7. **How is pain of malignant origin treated?**

   Pain of malignant origin should be treated aggressively with a multiple therapeutic approach. This approach should initially be pharmacologic with introduction of short- and long-acting opioid preparations and some adjuvants. Adjuvants should be chosen according to the symptomatology and their side-effect profile. For example, nonsteroidal antiinflammatory drugs (NSAIDs) and steroids are very useful in the treatment of bone pain from primary or metastatic disease; anticonvulsants and tricyclic antidepressants (TCAs) can be used in the treatment of neuropathic pain from compression or from previous interventions such as chemotherapy or radiation therapy.

   Diagnostic nerve blocks can be followed by either chemical or radiofrequency ablation procedures. For malignancies located in the abdomen, celiac plexus chemical ablation can be attempted; for malignancies located in the pelvis, a superior hypogastric plexus block can be beneficial; and perineal pain can be treated with a ganglion impar ablation. With the introduction of sophisticated intrathecal delivery systems, neuraxial ablative procedures are becoming less popular but are still very useful. As mentioned, intrathecal delivery systems and long-term epidural catheters can be used to deliver opioids, local anesthetics, and other potentially beneficial drugs to the neuraxis and therefore improve the patient's condition and decrease the side effects from other medications. Finally, radiation therapy and chemotherapy can also improve pain symptoms by reducing the extent of the disease.

8. **Define CRPS I and II. What nerve blocks are commonly used to treat these conditions?**

   CRPS stands for *complex regional pain syndrome*. It is a painful condition usually centered in an extremity in which different degrees of sympathetic dysfunction can be identified. CRPS usually presents with spontaneous pain, hyperalgesia, hyperpathia, and allodynia that is not restricted to the territory of a single nerve. Sympathetic dysfunction presents as variations in regional blood flow that can cause edema and cyanosis. Localized sweating and trophic changes in the skin and nails of the affected part of the body can be seen as the disease progresses. CRPS I (formerly known as RSD) can follow minor trauma, venipuncture, or carpal tunnel surgery; sometimes no identifiable cause can be found. CRPS II (formerly called causalgia) follows damage to a peripheral nerve. Sympathetic blocks are very useful since they can facilitate physical therapy and help the patient regain some function in the affected extremity. Upper-extremity sympathetic denervation is accomplished by blocking the stellate ganglion; for lower-extremity sympathetic block, a lumbar sympathetic block is performed.

9. **How is neuropathic pain treated?**

   Medical management that includes anticonvulsants and TCAs has been shown to improve symptomatology. Methadone, due to its N-methyl-D-aspartate receptor antagonism, is probably the most useful opioid in the treatment of neuropathic pain. Other agents such as clonidine and mexiletine have also been used successfully. Injection of local anesthetics and steroids has a role in the treatment of isolated peripheral neuropathies. The introduction of peripheral and spinal cord stimulators is now an accepted therapy for very complex problems such as postlaminectomy pain syndromes and CRPS types I and II.

10. **Define myofascial pain syndrome.**

    Myofascial pain syndrome is a group of muscle disorders characterized by hypersensitive areas called *trigger points* that can occur in more than one muscle group. When trigger points are mechanically stimulated, they are painful and refer pain to an area called the *reference zone*. This reference zone does not correlate with any dermatome or peripheral nerve innervation area.

11. **Define fibromyalgia.**

    Fibromyalgia is a chronic pain condition characterized by widespread musculoskeletal pain, aches, and stiffness, soft-tissue tenderness, general fatigue, and sleep disturbances. The most common sites of pain include the neck, back, shoulders, pelvic girdle, and hands, but any body part can be involved. Fibromyalgia patients experience a range of symptoms of varying intensities that wax and wane over time.

12. **How is fibromyalgia managed?**

New research shows that fibromyalgia very likely has a central nervous system component. This theory helps explain the widespread nature of the patients' symptoms and its association with sleep disturbances. Pregabalin is the only Food and Drug Administration–approved medication for the management of fibromyalgia. In a randomized, double-blinded, placebo-controlled study, monotherapy with pregabalin showed statistically significant benefit in mean pain scores and Patient Global Impression of Change (PGIC). Aerobic conditioning and management of underlying depression are also very important in the management of these patients.

13. **List possible etiologies of low back pain.**

Low back pain can arise from multiple anatomic structures located in the lower back; these include the following:
- Muscle strain in the paravertebral muscles or quadratus lumborum
- Posterior elements of the vertebral column such as the facet joints and ligamentous structures
- Anterior elements such as vertebral compression fractures and damage to the annulus fibrosis of the intervertebral disc
- Vertebral canal and foraminal stenosis, which can cause myelopathy or radiculopathy, respectively
- Sacroiliac joint dysfunction

14. **What is the rationale behind the use of epidural steroids in the treatment of radicular symptoms associated with a herniated disk?**

Radiculopathy is pain that is present as a result of either mechanical or chemical (most of the time both) irritation of a nerve root and can lead to pain and edema of the same nerve. The site where this usually occurs is the neural foramen. Local injection of steroids will decrease the amount of time needed to recover from an acute episode of sciatica by four mechanisms:
1. Decreasing the inflammation of the nerve root due to the antiinflammatory properties of the steroids
2. Dilution of chemical irritants coming from a ruptured disc
3. Nerve membrane stabilizers
4. Inhibiting action of phospholipase A2

15. **Explain the gate theory of pain.**

In 1965 Melzack and Wall proposed that the substantia gelatinosa in the spinal cord was the primary gate in the transmission of noxious and nonnoxious stimulus to the central nervous system. The pain gate is opened by information coming from slow unmyelinated C fibers and closed by the impulses from faster myelinated fibers such as A-β. Since pain is transmitted by slow A-δ and C fibers, they reason that, by activating faster fibers such as the ones that transmit proprioception, the gate will be closed, and the pain symptoms will improve. A practical application is the use of transcutaneous electrical nerve stimulation units and spinal and peripheral nerve stimulators for the treatment of pain.

16. **Name some indications for the use of spinal cord stimulators.**

The most common indication for use of spinal cord stimulation in the United States is in the treatment of postlaminectomy pain syndromes. In Europe the most common indication is in the treatment of peripheral vascular disease. Among other uses are CRPS I and II, arachnoiditis, and intractable angina pectoris.

17. **What are the most common medications used for intrathecal delivery via implantable delivery systems?**

The most common medications used in the implantable delivery systems are opioids in general and morphine and hydromorphone in particular. Local anesthetics are used, usually in combination with an opioid for the treatment of malignant pain. Baclofen is used for the treatment of spasticity and painful muscle contractions. Clonidine is used for the treatment of neuropathic pain. Recent studies have explored the potential for the use of ketamine, neostigmine, and some calcium channel blockers.

KEY POINTS: CHRONIC PAIN MANAGEMENT

1. Chronic pain is best treated using multiple therapeutic modalities. These include physical therapy, psychological support, pharmacologic management, and the rational use of more invasive procedures such as nerve blocks and implantable technologies.
2. Patients suffering from cancer pain often exhibit complex symptomatology that includes various forms of nociceptive and neuropathic pain.
3. In patients suffering from chronic pain, underlying psychological/psychiatric conditions should be addressed if any meaningful recovery is to be achieved.
4. Neuropathic pain is usually less responsive to opioids than pain originating from nociceptors.

WEBSITE

International Association for the Study of Pain: http://www.iasp-pain.org

SUGGESTED READINGS

Cameron T: Safety and efficacy of spinal cord stimulation for the treatment of chronic pain: a 20-year literature review, J Neurosurg 100(3 Suppl):254–267, 2004.

Mease PJ, Russell IJ, Arnold LM, et al: A randomized, double-blind, placebo-controlled, phase III trial of pregabalin in the treatment of patients with fibromyalgia, J Rheumatol 35:502–514, 2008.

Melzack R, Wall P: Pain mechanism: a new theory, Science 150:971, 1965.

Vranken JH, van der Vegt MH, Kal JE, et al: Treatment of neuropathic cancer pain with continuous intrathecal administration of S+ ketamine, Acta Anesthesiol Scand 48:249–252, 2004.

INDEX

Page numbers followed by "f" indicate figures, "t" indicate tables, and "b" indicate boxes.

Surgery *(Continued)*
 as myocardial ischemia risk factor, 189
 in patient with high blood pressure, 192
 use of herbal medications before, 322–323
Surgical blockade, with epidural anesthetic, 412
Sweating
 drug-induced, 180
 hyperthermia-related, 180
Sympathetic blockade, after epidural anesthetic
  initiation, 408
Sympathetic ganglia, names and location of, 9
Sympathetic nervous system (SNS), anatomy of, 9,
  10f, 10t
Sympathomimetic amines, intracellular intermediary
  in, 103
Sympathomimetics
 definition of, 12
 as hyperthermia risk factor, 180
 intravenous, for hypotension, 399
 perioperative use of, 12
Syncope, pulmonary hypertension and, 248
Syndrome of inappropriate antidiuretic hormone
  (SIADH), 29
 disorders associated with, 29
 as hyponatremia cause, 33–34
Systemic hypertension (HTN), as heart failure cause,
  194
Systemic vascular resistance (SVR), in hypertension,
  166
Systolic dysfunction, 195f, 197

T

Tachycardia
 after epidural anesthetic initiation, 408
 as blood transfusion indicator, 38
 electroconvulsive therapy-related, 455–456
 hyperthermia-related, 180
 medications for, 457
 postoperative, 184
Tachyphylaxis
 ephedrine and, 12–14
 nitrovasodilators-related, 105
Tachypnea, in acute respiratory distress syndrome
  patients, 243
Tamponade, cardiac, 326–327
 as perioperative hypotension cause, 168
Tapentadol, 462–463
Temperature, as physiologic variables alter in
  somatosensory-evoked potentials, 442
Temperature compensation, 121–122
Temperature disturbances, 177–180, 179b
Temperature regulation
 effect of spinal anesthesia on, 400
 in neonates, 340
Terbutaline
 as asthma treatment, 226, 227t
 as chronic obstructive pulmonary disease
  treatment, 237t
Terlipressin, for hepatorenal syndrome, 258
Terminal ganglia, 9
"Tet spell", 350, 358
Tetracaine
 maximum safe dose of, 98t
 potency of, 98t

Tetralogy of Fallot, 350, 357
Theophylline
 as asthma treatment, 226–227, 227t
 as chronic obstructive pulmonary disease
  treatment, 237t
Thermal burns, 330–335
Thermogenesis, 179
Thermoregulation, 177–180
Thiazides, as diuretic, 270t
Thiopental. *see* Sodium thiopental
Third-space losses, 32
Thoracic duct, central venous catheterization-related
  puncture of, 159
Thoracic paravertebral analgesia, 418
Thoracic paravertebral block, 418
Thoracic surgery, lung isolation, 434
Thoracoscopic procedure, 451
Thoracotomy, mortality/morbidity associated with,
  236t
Thorpe tubes, 120
Thrombin time, preoperative, 117
Thrombocytopenia, 46–47, 401
 cirrhosis-related, 259
 preeclampsia-related, 378–379
Thromboelastography (TEG), 49, 50f, 117
 in clotting process, 264
Thromboembolism
 central venous catheterization-related, 157b
 perioperative prophylaxis against, 117
Thromboendarterectomy, for pulmonary
  hypertension, 251
Thrombolytic therapy, regional anesthesia and,
  400
Thromboxane A2 (TXA2), 45
Thyroid function tests, 305–309, 306t
Thyroid hormone replacement therapy, 305–306
Thyroid hormones, 305–309
 inotropic effect of, 107
Thyroid-stimulating hormone, 305, 306t
Thyroid storm (thyrotoxicosis), 306
Thyroidectomy
 complications of, 306–307
 surgical subtotal, 306
Thyroiditis, Hashimoto, 305
Thyrotoxicosis (thyroid storm), 306
Thyroxine, 306t
Tibial arteries, posterior, as arterial pressure
  monitoring cannulation site, 171
Tibial nerves, 418
 posterior, characteristic peaks for evaluation of,
  441t
Tidal volume, 61, 62f
 on anesthesia ventilators, 127
 during extubation, in obese patients, 312t
 fresh gas flow rate and, 127
Tissue Doppler, in diagnosis of diastolic dysfunction,
  199, 199f
Tobacco use, as postoperative pulmonary
  complication risk factor, 116t
Tocolytics, 382t
Tonicity, regulation of, 27
Topical agents, for acute pain treatment,
  460–461
Total body surface area (TBSA), of burn injuries,
  333, 334t